Diagnostic Hematology

Norman Beck

Diagnostic Hematology

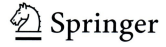 Springer

Norman Beck
University of Pretoria
Hillcrest, Pretoria
South Africa

ISBN: 978-1-84800-282-1   e-ISBN: 978-1-84800-295-1
DOI 10.1007/978-1-84800-295-1

British Library Cataloguing in Publication Data
A catalogue record for this book is available from the British Library

Library of Congress Control Number: 2008938340

Printed on acid-free paper

Springer Science+Business Media
springer.com

Foreword

This book is intended for those who have to deal with clinical hematological problems. It is designed and written in such a way that the information on hematological problems is constantly put into the clinical context in which they occur.

The author has extensive experience not only as a clinician evaluating patients in the clinic but also as a laboratory hematologist. This book reflects this integration of clinic and laboratory but written with a bias toward the clinic in a language that will appeal to clinicians. There are a number of relatively new ways of looking at hematological problems that, in many ways, enhances understanding.

Every effort has been made to make sufficient basic and clinical knowledge available to keep the interest of the reader. A textbook is probably only as good as if and how it is read. This book will contribute to filling the gap that sometimes exists between basic science and clinical medicine.

James A. Ker
Professor of Medicine
Faculty of Health Sciences
University of Pretoria

Many years' experience teaching undergraduates and postgraduates in both hematology and internal medicine and daily consultation with colleagues both in hospital and private clinical practice have brought home very clearly the problems experienced by most students (and practitioners) in the approach to hematological problems and the interpretation of hematology reports. Indeed, there often seems to be a psychological block with respect to hematology and its tests that I am at a loss to understand. Most probably, this has something to do with the traditional status that hematology has had within the medical field. Together with clinical chemistry, microbiology, and immunology, hematology was traditionally regarded as part of "clinical pathology." However, "clinical" in this context was (and is) something of a misnomer: these subjects were hardly clinical in the typical sense of the word – they merely represented the laboratory results as applied to disease processes; there was no sense of a clinical approach involved.

Thus, hematology was for decades regarded as, and taught as, a purely laboratory subject; today, as it is emerging as a clinical specialty in its own right, this approach is no longer sufficient. However, habits, including habits of thinking and approach, die hard, and the laboratory mind-set is still predominant as far as teaching material is concerned. Even the most up-to-date clinical primers do not include adequate descriptions of clinical methods as applied to blood diseases, it apparently being taken for granted that these are irrelevant.

Also, hematology is difficult to teach at the undergraduate level. The curriculum is necessarily fragmented across different years of study, and often separated considerably in time. Understanding hematology requires insight into several distinct aspects: applied physiology, generally taught early; an understanding of the essential pathological processes involving the blood is taught somewhat later (if at all); the (necessarily) strong laboratory aspect is generally taught more or less concurrently with other clinical pathology topics, such as clinical chemistry and immunology. By the time the student is faced with blood diseases in the wards, the laboratory/pathological bias is well entrenched. It is thus difficult for the student to get an integrated view of the subject. The unspoken assumption, often reinforced by clinical tutors trained in the traditional perspective, is that blood tests are all that are required for a diagnosis in blood diseases.

The result has been that clinical expertise in blood diseases is generally poor. This is reflected in the importance given to the examination of the hematological system in most student primers. The hematological system, by and large, is almost completely neglected. Such relevant features such as pallor, jaundice, bleeding, and splenomegaly are dealt with either in passing or in relation to another system or as part of the "general examination." It is almost as though it is taken for granted that the hematological system cannot be assessed clinically – and yet, as demonstrated later in the book, it is in very many cases impossible to reach a complete hematological diagnosis without clinical assessment.

A further factor making things difficult for the gaining of a sensible holistic approach to diagnosis in blood (and other) diseases is the modern trend to rely on statistics to make one's judgments. Apart from dehumanizing medicine, this approach is generally unsuccessful in the interpretation of the first-line tests in hematology (although of great value in the evaluation of subsequent confirmatory tests).

There is no substitute for the clinical approach in the final assessment and management of any patient's disease, of whatever nature. No matter what the laboratory says, the final evaluation and judgment must come from the clinician. Even with adequate interpretation of the tests as such, they **CANNOT PROVIDE A COMPLETE CLINICAL ANSWER**. For example, consider **PURPURA**. The knee-jerk reaction to purpura is to order (at least) the full blood count (FBC), as if there is no point in thinking about it clinically, and allowing the lab to take the diagnosis further. There are two serious critical comments:

a. The diagnosis of purpura itself is entirely clinical – there is no laboratory test that can do this for you. And if you are wrong, you have wasted the patient's money and time by ordering the tests.
b. Even if you are correct in your clinical diagnosis, you may still be wasting valuable time by ordering standard lab tests, since the commonest causes of purpura in a hospital patient probably are sepsis and drug toxicity. These may need urgent therapy and **any** blood tests (apart from blood cultures) may have to be postponed.

Alternatively, the doctor sees a boy of 10 with what appears to be purpura on his buttocks and down the back of his legs; a proper examination reveals numerous sore joints and blood and protein in the urine; he realizes that that this is most probably not purpura but vasculitis and that he is dealing with the Henoch–Schönlein syndrome. What value would the FBC and hemostatic screen be in this case, except where the diagnosis of vasculitis is uncertain and the discovery of a thrombocytopenia would be very helpful?

Effective, patient-centered care of hematological patients requires, as with all other patients, a comprehensive clinical insight into these disease processes, i.e., an integrated clinical and pathological approach. Added to these problems is the fact that the number of laboratory tests has increased explosively, and the laboratory simply does not have the time to attempt more than a brief, generalized, and, increasingly, an automated interpretation of the results. Thus, the onus of clinical interpretation necessarily falls more and more on the attending clinician, whose grounding in clinical hematology is too often inadequate, for the reasons mentioned.

As mentioned above, hematology is emerging as a clinical specialty in its own right. The training of hematology residents today includes extensive clinical exposure (indeed they are expected to handle the clinical aspects themselves), while training of residents in internal medicine requires considerable knowledge of hematology and its reports. Achieving an integrated approach would be made immeasurably easier by a book presenting the subject in a fully integrated, clinical way. This then has been the motivation for this book. Properly, this approach should be taught to students as well.

There is no shortage of hematological texts, some of them very good, and it would be presumptuous and self-indulgent to add to them without clear justification. However, practically all of the student-orientated texts tend still to teach hematology from a formal and largely static laboratory perspective, and the reports emanating from the laboratory tend to reinforce this. Many of the "Crash Course" types of hematology book on the market have (at least) two major weaknesses: they considerably oversimplify the subject, contributing to the very mechanistic and almost anti-intellectual approach to blood diseases and especially to the FBC and hemostatic screen; and they tend to concentrate on primary blood diseases, whereas in practice most abnormalities of the blood and in the FBC are secondary to disease outside the system – that is to say, they work primarily from a pathological and not from a clinical viewpoint. The FBC is one of the most common and valuable tests in use; while it is not a particularly expensive test, it is generally speaking poorly interpreted, and the potential wealth of information that can be gleaned is missed.

The approach described in this book is different from that in most student texts, and has been very successful in practice. I start almost from scratch, but omitting many of the "basics" such as the details of hematopoiesis and laboratory technology, which are hardly relevant to the practising clinician and the student in the wards, and are primarily of interest to the hematologist and sometimes to the clinical specialist. Considerable emphasis is given to the clinical history and examination, and the interpretation of the clinical patterns thus exposed. Hopefully it will overcome many of the traditional problems experienced in practical diagnostic hematology.

All the practical essentials are covered, and effectively this book contains all the information the student will ever need, apart from details of therapy (until and unless they enter certain specialties).

The book is restricted to adult hematology, for practical reasons. While there are considerable areas of similarity between adult and pediatric hematology, there are also very significant differences. Thus, the only congenital diseases discussed in this book are those that can present after childhood and occasionally those that pose a significant problem in adult practice. Generally, these are discussed only briefly. Often with these the assistance of a hematologist would have to be sought anyway. Sometimes even the hematologist may have to further consult someone sub-specializing in pediatric hematology.

Pretoria, South Africa   Norman Beck

Acknowledgments

No modern medical book can be written without a huge amount of input from colleagues. I mention elsewhere in the book that the Full Blood Count represents and can be seen as a resultant of many interacting processes. I find myself in the same position, with respect to all the assistance, advice, and encouragement I have received. It is impossible to mention, even to know the thousands of patient and dedicated workers in the field whose work I have had the temerity to distil and reproduce. I doff my hat to them in deep respect. Specifically however I gratefully mention some names:

Ingram Anderson, Lindsay Anderson, Ronald Anderson, Ernest Beutler, Liesl de Wet, Anthon Heyns, Peter Jacobs, James Ker, Nick Laage, Louis Lombaard, Patrick Mac-Phail, Barry Mendelow, Johan Nieman, Roger Pool, Neels Potgieter, Jan Pretorius, Andre Swart, and Antoine van Gelder.

I have borrowed shamelessly from the various seminars and lectures given by, and informal discussions with, residents in the various departments in the medical school.

With respect to the cases presented, about 90% derive from my private practice (where it is easier to follow up and investigate difficult problems). Most of the rest are hospital cases, but one very interesting one (Case #65) came from Sadique Jina – thank you.

Riana Cockeran, Helen Steel, and Annette Theron were of huge help to me with many of the graphics.

My editors at Springer with enormous professionalism guided me through the labyrinth of getting a book like this into print.

Gillian Nineham and John Harrison – without your massive efforts on my behalf this project would never have got off the ground.

Finally to my long-suffering family – sorry for the times of neglect and neurosis.

To all the above, I can only give you my heartfelt thanks. Needless to say, the errors are all mine.

Contents

Abbreviations

ALL	Acute lymphoblastic leukemia
AML	Acute myeloblastic leukemia
AMML	Acute myelomonocytic leukemia
ANLL	Acute non-lymphocytic leukemia
APL	Acute promyelocytic leukemia
CCF	Congestive cardiac failure
CLL	Chronic lymphocytic leukemia
CML	Chronic myelocytic leukemia
CMML	Chronic myelomonocytic leukemia
CRP	C-reactive protein
DAT	Direct Antiglobulin Test (Coombs)
DDAVP	1-Deamino-8-D-arginine vasopressin
DIC	Disseminated intravascular coagulation
ESR	Erythrocyte sedimentation rate
ET	Essential thrombocythemia
FAB	French–American–British (classification)
FBC	Full blood count
G6PD	Glucose-6-phospate dehydrogenase deficiency
GP	General practitioner (equivalent to medical practitioner/family practitioner/family doctor/generalist)
GvHD	Graft-versus-host disease
Hb	Hemoglobin
HCL	Hairy cell leukemia
Hct	Hematocrit
HD	Hodgkin disease
HS	Hereditary spherocytosis
HUS	Hemolytic-uremic syndrome
IgA	Immunoglobulin A
IgE	Immunoglobulin E
IgG	Immunoglobulin G
IgM	Immunoglobulin M
ITP	Immune (or idiopathic) thrombocytopenic purpura
JCML	Juvenile chronic myelocytic leukemia
MCH	Mean cell hemoglobin
MCHC	Mean cell hemoglobin concentration
MCV	Mean cell volume
MDS	Myelodysplastic syndrome/s
MF	Myelofibrosis
MM	Multiple myelomatosis

MPD	Myeloproliferative disorder/s
NHL	Non-Hodgkin lymphoma
NRBC	Nucleated red blood cells
PC	Platelet count
PLT	Platelet/s
PNH	Paroxysmal nocturnal hemoglobinuria
PT	Prothrombin time
PTT	Partial thromboplastin time
PV	Polycythemia vera
RBC	Red Blood Cell
RCC	Red cell count or Red Cell Concentrate
RDW	Red cell distribution width
SAA	Serum amyloid A
TTP	Thrombotic thrombocytopenic purpura
vWD	von Willebrand disease
vWF	von Willebrand factor
WBC	White Blood Cell
WCC	White cell count

Preliminary Concepts

A good beginning makes a good ending.
(14th century proverb)

This book is aimed primarily at students and family practitioners, and the approach is as simple, straightforward, and user-friendly as possible. Feedback, however, has been such that it is clear that clinical residents and even consultants will find the book useful. This book will cover 95% of the general caseload if not more, and readers will understand that more complex cases will need to be referred. (Note that the **EXPERT** level, that of the hematologist, is not covered at all). The major focus in this book is on clinical and laboratory diagnosis; thus only the irreducible minimum of **BASIC** knowledge is presented to this end. This basic knowledge must, however, be known well so as to avoid shotgun approaches on the one hand and an unthinking algorithmic approach on the other.

There are several essential preliminary issues that need clarification:

1. *The nature of modern hematology. Hematology has changed considerably in the last decades and is becoming an essentially clinical subject, requiring a quantum shift in thinking.*
2. *The general overview of the types of blood disease in relation to the essential blood tests required, without which diagnosis of these diseases is usually impossible.*
3. *Certain practical issues with respect to the problems and limitations commonly found in practice.*
4. *Nomenclature in hematology is very unsystematic. To know what we are talking about, it is essential to have clarity in this regard.*
5. *Conventions adopted in the text.*
6. *A brief outline of the chapters.*

Modern Hematology in Context

Hematology has changed considerably over the last few decades. Greater knowledge has enabled far more conditions to be treated than before. The advances in molecular medicine in particular have been astonishing.

Secondly, before the days of mass travel and migration, the practitioner could conveniently concentrate on (and remember) only those conditions that were prevalent in his community. Today, however, the practitioner can be faced with any number of diseases not endemic to the community, and he must perforce at least be aware of the basic principles underlying their diagnosis. Thus the practitioner in say northern Scotland can easily be faced with conditions such as tropical eosinophilia, African-type G6PD deficiency, and sickle disease. This book therefore is very general in scope. The user must use considerable discretion in what he skims over and what he concentrates on.

Thirdly, as in medicine as a whole, clinical epidemiology is gaining greater and greater significance in practice. This is particularly so in hematology, since it is so dependent on tests.

Finally, hematology is emerging as a primarily clinical specialty. This has not been plain sailing, since it has had to do battle with a centuries-old mind-set where it has been taken for granted that diagnosis of blood diseases is via the laboratory. Originally this was quite understandable: in view of the paucity of clear and clinically definable

O.N. Beck, *Diagnostic Hematology*, DOI 10.1007/978-1-84800-295-1_1,
© Springer-Verlag London Limited 2009

signs and symptoms, there was little in the way of a body of clinical knowledge developing in blood diseases. The emergence of modern clinical medicine as a scientific endeavor initially came about when intensive necropsy studies and the associated clinical features were correlated. These had little to contribute to hematology. **THE HEMATOLOGICAL SYSTEM IS RELATIVELY INACCESSIBLE CLINICALLY,** unlike most other systems. It is interesting to place clinical entities in hematology, as we know them today, into a historical perspective and to note how few of these were recognized as such before the advent of modern blood tests. Some examples are as follows:

1. **CHLOROSIS.** This strange condition, hardly ever seen today, was correctly linked to iron deficiency in the 1830s. The nature of the clinical presentation was (and is) obscure.
2. **PERNICIOUS ANEMIA.** The clinical features were well described by Addison in 1855. However, there was no understanding of the condition until Cohnheim found specific morphological changes in the marrow ±20 years later; Ehrlich described the histological changes shortly thereafter. In 1883, Manson empirically discovered the utility of raw liver in this condition.
3. **HYPERSPLENISM.** In 1882 a group of conditions characterized by decreased cell counts in association with a large spleen was described. There was little understanding of pathological processes that could cause this picture, and they were lumped together with other conditions causing splenomegaly such as hemolytic anemias, myelofibrosis, and so on.
4. **PAROXYSMAL COLD HEMOGLOBINURIA.** This was identified in 1868 and differentiated from the hemoglobinuria of trauma. It was later associated almost exclusively with tertiary syphilis, and today with viral infections, mainly in children.
5. **BLEEDING DISORDERS.** As far as these are concerned, their history goes back very much further – to the time of the ancient Israelites. This history is long and fascinating. Only a few highlights are presented:

   (a) Hemorrhagic purpura was described by Werlhof in 1735. Its nature was completely unknown, the platelet never having been seen.
   (b) A hemorrhagic disposition existing in certain families was described by Otto in 1803; its modern name – hemophilia – was coined by Hopff, a student of Schönlein in 1828. The prolonged coagulation time was **NOT** recognized.
   (c) In 1935 and 1936, it was shown that the prothrombin time (PT) was reduced in various jaundiced patients. The PT had been developed in 1935 by Quick et al. Quick predicted that bleeding in jaundiced patients was probably caused by a lack of vitamin K. This was rapidly confirmed.

There was very little insight into what exactly was the nature of the disease processes. Clinical features in blood diseases were considered as vague and misleading. The more precise identification of various diseases of the blood by noting laboratory-derived changes in the blood seemed to show that any clinical features present would not have permitted clinical diagnosis as revealed by the test. This is all the more understandable when one considers the nature of the system itself: it consists of a fluid tissue – blood – that flows through all the other organs, including those organs that maintain this fluid. As it flows, the blood affects and is affected by all the tissues, healthy or otherwise, through which it flows. But there are no direct clinical means by which one can examine this fluid.

Thus it was inevitable that the conclusion was reached that the traditional clinical methods used in most other branches of clinical medicine were irrelevant in blood diseases. We can refer to this as the **LABORATORY BIAS.**

And of course this bias still tends to be perpetuated in teaching. The diagnostic utility of blood tests is taught to students separately, usually by laboratory hematologists, who often tend to be very scientifically orientated: the concept of clinical judgment in the choice and interpretation of tests is rejected by some of them, held as being subjective and unscientific. Thus they attempt to make an exact science out of laboratory medicine, without reference to the context in which it is used. Laboratory findings are sometimes presented, sometimes very subtly, as the **PRIMARY** presentation of disease, with the clinical features regarded as semi-confirmatory, instead of the other way around. This type of bias has inevitably worked its way through into the thinking of many students and is perpetuated as such when they themselves become teachers.

The same bias is sometimes extended to morphological comment on reports, this being regarded by many as subjective and inherently subject to error – measured results are automatically regarded as more reliable (a most dangerous conclusion!). One cannot, for example, measure with an instrument the presence of spherocytes (yet), and therefore it is held that osmotic fragility and other tests are far more reliable. Yet these tests take a lot of time (and money), and the experienced morphologist will diagnose spherocytes in most cases by looking at the smear for less than a minute.

Why then bother with a clinical approach to blood diseases?

1. Laboratory diagnosis is by no means infallible. In good hands a laboratory diagnosis is very good as far as it goes, but it very often does not – and cannot – go far enough.

2. Patients expect – and appreciate – a holistic patient-centered approach to their problems, particularly in view of the modern impersonal HMO type of trend in patient care.

3. While **INITIAL** access to the hematological system, in the sense of enabling a pathological definition of the disease process, is still by means of blood tests in the vast majority of cases, several major factors stress the strong contribution that clinical assessment makes. The three most important are

    (a) The actual suspicion that the patient has a blood disease, which would then prompt further, more directed investigation, is an entirely clinical assessment.

    (b) Once the first-stage diagnosis is made by means of a blood test, subsequent identification of the pathological process involved is a highly clinical activity, as will be discussed in Chapter 5.

    (c) Monitoring the patient's progress cannot be done exclusively by repeated blood tests.

4. It has been shown quite clearly that examining other organs and tissues can provide considerable clinical insight into the nature of the blood, indeed complementing (and sometimes negating) the laboratory findings. Clinical assessment of organs and tissues in all fields usually involves two groups of methods: the direct and the indirect. For example, in the assessment of suspected lung disease, the standard examination of the chest provides direct evidence, while the presence of central cyanosis, a flapping tremor, and so on will provide indirect evidence (i.e., changes in organs outside the chest). In blood diseases, virtually **ALL THE EVIDENCE IS INDIRECT**. The systematic description of changes in the other organs has provided a significant database of features that are valuable in the assessment of blood diseases. Those wishing to learn these features have great difficulty, however, since the application of the relevant clinical methods is largely ignored in teaching scripts, certainly in the sense of a systematic presentation, reflecting the **LABORATORY BIAS**.

Note that the experienced clinician is perfectly prepared to rely on his own clinical judgment in conditions such as dysdiakokinesis or tension pneumothorax. Yet, with a perceived blood disease, he seems prepared to surrender his judgment.

In the rest of this book a sensible clinical/laboratory approach to diagnosis of blood diseases will be shown to be possible and indeed desirable.

The central theme of this book is the concept of an integrated clinical and laboratory approach to hematological disorders, including changes in the blood secondary to disease in other systems. It will be shown by explanation and many practical examples that this approach will resolve most of the problems experienced. All that is required is a willingness to adopt an integrating mind-set.

The Broad Types of Hematological Disease and Their Tests

It is important that two points be understood:

1. Most abnormalities in the hematological system and its tests are due to disease in other systems.

2. It is practically impossible to diagnose most disorders that affect the blood without laboratory tests.

It is important to place these in perspective, and one way of characterizing blood diseases is, logically, in terms of the tests that most prominently show abnormalities. The two tests that have emerged as the **BASIC**, first-line tests are the full blood count (FBC) and the hemostatic screen. It is important to see the power and scope of these indispensable tests; they with their clinical correlates, particularly the FBC, are hence the main focus of this book. However, contrary to what very many people think, these tests are generally pretty useless without proper interpretation – and effective interpretation of these tests is not trivial, relying considerably on clinical input and expertise.

Blood Diseases Characterized Essentially by Changes in the FBC

Here we can broadly identify three groups:

1. FBC changes reflecting diseases that only incidentally affect the blood and where the FBC picture is purely reactive or responsive. Examples are the neutrophilia of acute bacterial infection; the anemia, thrombocytosis, and reticulocytosis secondary to acute blood loss; erythrocytosis secondary to chronic hypoxia. The changes in the bone marrow are primarily reactive

and do not indicate any disease of the marrow or the blood per se. For our purposes we will refer to these disorders as **REACTIVE**. These are **COMMON**. They are particularly significant in that the appearances sometimes can mimic, often very closely, true hematological disease.

2. FBC changes reflecting diseases outside the blood system but where there is a secondary deleterious effect on the marrow or the blood itself. Examples are iron-deficiency anemia due to chronic bleeding from a malignant lesion in the colon; hemolytic anemia due to autoantibodies to normal red cells. For our purposes we will refer to these disorders as **SECONDARY**. These are **COMMON.**

3. Primary disorders of the marrow or developing blood cells. Examples are leukemia; hereditary spherocytosis. For our purposes we will refer to these disorders as **PRIMARY** or **TRUE** blood diseases. These are **UNCOMMON.**

Diseases Characterized Essentially by Changes in the Hemostatic Screen

Here again we can broadly identify three groups:

1. Changes reflecting diseases that only incidentally affect the blood and where the reaction is purely reactive or responsive. Important examples are the raised factor VIII levels that can occur as an acute phase reactant, and raised platelets as a result of splenectomy. These changes are essentially reactive and do not indicate any disease of the hemostatic mechanisms per se (although hypercoagulability is theoretically possible in the above cases). For our purposes we will refer to these disorders as **REACTIVE**. These are relatively **RARE**.

2. Changes in the hemostatic system reflecting diseases outside the system but where there is a secondary deleterious effect on the liver, the endothelium, the marrow, or the blood itself. To mention just a few examples,

   (a) Liver failure for any number of reasons.
   (b) Adsorption of coagulation factors, notably factor X, by abnormal proteins, leading to a bleeding disorder.
   (c) Autoantibodies to platelets or coagulation factors.

   For our purposes we will refer to these disorders as **SECONDARY**. These are **COMMON**.

3. Primary disorders. Examples are hemophilia, myelodysplasia. For our purposes we will refer to these disorders as **PRIMARY** or **TRUE** hemostatic diseases. These are relatively **UNCOMMON**.

Problems and Limitations Found in Practice

Training in the laboratory sciences tends not to prepare the student for post-graduate realities. Practice in the big wide world is different from that in the teaching hospitals. Those going out into independent (i.e., non-institutional) practice usually have to make considerable adaptations to their thinking. One of the issues is the ordering of **ROUTINE** tests, a common tendency in teaching hospitals. In practice, the cost implications become significant. Tests done as a routine have a very low clinical yield: ±2%. This applies to the FBC as well but only when it is requested without a clinical suspicion of a hematological disorder or of a possible disorder in another system where an abnormality in the FBC is known to occur secondarily and relatively frequently.

Routine Screening Tests In general, routine screens performed to try to identify disease are discouraged. Statistically, it can be shown that if a sufficient number of tests are performed on an (apparently) healthy patient at any one time, the result of one (or more) is going to be false, and even perhaps outside the reference range, occasioning unnecessary expense, not to say alarm for the patient. This phenomenon has prompted one cynic to remark that *The normal patient is one who has been insufficiently investigated* (!) Broadly speaking, routine tests, if done, should be done for medico-legal rather than clinical reasons.

The epidemiology of blood diseases too is very different in general practice. Consider, for example, anemia: over half of all hospital patients are anemic; identifying the nature of their anemia can be of great assistance in the management of their conditions. But in family practice, anemia is much less common, and one simply cannot do routine FBCs on all patients in family practice (bearing in mind that mild anemia and often even moderate anemia are very difficult to detect or even suspect clinically especially when the clinical focus is on another system).

What is needed is a high index of clinical suspicion and perspective; and this clinical insight tends to be neglected in teaching. This is a significant problem, especially in private general practice. The good family practitioner requests about 25 FBCs per week (out of an average patient load of say 200 per week) and faces a serious problem: many laboratories, particularly many private and many small public laboratories do not or cannot offer, as a routine, a professional morphological opinion or clinical comment. The GP is thus constrained to interpret the numerical results and **FLAGS** himself, and this requires a lot of expertise, which again is hardly touched on in teaching. This important issue is discussed in Chapter 2.

Nomenclature

One of the major problems in medicine is confusing, illogical, and archaic terminology. We are stuck with this because meaning is determined by common usage. In hematology, the culprits are largely the names given to changes in the cell concentrations – which happen, as you will see later, to be first-stage diagnoses, and improper usage can have serious consequences.

The problem can lie in the **STEM** or in the **SUFFIX**. Uncontroversial words, stems, or suffixes are

1. **ANEMIA** (although it actually means **WITHOUT BLOOD!**)
2. **LEUKO-**, the stem for white cells
3. **MONO-**, the stem for monocytes
4. **EOSINO-**, the stem for eosinophils
5. **BASO-**, the stem for basophils
6. **LYMPHO-**, the stem for lymphocytes
7. **THROMBO-**, the stem for platelets
8. **-PENIA**, a suffix meaning a decrease in

Problems in nomenclature arise with the use of some stems and with most of the suffixes. These problems are with

1. **NEUTRO-**, whereas many prefer **GRANULOCYTO-** or sometimes **GRANULO-**. In fact, **GRANULO-** is not a synonym for **NEUTRO-**, since the term **GRANULOCYTES** embraces neutrophils, eosinophils, and basophils.
2. The suffix **-CYTOSIS** is used in certain circumstances, while **-CYTHEMIA** and **-PHILIA** are used in others. **-CYTOSIS** refers primarily to a benign increase in that particular cell type, although irregular use is common. Examples include
   (a) Thrombocytosis, referring to a benign increase in circulating platelets
   (b) Leukocytosis, referring to a benign or malignant increase in circulating white cells

Table 1.1 Common Terms in Hematology

Name	Meaning
Leukocytosis	Benign or malignant increase in leukocytes
Leukopenia	Decrease in the total white cell count
Neutrophilia	Benign (usually) increase in neutrophils
Neutropenia	Decrease in neutrophils
Monocytosis	Benign (usually) increase in monocytes
Monocytopenia	Decrease in monocytes
Lymphocytosis	Benign or malignant increase in lymphocytes
Lymphopenia	Decrease in lymphocytes
Eosinophilia	Benign (usually) increase in eosinophils
Eosinopenia	Benign (usually) decrease in eosinophils
Basopenia	Decrease in basophils
Thrombocythemia	Malignant increase in platelets
Thrombocytosis	Benign increase in platelets
Thrombocytopenia	Decrease in platelets

-CYTHEMIA is generally used to refer to a malignant increase in a particular cell line, as in **THROMBO-CYTHEMIA**, but on the other hand the term **POLY-CYTHEMIA** can refer to both benign or malignant increase in red cells or of all three cell lines (this important issue is discussed below). Another suffix used for increases in some of the components is **-PHILIA**, which is a misnomer, but is hallowed by widespread and ancient usage. This also applies to the two words **HEMOPHILIA**, meaning **LOVE OF BLEEDING**, and **THROMBOPHILIA**, meaning **LOVE OF CLOTTING**.

For a summary see Table 1.1.

There are four terms that are particularly controversial and where clarity is essential: basophilia, polycythemia, erythrocytosis, and pancytopenia.

Basophilia

Note that there is no mention in Table 1.1 of increase in basophils. The term **BASOPHILIA** is not to be used without qualification. When there is a reticulocytosis, in the ordinary blood smear the reticulocytes will be seen as purplish-staining red cells. This is frequently called **DIFFUSE BASOPHILIA** and has nothing to do with the leukocytes of that name. **POLYCHROMASIA** is far preferable, but usage of **DIFFUSE BASOPHILIA** is too widespread to ignore it. Thus when we want to talk of an increase in basophils – the leukocytes – to avoid possible confusion, we should use the term **BASOPHIL LEUKOCYTOSIS**, and **NOT** simply **BASOPHILIA**.

Polycythemia and Erythrocytosis

These terms are the sources of considerable confusion and irregular usage. Some clinicians use these terms more or less interchangeably, but there are many variations. For example,

1. Some (the better informed) seem to use **POLYCYTHE-MIA** for the myeloproliferative (malignant) condition and **ERYTHROCYTOSIS** for all the others.
2. Others seem to eschew the term **ERYTHROCYTOSIS** and divide **POLYCYTHEMIA** into **PRIMARY** (the malignant form) and **SECONDARY**.

One problem (among several) with the various classifications is that, as so often occurs in medicine, the identified classes are not discreet – i.e., there is considerable overlap.

A brief historical context may assist. When, over 100 years ago, the first patients with plethora (and which, according to Osler's description, were almost certainly what we would today call polycythemia vera (PV)) were described, the increase in hematocrit (Hct), and later in the red cell count (RCC), was recognized, and thus the term **POLYCYTHEMIA** came to be used in all cases presenting with plethora and with an increase in hematocrit (and when the technology became available, an increase in most cases of hemoglobin (Hb)). With increasing experience, however, it was realized that the condition or finding as described could represent different entities:

1. Classical polycythemia vera. When, in addition to the raised RCC (and hematocrit (Hct)), the white cell count (WCC) and platelet count (PC) were also found to be increased, the term continued to be applied without further difficulty. And indeed, this type of presentation was easily understood and in itself was initially the source of no controversy. As the nature of PV became clearer, it came to be recognized as one of the chronic myeloproliferative disorders (a malignancy).
2. Later it became clear that some cases of PV, especially in the early stages, **PRESENTED ONLY WITH A RAISED HCT**. This became a problem when it was realized that there were many other causes of a raised Hct, most of them **NOT MALIGNANT** – clearly a crucial distinction.
3. The plethora and raised Hct in cases with chronic chest disease were also recognized quite early. These were seen as a physiological response to tissue hypoxia. It came to be referred to, confusingly, by two different terms, **ERYTHROCYTOSIS** and **SECONDARY POLYCYTHEMIA** (with PV then being referred to as **PRIMARY POLYCYTHEMIA**).

4. Polycythemia and plethora were quite early recognized as (benign) characteristics of Cushing syndrome.
5. A further complication arose when the apparent increase in red cells due to decreased plasma water was recognized:

   (a) The form associated with acute dehydration was easy to understand, since it was due to hemoconcentration and did not represent any change in actual red cell mass. Most cases were found to have only an (apparent) increase in Hct. However, occasionally, and confusingly, all three cell lines could be increased in the short term, requiring extra care in assessment.

   (b) A strange condition was found to be associated, at least in part, with chronic loss of plasma water. This condition passed through several incarnations as far as the name was concerned, such as Gaisbock syndrome, stress polycythemia, and currently **APPARENT ERYTHROCYTOSIS**. There is evidence, however, that the pathogenesis is more complex than first thought, at least in some cases.

6. Finally, a number of unusual causes of erythrocytosis were recognized, some of which had features suggestive also of a possible malignant process, but in other cases of an unusual pathogenesis, such as in smokers' erythrocytosis.

None of these problems would, however, be important were it not for the fact that precise clinical diagnosis (which requires precise naming) is essential for rational therapy.

In all of the above except in cases that have been treated, the hematocrit is raised, and a common point of departure with most clinicians and some hematologists is to lump all these cases as **POLYCYTHEMIA**, defined by a raised hematocrit, and then to further characterize the nature, dividing them into primary and secondary. This is reasonable but it turns out that the formal investigation of such cases is very elaborate (and expensive), and the practical clinician will always look for features that will save time and make his life and that of his patient easier. And one major feature in this regard is that **THE RANGE OF CAUSES OF A POLYCYTHEMIA WHERE ALL THREE CELL LINES ARE INCREASED AS OPPOSED TO ONLY A RAISED HEMATOCRIT IS VERY MUCH NARROWER AND HENCE EASIER (AND CHEAPER) TO INVESTIGATE AND TYPE.**

The policy thus adopted in this book (and which is found among growing numbers of hematologists) is to use the term **POLYCYTHEMIA** for an increase in all three cell lines and **ERYTHROCYTOSIS** to refer to an

Table 1.2 Common Terms in Hematology

Name	Meaning
Polycythemia	Increase in all three cell lines
Erythrocytosis	Increase in the hematocrit alone
Basophil leukocytosis	Increase in the basophils (leukocytes)
Pancytopenia	Decrease in all three cell lines

increase in red cell numbers **AND/OR** in hematocrit, whether the latter is a true increase in red cell mass or not (i.e., an **APPARENT ERYTHROCYTOSIS**). It will be seen in Chapters 16 and 17 that this distinction considerably simplifies the investigative process.

Pancytopenia

A rather odd problem exists with this term. It means an abnormal reduction in all three cell lines. The problem lies in the fact that most people relate the peripheral cell count to marrow function only, and thus to cells produced directly by the marrow. But what about the lymphocytes, which are only partly dependent on marrow function? If all the cells of myeloid origin are reduced, but the lymphocyte count is on the high side, this could push the total white cell count into the normal range. Is this still a pancytopenia? There is no clear answer to this; just bear the controversy in mind.

Thus we can complete Table 1.1 – see Table 1.2. Further notes on Table 1.1:

1. Strictly, a malignant increase in white cells is called leukemia (actually an archaic term). Sometimes, when suspecting a chronic leukemia, one is not always sure of the nature of the increase until further investigations are done. **LEUKOCYTOSIS** then is a convenient term to describe the picture until clarity is reached.
2. The accuracy of the eosinophil count is dependent upon the method of counting, and thus the level of laboratory. Electronic counters count thousands of cells, and thus an accurate eosinophil count can be produced. In manual counting, however, the usual way to do an eosinophil count is to use the total white count and the differential count to work out the eosinophil count. This means that usually only 100 white cells are counted. By chance, with even a normal eosinophil count, one may come across **NO** eosinophils. When the count is decreased, this trend is accentuated. Thus, in level 1 laboratories (see later), the reference range for eosinophils is (or should be) given as $0–450×10^9$/l, whereas in other laboratories, it is 40–450.

3. What was said about eosinophils is even more relevant to the basophil count, since basophils are even more scarce than eosinophils.

Conventions Adopted

This book consists of **FACTS, DISCUSSIONS,** and **PRACTICAL EXAMPLES**. Certain passages are of particular importance and marked as such in the margins with the icon: **!**

This represents one or more facts to be taken **PARTICULAR** note of and to be studied, **UNDERSTOOD**, and **REMEMBERED**.

When the icon is found next to the **HEADING** of a section, then the significance of the emblem applies to the whole section.

During their training students are used to first-class laboratory facilities. After their training, however, they may find themselves in very different circumstances, such as severely under-funded rural or field hospitals. In this book we use laboratory results for teaching purposes extensively; to cater for the variety of laboratories the reader may one day be associated with, four levels of laboratory have (fairly arbitrarily) been defined and from which these examples will be drawn. Where the level of a laboratory is not stated, it is assumed to be a level 4 lab.

LEVEL 1. This is a very basic laboratory. The range of tests is limited and the technology is manual and fairly primitive.
LEVEL 2. This laboratory would have one of the earlier types of particle counters, with a generally larger margin for technical errors than with today's instruments. The other tests would mainly still be done manually, including the differential count of the leukocytes. The range of tests done is limited.
LEVEL 3. This is a reasonably modern laboratory with instruments of a 10- to 15-year vintage. The differential count is to varying degrees automated (with varying accuracy) and frequently only a 3-part (automated) differential count will be available.
LEVEL 4. This is a modern, fully equipped laboratory.

Note also that laboratory hematologists and pathologists vary considerably in their special interests, background, and experience. The level of laboratory has an effect; a level 1 laboratory may only have a general pathologist, perhaps on a part-time basis. The user should tailor her expectations accordingly.

CONVENTION WITH RESPECT TO THE PRACTICAL EXAMPLES. To make discussion easier and more relevant, abnormal results are printed in **RED**.

A Brief Overview of the Contents

Chapter 2 is an essential introduction and overview of the blood system and the first-line tests used in this system, purely from the clinical and general point of view.

Chapter 3 provides an overview of the difficulties arising from using these tests, as well as an introduction to modern clinical epidemiological approaches to diagnosis.

Note that most of Chapters 2 and 3 are for background reading; much of the material has been covered in the pre-clinical years, but is presented here from a purely clinical point of view. A grasp of the concepts is far more important than remembering the facts. These chapters essentially provide the basis of a rational understanding of the tests used in hematology. The emphasis is from the viewpoint of the practicing clinician, in an attempt to counteract the confusion and uncertainty that pervades the minds of many colleagues when it comes to blood diseases.

Chapters 4 and 5 represent a major departure from traditional teaching sources in hematology. The blood interacts with all the other systems and, not surprisingly, clinical features suggesting blood disease are found by examining other systems; by the same token, disease of other systems commonly affects the blood; the consequent changes in the blood may be sufficiently specific to suggest the nature of the other systemic disorder. Thus Chapter 4 presents a summary of the clinical interactions between the blood and other systems, to facilitate diagnosis, therapy, and prognosis. It thus also presents an overview of the hematological aspects of particular systems, of value to specialists in the relevant fields.

Chapter 5 presents a practical clinical approach to hematological diagnosis, to a large extent using the data from Chapter 4, and forms the basis for what follows thereafter. Much of this chapter is a recapitulation of basic clinical science but from the perspective of the blood; readers needing a grounding in or a refresher of the basic clinical methodology will find this chapter especially useful.

Chapter 6 presents a formal but highly practical diagnostic approach to the first-line tests.

Chapter 7 discusses some very important considerations about anemia in general.

Chapters 2–7 conclude with a series of quick tests of comprehension.

Each chapter from Chapters 8 to 23 presents and discusses a particular type of hematological presentation, with case studies, tutorials, and exercise cases. These tutorials make no claim to completeness, the intention has been only to provide enough theoretical knowledge to enable the problem being discussed to make sense and to provide a springboard for thinking about similar cases. THE MAIN METHOD OF TEACHING IS VIA CASE STUDIES. This approach is in direct contrast to the usual formal textbook style of teaching of hematology to undergraduates. The cases chosen reflect a wide variety of presentations and a wide variety of causes. Many of these teaching cases are of diseases outside the hematological system.

Further Reading

Loudon ISL. Chlorosis, anemia, and anorexia nervosa. Br. Med. J. (1980) 281: 20–27.

Werlhof PG (1933). Opera medica. In Jones HW, Tocantins LM. The History of Purpura Haemorrhagica. Ann. Med. Hist. 5: 349.

Otto JC (1803). An account of an hemorrhagic disposition existing in certain families. Med. Reposit. 6: 1.

Quick AJ, Stanley-Brown M, Bancroft FW (1935). A study of the coagulation defect in hemophilia and in jaundice. Am. J. Med. Sci. 190: 501.

Knowledge is an essential prerequisite to performance.
(J.H. Hertz)

Preview *It is often only after having entered professional practice that the importance of hematology and of hematological reports are realized, and by then it can be very difficult to catch up. It will be seen that an integrated clinical/laboratory approach to hematology reports is essential. For this, an understanding of six basic topics is required and these then are the study themes of this chapter:*

a. The nature of the blood cell system. Physiologically it must be seen as a balanced homeostatic system.
b. (Very) basic pathology of the hematopoietic system.
c. The nature of the major first-line test in hematology – the FBC.
d. The critical importance of morphology.
e. Sub-components within the red cell circulation: nutrients.
f. The nature of the second first-line test in hematology – the hemostatic screen. This includes

> *i. The nature and mechanism of hemostasis.*
> *ii. Procoagulant, anticoagulant, and fibrinolytic processes.*
> *iii. The basic pathology of the hemostatic processes.*
> *iv. General disorders of hemostasis.*

Hematology and hematological reports are essentially straightforward and easy to grasp and use, given a simple change in mind-set, which entails the development of an integrated clinical and laboratory approach.

!

It will be seen that with an integrated approach, the interpretation of the first-line tests is straightforward and logical. Indeed, the intellectual methodology used in an effective interpretation of the FBC is very akin to the clinical process itself. It is essential, however, that the dynamic nature of the blood system be understood, particularly the fact that the blood pervades all the tissues, affecting them and being affected by them. Indeed, the blood should be seen as a barometer as to what is going on in the tissues.

Since the blood itself – a fluid tissue – is not susceptible of clinical examination, examination of the other organs frequently will indicate, albeit indirectly, changes in the blood. This fact is the primary mechanism that permits clinical examination of the system. **THIS IMPLIES, HOWEVER, THAT THE INTERACTION OF THE BLOOD WITH THE TISSUES MUST BE WELL UNDERSTOOD. SEE CHAPTER 4.**

The Nature of the Blood System

Figure 2.1 depicts how the blood system integrates with the whole.

This shows the basic functions of the blood in the broadest terms:

O.N. Beck, *Diagnostic Hematology*, DOI 10.1007/978-1-84800-295-1_2,
© Springer-Verlag London Limited 2009

Fig. 2.1 The interaction of blood cellular elements and proteins with the tissues

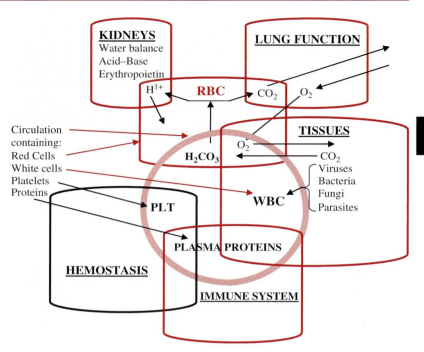

1. **THE RED CELLS:** The provision of oxygen to the tissues and the removal (and buffering) of CO_2 and H^{1+} (in part) from them. Bear in mind that there are ±75 trillion cells in the adult body, of which **FULLY ONE THIRD ARE RED CELLS** (for oxygenation).
2. **THE WHITE CELLS:** The detection and combating of infection (and malignancies) anywhere.
3. **THE PLATELETS:** The sealing of any breaches in the circulation.
4. **PLASMA PROTEINS (VARIOUS):** Cooperation with white cells and platelets to achieve specific functions to do with the integrity of the vessels and the integrity of the organism as a whole (i.e., defense mechanisms).

Note that the functions of the red and white cells, and many of the plasma proteins, are ultimately concerned with **ACTIVITIES OUTSIDE THE CIRCULATION**.

There are two fundamental principles about the system that once understood should enable a more meaningful insight into the reports – primarily of the FBC. (The dynamics of the plasma protein elements of the hemostatic system are not nearly as significant as with the FBC. These are briefly discussed separately, toward the end of the chapter).

1. The FBC should not be seen only as set of static results, but as the dynamic resultant of numerous interacting processes. The FBC is in most cases quite straightforward, given some basics. There is a tendency, however, to try to evaluate each of the reported results separately, and to see the FBC as relatively stable and mono-dimensional. This is incorrect. The potential information it can yield can be markedly increased if interpreted with the dynamics in mind. For example, huge numbers of red cells are being produced and destroyed every second; even a small temporary interference with any of these processes can cause dramatic changes. Also,

   a. Some of the reported entities are interdependent functionally; a change in one may be associated with changes in others, producing different **PATTERNS**.
   b. Patterns may also be generated by the coexistence of independent changes in many of the reported entities.

2. It is a summation at one point in time (the time the blood was drawn) of numerous interacting processes, with the different cell lines having completely different functions, having different life spans, and reflecting different stresses as well as bone marrow, splenic and other functions. (Indeed, the FBC is referred to as a single test only because it is performed on one sample on a single instrument (except in level 1 labs.)).

3. These interacting processes all act in terms of a homeostatic balance between production and disposal of cells (and of hemostatic factors). The efficacy of this

Table 2.1 The red cell snapshot

PERIPHERAL BLOOD.	Coming from: BONE MARROW 1 to 120 days earlier	Going to: BLOOD, SPLEEN, BONE MARROW; OR BLEEDING OR IV HEMOLYSIS. 0–120 days later
THE RED CELL SNAPSHOT.	Production and Release:	
RCC Hb Hct MCV MCH MCHC RDW Retics ESR SHAPE, etc.	Stem cells Rate of proliferation Healthy stroma Iron - Adequate diet, stores - Adequate incorporation into heme Vit B$_{12}$ and folate - Adequate diet, stores EPO, hormones, etc.	Breakdown in spleen with production of bilirubin and re-circulation of iron - Normal rate - Increased rate Bleeding with loss of iron etc. Intravascular hemolysis with loss of iron.

Table 2.3 The platelet snapshot

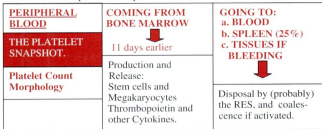

PERIPHERAL BLOOD	COMING FROM BONE MARROW	GOING TO: a. BLOOD b. SPLEEN (25%) c. TISSUES IF BLEEDING
THE PLATELET SNAPSHOT.	11 days earlier	
Platelet Count Morphology	Production and Release: Stem cells and Megakaryocytes Thrombopoietin and other Cytokines.	Disposal by (probably) the RES, and coalescence if activated.

balance both depends on and determines the health of the system.

The FBC represents both **CHANGES IN SPACE** and **CHANGES IN TIME,** and it can be seen as **A SET OF DIFFERENT SNAPSHOTS (SPACE),** one for each of the cell types, of several dynamic and frequently changing processes occurring in **TIME,** and **WITH ALL THE SNAPSHOTS COALESCED INTO ONE REPORT.** From the dynamic point of view, we first consider each cell line separately (Tables 2.1, 2.2, and 2.3).

The red cells have the longest survival, a little less than 120 days. Therefore, a little less than 1% of cells in circulation are **NEW,** i.e., reticulocytes, and erythropoietic activity is most conveniently assessed by the **RETICULOCYTE COUNT,** done by using special stains. Reticulocytes (retics) are the earliest circulating form of the red cells. To assess the degree of reticulocytosis, the count must be related to the number of circulating red cells. Even without the retic count, the number can be estimated on the ordinary stained film, since the retics stain darker than the red cells, and this is called **DIFFUSE BASOPHILIA.** Breakdown of red cells normally occurs in the spleen, with the resultant production of

unconjugated bilirubin, the level of which together with some other measurements is used to assess the breakdown rate.

Another perspective about the red cells is valuable: first, of the 75 **TRILLION** cells in the body, fully one third (i.e., 25 **TRILLION**) are red cells; second, 2,500,000 red cell are broken down every **SECOND,** and correspondingly 2,500,000 red cells (actually reticulocytes) are produced every second.

Survival varies considerably with the different **WHITE CELL** types, of which there are two broad groups: the myeloid cells produced only in the marrow and the lymphoid cells which are only initially produced in the marrow; subsequent production is complicated by their involvement in the immune system.

NEUTROPHILS. Their survival in the circulation is about 15 hours, and they die in a day or two, unless apoptosis is inhibited by certain pro-inflammatory factors. Frequently, especially in bacterial infections, earlier forms appear in the blood, and this is known as a **LEFT SHIFT,** which is generally and sometimes incorrectly interpreted as meaning increased production. Nor does its absence preclude increased production. Also, nor do increased numbers of circulating neutrophils necessarily mean increased production: about half of them at any one time are adherent to the endothelium (**MARGINATION**); these can be mobilized by stress, infection, etc., with a near-doubling of the count without increased production.

No routine methods to assess production rate exist. Immature forms and certain morphological changes can only be suggestive of increased production.

MONOCYTES. Their half-life in the circulation is ± 17 hours, whereupon they enter the tissues. **LYMPHOCYTES.** There are three groups of these, with sub-types: the T-cells, B-cells, and N(atural) K(iller) cells. Their life span can be measured in days, unless stimulated to become memory cells.

EOSINOPHILS have a survival of ± 6 hours in the circulation, whereupon they enter the tissues. **BASOPHILS** survive in the circulation for probably a few days, whereupon they enter the tissues.

Table 2.2 The white cell snapshot

PERIPHERAL BLOOD	COMING FROM: BONE MARROW Hours to 14 days earlier	GOING TO:BLOOD. TISSUES OR APOPTOTIC DEATH Hours to days later
THE WHITE CELL SNAPSHOT	Production and Release: Stem Cells Cytokines	Disposal: Apoptosis or digestion (tissues)
WCC Neutrophils Monocytes Eosinophils Basophils Precursors Lymphoid cells Morphology	COMING FROM LYMPHOID TISSUES	TRAFFICKING IN AND THROUGH THE LYMPHOID TISSUES
	Production and Release: Stem Cells, Stimulated lymphocytes, Cytokines. Antigenic stimulation.	Disposal by Apoptosis

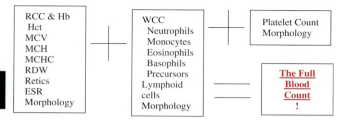

Fig. 2.2 The integrated snapshots

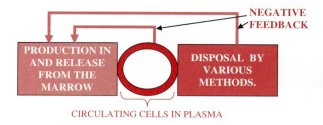

Fig. 2.3 Diagram of the hematological system and its controls

Platelets sequestered in the spleen can be released rapidly by an acute stress response (**FLIGHT OR FIGHT**), etc. This causes a dramatic and short-lived increase in the platelet count.

Now imagine the three snapshots coalesced (Fig. 2.2).

The largely independent cell lines can show considerable interactions from the clinical point of view. Thus, acute post-hemorrhagic anemia is typically accompanied by thrombocytosis; malaria, which causes a hemolytic anemia, is typically accompanied by thrombocytopenia.

> *The most critical conceptual tasks, however, are to see the system as balanced, and to see disturbances or changes in counts in terms of disturbances of this balance.*

The Hematological System Is a Balanced System

Essentially, this refers to the balance between production and disposal or utilization. Physiologically, the blood cells form a balanced system, reflecting homeostatic mechanisms. Thus marrow production, by a feedback mechanism, attempts to adjust itself to the tempo of disposal (so as to maintain a satisfactory level of Hb), but with the following provisos:

1. Production tends to **INCREASE** with **INCREASED** disposal. Increased disposal can occur in the circulation or in the tissues or spleen.
2. It is a one-way adaptation – disposal will not increase or decrease to match increased or decreased production respectively.

Production can thus be decreased, normal, or increased. It would be very useful to be able to assess the rate of production; unfortunately, techniques for this are not easily available, with one exception – the reticulocyte count. Thus from the red cell point of view, we have a convenient method of assessment of marrow activity, and

by extension, how effective attempts at compensation are. Granulocyte precursors and large platelets cannot be used as reliably for white cell and platelet production. Since anemia is by far the commonest disorder of blood, the retic count is extremely useful in practice.

Figure 2.3 shows the basic functional component sites, with control mechanisms.

To see this mechanism in another way, emphasizing the fact that the peripheral count is (normally) controlled by the rate of production, which is in turn controlled by the rate of disposal, see Fig. 2.4.

The normal reticulocyte count (in the presence of a normal Hb) reflects normal production and breakdown.

PATHOLOGICALLY, NUMEROUS EVENTS CAN OCCUR:

1. **THE BALANCE TIPS TOWARD PRIMARY DECREASED PRODUCTION.** There is no possibility of a compensatory decreased disposal. This is illustrated in Fig.2.5.

   Note on Fig. 2.5:

   Disposal is normal only in the sense that such cells reaching the disposal mechanism are disposed of at the normal rate. Since there are fewer cells, **TOTAL**

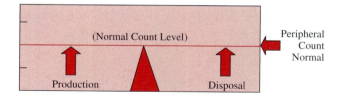

Fig. 2.4 The Physiological Balance

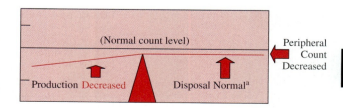

Fig. 2.5 Decreased Production

Table 2.4 Example of recent bone marrow aplasia

	Value	Units	Low	High
Erythrocyte count	3.99	$\times 10^{12}$/l	3.8	4.8
Hemoglobin (Hb)	12.8	g/dl	12	15
Retic count %	**0.21**	%	0.25	0.75
Retic absolute (abs.)	**8.4**	$\times 10^9$/l	30	100
White cell count	**1.45**	$\times 10^9$/l	4	10
Neutrophils abs.	**0.41**	$\times 10^9$/l	2	7
Lymphocytes abs.	1.00	$\times 10^9$/l	1	3
Platelet count	**7.0**	$\times 10^9$/l	150	400

disposal decreases. Since production is defective, breakdown products that are normally re-utilized and not excreted (e.g., iron), will **ACCUMULATE.** The decrease in the peripheral count is **GRADUAL**, with the rate of decline dependent upon the life span of the cells involved. Since this differs among the different cell types, those that are short lived will decrease sooner than say the red cells, which (apart from memory lymphocytes) have the longest life span. The reticulocyte count will be decreased, reflecting the degree of bone marrow suppression even if, in certain cases, the red cell count is normal or near normal. Thus a recent bone marrow aplasia could present with a leukopenia and thrombocytopenia with **NORMAL** Hb, e.g., in the case (Table 2.4) of a young woman who 20 days before had severe hepatitis with severe bone marrow aplasia, and presents now with purpura.

Note: the normal red cell indices and normal lymphocyte count; the decreased reticulocytes, decreased neutrophils, and decreased platelets; that decreased **PRODUCTION** of red cells is characterized by decreased reticulocytes.

2. **THE BALANCE TIPS TOWARD PRIMARY INCREASED PRODUCTION.** There is no possibility of a compensatory increased disposal, with thus an absolute increase in the relevant cell line(s). This can be found in leukemia, thrombocythemia, and so on. See Fig. 2.6

Again, disposal is normal only in the sense that such cells reaching the disposal mechanism are disposed of at the normal rate. Where the red cells are involved, **THE RETICULOCYTE COUNT** could be increased or within the normal range depending on the speed at which the process develops.

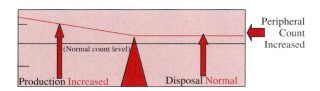

Peripheral Count Increased

Production Increased   Disposal Normal   (Normal count level)

Fig. 2.6 Increased Production

3. **THE BALANCE TIPS TOWARD PRIMARY INCREASED DISPOSAL. THIS SITUATION IS COMMON, AND IT IS MORE DIFFICULT TO UNDERSTAND BECAUSE THE MARROW NORMALLY ATTEMPTS TO COMPENSATE FOR PERIPHERAL LOSS, DESTRUCTION, OR INCREASED FUNCTIONAL REQUIREMENTS.** Compensation may be complete or incomplete, and the normal marrow gradually increases in cellularity proportional to the requirements. The problem is to assess (or even suspect) increased compensatory production, and the role of the FBC in this regard is particularly important. Where the red cells are involved, the reticulocyte count will be increased depending on how efficacious the compensation is.

a. **INCOMPLETE,** i.e., partial compensation. Here there will be a peripheral cytopenia despite the attempt at compensation. Variants of this situation are depicted in Fig. 2.7.

Assuming that we measure red cell marrow production by the reticulocyte count, there are three possible marrow reactions. They are shown as (1), (2), (3) in Fig. 2.7.

(1): Production is clearly subnormal. The FBC fragment in Table 2.5 is from a patient with hemolytic anemia.

The anemia is also accompanied by a retic lower than normal, and there is thus something wrong with the marrow.

(2): Here production is at a level consistent with normal breakdown. However, it would be incapable of restoring the Hb to normal as

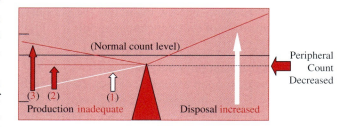

(Normal count level)   Peripheral Count Decreased

(3) (2)   (1)

Production inadequate   Disposal increased

Fig. 2.7 Compensated Production

Table 2.5 Example of a hemolytic anemia plus defective marrow

Red cell count	2.47	$\times 10^{12}$/l	3.8	4.8
Hemoglobin (Hb)	**7.4**	g/dl	12	15
Retic count %	**0.21**	%	0.25	0.75
Retic Absolute (abs.)	**5.2**	$\times 10^9$/l	30	100
White cell count	8.91	$\times 10^9$/l	4	10
Normoblasts	**11**	/100 WBC	0	0
Platelet count	351.0	$\times 10^9$/l	150	400

long as destruction continues. The absolute retic count would be say around 50.

(3): Production is above normal but still insufficient to restore the Hb in a reasonable time. The retic count would be say around 110.

b. **COMPLETE,** i.e., fully effective, maintaining a normal cell concentration. The reticulocyte count would be appropriate (see later).

There are several disease processes to do with increased disposal of cells; the most important from the clinical point of view are

a. **PREMATURE DESTRUCTION OF BLOOD CELLS** because of some abnormality in the cells themselves. In effect, it means that the normal life span is reduced.

b. **AN INCREASE IN THE NORMAL CULLING OF NEWLY FORMED BLOOD CELLS BY THE MARROW** (see later). The result is, effectively, that very active hematopoiesis is incapable of being translated into an equivalent number of cells in the periphery.

c. **DESTRUCTION OR SEQUESTRATION OF NORMAL BLOOD CELLS** by a diseased spleen.

These conditions are discussed under **PATHOLOGY** below.

4. **THE BALANCE TIPS TOWARD PRIMARY INCREASED DEMAND.** The physiology is very similar to point (3). For example, an increased demand for red cells tends to occur in hypoxia; an increased demand for neutrophils tends to occur in bacterial infections; an increased demand for platelets tends to occur in acute hemorrhage.

In summary, the bone marrow maintains the peripheral blood concentration of cells depending upon:

1. The **DEMAND** or **RATE OF DISPOSAL**.
2. **BUT** within certain physiological limits.
3. **AND** dependent upon a number of factors: A healthy bone marrow, both in terms of the progenitor pool and the stroma; normally responsive humoral factors such

as cytokines, certain systemic hormones, and the like; and sufficient supplies of essential nutrients, notably iron and folate.

Figure 2.8 provides another view of the red cell dynamics.

The Basic Pathology of the Hematological System

In most general clinical situations, the clinical features are usually enough to enable one to identify the site and very often the general nature of the pathology. In hematology, this type of process is seldom feasible except in a very general sense. The first-line tests have dramatically changed the situation and allowed us to study the possible pathogenetic mechanisms, supplementing the traditional clinical approach. Thus, just as an absent knee-jerk can reflect more than one underlying pathology, so does say neutrophilia, which could reflect an acute infection, or a reaction to a malignancy or be part of a malignancy. From the clinician's point of view, it is best to discuss the pathology of the system in terms of the production and disposal of blood cells and/or hemostatic elements; the pathology of the blood cell system and of the hemostatic system is discussed separately. Note that in Chapter 4, the relevant pathology of the other systems vis-à-vis the blood is explored.

The Importance of Pathology in the Diagnosis In scientific medicine, we search for the underlying pathology commencing, properly, with the traditional clinical approach. The basic assumption is *clinical features reflect the underlying pathology.* But this reflection is not straightforward: it is true that there are times when a single feature is of such significance that the diagnosis is immediately clear, but too often one pathology, perhaps at different sites, can be reflected in different clinical features, and different pathologies can be reflected in the same or similar clinical presentations. The same considerations apply in the interpretation of many tests, especially the FBC. The classical solution is to identify associated features as patterns, or syndromes, as differentiating features of the actual underlying pathology (the development and refinement of this process has been going on at least since the time of Hippocrates). Thus a mid-diastolic murmur has other causes besides mitral stenosis; *associated features* either tend to confirm or negate your impression of mitral stenosis. And it is no

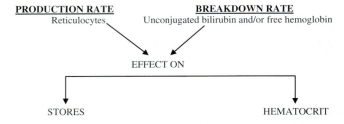

Fig. 2.8 Global dynamics of the red cell system

accident that the common, usually successful, approach to the first-line tests is similarly based on various *patterns* found in the results, and with the same caveats: thus for example not all leuko-erythroblastic reactions reflect an underlying bone marrow malignancy; not all bone malignancies will show such a reaction. It is clear that the pattern is of overriding importance – the total clinical pattern.

The Pathology of the Blood Cell Sub-system (Clinical View)

In studying the basic pathology of this system, it is convenient to use a simplified representation of the system as a whole. Please bear the diagram as shown in Fig. 2.9 in mind: in the broadest terms, it represents the functioning of the system in health and disease – it will be elaborated upon and referred to later in this book. In this diagram, there is no indication of any control or feedback mechanisms. For many students, the hematological system is simply as is represented in this diagram, without any recognition of these feedback or control mechanisms, affecting most of the components of the blood, and thus making the interpretation of the FBC too simplistic. But to explain the pathology, this schema is satisfactory.

Essentially, the production system in the bone marrow consists of huge sets of precursor cells, functioning within a supportive matrix called the stroma; this support is more than merely physical – it has vital roles in stimulating and managing hematopoiesis.

The disposal/utilization aspect is mainly to do with pathology in the spleen, the marrow, and the liver, although disposal can also occur within the circulation.

Types of Pathological Abnormality Affecting the Blood Cell Sub-system

1. Disorders of the plasma affecting concentrations of cells.
2. Production of abnormal cells.

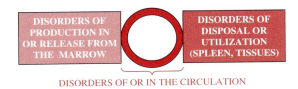

Fig. 2.9 Basic diagram of the hematological system

3. Quantitative disorders of production.

   a. Decreased production.
   b. Increased production: primary and secondary (reactive).

4. Qualitative disorders of blood cells.
5. Disorders of the circulation affecting the blood cells.
6. Disorders of the spleen and increased destruction or sequestration of cells as a result of splenic enlargement
7. As a subset of points (4) and (5): Disorders of survival of blood cells, mainly red cells.
8. As a subset of (2), (4), and (6): Disorders of hemoglobin.

Disorders of the Plasma

Of relevance here are

1. **THE ABSOLUTE AMOUNT OF PLASMA WATER**. This causes dilution or concentration effects on the blood cell numbers. The effects of dehydration and of expansion of the intra-vascular water space are not trivial. Both can have significant effects on many values in the FBC, and their interpretation. Dehydration is further discussed in Chapter 4. Important causes of expansion of the plasma water are fluid overload, congestive cardiac failure, and the syndrome of inappropriate secretion of ADH.
2. **DISORDERS OF PLASMA PROTEINS**, particularly when these are increased, due to reactive or malignant proliferation of certain of the blood cells. The effects on water volume, electrolytes, and cell counts and size can be significant, particularly since they can lead to false results.
3. **THE VAST MAJORITY OF COAGULATION FACTORS**, factors controlling the coagulation process, and the factors responsible for and controlling the breakdown of fibrin clots, are plasma proteins. These belong to the hemostatic system.

Quantitative Disorders of Production of Blood Cells

1. **FAILURE OF PRODUCTION OF NEW CELLS**. This may be due to

   a) **A DEFECT IN THE HEMOPOIETIC ELEMENTS** in the marrow. This in turn can be due to

i. Damage to the precursors themselves, as may be found with physical destruction (e.g., radiation), antibodies, or idiopathic

ii. Marrow necrosis (e.g., in sepsis, collagen disease)

iii. Myelodysplasias (see below)

iv. Defects in the necessary stimulatory growth factors. These factors can be

- Extrinsic to the marrow, such as erythropoietin (EPO) and various hormones (see later)
- Intrinsic to the marrow, which may be derived from the hemopoietic cells themselves or from the stroma

v. Lack of essential nutrients, notably iron, folate, and vitamin B_{12}.

b) **INFILTRATION OF THE MARROW.** This may be due to

i. Fibrosis (called **MYELOFIBROSIS**, and this can be primary (a malignant condition) or secondary)

ii. Primary (hematological) malignancies. While these usually produce large numbers of malignant cells in the peripheral blood, very often the production of normal hemopoietic cells is decreased. These can be

- Acute leukemias and the high-grade lymphomas
- Chronic leukemias and the low-grade lymphomas

iii. Metastatic malignancies

iv. Chronic inflammatory processes and storage diseases.

c) **HEMOPHAGOCYTOSIS (HPS).** This is characterized by proliferation of macrocytes in the marrow, liver, spleen, and lymphoid tissues, with phagocytosis of blood cells and their precursors. There are two broad groups: **INFECTION-ASSOCIATED HPS,** typically due to viruses, such as CMV, tuberculosis, and fungal infections, and it is quite frequent though under-diagnosed in the critically ill with septic shock; and **MALIGNANCY-ASSOCIATED HPS,** usually lymphoma.

2. **PRODUCTION OF INCREASED NUMBERS OF CELLS.** This may be because of

a) **REACTIVE** hyperactivity, such as a (normal) reaction to hypoxia, peripheral infection, bleeding, and so on. Reactive hyperactivity should be suspected

if there is an increase in one cell line only. This is further explained later.

b) **MALIGNANT TRANSFORMATION,** i.e., the myeloproliferative and lymphoplasmaproliferative disorders, either acute or chronic. Malignant hyperactivity should always in the first instance be suspected when there is an increase in more than one cell line – indeed, it suggests that the increase has originated in one of the early precursor cells.

THE LYMPHOPLASMAPROLIFERATIVE DISORDERS include the plasma cell dyscrasias, discussed in Chapter 22; and the lymphomas and lymphoid leukemias, discussed in Chapter 15. Classification of these is very difficult and requires highly specialized techniques and knowledge.

THE CHRONIC MYELOPROLIFERATIVE DISORDERS include chronic myelocytic leukemia (CML), essential thrombocythemia (ET), primary myelofibrosis (PM), and polycythemia vera (PV). One characteristic feature of these is the tendency to transform into acute leukemia, but this is much more common with some than with others. Another is that any one of them may change into the other, again more frequently with some than with others: for example, ± 25% of PV convert into PM eventually, while this is very rare with CML. Myelofibrosis also very rarely converts into another form. There also is a group of these conditions that cannot be satisfactorily pigeonholed, and are termed **UNDIFFERENTIATED CHRONIC MYELOPROLIFERATIVE DISORDER**; in these cases, eventually one of the four types becomes dominant.

3. **DISORDERED PRODUCTION OF BLOOD CELLS.** Many blood diseases have as part of their pathology an effect on the quality of the cells being produced. The effect of this is generally a shortened life span.

a. **DISORDERED PRODUCTION OF BLOOD CELLS AS A RESULT OF INTRAMEDULLARY DESTRUCTION.** This is an overlap category between quantitative and qualitative disorders. There is a large group of disorders where the cells produced are **STRUCTURALLY AND/OR FUNCTIONALLY ABNORMAL**, and as a result the marrow tends to destroy many of them before release into the blood. This is known as **INEFFECTIVE ERYTHROPOIESIS.** These comprise three groups of conditions: megaloblastic anemia, the myelodysplasias, and the hemophagocytic syndrome.

MEGALOBLASTIC ANEMIA. Here, because of defective DNA synthesis, the cells are so abnormal that they are to a large extent destroyed in the marrow, resulting in peripheral cytopenia and marked morphological changes.

THE MYELODYSPLASTIC SYNDROMES. There are two broad groups:

i. The hereditary myelodysplasias: these are seldom of importance in adult medicine.

ii. The acquired myelodysplasias (or myelodysplastic syndromes or MDS). This is a disparate group of disorders whose obvious common feature is dysplastic changes in the blood cell precursors, affecting the FBC appearances. They are usually primary and tend to be pre-malignant. For two reasons, a brief discussion of these is necessary:

  – While they are uncommon, their incidence is undoubtedly increasing, particularly in the First World.
  – They enter into the differential of a great many FBC findings and clinical blood disorders.

The conditions included in the myelodysplastic syndromes are

– **REFRACTORY ANEMIA.** This is actually a very old term, used originally for any chronic anemia that did not respond to hematinics. Many of these cases were later recognized to be what came to be known as an **ANEMIA OF CHRONIC DISORDERS**. Currently, the term is used for a refractory anemia where dysplastic changes are seen in the precursor cells (predominantly the red cell precursors) in the marrow (and generally associated with erythropoietic hypoplasia) and with less than 1% blasts; and a variety of abnormal appearances in the peripheral blood, again mainly affecting the red cells.

– **REFRACTORY ANEMIA WITH RINGED SIDEROBLASTS.** This is effectively a synonym for sideroblastic anemia. The features are essentially the same as under refractory anemia, but with >15% ringed sideroblasts (normoblasts containing iron granules in a ring around the nucleus).

– **REFRACTORY ANEMIA WITH EXCESS BLASTS.** The features are essentially the same as in refractory anemia, but with 5–19% blasts in the marrow but <5% blasts in the blood.

– **REFRACTORY ANEMIA WITH EXCESS BLASTS IN TRANSFORMATION.** The features are essentially the same as in refractory anemia, but with 20–29% blasts in the marrow (but still <5% blasts in the blood).

– **CHRONIC MYELOMONOCYTIC LEUKEMIA.** This is the only MDS with splenomegaly. The bone marrow shows <30% blasts and the blood shows $>1 \times 10^9$/l monocytes.

Note that these disorders are not always accompanied by pancytopenia. There are other classifications of the MDS; cytogenetic studies have identified some clear subsets, such as the 5q⁻ syndrome characterized by thrombocytosis and a good prognosis (relatively). Cytogenetics and immunophenotyping will undoubtedly eventually replace the above classification. For the time being and for the general user, however, this classification is sufficient.

The characteristics of the MDS are diverse, and related to four aspects:

– **THEIR MORPHOLOGY.** They are always (at present) identified in the first instance by morphological changes. These can be subtle, and it is important that they not be missed.

– **THEIR FUNCTIONING.** They tend to be ineffective to variable degrees in respect of their proper functions.

– **THEIR DISPOSAL.** They all tend to have reduced life spans, by various mechanisms.

– **THEIR FREQUENT OVERT MALIGNANT TRANSFORMATION** (usually to acute myeloblastic leukemia).

b. **DISORDERED PRODUCTION AS A RESULT OF CERTAIN CLONAL DISORDERS.**

The only disorder of significance here is paroxysmal nocturnal hemoglobinuria, and a brief mention is included only because it enters into the differential of some more common presentations. It is a strange condition with many different possible presentations, depending at which stage of hematopoiesis the clonal disorder becomes manifest. Thus there may be various combinations of aplastic anemia, chronic intravascular hemolysis tending to present as iron deficiency, and/or a hypercoagulable state (the Budd-Chiari syndrome seems to be a particularly common presentation). Of interest is that, in cases with aplasia, there is usually an accompanying **RETICULOCYTOSIS**.

Qualitative Disorders of Blood Cells

These may be hereditary or acquired, and it may affect any of the cell types.

1. **QUALITATIVE DISORDERS OF THE RED CELLS**. These are almost all hereditary, the only exception being paroxysmal nocturnal hemoglobinuria. They are discussed below under **DISORDERS OF SURVIVAL**.

2. **QUALITATIVE DISORDERS OF THE WHITE CELLS**. These are rare, and briefly discussed in Chapter 22: IMMUNE DEFICIENCIES AND THE IMMUNOPROLIFERATIVE DISORDERS, since their primary effect is a form of immune deficiency.

3. **QUALITATIVE DISORDERS OF THE PLATELETS**. These may be hereditary or acquired. Acquired platelet dysfunction is found in a large number of conditions, predisposing the patient to a bleeding tendency. These include renal failure and liver failure; the commonest causes of platelet dysfunction however are drugs, such as aspirin and non-steroidal anti-inflammatory drugs.

Disorders of Circulating Blood Cells

BLOOD CELLS MAY BE SUBJECT TO SECONDARY INSULTS IN THE CIRCULATION, such as attachment of antibody, physical destruction, chemical or toxic damage, with the cells themselves otherwise normal; or they may have some predisposing condition that renders them unusually susceptible to these secondary insults. Some diseases, such as septic shock, can result in swelling of the endothelium, narrowing of the capillary lumen, and consequent increased stress on the cells.

Disorders of the Spleen: Hypersplenism. An Introduction to Hemolysis

So important is the spleen to the blood that its pathology and pathophysiology must briefly be reviewed. The functions of the spleen are

1. **CULLING**. In brief, as red cells get old, they lose enzymes (of which they have a finite supply to begin with); they thus lose their ability to generate ATP, and because of this lack of energy can no longer adapt to and repair damage from the stresses they undergo in the circulation. In addition, they (are said to) lose tiny layers of their membrane with passage through narrow capillaries, exposing deeper antigens to which circulating IgG can attach. The sum total of these processes is that the red cell becomes permanently deformed and

more rigid, often (or perhaps always) with attached antibody. The spleen recognizes these cells as abnormal (mainly because they can no longer easily traverse the endothelial clefts in the red pulp of the spleen, and they are removed by the splenic macrophages. The exact mechanism is still uncertain, but the intact specialized microcirculation of the spleen is of fundamental importance). Two points have relevance:

a) The flow of blood through the spleen is very slow, allowing greater time of contact between the blood cells and the splenic macrophages (which are extravascular, lining the sinusoids). Note that these macrophages preferentially bind IgG-coated red cells (as opposed to IgM-coated cells); this is of great significance in understanding the different types of immune hemolysis. See below and Chapter 4.

b) Abnormal and damaged red cells will be destroyed in the spleen before their due date.

The breakdown of red cells leads to the release of red cell contents. Some of these are retained, completely or in part: iron is all recycled (unless the breakdown is intravascular); amino acids are largely returned to the pool; and some of the folate is recycled. The breakdown of heme results in the formation of (unconjugated) bilirubin, which circulates as such, and in the liver is conjugated. The spleen is the major ultimate source of the bilirubin in the blood (10% comes from the bone marrow, as described below). Most other catabolites are excreted.

2. **IMMUNE FUNCTION**. This is particularly relevant to a number of infections, such as pneumococcal and hemophilus infections, and malaria.

3. **STORAGE**. The spleen stores large numbers of platelets and granulocytes (and in a virtual sense, red cells). These are immediately available in times of acute stress – part of the **FLIGHT-OR-FIGHT** reaction.

It follows that many disorders of the spleen will be followed by hematological changes. The following are the commonest causes of splenic pathology:

1. **CHRONIC CONGESTION** – venous outflow obstruction usually as a result of cirrhosis and portal hypertension.

2. **INFILTRATIONS**, such as sarcoidosis, amyloidosis, Gaucher disease, lymphoma, hairy cell leukemia, and metastatic carcinoma.

3. **MYELOPROLIFERATIVE DISORDERS**.

4. **WORK HYPERTROPHY**:

a) **CHRONIC IMMUNE STIMULATION**, such as with infective endocarditis or Felty syndrome.

b) **RED CELL DESTRUCTION**, as in hereditary spherocytosis, etc.

HYPERSPLENISM. Any cause of an enlarged spleen may be associated with increased sequestration or destruction of **NORMAL** blood cells. The resultant cytopenia is not typically accompanied by a hypercellular marrow; this probably indicates that, in most cases, the blood cells are not so much destroyed as sequestered.

Disorders of Survival of Blood Cells

There are four major processes involved in the disposal of blood cells once they have been produced: apoptosis; marrow culling of a percentage of newly formed cells; destruction and/or sequestration of normal blood cells by a diseased spleen; and destruction of effete cells by the spleen and to a much lesser extent the liver. These processes may be increased in various conditions.

1. **APOPTOSIS** is a normal process where aged (nucleated) cells undergo programmed involution and death. Apoptosis can be inhibited or stimulated in certain cells by many cytokines. Its status as a pathological process is still poorly defined.
2. **MARROW PATHOLOGY AFFECTING PRECURSORS.** There are two basic abnormal processes here (it will be seen that there is some overlap with **QUANTITATIVE DISORDERS OF PRODUCTION OF BLOOD CELLS** above):
   a. **PHYSIOLOGICALLY**, about 10% of newly produced cells are destroyed in the marrow, presumably as a form of quality control, and in the process contributing to the circulating bilirubin. Pathologically, this may be increased, usually due to the cells produced being very abnormal, with the effect therefore of a highly active marrow and peripheral cytopenia; the condition is then called **INEFFECTIVE ERYTHROPOIESIS**.
   b. **HEMOPHAGOCYTOSIS**. Here, cells in the marrow are attacked by increased numbers of activated macrophages. There are various syndromes and causes, both benign and malignant, which are discussed in Chapter 13.
3. **PRIMARY DISORDERS OF THE SPLEEN** affecting circulating blood cells, causing **HYPERSPLENISM.**
4. **DESTRUCTION OF EFFETE CELLS BY THE SPLEEN** and to a much lesser extent the liver. The spleen plays significant roles in the physiology of the blood cells. One of them is the removal from the circulation of effete and abnormal red cells. Clearly therefore, the most common sequel of the production of qualitatively abnormal red cells and of physical or chemical damage to red cells in the circulation (including the attachment of antibody) is early removal of the abnormal cells from the circulation by the spleen. This process is called **HEMOLYSIS**.

The Pathology of Hemolysis

Hemolytic anemias are a difficult topic to teach to undergraduates in an easily comprehensible way, although they are not difficult to understand once clarified and as long as a number of problems with hemolysis are understood:

1. **HEMOLYTIC ANEMIAS** are commonly and misleadingly defined as anemias that result from an increase in the rate of red cell destruction. This definition is only accurate where hemolysis is the primary, major disorder; this state is then correctly called hemolytic anemia. This is rare and often discussed very cursorily. But a reduced life span of red cells occurs as a secondary phenomenon in the pathogenesis of many other red cell diseases, such as the anemia of chronic disorders and thalassemia, which are not considered nor approached as hemolytic disease; in these cases, the contribution of reduced red cell life span is overshadowed by the other processes and thus frequently overlooked. Indeed their effects can considerably complicate the interpretation of the disease process in question and of the laboratory results. It is therefore necessary that the practical essentials of hemolysis be known.
2. **ACUTE HEMOLYTIC DISORDERS** are generally quite easy to recognize or at least suspect. But there are a number of **CHRONIC HEMOLYTIC PROCESSES** that easily can be overlooked or misdiagnosed as something else. However, these odd presentations are not difficult to spot once one is aware of their existence; they are discussed in Chapter 4.
3. **IMMUNE HEMOLYSIS** is a prominent cause of acute (and occasionally chronic) hemolysis; it is however a complex process and is often grossly oversimplified – or presented in unnecessary detail. The process is outlined in Chapter 5.
4. There are exceptions to most of the processes and presentations described.
5. The Coombs test (most commonly the direct antibody test) is used to confirm the diagnosis of an immune-mediated hemolysis.
6. **NON-IMMUNE-MEDIATED HEMOLYSIS** has a great many causes. They are discussed in Chapter 10. In brief, they may be categorized as

a. **HEREDITARY**. These may be due to

   i. Red cell membrane disorders, such as hereditary spherocytosis
   ii. Red cell enzyme deficiencies, such as G6PD deficiency
   iii. Abnormal hemoglobins, such as sickle disease.

b. **ACQUIRED**. This is a mixed bag of causes, such as

   i. Red cell fragmentation syndromes such as disseminated intravascular coagulation (DIC) and pre-eclampsia
   ii. Certain infections, such as due to clostridia and malaria
   iii. Chemical and physical agents, such as burns, industrial poisons, near-drowning in fresh water
   iv. Paroxysmal nocturnal hemoglobinuria.

What Are the Specific Mechanisms of Hemolysis?

There are broadly two sites for the removal of **PATHOLOGICALLY DEFECTIVE OR COMPROMISED RED CELLS** from the circulation: the spleen and the circulation. These have very different characteristics. In certain disease situations, the liver also can play a large role in the culling of abnormal red cells.

In the circulation, the process is obviously intravascular. True lysis of red cells, i.e., where the red cell membrane is disrupted and the cell contents released into the plasma, is uncommon. There are two basic mechanisms of true lysis:

1. **PHYSICAL OR CHEMICAL DISRUPTION OF THE MEMBRANE**, such as in burns, near-drowning in fresh water, many chemicals, some infections such as clostridia, and, of course, DIC. The pathogenesis of DIC is discussed later in this chapter.
2. **ATTACHMENT TO THE CELL MEMBRANE OF CERTAIN TYPES OF ANTIBODY** is followed by the activation of complement, the formation of the membrane attack complex (MAC) on the surface, and true intravascular lysis. This is essentially a Type II (cytotoxic) immune response.

In the spleen, hemolysis is mediated by macrophages and occurs **EXTRAVASCULARLY**, since in the red pulp the walls of the sinusoids are in part formed by macrophages. Note that the term **HEMOLYSIS** in these circumstances is not strictly accurate – a more correct term would be red cell phagocytosis; however, **THE CLINICAL EFFECT** is indeed the breakdown of red cells. **EXTRAVASCULAR HEMOLYSIS** is the commonest mechanism. It is basically an exaggeration of the normal culling process and clearly is due to the presence of increased numbers of abnormal red cells. Thus one finds increased bilirubin levels, pallor, an enlarged spleen, and a tendency for the marrow to be hypercellular because of attempts at compensation.

There is a third mechanism, however, which is a combination of extra- and intravascular hemolysis. This is due to the attachment to the cell membrane of certain types of IgM and IgG **WITHIN THE CIRCULATION**; complement is then activated, but activation does not proceed beyond the point of C3. C3 is then converted by the red cell membrane into another form. Red cells thus sensitized are sequestered (not phagocytosed) by the Kuppfer cells in the liver which have specific receptors for this form of C3. This form of C3 is then cleaved by the Kuppfer cells, leaving an inactive form on the surface, and the red cell is returned to the circulation. However, when IgG is also present on the surface, phagocytosis of these cells can occur in the spleen and the liver.

Note that, even in the case of true lysis of circulating red cells, debris – such as bits of cell membrane, etc. – will be cleared extravascularly. Even in the normal patient, culled effete red cells frequently have attached antibody on their surface; this is normal IgG in the plasma and attachment occurs because repeated passage through narrow capillaries has exposed deeper antigens in the red cell membrane.

It is thus clear that in one way or another, antibodies play a large part in the understanding of hemolysis. A brief overview of red cells antigens and antibodies will be found in Chapter 4, including a discussion of the tests used to diagnose their presence.

Disorders of Hemoglobin

These may be qualitative or quantitative.

1. **QUALITATIVE**. These are generally hereditary but may be acquired.

   a. **HEREDITARY** causes are called the hemoglobinopathies, of which there are a very large number. They generally present as an extravascular hemolysis but with some of them there are additional effects, such as endothelial and tissue damage, as in sickle disease, or in the case of hereditary methemoglobin, defects in oxygen transport accompanied by pigmentary changes. Another type of hemoglobinopathy is associated with abnormalities in oxygen affinity. See Chapter 17.
   b. **ACQUIRED** causes include other forms of methemoglobinemia, sulfhemoglobinemia, and carboxyhemoglobinemia.

2. **QUANTITATIVE.** These too are generally hereditary but may be acquired.

   a. **HEREDITARY** causes are the thalassemias, discussed elsewhere.

   b. **ACQUIRED** causes include lead poisoning and other causes of interference with heme synthesis.

Notes on Two Important Hemoglobinopathies *Two abnormal Hb genes originated in West Africa, namely HbS and HbC. In the heterozygous form, these are relatively mild, often asymptomatic. They emerged and survived because of the partial protection they offer to the patient with respect to malaria (of interest is that two other genetic changes were also encouraged by malaria – G6PD deficiency and thalassemia). The problems emerge when they are homozygous.*

HbSS (or sickle) disease is usually devastatingly serious. Apart from the anemia that is found, the major pathology is due to microvascular damage, since the sickled cells are very rigid and damage the endothelium, resulting in tissue destruction (in the case of the spleen) and micro-infarcts in soft tissues and bone, producing the classical crises.

HbCC disease. This is not usually as serious as HbSS disease. It is characterized by a chronic extravascular hemolysis and the blood shows marked target cell formation, with condensation and crystallization of Hb in the red cells.

The pathology of the hemostatic system is discussed later in the chapter, since it will be more meaningful once the physiology of hemostasis is clear.

The Nature of the First-Line Tests in Hematology

With respect to the two first-line tests, difficulties are experienced with both, but in different ways. The hemostatic screen consists of a relatively small group of exploratory tests. The difficulties with the hemostatic tests arise from the confusion about the nature of hemostasis (as taught until quite recently). Fortunately, these difficulties have (largely) been resolved, but older colleagues still remember the confusion of their student days. Hemostasis and the hemostatic screen are discussed separately toward the end of the chapter.

The FBC on the other hand is a complex investigation consisting usually of 21 parameters and (if you are lucky) a morphological and clinical commentary. It is potentially very rich in the information it can yield **IF AND ONLY IF** interpreted properly by the clinician. (Even in cases where a full-fledged commentary is provided by the laboratory, the report must, to a greater or lesser extent depending on the type of diagnosis, be re-interpreted by the person actually responsible for the patient.)

A Brief Look at Laboratory Tests, with Particular Reference to the First-Line Tests in Hematology

It is valuable to see the hematological tests in the context of other laboratory tests. Basically, there are four types of test:

1. **SCREENING TESTS.** With few exceptions these are not recommended without the presence of suggestive signs and/or symptoms. One strong exception is the ANA test – systemic lupus erythematosis (SLE) is rarely if ever present when this test is negative (although it is too sensitive, with many false positives – sensitivity and other operating characteristics are discussed in Chapter 3). Urinalysis is unique in some respects: it is often very difficult to even suspect kidney disease (as well as some metabolic diseases) without a (more or less routine) urine examination.

2. **TESTS CONFIRMING A DIAGNOSIS**, for example confirming the clinical suggestion of iron deficiency anemia. The vast bulk of laboratory tests are (or should be) regarded as confirmatory tests, or indeed tests that merely support a clinical diagnosis – tests to support or exclude a provisional clinical diagnosis.

3. **TESTS ASSESSING PROGNOSIS.** Very few tests are of value in this regard, for example testing for Jo-1 in myositis.

4. **MONITORING PROGRESS.** These are tests that are not sensitive enough for diagnostic purposes but are quite adequate for follow-up purposes. Most of the tumor markers, for example, fall into this class.

To return to the first-line tests in hematology:

1. The hemostatic screen is never used as a screening test. It is only requested when there is clinical evidence or a strong suggestion of abnormal bleeding. Elements of the screen are, however, used for monitoring, in certain circumstances.

2. The FBC, however, can occupy different diagnostic roles – either as a confirmatory/supportive test for a

preliminary clinical diagnosis or actually making the diagnosis (i.e., clinical features are minimal or vague). Because of the relative clinical inaccessibility of the blood system, one resorts to a FBC at the slightest suspicion of blood disease, and in this sense the FBC can be considered a part of the clinical examination, and its successful interpretation is thus as important a clinical enterprise as the approach to say a swollen joint, particularly since the majority of abnormal FBCs are found in non-hematological disease. Compare the value of the FBC in the following typical presentations:

a. A young female patient with clinical features suggestive of acute appendicitis. Typically, the only contribution the FBC would make in the typical case is the finding of a mild neutrophilia (i.e., **REACTIVE**); the FBC plays no part in the diagnosis of appendicitis per se.

b. A middle-aged fit man suddenly started feeling tired. His detailed history was entirely unproductive and on thorough examination the only positive feature was some pallor. There are NO features whatsoever to assist in the diagnosis. **HERE THE FBC HAS ANOTHER ROLE ENTIRELY – TO AID IN FINDING THE PATHOLOGY,** not simply confirming a clinical diagnosis.

The First-Line Tests

Access to the hematological system is primarily by means of the first-line tests.

Blood is a complex mixture of cells and molecules. In practice, the most common aspects investigated are the cells – counting and sizing them, and the hemostatic proteins – largely measured in terms of their function.

The hemostatic screen is a fairly straightforward set of tests, largely functional in nature (see later in the chapter). The FBC by contrast is a complex set of results and requires extensive discussion, especially since the FBC is central to the diagnosis of most blood diseases.

By way of introduction: firstly, the FBC is traditionally done on venous blood from an arm vein. It is sometimes assumed that this reflects the composition of the blood throughout the body. This is false: apart from the known differences between arterial and venous blood, it is well established that there are differences between limb blood and blood in the splanchnic circulation; in pathological circumstances, notably sepsis, this difference can be marked. This is potentially of great importance in the critically ill. Secondly, the FBC is not primarily a set of function tests but essentially tests changes in anatomical structures. It contains data of two types: the **CONCENTRATION** (as well as the average sizes of RBC and platelets) of cells suspended in the plasma; and their **MORPHOLOGICAL APPEARANCE**. Thirdly, the concentration of cells (i.e., the number counted) reflects the balance between two factors: the number of cells per unit volume of blood, and the volume of plasma per unit volume of blood. Thus the challenge in interpreting the FBC when dealing with a blood disease, whether suspected or identified, is to make clinical decisions of an essentially patho-physiological nature (i.e., to attempt to evaluate underlying **FUNCTIONAL** change) based upon laboratory reports that are essentially **ANATOMICAL** in origin. Since similar changes in the FBC are typically caused by more than one underlying pathology, getting to the true nature of the pathology requires

1. A recognition of any pattern of changes in the FBC
2. Close integration of these findings with the clinical features
3. Proceeding to further tests suggested by this integral evaluation.

The Proper FBC Report Consists of

1. Counts and various measurements of the cells
2. Assessment of morphology by a hematologist
3. A provisional interpretive comment.

Modern instruments cannot replace the morphological assessment or comment. It is the clinician's responsibility to re-interpret the report in the light of the clinical presentation.

Understanding the FBC

This requires a certain amount of insight into what the different parameters represent physiologically. To refresh some basic concepts:

THE BLOOD CELLS ARE SUSPENDED IN PLASMA. The volume of plasma (particularly the water content) is controlled independently of the blood cells. All the counts (and most of their derived indices) are expressed as **CONCENTRATIONS**; thus a change in the water content of plasma will change the concentration of the cells, possibly causing, for example, an **APPARENT** anemia or erythrocytosis. However, the significance of **MORPHOLOGICAL** changes are not primarily dependent on the concentration – it lies in their presence and severity (another important advantage of the morphology).

The FBC is not a single test and has numerous constituents, in many respects unrelated to each other biologically. The fact that the FBC consists of so many more or less independent components presents a great challenge in clinical interpretation. Each measurement, calculation, and described change in the FBC represents the resultant of several interacting processes both in **TIME** and in **SPACE**.

The Constituents of the FBC and Their Clinical Significance

1. **THE RED CELL (ERYTHROCYTE) COUNT** (RCC).
2. **THE WHITE CELL (LEUKOCYTE) COUNT** (WCC), with a differential count of the various types of leukocyte, expressed in absolute numbers, in the same units as the WCC.
3. **THE PLATELET COUNT** (PC).

These counts represent the balance between production and loss or destruction. However, we are referring to production not so much at that point in time, but **AT THE TIMES THAT THOSE CELLS WERE FIRST MADE** (and since they all have different life spans, the cells one counts can be of any age within that cell line's life span). The rate of destruction may be normal, increased, or decreased. The balance between production and destruction or loss (i.e., what is actually happening) cannot reliably be assessed with one count only.

Originally, these counts were done by various manual, low-tech means, still to be found in any level 1 laboratory. Indeed, the first FBCs were simply that – counts per cubic mm of red cells (RBC), white cells (WBC), and platelets (PLT), together with a morphological assessment of the stained smear which included a differential count of the different types of white cell. The counting was done in glass chambers. The variation was large, even in the best hands, being in the order of 15% for RBC and WBC, and 20 to 25% for PLT.

These three counts were (and are) of mixed usefulness. Diseases of white cells and later platelets were fairly well characterized early on, these being relatively straightforward, diagnosis depending on the counts and the morphological appearances. The variation in WCC

and PC encountered with manual methods made little practical difference to the diagnosis. It was in this way that the largely morphological bias in classification and characterization of blood diseases came about as well as the view that blood diseases are largely a laboratory activity.

However, red cells were another story altogether. First, a variation of 15% in a red cell count of say 5.0 million/cubic mm, with a **NORMAL** range of say 4.64–5.67 million/cubic mm, is of major significance, and could push the patient into say the anemic range erroneously. Secondly, the red cell count per se gives very little information on the nature of an anemia (by far the commonest presenting feature in blood disease – and indeed of very many general diseases). While the morphology of the red cells on its own can on occasion be very informative, this requires considerable experience. Thus, before the days of electronic counters with their ability to measure the size of red cells, the hemoglobin and hematocrit estimations (with far less variation) were instead the preferred measurements of red cell functionality and these were used, with mixed success, to evaluate the nature of anemia, rather than the red cell count.

The Red Cells

1. **HEMOGLOBIN (HB)**. This is done photometrically.
2. **THE HEMATOCRIT (HCT)**, (or packed cell volume (PCV)) in level 1 laboratories is done by centrifugation, and in the others it is either a calculation based on the red cell count and average size of the red cells or using another technology, a quasi-direct measurement.
3. **MEAN CELL HEMOGLOBIN CONCENTRATION (MCHC)** is the ratio of the Hb to the Hct and is a measure of how much Hb is **PACKED** into the average cell.

   THE HEMOGLOBIN AND HEMATOCRIT ESTIMATIONS REPRESENT THE AMOUNT OF CIRCULATING HEMOGLOBIN. THE RCC DOES NOT DO THIS, SINCE IT DOES NOT NECESSARILY BEAR ANY RELATIONSHIP TO THE HCT OR HB, BECAUSE OF MARKED VARIABILITY IN RED CELL SIZE AND THEREFORE HB CONTENT. Since hemoglobin is the carrier of oxygen to the tissues (the primary function of red cells), the hemoglobin and hematocrit estimations represent a more functional assessment than does the red cell count.

4. The advent of electronic counters was a major advance. Not only could the RCC be estimated very accurately, but the average size of the red cells could be measured – an important advance since it had long

been suggested by Wintrobe and others that a sensible approach to anemias was in terms of the average size of the red cells, i.e., whether they were micro-, macro- or normocytic. Thus there came into being the **MEAN CELL VOLUME (MCV)**. This is a direct measurement on most instruments. To repeat, it supplies only the average size of the red cells, and says nothing about the range or variation of their sizes. The actual size of the red cells is a resultant of many interacting factors, and the MCV as the average red cell size represents one or more of several mutually interactive processes. Note that this average size includes that of the reticulocytes (retics); since retics are larger than red cells, an increase in retics will increase the MCV.

5. A modern refinement is the **RED CELL DISTRIBUTION WIDTH (RDW)**, which is a **MEASUREMENT OF THE VARIATION IN SIZE OF THE RBCs,** and attempts to give a figure to the degree of **ANISOCYTOSIS,** this being a morphological term indicating how much the cells vary in size. It has become increasingly clear that an increased RDW, even in the presence of an otherwise completely normal count, is cause for concern, and the smear MUST be examined.

6. From the RCC and Hb, another valuable parameter can be derived, the **MEAN CELL HEMOGLOBIN (MCH)**, which is the ratio of Hb to RCC.
    THE MCH REPRESENTS THE AMOUNT OF HB PER CELL ON AVERAGE.

The White Cell Series

Normally the leukocytes in the peripheral blood comprise five types of cell:

1. The neutrophils.
2. The eosinophils. ⎫ These three comprise the
3. The basophils.   ⎬ granulocytes.
4. The monocytes.
5. The lymphocytes.

How these are counted is very technology dependent. In level 1 labs, this is done by looking at a stained smear and physically counting each type of cell. Normally only 100 total cells are counted. The count of each type of cell is thus first expressed as a percentage; then by using the total white cell count, the **ABSOLUTE NUMBERS OF CIRCULATING CELLS** are expressed. **THIS IS BY FAR THE MOST VALUABLE WAY OF EXPRESSING THE NUMBER OF THE DIFFERENT WHITE CELLS.** This very important issue is further discussed in Chapter 15.

The Platelets

The platelet count also is technology dependent. In levels 1 and 2 labs, it is done manually with a large coefficient of variation. At the other levels, the instrument count is usually very accurate **IF**

1. The platelets are evenly distributed. There are many causes of uneven distribution and will be discussed in a later chapter.
2. There is not a significant number of red cell fragments lying around. The automated counting of platelets depends on their small size. Thus all cells below a certain size threshold are counted as platelets.

THUS PLEASE REALIZE THAT THE INSTRUMENTS USED FOR BLOOD COUNTING ARE NOT INFALLIBLE!

The Role of Blood Film Morphology

PRIMARY blood diseases can be very complex, and the FBC reports of these cases always require expert assessment, comment, and suggestions for further investigation. However, when it comes to the FBC changes in **SECONDARY** and **REACTIVE** disorders, **THERE EXISTS A MISCONCEPTION THAT THE MORPHOLOGY ADDS VERY LITTLE VALUE TO THE FBC.** In our unit, we have estimated that insightful morphological assessment adds significant value in about one third of cases (**SIGNIFICANT** in this context implies that without morphological assessment an important amount of time would have been lost in unnecessary further investigations). Minor changes in the shape of the red cells can be enormously helpful, e.g., in a case with a raised MCV, the shape of the macrocytes can point either to megaloblastosis or to liver disease/alcoholism/hypothyroidism, possibly saving a lot of unnecessary other tests. Certain morphological patterns are characteristic. These can be identified in a very short time by an experienced eye, and not at all by an instrument. In addition, many functional states can be suspected: **DIFFUSE BASOPHILIA** (also called **POLYCHROMASIA**) indicates a reticulocytosis, and thus increased red cell production (and, indeed, other things being equal, a more or less functional marrow); certain abnormal shapes are implicated in poor oxygen delivery to the tissues.

HOWEVER, MORPHOLOGICAL ASSESSMENT OF THE SMEARS AND DIAGNOSTIC COMMENT IS BECOMING INCREASINGLY UNCOMMON.

1. The FBC is an extremely popular and common test, and hence there are very large numbers of FBC requests in modern laboratories. The laboratories have had to automate to handle the volume. It has become impossible for slides of every FBC to be examined by a hematologist or even a senior technologist. Studying smears is a time-consuming operation, and hematologists are very expensive.

2. Fortunately, the manufacturers have expanded the capabilities of the instruments, recognizing the pressure under which hematologists work. **MODERN COUNTERS CAN DETECT CERTAIN GENERAL ABERRATIONS WHICH HAVE BEEN CORRELATED WITH CERTAIN MORPHOLOGICAL CHANGES**, and have been programmed to display low level comments – **FLAGS, ORIGINALLY INTENDED AS PROMPTS TO THE HEMATOLOGIST TO LOOK AT THE SMEAR**.

    Since 70–80% of bloods in private practice are entirely normal, this saves an enormous amount of work. However, problems remain:

    a. The other 20 or 30% of bloods submitted.
    b. The far higher percentage of abnormal FBCs in tertiary institutions.
    c. Abnormalities can be detected under the microscope with a completely normal count, as for example with exposure to lead.

There is also no doubt that these instruments can be seriously wrong in certain circumstances. For example, one of the instruments on the market, after an extensive evaluation, was found to perform satisfactorily in most circumstances. However, in patients recovering from aplastic anemia, there was a tendency to produce falsely low monocyte counts and falsely high neutrophil counts – and only a small minority of these were flagged as abnormal by the instrument. The consequence was that these patients were refused financial support for growth factors. The problem could so easily have been obviated by a morphological check.

All in all, morphological assessment of blood films is essential in cases of

1. Leukopenia
2. Leukocytosis
3. Thrombocytosis
4. Thrombocytopenia
5. Anemia of unknown etiology
6. A moderately to severely raised RDW even in an otherwise normal count
7. A moderate to severe left shift with a normal WCC
8. The presence of nucleated RBCs.

The Value of Good Morphological Assessment

1. Many blood diseases can confidently be diagnosed, or at least strongly suspected, on the morphology. This can save a great deal of time, money, and even discomfort for the patient (see Chapter 5 for examples).
2. There are some diseases where the FBC can be completely normal and only the morphology will show abnormalities, such as lead poisoning.
3. It has been pointed out that the absolute amount of plasma water affects the counts and many of the measurements in the FBC, which may produce spuriously abnormal results. Plasma water does not affect the morphology, and this may be of assistance in such cases.
4. The presence in a report of an obviously careful morphological assessment indicates that the FBC as a whole was looked at by a professional.

Consider case #1 (see Table 2.6). It is open to an oversimplified and dangerous misinterpretation without a **GOOD MORPHOLOGICAL COMMENT**.

CASE #1

Table 2.6

Patient	Age	Sex	Race	Altitude
Mr B V	56	M	W	5,000 ft

He is a 56-year-old electrician. He has been fit all his life. Two weeks ago he suddenly started feeling tired. His family doctor examined him thoroughly and the only positive feature was obvious pallor. A FBC report accompanied the patient.

	Value	Units	Reference range Low	High
Red cell count	3.25	$\times 10^{12}/l$	4.77	5.83
Hemoglobin (Hb)	8.5	g/dl	13.8	18.0
Hematocrit (Hct)	0.25	l/l	0.42	0.53
Mean cell volume	**78.3**	fl	80	99
Mean cell Hb	**26.2**	pg	27	31.5
Mean cell Hb conc.	33.4	g/dl	31.5	34.5
Red cell dist. width	**23.2**	%	11.6	14
White cell count	**2.13**	$\times 10^9/l$	4	10
Neutrophils	66.1	%		
Lymphocytes	29.1	%		
Monocytes	3.1	%		
Eosinophils	1.1	%		
Basophils	0.6	%		
Neutrophils abs.	**1.41**	$\times 10^9/l$	2	7
Lymphocytes abs.	**0.62**	$\times 10^9/l$	1	3
Monocytes abs.	**0.07**	$\times 10^9/l$	0.2	1
Eosinophils abs.	0.02	$\times 10^9/l$	0.02	0.5
Basophils abs.	0.01	$\times 10^9/l$	0.02	0.1
Platelet count	151.2	$\times 10^9/l$	150	400
Red cell morphology Anisocytosis, microcytosis, elliptocytosis.				

The family practitioner was very experienced and hematologically insightful (and, one likes to think, well trained). He suspected that there was more to this FBC than simply a microcytic anemia, since clinically he found nothing to suggest any of the common causes of a microcytic picture, i.e., iron deficiency, obvious chronic disease or thalassemia. In fact, he found no positive clinical features at all. The FBC, apart from showing microcytic red cells, showed a subtly confusing pattern. He suspected that the lab had not performed a proper morphological assessment, and in particular, he found the high RDW to be extremely significant. He referred the patient. The FBC was repeated and reported on in our unit. It was noticed that the counts and derived values differed very little, with the exception of the white cell differential (see Table 2.7). It was the morphological assessment that provided the answer – or at least a rational path to the answer.

Blast > Promyelocyte > Myelocyte > Metamyelocyte > Band cell > Mature granulocyte.

Note the following in the above count:

1. It is obvious that in the original laboratory the film was not examined by a pathologist: he would have seen the dysplastic changes and the blasts virtually at a glance. It is questionable also whether the final report was checked by a hematologist – the very large RDW (see later) would immediately have alerted him to look at the film.

2. It is equally clear that the film was briefly examined by a technologist, because, while anisocytosis and microcytosis can be generated by the instrument as flags, elliptocytosis requires a look. However, probably due to pressure of time, the leukocytes were not looked at, and thus the dysplasia and blasts were not spotted.

3. The differential count done in our unit was clearly done manually, since the percentage figures for the white cells are in whole numbers and not decimals as produced by the automated counter; the reason for this is that automated counters count thousands of cells while manually only 100 are counted. (In general, this is a useful tip to see whether an abnormal FBC involving leukocyte abnormalities was assessed morphologically by a hematologist or technologist).

An uninformed family doctor (and indeed many specialists) could (and probably would) have been primarily impressed by the microcytosis, would have decided that he was dealing with an iron deficiency,

Table 2.7

	Value	Units	Reference range Low	Reference range High
White cell count	**2.07**	$\times 10^9/l$	4	10
Neutrophils	68	%		
Band cells [a]		%		
Lymphocytes	20	%		
Monocytes	3	%		
Eosinophils		%		
Basophils		%		
Neutrophils abs.	**1.41**	$\times 10^9/l$	2	7
Band cells abs.[a]	0		0	0
Lymphocytes abs.	**0.41**	$\times 10^9/l$	1	3
Monocytes abs.	**0.06**	$\times 10^9/l$	0.2	1
Eosinophils abs.	**0.00**	$\times 10^9/l$	0.02	0.5
Basophils abs.	**0.00**	$\times 10^9/l$	0.02	0.1
Blasts	**9**	%	0	0
Normoblasts	0	/100 WBC	0	0
Platelet count	143.3	$\times 10^9/l$	150	400
Morphology		The red cells show anisopoikilocytosis with prominent elliptocyte formation. Dysplastic changes in the neutrophils are seen. There are 9% blasts present. The picture is very suggestive of myelodysplasia.		

[a]Band cells are the developmental form immediately perceding the mature granulocyte. Since they are relevant in later FBCs, the stages of development are given in the box alongside.

and have prescribed iron. He might have been reinforced in this opinion were he to remember that elliptocytosis is a frequent finding in iron deficiency. When the anemia did not respond to oral iron, he might have been tempted to give parenteral iron. You will see later that myelodysplasia is characterized by iron **OVERLOAD**, with poor utilization of iron causing poor hemoglobinization and thus microcytosis: oral iron therapy is useless and potentially dangerous, and parenteral iron therapy is absolutely contra-indicated.

From innumerable cases of personal feedback, it is clear that the clinician is being left high and dry, to the disadvantage of the patient.

This issue (of morphological and clinical comment on FBCs) is a serious dilemma for most big clinical laboratories. Note that quality laboratories, both public and private, do exist. The author knows of at least one huge laboratory where a serious effort is made to look at the smear of every single FBC – usually this takes 10 or so seconds at the most, and the experienced eye will almost always pick up pointers that would induce him to study the smear further. This is entirely acceptable. Relying on the instruments to pick up abnormalities **TO TRY TO SCREEN OUT NORMAL BLOODS, SUCH THAT THEIR SLIDES DO NOT NEED EXAMINING,** is an acceptable and justifiable motivation.

Shortcuts, however, are not, and what unfortunately is happening is that undue reliance is often placed on the interpretive capabilities of these instruments, such that fewer and fewer slides are being examined, including many that should be. Such flags that are present are reported as such, in place of a morphological assessment, and it is expected from the referring doctor to evaluate the blood and its cells from the numerical results and the flags – which he usually cannot and he has to resort to what he remembers and what he has seen recently. The flags can be misleading, particularly when couched as semi-quantitative comments at the end of the report, such as **MACROCYTES + +.** If multiple flags are reported, these can be confusing and apparently contradictory, such as **MACROCYTES + + +** as well as **MICRO-CYTES + +.** It is sometimes questioned how this type of report can come about, e.g., one reporting both microcytes and macrocytes: these instruments measure thousands of cells, and can pick up **TAILS** of small and large cells that may be discounted by careful examination; the instrument's computer will, however, report these tails. This issue is particularly important with the normocytic anemias, and is further discussed in Chapter 6. The author was astounded to hear from outstanding clinical internist colleagues that they too were under the impression that these **COMMENTS** were the result of a proper morphological assessment. They were left very disillusioned after the facts were explained.

What then is the poor clinician to do? It is his right to demand from the laboratory that a smear be examined. Nevertheless, in the absence of this, a good insight into the FBC often permits a reasonable conclusion.

HAVING SAID ALL THIS, EVEN A FULL MORPHOLOGICAL COMMENT CAN USUALLY ONLY BE REGARDED AS CONTRIBUTORY SINCE THE PARTICULAR CLINICAL SITUATION OF THE PATIENT CANNOT USUALLY BE TAKEN INTO ACCOUNT BY THE PATHOLOGIST.

The Reticulocyte Count *To summarize all of the above in terms of practical diagnosis, it can be seen that the reticulocyte count is a very valuable measure of assessment of the rate of production of the red cells, and therefore the efficacy of the marrow in terms of adapting to anemia. Thus the reticulocytes reflect erythropoiesis and therefore the health of the*

marrow. The reticulocyte count must be interpreted with this in mind.

To oversimplify, if the disease causing the anemia is inside the marrow, the reticulocyte count is decreased; if the disease causing the anemia is outside the marrow, the reticulocyte count is increased.

The Subcomponent Red Cell Circulations

Essential Nutrients Required by the Blood System

Figures 2.10, 2.11, 2.12, and 2.13 depict changes in **TIME AND SPACE** of circulations of different nutrients. Seeing them as circulations assists considerably in understanding deficiencies. The numbers given are those for a 70 kg adult male. Figure 2.10 provides the context for the display of the three most vital nutrients.

The Body Iron Circulation

Gender is responsible for **CLINICALLY SIGNIFICANT DIFFERENCES** in iron status. Females are under constant threat of iron deficiency. The distribution of iron is shown in Table 2.8 for First World countries – it is far worse in the Third World. Figure 2.11 depicts the body iron circulation.

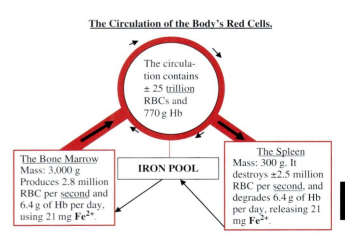

Fig. 2.10 The red cell circulation

Table 2.8 Body iron content

	Male (g)	Female (g)	% of total
Iron in hemoglobin	2.4	1.7	65
Easily available storage iron (ferritin)	0.65	0.2	22
Unavailable storage iron (hemosiderin)	0.35	0.1	13
Total body iron	3.5	2.0	100

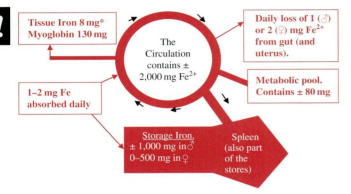

Fig. 2.11 Circulation of body iron

Notes on Fig. 2.11

1. All the **IRON RELEASED BY BREAKDOWN OF RED CELLS** is re-utilized in the production of new red cells.
2. Very small amounts of iron are **LOST THROUGH DESQUAMATION OF THE SKIN AND GUT, AND IN THE MENSES**. This loss must be replenished by absorption from the diet. The average Western diet contains 10–20 mg iron per day, but normally only 1–2 mg/day are absorbed.
3. **DIETARY IRON** is in the form of
   a. **HEME IRON**, as found in red meat and so on. This is absorbed very efficiently. Since it is already in the ferrous form (the form in which iron is absorbed), it does not need reducing substances in the gut (e.g., HCl or ascorbate). HCl **IS** however required for the digestion of the protein containing the iron.
   b. **INORGANIC IRON**, found in dairy products, greens etc. (and only in small amounts), and of course many kinds of iron tablets. This is absorbed inefficiently, and being in the ferric form, needs reduction by acid in the gut for absorption.
4. **THE ABSORPTION OF IRON** is very complex and is discussed further in Chapter 4.
5. **STORAGE IRON** exists in two forms. In the iron-replete individual, about $^2/_3$ is ferritin, water soluble, and easily mobilized. The other $^1/_3$ is hemosiderin, water insoluble, with a much slower mobilization and circulation.

6. If no iron whatever is ingested or absorbed, the storage iron will be utilized. In a male, it will take about 6 months for iron deficiency to develop; in a female it will be much shorter, depending on
   a. Age of menarche (i.e., whether she has time to build up stores from the age of about 11 – before this age, both boys and girls have no iron stores because of rapid growth).
   b. The number of pregnancies, time between pregnancies, and iron supplementation during pregnancy.
   c. Diet and normal absorption.
   d. Gynecological problems leading to menorrhagia.
7. Thus decreased iron stores leads to decreased production of red cells. The opposite is not true – increased iron stores do not lead to increased production of red cells (it is surprising how often this is assumed).
8. Note * the small amount of **TISSUE IRON** – this is iron mainly in iron-containing enzymes, e.g., the cytochromes in the mitochondria. It is instructive to realize that the huge amounts of oxygen (600 L/day) transported in Hb containing (in toto) huge amounts of iron, which is found in 25 **TRILLION** RBCs (one third of the body's cells) is primarily required to supply mainly these enzymes (containing so little iron), for their generation of ATP.
9. There are still many unanswered questions about iron metabolism and absorption, iron deficiency, and iron malutilization.

The Body Vitamin B$_{12}$ Circulation

Body vitamin B$_{12}$ circulation is depicted in Fig. 2.12. Total body vitamin B$_{12}$ is about 4 mg.
   Notes on Fig. 2.12.

1. Vitamin B$_{12}$ is found only in **FOODS** of animal origin (and bacteria).
2. **ABSORPTION** of vitamin B$_{12}$ is complex and further discussed in Chapter 4:

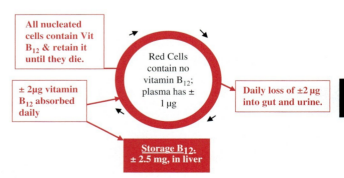

Fig. 2.12 Circulation of body Vitamin B$_{12}$

Notes on Fig. 2.12

a. Ingested vitamin B_{12} is bound to intrinsic factor, secreted by gastric parietal cells.
b. The vitamin B_{12}/intrinsic factor complex travels to the distal ileum where the complex is deconjugated and the vitamin is absorbed.

3. The normal **STORES** of vitamin B_{12} are enormous, sufficient for 4 years.

The Body Folate Circulation

Body folate circulation is depicted in Fig. 2.13. Total body folate is about 10 mg.

Notes on Fig. 2.13.

1. **DIETARY SOURCES** can be classified into:

   a. **GREEN VEGETABLES**. The folate in these is destroyed easily by cooking.
   b. **YEAST AND LIVER**. The folate in these is not destroyed by cooking.
   c. **HUMAN AND COW'S MILK REQUIRE A SPECIAL MENTION.** These milks contain folate binding protein (FBP). This concentrates folate and protects it from oxidation and proteolysis by pancreatic enzymes.
   d. **SOME DIETS ARE FREQUENTLY POOR IN FOLATE.** These can be seen in a number of conditions: anorexia nervosa, bulimia, some weight-loss diets, and some special diets or foodstuffs such as those for phenylketonuria and maple syrup disease, and goat's milk.

2. **FOLATE DEFICIENCY** (and thus megaloblastic anemia) is the most rapidly developing of all the nutritional anemias, for the following reasons:

   a. **THE STORES** (mainly in the liver) will last for only 3–4 months in the absence of any folate ingestion (compare with up to 6 months for iron and 4 years for vitamin B_{12}).

b. **MALABSORPTION** is a serious problem, particularly in various parts of the world, and is further discussed in Chapter 4.

   Note that in many forms of malabsorption, folate loss is particularly rapid, since folate will not be reabsorbed in the enterohepatic circulation.

c. **DRUGS ACTING AS FOLATE ANTAGONISTS** (but very much dosage dependent), such as

   i. Some anticonvulsants notably carbemazepine
   ii. Many chemotherapeutic agents:

   - Methotrexate, which is commonly used in non-malignant conditions as well, albeit generally in very low dosage.
   - Purine antagonists such as 6-mercaptopurine and azothiaprin: these rapidly lead to the development of megaloblastosis and later aplasia.
   - Pyrimidine antagonists such as 5-fluorouracil, with effects as with purine antagonists.
   - Deoxyribonucleotide inhibitors such as cytosine arabinoside, and intercalating agents such as doxorubicin and mitoxanthrone.

d. **INTERFERENCES WITH FOLATE METABOLISM** are common:

   i. Pregnancy has very large demands for extra folate – 5–10 times normal in the 3rd trimester, and much more with multiple pregnancies.
   ii. Alcohol has complex effects on folate (and vitamin B_{12}) absorption, as well as having direct toxic effects on the marrow.
   iii. Orotic aciduria, a rare inborn error of metabolism.
   iv. Any cause of cellular hyperactivity will consume increased amounts of folate, such as in hyperactivity of the bone marrow, infections, and cancers.
   v. Exfoliative skin disorders need a special mention: in severe cases up to ¼ of daily requirements of folate can be lost; in addition methotrexate is a common form of therapy. It is advisable to administer folate before commencing therapy as well as during the course of treatment.

A Word of Warning Regarding Some Serum Levels

Vitamin deficiencies in the presence of normal vitamin levels seem to be more common in the elderly than previously believed. Functional vitamin B_{12}, B_6, and

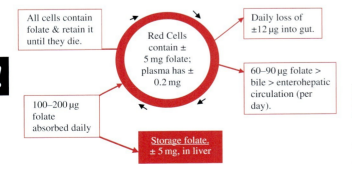

Fig. 2.13 Circulation of body folate

folate levels were assessed by advanced biochemical techniques involving their metabolites; the majority of elderly patients were shown to be effectively depleted of these vitamins.[1] For these special techniques in your elderly patients, it is suggested that you consult the laboratory.

Hemostasis and the Hemostatic Screen

Hemostatic test reports are relatively simple at the general level, as long as some basic physiological facts are understood.

Disorders of hemostasis tend to be glossed over by most people not working in the field; there is a tendency to think of them as rare and esoteric. The inherited bleeding disorders (which seem to be what most focus on) are indeed rare, but in fact bleeding disorders in general are relatively common.

The basic physiology is discussed somewhat more elaborately than usual, for two reasons:

1. The modern synthesis is much simpler than before.
2. Hypercoagulability due to defects in the hemostatic control system is assuming greater and greater importance – thrombotic disorders still account for the largest cause of mortality and morbidity in developed countries. However, to understand the hypercoagulable states, one must understand the mechanisms of natural anticoagulation (since very many of these disorders are the result of defects in these mechanisms); and to understand natural anticoagulation, it is necessary to understand the mechanism of coagulation in fairly great detail.

The older generations of doctors were considerably confused by the physiology of blood coagulation, as taught right up to circa 1990:

1. Theories propounded to explain an apparently very involved process have been inordinately complex; they have been offered for at least 200 years, but it is only in the last 2 decades that true clarity is being reached; unfortunately, many of our older colleagues remember the confusion of their student days, and are strongly put off by the topic. The modern synthesis is very close indeed to the truth, and, as is so often the case, the explanation is very much simpler and more straightforward than it used to be.

2. It used to be held that the coagulation cascade could be initiated either by the extrinsic pathway (tissue factor – factor VII) or by the intrinsic pathway (factor XII and a foreign surface). It is now well established that TF-VII is the **INITIATOR**, and the so-called intrinsic pathway normally is primarily concerned with **AMPLIFICATION** of the process.

3. Hemostasis was understood as occurring in distinct stages:

   a) Typically first the platelet plug (plus vasoconstriction)
   b) Followed by coagulation
   c) Then dissolution of the clot and healing
   d) The tight coupling of the processes of coagulation, anti-coagulation, and fibrinolysis was not made clear.

It was taught that the role of the platelet was clearly separate from that of the coagulation mechanism. This was perfectly understandable in view of certain clinical observations and the primitive tests available at the time: a typical wound would stop bleeding fairly quickly (shown to be due to a combination of vasoconstriction and platelet plugging), and only later would a visible clot be observed; in the same way, the bleeding time measuring the former two would be seen to much shorter than the whole blood clotting time (a forerunner of the thromboplastin-based tests of today). Yet, over 30 years ago, identifiable fibrin strands were demonstrated by electron microscopy within 30 s of the inflicting of a wound. (Note that in some pathological conditions, initiation of coagulation need not be TF-VII – see the discussion on DIC in Chapter 18.)

The modern synthesis is much simpler – and integrated. Nevertheless, there still are problems, the most notable being that the basic scenario is still the idealized damage to the vessel. There are many variables in the manifestation of the coagulant process, depending on

1. The availability of **NORMAL AMOUNTS OF NORMAL HEMOSTATIC MOLECULES**.
2. **THE AMOUNT OF TISSUE AND VASCULAR DAMAGE**, even physiologically.
3. **THE TYPE OF INJURY**. For example, abrasions bleed differently from the bleeding found in lacerations. Different vessels are damaged in different circumstances.
4. **THE EFFECT OF LOCAL BLOOD FLOW**. Clots occurring in vessels exposed to high frictional forces (shear forces – see later) contain large numbers of platelets (**WHITE THROMBI**), enabling the clot to

withstand these forces; whereas clots in low flow situations such as veins have far fewer platelets and contain large numbers of red cells (**RED THROMBI**).

5. **THE AMOUNT OF ELASTIC TISSUE AND THE DENSITY** of the connective tissue in the damaged area.
6. **LOCAL PRESSURE FACTORS**. For example, bleeding into a joint or spinal cord will tend to be arrested quite soon by the structures, as opposed to say into the lesser sac. In general, bleeding into the tissues will cause increased tissue pressure and further retard blood flow in the area.
7. **THE TYPE OF SURFACE IN QUESTION**. For example, the peritoneum as contrasted with the skin on the soles of the feet.
8. **THE AMOUNT OF ARTERIAL DAMAGE.**

We will remain with a somewhat idealized, generalized scenario; even the simpler modern explanation can be further simplified for practical purposes.

The Critical Biological Importance of Hemostasis
The circulation of the blood is essential for all tissue functioning – indeed, it is essential for the classical homeostatic mechanisms to operate. To maintain this circulation, the heart requires a certain blood volume for proper functioning (Starling's Law). It is therefore perfectly understandable that mechanisms to prevent, minimize, and ultimately restore loss of blood (i.e., to maintain the blood volume) from the circulation have been very well preserved in evolution. And here the hemostatic mechanism, in its role of producing a thrombus, plays a literally vital role. It also follows that the thrombus thus produced must be limited to the site of injury, i.e., the rest of the blood must remain fluid. Once the defect is healed, the thrombus must be eliminated so as to restore normal flow to that area. In other words, the hemostatic mechanism must be tightly controlled, so that it is limited to the site of the defect, and, once this is healed, the clot disappears (by the process of fibrinolysis). Again there has been a tendency to refer to natural anticoagulation and fibrinolysis as subsequent stages of the process. In fact, these processes occur at more or less the same time.

Testing the hemostatic system is fairly straightforward. However, a problem with hemostasis and its control is that **THE TESTS CANNOT BE UNDERSTOOD AND PROPERLY UTILIZED WITHOUT A BASIC UNDERSTANDING OF THE PHYSIOLOGY.**

It is convenient to talk about **PROCOAGULANT, ANTICOAGULANT, AND FIBRINOLYTIC PROCESSES,** as long as one bears in mind at all times that these are **NOT CLEARLY SEPARATE IN TIME.** Under physiological circumstances, hemostasis is only activated when blood vessels are damaged. When this happens:

1. The blood is exposed to substances with which it does not usually come in contact.
2. The endothelium is necessarily damaged as well – and the endothelium is an important source of activation of hemostasis.
3. All the component processes of hemostasis are activated at almost the same time.

Figure 2.14 illustrates the close interaction of the processes.

Notes on Fig. 2.14:

1. The immediate response is the activation of the procoagulant processes.
2. Soon after (very soon indeed) the natural anticoagulant and fibrinolytic mechanisms are stimulated.
3. The activation of the procoagulant processes leads to the formation of a fibrin clot.
4. The natural anticoagulants very soon start antagonizing, and in the process damping down and controlling, the process of coagulation.
5. Very soon after fibrin is formed, the fibrinolytic process starts to break down, and in the process control, the formation of fibrin.

Within the context displayed by Fig. 2.14, we now discuss each process separately.

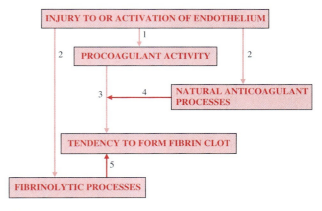

Key
→ indicate stimulatory, activating, and/or converting processes.
→ indicate inhibitory, deactivating, and/or destructive processes.

Fig. 2.14 Interaction of procoagulant, anticoagulant and fibrinolytic processes

> !
>
> **The Procoagulant Aspect of Hemostasis**
>
> *1. There are three basic anatomical elements.*
> *2. There are three basic processes.*

The Three Anatomical Elements (or Groups of Elements)

These all cooperate closely and are

1. **THE PLATELETS.** These are activated by contact with sub-endothelial collagen or ADP released from other platelets upon activation, form the initial plug that together with vasoconstriction tend to stop the bleeding, and form a template upon which many coagulation factors will subsequently assemble.
2. **THE VESSEL WALL, ESPECIALLY THE ENDOTHELIUM.** This performs numerous vital functions, including vaso-constriction and contributing to many aspects, including fine control, of all the hemostatic stages.
3. **CERTAIN PROTEINS.** From our point of view, we can group these into three, the coagulation factors, the natural anticoagulants, and the pro-fibrinolytic proteins. All of these (physiologically) work in close conjunction with receptors on the endothelium and with stimulatory and inhibitory factors produced by the endothelium (the endothelium plays the central role in the control of the entire process).

The Procoagulant Factors Are of Three Types

1. **PROTEOLYTIC SERINE PROTEASES.** These are activated either by contact with sub-endothelial structures (just like the platelets), or by other, previously activated proteases prior in the sequence. In some of these, vitamin K plays a critical role. See below.
2. **STRUCTURAL PROTEINS** such as fibrinogen. This is almost the final step in coagulation, since it gives rise to fibrin, which, together with the platelets, forms the **STRUCTURAL BASIS** of a coagulum.
3. **CO-FACTORS.** These are of two types:

   a) **TISSUE FACTOR**, which is anchored to specific cell surfaces.
   b) **FACTORS V AND VIII**, circulating as unactivated pro-factors.

The net effect of the above is to consolidate the platelet plug by forming a coagulum in and around the platelets.

It is still taught that these proteases work according to a simple cascade, by which means the process is amplified to produce relatively vast amounts of end product (in this case, fibrin). This concept is no longer fully appropriate, as will be shown a little later.

The Role of Vitamin K

Vitamin K is essential for post-production modification of six hemostatic factors. These are II, VII, IX, and X (**1927** for easy remembering): procoagulant; and proteins C and S: natural anticoagulant. Without vitamin K, the liver produces inactive molecules called PIVKAs (**P**roteins **I**nduced by **V**itamin **K** **A**bsence). Developing deficiency or antagonism of vitamin K will affect all these factors, starting with those with the shortest half-life, i.e., protein C, then factor VII, then progressing steadily. Clearly the full effect of deficient vitamin K will only be seen when the production of the factors with the longest half-life is affected. At the same time, levels of PIVKA will rise progressively. The following aspects of vitamin K patho-physiology have relevance:

1. **STORES**: These are minimal, supplying sufficient vitamin K for usually only a few days, up to a maximum of a week. Therefore vitamin K deficiency will develop within days of absent effective supply.
2. **ADULT DAILY REQUIREMENT:** about 0.25 µg/kg. Normal **SUPPLY** derives from

   a) **THE DIET:** green leafy vegetables, milk, various vegetable oils.
   b) **NORMAL COLONIC INTESTINAL FLORA.** The extent to which absorption occurs from the colon is uncertain, as thus is the contribution of colonic flora to normal levels.

3. **ABSORPTION**: Vitamin K is a fat-soluble vitamin, and thus is impaired in any type of cholestatic disease, and many types of steatorrhea leading to malabsorption (and of course bowel resection). Some other bowel diseases such as Crohn disease, cystic fibrosis, and fistulae tend to lead to sub-clinical deficiency, with raised PIVKAs but usually a normal prothrombin time.
4. **DRUGS**: The coumadin-type anticoagulants inhibit certain pathways of vitamin K metabolism, causing effective deficiency. However, their effect on vitamin K metabolism is variable. Important factors are

   a) Patient age.
   b) The diet.
   c) The presence of some other drugs that interfere with coumadin binding and metabolism (see Appendix

A). Broad-spectrum antibiotics may also cause vitamin K depletion; the old explanation that this is due to eradication of colonic bacteria seems less and less likely – in truth, the mechanism has not convincingly been explained.

The Three Procoagulant Processes

1. **VASOCONSTRICTION**
2. **PLATELET PLUG FORMATION**
3. **COAGULATION.**

With each of these elements, one can speak of different phases of the global process – **INITIATION, AMPLIFICATION, CONSOLIDATION, AND RESOLUTION.**

The Initiation of Hemostasis

This is normally triggered by an injury to the endothelium. This produces a gap in the tissues that is immediately filled with blood from the damaged vessel(s). See Fig. 2.15. The two primary activations are those of the platelets and of factor VII.

The blade cuts through the tissues, through the sub-endothelium, and then through the endothelium, producing a gap. The blade is withdrawn, and blood immediately fills the gap. See Fig. 2.16.

The immediate response is vasoconstriction, which initially is myogenic in origin. Within the blood filling the site of trauma there are two extremely significant

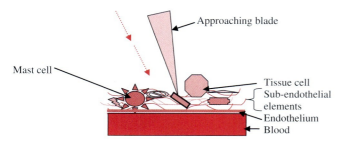

Fig. 2.15 Impending tissue trauma

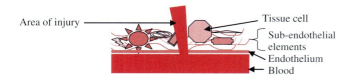

Fig. 2.16 Trauma to tissue and blood vessel

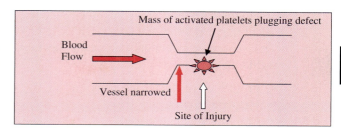

Fig. 2.17 Vasoconstriction and platelet plug formation

elements: **THE PLATELETS** and **FACTOR VII**, and these are the **INITIATORS OF HEMOSTASIS**, and they do this via **CONTACT** with elements in the sub-endothelium.

These two **INITIATORS** will be discussed separately, but bear in mind that **THEIR ACTIVATION OCCURS SIMULTANEOUSLY**.

THE PLATELETS (AND VASOCONSTRICTION, discussed together with the platelets, since platelets considerably enhance initial vasoconstriction). Figure 2.17 summarizes these processes.

1. **THE VESSEL AROUND THE SITE OF INJURY NARROWS DUE TO**

   a. **EFFUSION OF BLOOD INTO THE TISSUES,** raising the interstitial pressure, tending to compress the vessel.
   b. **VASOCONSTRICTION.** This results from two processes:

      i. Reflex (myotonic) spasm
      ii. Release of vasoactive substances from the platelets, primarily serotonin and thromboxane A2.

2. **PLATELET PLUG FORMATION. THERE ARE THREE PHASES:**

   a. **ADHESION OF PLATELETS TO ENDOTHELIUM** around the injury. This happens within 1–2 s. There are numerous adhesion proteins involved here, including von Willebrand factor (this is found in the sub-endothelial space, where it was secreted by the endothelial cell in health, and also from release from the Weibel–Palade bodies from damaged endothelial cells). Platelet adhesion is followed by
   b. **ACTIVATION OF PLATELETS** within 15–20 s. This is initially reversible. It results in a number of metabolic reactions which lead to

      i. Shape change
      ii. Release of substances from within the platelet, most of which, in one way or another, facilitate platelet plug formation and subsequent stabilization by coagulation. One of the earliest is

arachidonate release from the membrane leading to the formation of **THROMBOXANE A$_2$**.
This substance has many important functions,
including

- Promotion of the release reaction
- Vasoconstriction (see 1b)
- Promotion of aggregation

iii. Aggregation of platelets to each other (sticki-
ness). In this process, additional platelets are
recruited to the site of injury from the circulation, mainly due to the release of ADP from
activated platelet granules. In the processes of
adhesion and aggregation, the platelet membrane is altered with exposure of deeper portions of the membrane.

c. **EXPOSED MEMBRANE PHOSPHOLIPIDS** are
now available to take part in two important processes in the coagulation pathway:

i. The activation of factor X (to form Xa).
ii. The formation of thrombin from the interaction
of factors Xa, Va, and II.

d. The surface platelet receptor GPIIa-IIIb is the major
platelet integrin. It forms a bridge between the cytos-
keleton and the polymerized fibrin formed by the
coagulation process. This receptor is important
because it is the target of very many drugs being
developed to decrease platelet function in many
hypercoagulable states, notably in heart disease.

**Factor VII (as the Physiological Initiator
of the Coagulation System)**

This too is activated by contact with a sub-endothelial
substance, in this case tissue factor, a phospholipid material
forming a perivascular sheath and secreted by the endothelium. (Note that monocytes too can secrete tissue factor,
and this undoubtedly plays a part in **ABNORMAL** clotting.) In this early stage of activation, activated VII, i.e.,
VIIa, now activates a small amount of IX in the circulation
as well as some X. (All activated factors are designated as
such by an **a** after the basic factor number.) IXa in turn
further activates X. Xa now attaches to the sub-endothelium, especially the phospholipid of exposed tissue cell
membranes, and where it binds passing Va. This **COM-
PLEX** now activates a small amount of passing prothrombin (factor II) to produce a small amount of thrombin. The
initiation phase is summarized in Fig. 2.18.

Figure 2.18a shows factor VII making contact with the
exposed collagen in the injured part of the endothelial

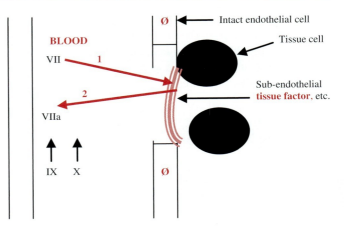

Fig. 2.18a First stage of coagulation

surface. Here it becomes activated and re-enters the
blood in the vicinity. Here it awaits contact with some
factor IX and X passing by.

Figure 2.18b shows factor VIIa activating both factor
IX and X. Factor IXa further activates factor X.

In Fig. 2.18c, Xa now attaches to the sub-endothelium,
especially the phospholipid of exposed tissue cell membranes, and where it binds Va. This complex now activates a small amount of passing prothrombin (factor II)
to produce a small amount of thrombin.

**THIS IS THE END OF THE INITIATION
PHASE.** Only small amounts of activated factor are
produced. There may be micro amounts of thrombin
and perhaps a strand or two of fibrin present, but as
yet no significant amount of thrombin have been
formed.

What Fig. 2.18c does not show is the mass of activated
platelets filling the gap, with plasma between. This is
shown in Fig. 2.19

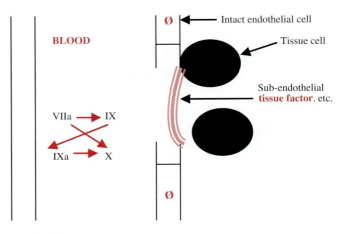

Fig. 2.18b Second stage of coagulation

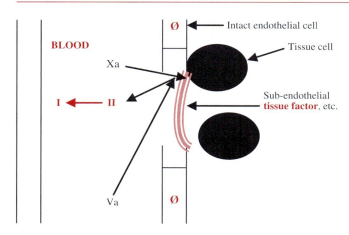

Fig. 2.18c Third stage of coagulation

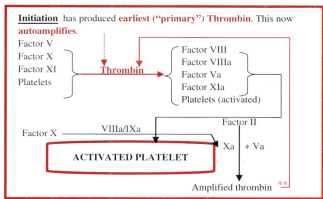

Fig. 2.20

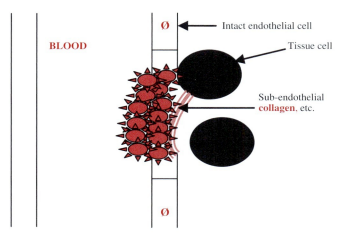

Fig. 2.19 Mass of platelets plugging defect

Try to superimpose Figs. 2.18 and 2.19 in your mind – doing it on paper is very messy. The net result, however, is shown in Fig. 2.21.

Thus the end point of the initiation phase is the appearance on the exposed sub-endothelium of **ACTIVATED FACTOR X BOUND TO Va (FROM THE PLASMA)**, as well as a mass of activated platelets. This stage is critical, and different paths may now be followed in different circumstances and disease states; these will be discussed later. The two sets of elements – the activated platelet plug and the Xa–Va complex on the sub-endothelium – now cooperate closely in the next stage – **AMPLIFICATION**. See Fig. 2.20.

The Amplification and Consolidation of Hemostasis

Figure 2.20 illustrates the amplification of thrombin production. It can be followed by tracing the thin red line backwards.

1. Small amounts of thrombin produced at initiation activate circulating factors VIII, V, and XI, as well as local platelets.
2. Factor XIa converts circulating IX to IXa; this then binds to activated platelets along with factors VIIIa and Va.
3. The factor VIIIa/IXa complex activates X on the surface of the activated platelets, which together with Va convert factor II (prothrombin) to thrombin, which once again activates more XI.
4. Stages (2) and (3) repeat continually, producing large amounts of thrombin (the **THROMBIN BURST**). Other effects of the thrombin produced:

   a) It catalyzes the activation of factor XIII to XIIIa. This is critically important for stage (6).
   b) It stimulates the release of plasminogen activator from the healthy endothelial cells around the area of hemostasis, with the resultant production of plasmin from circulating plasminogen.
   c) The presence of thrombin causes the activation of the natural anti-coagulant system, at a very low level.
   d) It activates more platelets.

5. Thrombin converts fibrinogen to fibrin.
6. XIIIa splits off fragments from fibrin, eliminating the negative charges on the surface, and thus permitting the spontaneous polymerization of fibrin into long, stable strands. This fibrin, having been formed on the surface of activated platelets that are plugging the vascular defect, and on the edges of the defect, thus binds the platelets firmly together and to the edges of the injury (see Fig. 2.21). The formation of stable fibrin is discussed later.

Figure 2.21 shows the platelet plug reinforced by fibrin strands, which also bind the plug to the adjacent endothelium.

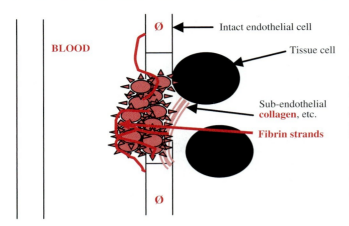

Fig. 2.21   Final stage of hemostasis

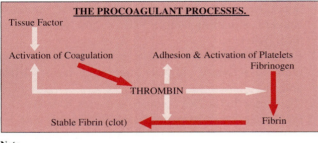

Note

These arrows ➡ indicate conversion processes.
These arrows ➡ indicate activating, catalytic processes.

Fig. 2.22   The basic physiology of coagulation

It is worth noting that the process from thrombin to stable fibrin occurs in less than 5 s. Figure 2.22 summarizes all of the above.

Were the above process to continue, widespread, catastrophic coagulation of the blood would occur. The procoagulant process must be limited in two ways: it must remain localized to the area of vascular damage, and it must be halted and the clot removed once healing has occurred. In effect, this means that as soon as intact endothelium is encountered, the process is stopped. This is the responsibility of the **NATURAL ANTICOAGULANT** and the **FIBRINOLYTIC PROCESSES**.

The Natural Anticoagulant Aspects of Hemostasis

There are three separate mechanisms to this aspect, and they all are to do with control of the production and function of thrombin.

1. Circulating antithrombin
2. The protein C/thrombomodulin mechanism
3. Tissue factor pathway inhibitor activation.

The natural anticoagulants are in operation virtually immediately after the injury, and serve to tightly control and modulate the coagulation process, and limit it to the site of the injury: **IT IS IMPORTANT FOR BLOOD FLOW TO BE MAINTAINED TO ALL AREAS WHERE THERE IS NO BREACH.** Thus control of the **GENERATION OF THROMBIN ONLY AT THE SITE OF INJURY** is critical to smooth and appropriate hemostasis, and the mechanisms involved are very effective (it is also important that something of these mechanisms be known, since abnormalities can indeed lead to serious thrombotic sequelae (discussed in Chapter 21).

There are several fundamental methods by which control and localization of hemostasis are achieved. They all are to do with

1. The control of thrombin levels locally. These mechanisms are illustrated diagrammatically in Fig. 2.23.
2. Destruction of fibrin and clotting factors outside the area of injury
3. Clot retraction and dissolution.

Understanding the control of thrombin levels is complicated by the fact that thrombin is not only required for fibrin formation: it is also required for the activation of V, VIII, XIII and of platelets, as well as for the stimulation of plasminogen production from the endothelium. Indeed, it has been claimed that by the time fibrin formation sufficient to clot the wound has been formed, about 50% of the generated thrombin is still present (as well as about 90% of the Xa). Presumably therefore the residual thrombin is concerned with these other functions – and it must occur very quickly, since the mean survival of a thrombin molecule is in the order of 20–25 s. This is the time taken for surplus thrombin (and unused Xa) to be inactivated.

The Control of Local Thrombin Levels

It can be seen that the methods to control thrombin levels and production are

1. **ANTITHROMBIN** complexes with thrombin, thereby inactivating it, but in addition has other anti-coagulant actions, by inactivating XIIa, XIa, IXa, and Xa.
2. **THROMBOMODULIN**, on the surface of intact endothelial surfaces, binds both thrombin and **PROTEIN C** (and the binding to protein C is strongly enhanced by the protein C receptor on the endothelium). Within this bound complex, thrombin loses its procoagulant properties and becomes an anti-coagulant, by the process of activating protein C. Activated protein C, on the surface of activated platelets (where

Fig. 2.23 Control of thrombin formation

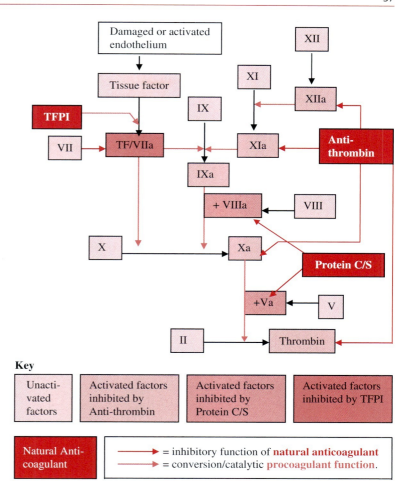

the coagulation process is going on), degrades Va and VIIIa, thus inhibiting further local coagulation. Note that proteins C and S also require vitamin K-dependent post-translational carboxylation for effect – this fact is important when considering coagulation disorders in liver disease and in instituting anti-coagulant therapy.

3. **TISSUE FACTOR PATHWAY INHIBITOR (TFPI).** The presence of thrombin stimulates its secretion from the endothelium. Despite its name, this does not inhibit TF alone, but only the TF-VIIa complex.

Destruction of Fibrin and Clotting Factors Outside the Area of Injury

There are several mechanisms:

1. Removal of activated coagulation factors by the liver

2. Removal of any particulate coagulant material happening to enter the circulation by the RE system

3. Dilution of clotting factors by the flowing blood.

Clot Retraction and Dissolution

It has long been known that clots retract in vitro. This is due to interaction between activated platelets caught up in the clot and the fibrin strands, and in the process strengthening the clot considerably. In vivo, the major value of clot retraction would appear to be producing resistance to the high frictional forces that are found – clearly this only applies to platelet-rich thrombi. To what extent this process assists in reducing the actual size of the thrombus and permitting or re-establishing flow in vivo is not known. The contribution is unlikely to be significant, particularly since the process can take up to an hour to occur, in vitro at any rate.

The dissolution of the clot by fibrinolysis is clearly of primary importance – see later.

> *The effect of all the above is either to keep the blood in the fluid state, to minimize any interruption in the flow, or to restore the fluid state as soon as possible after a leak is plugged. As mentioned, both the anticoagulant and fibrinolytic elements can be abnormally activated, causing potentially severe bleeding.*
>
> *On the other hand, a deficiency of any of these can result in a tendency to thrombosis. Aside from the contributory factors mentioned above, defects in these factors are usually hereditary. When heterozygous, there is a variable tendency to thrombosis, and when homozygous, they frequently lead to death from widespread thrombosis in infancy. These factor deficiencies have come to be seen as a major contributor to the very high incidence and prevalence of thrombo-embolic disease in clinical practice, and therefore an understanding of the mechanisms is essential.*
>
> *It is thus not surprising that close control of thrombin production is a major part of natural anticoagulation. This is summarized in Fig. 2.24.*

Thrombin Production and Its Control

> **The Fibrinolytic Aspect of Hemostasis** *Only a brief outline of fibrinolysis is given at the general level.*

As the name implies, fibrinolysis, by the production of plasmin, destroys fibrin, and is set in operation again virtually at the time of injury. It performs two evident functions:

1. It assists in controlling the process of coagulation at the site of injury.
2. It counteracts any tendency for fibrin formation to occur outside the site of injury.

The fibrin formed by the action of thrombin is not strong or functional. It is converted to stable fibrin by factor XIII. See Fig. 2.25. In the process, very important and clinically significant breakdown products are found.

Because the D-dimer test has achieved such clinical importance, something should be known about it. Deep vein thrombosis (DVT) and pulmonary thrombo-embolism (PTE) are common and important conditions (up to 1,000,000 cases per annum on a worldwide basis); they are also difficult to diagnose; they can be associated with significant morbidity and mortality; and the diagnosis must be made rapidly for any specific treatment to be

Fig. 2.24 Summary of thrombin physiology

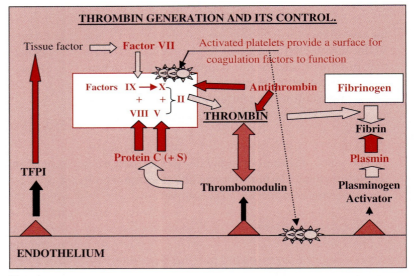

Note

These arrows	➡	indicate conversion processes.
These arrows	➡	indicate activating, catalytic processes.
These arrows	➡	indicate substances produced by endothelium.

Elements displayed in this color derive from the circulation.

Elements displayed in this color derive from the endothelium

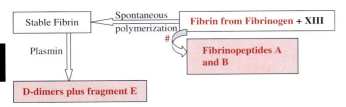

Fig. 2.25 Formation of stable fibrin

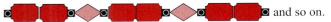 and so on.

Fig. 2.27 A strand of fibrin monomers

Fig. 2.28 D-dimer plus fragment E

D-dimer   Fragment E

worthwhile. Even more patients present with features clinically only **SUGGESTIVE** of DVT or PTE, particularly in general and emergency room practices. The gold-standard test – venography – has limitations: allergic reactions, technical expertise, and subsequent thrombophlebitis. Ordinary Doppler studies and ^{125}I-scanning are not sensitive or specific enough. B-mode Doppler studies with compression have very good sensitivity and specificity; however, the test is expensive and not always available. The major requirement therefore is for a sensitive test to **EXCLUDE** these conditions – only if such a test were positive, would this specialized Doppler examination be justified. The D-dimer test has been thoroughly investigated as such a method, and found to be extremely specific to **EXCLUDE** DVT. Interpretation of the D-dimer test is discussed in Chapter 21; a preliminary discussion of the physiology is necessary here.

The fibrin monomer consists of two **D DOMAINS** joined by an **E DOMAIN**, as shown in Fig. 2.26.

Under the influence of factor XIII, these monomers join to form the long strands of fibrin, as shown in Fig. 2.27.

The stable fibrin clot, once formed, is immediately under attack by the fibrinolytic process. It was seen in Fig. 2.24 that plasminogen activator is released from the endothelium in the presence of thrombin (and factor XII). This acts on circulating plasminogen, which in the mean time has been caught up in the thrombus, to be converted into plasmin, a very powerful fibrinolytic agent. Plasmin produces a number of by-products called fragments, which have potential clinical importance, in that they have anticoagulant activity; this is only of clinical relevance at very high (non-physiological) levels.

Plasmin breaks up the chain at the ◉ positions, in a progressive manner, ending up with D-dimers and fragment E, as seen in Fig. 2.28.

Note that in some pathological conditions, fibrinogen is broken down by plasmin. The product of this is called fibrin degradation products (FDPs). FDPs are not significantly increased in physiological thromboses. The interpretation of these tests is discussed later.

Fig. 2.26 A fibrin monomer

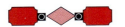

An Integrated View of Hemostasis

THE MECHANISMS OF HEMOSTASIS AND ITS CONTROL SHOULD BE SEEN IN THE CONTEXT OF A CONTROLLED AND BALANCED SYSTEM, COMPRISING PROCOAGULANT AND ANTICOAGULANT FACTORS, EACH IN TURN WITH THEIR OWN CONTROLLING MECHANISMS.

The dynamics of the hemostatic system are very different from that of the blood cell system. This system should be understood independently.

The concept of a balanced system in hemostasis is different from that with the FBC. In the FBC, the balance primarily refers to a balance between production and disposal of cells, such that the peripheral concentration of cells is kept within certain parameters, and includes various compensatory mechanisms to achieve this object. With hemostasis, the balance is between opposing processes for the maintenance of and correction of defects in vascular integrity. The hemostatic mechanism springs into a high state of activity when such injury occurs; otherwise is operates at a very low level indeed. This is fundamentally different from the state of affairs with the blood cells.

It is quite clear that the procoagulant, anticoagulant, and fibrinolytic processes need to operate seamlessly together. **THE ENDOTHELIUM PLAYS A MAJOR ROLE IN THIS SEAMLESS AND CONTROLLED INTERACTION.** Pathologically, any of the aspects may be triggered independently; very often this occurs in an explosive and uncontrolled fashion. In addition, endothelial disorders are associated with abnormalities of one or more of these aspects. Under physiological circumstances, it is always the procoagulant aspect that is the starting point of the complete process.

All the clotting processes are normally in a tightly controlled balance of pro-thrombotic and antithrombotic activities. Any disturbance in this control leads to excessive bleeding or excessive clotting (or occasionally both). By contrast, control mechanisms for the initial platelet aspect of homeostasis do not, as far as we know, exist.

Figure 2.29 summarizes this balanced, controlled system.

Note that the various controlling mechanisms can affect initiation of a process, control of the extent of a

Fig. 2.29 Summary of the balanced hemostatic system

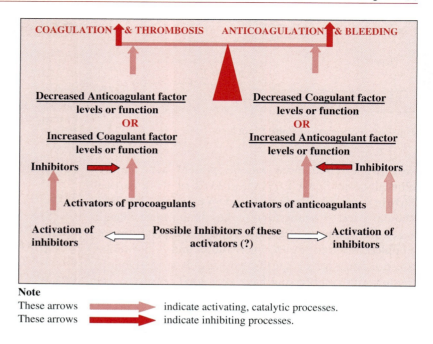

Note

| These arrows | → | indicate activating, catalytic processes. |
| These arrows | → | indicate inhibiting processes. |

process, and/or breakdown of the end product. They are also responsible for a graduated response.

A GOOD WAY OF ILLUSTRATING THE ABOVE AS AN INTEGRATED VIEW IS TO LOOK AT THE STATE OF AFFAIRS IN DIFFERENT DEGREES OF VASCULAR INJURY.

In **HEALTH**, there is a **TENDENCY** for the pro-thrombotic processes to be **VERY SLIGHTLY ACTI-VATED** because of normal mitotic replacement of endothelial cells, slight oozing from the gut, and the bumps and cuts of everyday life. Clearly this has to be tightly controlled, and therefore the anti-thrombotic and fibrinolytic mechanisms are also constantly very slightly activated. The amount of thrombin generated is tiny, and the circulating antithrombin can easily cope with this (the thrombin–antithrombin (TAT) complexes being cleared by the reticulo-endothelial system). Any fibrin formed as a result can easily be coped with by the local release of plasmin (the endothelium is essentially healthy, and the control measures are very efficient). So, this tendency to thrombosis is essentially limited to those areas where endothelial cells are breached, since, as a response to this tendency, the anticoagulant mechanisms are slightly and appropriately activated **IN THE GENERAL CIR-CULATION**, preventing thrombosis occurring else-where. **THUS, AS A WHOLE, THE BALANCE IS SHIFTED TOWARD THE ANTICOAGULANT SIDE, WHILE LOCALLY, IT IS SHIFTED TOWARD THE PROCOAGULANT SIDE.**

With **VASCULAR INJURIES**, a lot depends on the extent. With any type of vascular injury, stable fibrin is

clearly necessary; and excess thrombin (i.e., over and above that necessary to generate the appropriate amount of fibrin) must be available for the activation of XIII (as well as the stimulation of plasminogen activators in the endothelium).

1. **ANTITHROMBIN** is the first and primary mechan-ism to deal with excess thrombin. If the amount of antithrombin is sufficient (relative to the extent of the injury), the protein C/thrombomodulin and TFPI mechanisms are probably minimally activated and would play an insignificant role, if any. At the same time, a small increase in the amounts of D-dimers will occur due to activation of plasminogen to form plas-min (and any plasmin escaping from the area of injury is mopped up by α_2-anti-plasmin).

2. Should the injury be larger, the point will be reached, if injury is widespread enough, for the antithrombin mechanism to be overcome. The **PROTEIN C/ THROMBOMODULIN** mechanism, leading to inac-tivation of factors Va and VIIIa, and the **TFPI** mechanism, leading to the inactivation of the factor VII/tissue factor complex, now become very impor-tant to limit thrombin levels and production. Increased requirements for stable fibrin will lead to increased amounts of fibrinopeptides A and B (see # in Fig. 2.25); increased amounts of fibrin leads to t-PA being released from the endothelium and gen-erating plasmin within the thrombus. This is con-trolled by the production of α_2-anti-plasmin. Thus, the numbers of fibrinopeptides (FDPs A and B) and

D-dimers are still small. However, the larger the thrombus, the more D-dimers will be produced, and very widespread physiological thrombosis, such as a DVT involving say much of a lower limb, is associated with high D-dimer levels.

3. Any fibrin formed despite these control mechanisms (i.e., a more significant activation of procoagulation and therefore a more significant injury) is disposed of by the fibrinolytic system.

4. Under pathological conditions (e.g., DIC – and extensive injuries may lead to the development of DIC independent of infection), where thrombin and hence fibrin and plasmin production are considerably increased, both the anti-thrombin and α_2-anti-plasmin mechanisms are overcome, the level of circulating plasmin increases, and now fibrinogen (as well as fibrin) can be attacked by it. The levels of D-dimers now increase sharply (as do FDPs). In other pathological conditions, particularly with endothelial loss or dysfunction, various parts of the system may be activated independently.

It can thus be seen that the degree of anticoagulant and fibrinolytic function roughly parallels the degree of injury, and to an extent, the type of injury or disorder, other things being equal.

The Role of the Flow of Blood in Hemostasis

One of the major developments in the last few decades has been the recognition of the immense important role of the **FLOW OF BLOOD** in the hemostatic process (among other processes). At the general level, a very brief summary is sufficient.

Normally blood flows in streamlines (**LAMINAR FLOW**), i.e., in concentric cylindrical layers. The fastest flow is in the center column, slowing down toward the periphery, such that the most peripheral layer flows hardly at all. Each layer exerts a shearing (**DRAGGING**) force on the next one, and at the periphery, the shearing force is on the endothelium itself, with considerable potential effects on endothelial function including its hemostatic and its anticoagulant functions. The activation of vWF is prominently due to shear forces on the endothelium. The greater the velocity of flow, the more shearing there is because of more friction.

The red cells concentrate in the center, and the platelets and leukocytes are pushed to the periphery. Platelets are thus likely to collide with and adhere, virtually immediately, to any irregularities in the endothelium. Endothelial irregularities (such as a plaque) will produce turbulent flow patterns which promote thrombus formation, partly due to concentration of activated platelets and coagulation factors in areas where the endothelium is already dysfunctional or injured and producing numerous procoagulant factors and partly possible interference with natural anticoagulant mechanisms.

This is augmented by the decrease in flow rate that occurs in injured vessels; this is due to (at least) three factors:

1. Increased capillary permeability leading to hemoconcentration and therefore local concentration of hemostatic factors
2. The increased tissue pressure tends to constrict the vessels in the vicinity
3. Reactive vasoconstriction.

Other major effects of the nature of blood flow are to do with viscosity of the blood. There are many causes of hyperviscosity, which will be discussed in Chapter 22.

The Hemostatic Screen

From the foregoing, it could follow that testing the hemostatic system is very complex. Fortunately this is not so. There are some fundamental conceptual differences between the FBC and the hemostatic screen (HS). The FBC is a full-fledged first-line test of more or less all of the blood diseases, whereas the HS is used for a very restricted presentation – abnormal bleeding. Hemostatic disorders are broadly classified into bleeding and thrombotic (or hypercoagulable) disorders. Thrombotic disorders are discussed in Chapter 21.

The hemostatic screen is used essentially for the diagnosis of the bleeding disorders. From the purely clinical point of view, there are two very broad groups of bleeding disorder: the **PURPURIC** and the **COAGULATION DEFECT** disorders.

A Note About the Terms "Purpuric" and "Coagulation Defect" *These terms are unsatisfactory, yet it is difficult to think of alternatives. Their characteristics are detailed in Chapter 4. Briefly, purpuric bleeds need not show purpura but have a specific and identifiable way of bleeding. In the vast bulk of these cases, the coagulation factors are normal. The prototype cause is immune thrombocytopenic purpura.*

The bleeding characteristics of the coagulation defects are generally distinct from the purpuric bleeds, and the prototype cause is hemophilia. Hemophilia however is a rare cause of this pattern of bleeding. It is difficult to find a satisfactory term for this pattern of bleeding; "hemorrhagic" will not do – purpura is also hemorrhagic. For convenience, we refer to these as "coagulation defects."

While these two groups can often present as identifiably different conditions, there is a great deal of overlap: that is to say, the obvious purpuric bleed may have associated a coagulation disorder that is not clinically obvious but whose presence may change the diagnosis considerably; similarly a coagulation defect bleed may have in addition some of the features classically associated with the purpuric disorders. Since the therapeutic implications can be very different, this is a very important clinical distinction, and thus the HS assumes fundamental importance.

In consequence, it would seem at first glance that there is not much clinical diagnostic prowess required in the bleeding disorders. Besides, if one were going to do the HS with any and all types of bleeding, what would be the point in trying to identify the specific type of bleeding from the clinical features? This, however, is a shortsighted view. Liver disease, for example, is a well-known disorder that can produce a variety of bleeding manifestations, and indeed, in liver disease the full HS is necessary, for more reasons than simply the diagnosis of the bleeding disorder (for example, they are very good liver function tests).

1. The different results of the screen components may give a clear insight into the nature and severity of the liver disease.
2. They may reveal complications that might not have been suspected, like DIC.
3. They can have strong therapeutic implications.
4. They may contribute to a proper understanding of the patient as a whole.

The Components of the Hemostatic Screen

The emergence of the HS has been crucial to the understanding of the bleeding disorders, and this has been primarily because of their complexity. For generations of doctors, the physiology and pathology of hemostasis have been a source of confusion, and the diagnosis therefore has been left to the laboratories. The modern HS has taken decades of development to reach its current form, in tandem with huge amounts of research into the pathophysiology.

Before discussing the HS, bear in mind that it is common practice to consult the laboratory, then submit the tubes of blood that they prescribe, leaving the further elucidation to them. The HS from the point of view of the laboratory hematologist is not the same as that of the clinician. From the lab's point of view, the full screen consists of

1. **THE BLEEDING TIME (BT)** (which of course is done by the ward staff and is submitted along with the blood to the lab)
2. **THE PLATELET COUNT (PC), PLUS MORPHOLOGY OF THE PLATELETS**
3. **THE PROTHROMBIN TIME (PT)**
4. **THE PARTIAL THROMBOPLASTIN TIME (PTT)**
5. **THE THROMBIN TIME (TT)**
6. **FIBRINOGEN**
7. **(PLUS IN SOME CASES, A MORPHOLOGICAL ASSESSMENT OF THE BLOOD FILM).**

In the laboratory, the thrombin time and fibrinogen levels are usually done only if a particular pattern of abnormality in the BT, PC, PT, PTT is observed, or if the clinical features (which should accompany the request to the laboratory) are strongly suggestive of a more involved pathology. Since the reader, particularly the student, needs to know the basics of what the tests involve, a short description of these tests follows.

The Bleeding Time and the Platelet Count

The bleeding time measures primarily the first stage of hemostasis, i.e., the formation of the platelet plug. One important caveat however is that it is also prolonged in many pure vascular disorders – the longest bleeding time the author ever saw was in a case of scurvy. The test is performed by deliberately causing micro-circulatory injury, and seeing how long it takes for bleeding to stop, taking care to avoid clot formation (see Appendix C for the method). The time taken for the bleeding to stop is a summation of a number of factors – platelet plug formation, vasoconstriction, certain molecules such as von Willebrand factor, and the health of the micro-circulatory sub-endothelium. The standard bleeding time, even when using the simplate device, is not very sensitive. It is highly significant if it is prolonged (unless the cut was made into a dilated vessel or hemangioma) but false negatives are the problem. Note that as such it is a relatively nonspecific test for any particular cause, but is fairly sensitive for the presence of **ANY** of these factors, so long as they are severe enough; and this is adequate as a test because milder degrees are seldom of clinical importance.

Apart from the technical issues in causing the injury, a major reason for variation in results is that the vascular response is very dependent on activation of vWF in the local endothelium; this in turn requires significant shearing force to be applied to the endothelium by the flowing blood, in that way activating platelets as well as the endothelial reaction to injury. The injury in the ordinary test leads to a blood flow with very low shear rate. A far more sensitive technique has recently been developed: the PMA-100; this has been designed to mimic the effect of shear on platelet and vascular function, thus activating vWF. It is unfortunately not widely available.

Since the BT it measures both the integrity of the vessel and the platelet function, it is prolonged in

1. **A LOW PLATELET COUNT.** If the platelets are functionally normal, the count must be very low to cause a prolonged BT – less than about $20 \times 10^9/l$. **MORPHOLOGICALLY,** these platelets are normal; they may however be fairly large, and the general feeling in these cases is that they are young and very active.
2. **PLATELET FUNCTION DEFECTS.** These may be hereditary, as in storage pool disease, etc., or acquired as in myelodysplasia. Here the BT may be prolonged with a moderately low or even a normal platelet count. **THE MORPHOLOGY** of the platelets (and occasionally of other blood cells) may be very suggestive, notably in the hereditary forms. Note that

   a) The morphological changes are not necessarily confined to the platelets.
   b) These conditions may also have low platelet counts.
   c) These conditions are very rare, and no details will be given at the general level.

Numerous appearances are recognized:

   a) A group of conditions characterized by giant platelets, bizarre morphology, hypergranularity, and thrombocytopenia
   b) Hypo- or agranular platelets (grey platelets)
   c) Defective aggregation (seen in smears made from fresh (non-anticoagulated) blood only).

The PT and PTT

A certain amount of basic knowledge is required. Although these tests are classically associated with the coagulation mechanism per se, they can also be affected by some disorders of fibrinolysis, as well as by a number of disorders where there is no bleeding tendency at all. Many patterns are possible, and it is far preferable to understand them than try to memorize them. There are four critically important points to note in their usage:

1. These times can be normal or prolonged in different patterns, depending on the nature of defects in the coagulation mechanism – it will be remembered that coagulation is the third phase of hemostasis (after vasoconstriction and platelet plug formation).
2. Not all defects in the coagulation mechanism will lead to a prolonged PT and/or PTT. A high level of clinical suspicion is required to suspect and diagnose the others. They may be normal with very mild or subclinical defects.
3. The PT and PTT can be prolonged in defects that are not associated with excessive bleeding.
4. The PT and PTT can be prolonged in defects of the fourth stage of hemostasis, i.e., fibrinolysis.

Understanding the PT and PTT

This requires some preliminary concepts. Please refer throughout to Fig. 2.30. It will be seen that the **PHYSIOLOGY** represented here is different from that presented earlier; the diagram in Fig. 2.30 in fact represents the state of knowledge of the coagulation system right up to the 1990s, and it was used as a basis for the diagnostic tests as we still know them today. And even for today's diagnostic purposes, the schema is perfectly adequate.

In Fig. 2.30:

1. These blocks comprise: The Common Pathway
2. The common pathway can be activated either by:

   The Intrinsic Pathway **OR**
   The Extrinsic Pathway

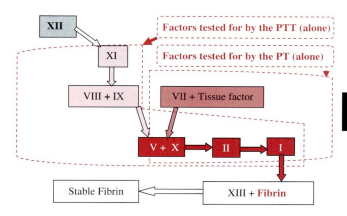

Fig. 2.30 The coagulation cascade (laboratory version)

Table 2.9 Factors and pathways tested by the PT and PTT

PT	PTT	Defective path	Factors deficient
Increased	Normal	Extrinsic	VII
Normal	Increased	Intrinsic	VIII, IX, or XI
Increased	Increased	Common	V, X, II, or I

3. **FIBRIN** is the end point of the testing procedures.
4. The PTT and PT measure different as well as overlapping parts of the pathways, as follows:

THE PTT

The PTT tests (is lengthened by) defects of XI, VIII, IX & V, X, II, I

In addition, the PTT is prolonged in deficiencies of a number of factors that do not predispose to a bleeding tendency, like prekallikrein, high molecular weight kinins, and XII (The latter are factors involved in the activation of factor XII, in the inflammatory sequences).

THE PT

The PT tests (is lengthened by) defects of VII & V, X, II, I

Note that the common pathway is **ALWAYS** involved in these tests. It is the activation of the common pathway by two distinct other pathways that give rise to the two tests, the PT and PTT.

To summarize therefore, see Table 2.9.

The Thrombin Time

In this test, excess thrombin is added to citrated blood and the time to clot measured. This is normally very short. The test essentially measures only factor I. Some unusual and very helpful patterns can emerge however.

Fibrinogen

Apart from the thrombin time, fibrinogen can be measured more directly. It can be measured immuno-chemically and functionally. The functional assays will indicate how much normal activity there is; the other method measures the amount of molecule present, regardless of how functionally effective it is. This gives an indication of abnormal fibrinogen molecules (the dysfibrinogenemias), which have assumed considerable importance in certain diseases. The important point to note is that one can have normal levels of fibrinogen (chemically) and yet have a functional defect.

> *Once the physiology of hemostasis and its control are understood, the formal pathology, albeit from a clinical standpoint, should be far easier to understand.*

The Pathology of the Hemostatic System (Clinical View)

The Functional Outline of the Hemostatic System

See Fig. 2.31

Most of the hemostatic factors are produced by the liver. The exceptions are

1. **THOSE PRODUCED BY THE ENDOTHELIAL CELL**: von Willebrand factor, thrombomodulin, tissue factor pathway inhibitor, plasminogen activator, plasminogen activator inhibitor.
2. **THOSE PRODUCED BY MEGAKARYOCYTES**: Factor V (also by the liver), von Willebrand factor.
3. **THOSE PRODUCED BY THE MARROW**: Platelets.

Types of Pathological Abnormality Affecting the Hemostatic Sub-system

Quantitative Disorders of Production of Hemostatic Factors

1. **THE LIVER MAY PRODUCE DECREASED AMOUNTS OF HEMOSTATIC FACTORS**, because of any number of diseases, usually chronic and affecting hepatocellular function. The hemostatic

Fig. 2.31 Basic diagram of the hemostatic system

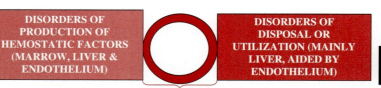

DISORDERS OF PRODUCTION OF HEMOSTATIC FACTORS (MARROW, LIVER & ENDOTHELIUM)

DISORDERS OF DISPOSAL OR UTILIZATION (MAINLY LIVER, AIDED BY ENDOTHELIUM)

DISORDERS OF OR IN THE CIRCULATION OR ENDOTHELIUM

!

factors may be procoagulant, anticoagulant, and fibrinolytic, with the logical consequences of such deficiency. The liver's role in transcarboxylation of certain factors may be diminished by cholestatic disorders; these are both procoagulant (factors II, VII, IX, and X) and anticoagulant such as protein C.

Occasionally **THE LIVER MAY PRODUCE INCREASED AMOUNTS OF HEMOSTATIC FACTORS**: some procoagulant factors react as acute phase reactants.

2. **THE ENDOTHELIUM**, under the influence of various processes such as shear stresses or activation secondary to inflammation, may produce increased or decreased amounts of von Willebrand factor, thrombomodulin, plasminogen, plasminogen activator, and plasminogen activator inhibitor. Under pathological circumstances, such as in sepsis, the endothelium may produce increased amounts of tissue factor.

3. **HEREDITARY DEFICIENCIES** of all the coagulation factors have been described. Hemophilia A (factor VIII) and hemophilia B (factor IX) are the commonest (by far).

4. The effect of liver disease on the **PRODUCTION OF PLATELETS** has been mentioned before.

5. **THEORETICALLY, ABNORMAL MEGAKARYO-CYTES,** such as found in myelodysplasias, could produce abnormal amounts of factor V and von Willebrand factor. This has not been thoroughly investigated.

Qualitative Disorders of Production of Hemostatic Factors

These may be hereditary or acquired.

1. **HEREDITARY DISORDERS OF QUALITATIVE PRODUCTION.** A number of abnormal molecules of various factors has been identified, such as abnormal fibrinogens. These often have distinct hemostatic sequelae.

2. **ACQUIRED DISORDERS OF QUALITATIVE PRODUCTION.** By far the most important here are some abnormal (and hemostatically ineffective) molecules produced as a result of vitamin K deficiency.

Disorders of Disposal of Excess Hemostatic Factors or Their Products

The reticulo-endothelial system and the liver play a major role in clearing the blood of the products of hemostasis. Defects will result in accumulation of factors and complexes, some of which have hemostatic effects as well.

The Pathogenesis of Disorders of Hemostasis

The disorders of hemostasis are in fact extremely complex and very many of them are very rare. The clinical features of the important ones are discussed in Chapter 4.

At the general level, we discuss the pathogenesis only of

1. *Bleeding disorders due to DECREASED COAGULANT FACTORS and PLATELETS, fairly extensively.*
2. *(Some) bleeding disorders due to (certain) INCREASED ANTICOAGULANT FACTORS OR FIBRINOLYSIS.*
3. *A brief introduction into thrombotic disorders due to DECREASED ANTICOAGULANT FACTORS.*

Bleeding disorders due to **DECREASED COAGULANT FACTORS AND PLATELETS** are easy to understand. In addition, however, there are numerous processes limiting or modulating thrombin or its function (thrombin formation is central to thrombosis) that are relevant here and have been discussed before. Important among these processes are numerous natural anti-coagulant mechanisms and fibrinolysis.

BLEEDING DISORDERS CAN THUS ALSO FOLLOW FROM INCREASED ANTICOAGULANT FACTORS OR PROCESSES, OR INCREASED FIBRINOLYSIS.

THROMBOTIC DISORDERS CAN FOLLOW FROM DECREASED ANTICOAGULANT FACTORS OR PROCESSES, OR DECREASED FIBRINOLYSIS.

Pathological Bleeding

THIS CAN RESULT EITHER FROM DEFECTS IN THE PROCOAGULANT MECHANISMS OR DEFECTS IN THE MECHANISMS CONTROLLING HEMOSTASIS, OR IN ABNORMAL FIBRINOLYSIS.

Defects in the Procoagulant Mechanisms

1. **PLATELETS**. The platelets must be of adequate number and normally functional.

a. **PLATELET NUMBERS.** There are numerous causes for decreased numbers of platelets, both congenital and acquired. No absolute figures can be given for platelet counts below which the patient will bleed. Apart from individual variation, a great deal depends on their functionality and hence the cause.

b. **PLATELET FUNCTIONS.** There are numerous causes for abnormal platelet function, both congenital and acquired. Assessing platelet dysfunction in the laboratory is a specialized activity, and will almost certainly only be available in level 4 laboratories.

c. Generally speaking, the most important causes of bleeding as a result of platelets disorders are

   MYELODYSPLASIA. In myelodysplasia, the platelet count may well be on the low side, but bleeding tends to be disproportionately severe because of functional defects in the platelets.

   APLASTIC ANEMIA. In aplastic anemia, the usual cause of bleeding is severe thrombocytopenia.

   LEUKEMIA. In the leukemias, both thrombocytopenia and functional platelet disorders may be responsible for bleeding.

2. **COAGULATION FACTOR DEFECTS.** Similarly, these can be hereditary or acquired. Hereditary causes are typically characterized by a defect in a single factor, whereas acquired causes may be characterized by deficiencies in multiple factors.

   The most common of **THE HEREDITARY BLEEDING DISORDERS** is von Willebrand disease. This is discussed below. However, the most common **SERIOUS** hereditary bleeding disorder is hemophilia A (factor VIII deficiency), followed by factor IX deficiency (hemophilia B, and which used to be called Christmas disease). After that, they are all extremely rare, with the exception of factor XI deficiency (also sometimes called hemophilia C) among Ashkenazi Jews.

   OF THE ACQUIRED CAUSES there are two significant clinical groups:

a) Those with defective production. These in turn are of two different groups:

   • **GENERAL LIVER DISEASE** leading to underproduction of all the factors.
   • **VITAMIN K DEFICIENCY-ASSOCIATED** defects.

   These are discussed under **COMBINED DEFECTS** below.

b) **THOSE DUE TO EXCESSIVE CONSUMPTION.** These are discussed under **COMBINED DEFECTS** below.

c) The abnormal plasma proteins in some of the paraproteinemias, e.g., myeloma, can adsorb onto their surface some of the coagulation factors – factor X seems to be particularly affected in this regard.

3. **COMBINED DEFECTS** (i.e., defects in both platelets and coagulation factors). There are three conditions that should be understood: von Willebrand disease, liver insufficiency, and disseminated intravascular coagulation (DIC).

   VON WILLEBRAND DISEASE is one of the commonest coagulation disorders. It is thus important to understand something about von Willebrand factor (vWF). vWF plays a fundamental part in the roles of both the platelet and coagulation processes. vWF is found in two forms:

1. A large multimeric form found within the endothelial cell in the Weibel–Palade bodies (involved in platelet adhesion). Release of vWF from the endothelium is facilitated by the shearing (frictional) forces on the endothelium caused by the blood flowing over it.
2. A form circulating in the plasma where its function is the transport of factor VIII.

There are various sub-types of von Willebrand disease, with very variable clinical and laboratory presentations. Suffice it to say that typically it is characterized by hemophilic-type bleeding of various degrees plus a functional platelet defect. It is thus associated with both purpuric and coagulation defect bleeding.

LIVER DISEASE. Since the liver manufactures most of the coagulation factors (and the natural anticoagulants), it is clear that liver disease will be associated with hemophilic-type bleeds. There are two broad groups of mechanisms by which liver disease is responsible for coagulation defects:

1. Underproduction of all the factors due to hepatocellular disease.
2. Interference with the carboxylation of factors II, VII, IX, and X, due to cholestatic disease.

In addition, however, thrombocytopenia is common in chronic liver disease, for a variety of reasons:

1. **PORTAL HYPERTENSION**, a common complication of chronic liver disease, can lead to an enlarged spleen with hypersplenism, which may lead to thrombocytopenia.
2. **CIRRHOSIS**, also a common complication of chronic liver disease, tends to be associated with thrombocytopenia because of chronic activation of the hepatic sinusoids being stretched around the cirrhotic nodules, resulting in irritation and activation of the endothelium lining the sinusoids.

The existence of underlying liver disease may be obvious, and the full HS would be indicated, including the D-dimer and FDP assays. However, sometimes it is not obvious, and one requires a considerable index of suspicion to investigate for these. Indeed, it is here that the clinical features of the underlying disease may be very helpful.

DISSEMINATED INTRAVASCULAR COAGULATION. The coagulation mechanism may become pathologically activated in many conditions, such as septic shock, leading to widespread intravascular coagulation. In the process, coagulation factors and platelets are consumed, leading, paradoxically, to bleeding.

The Pathogenesis of Disseminated Intravascular Coagulation *This is complex: in brief, the coagulation process is activated inside the circulation, leading to the consumption of platelets and coagulation factors and the deposition of fibrin on and across the endothelium; red cells striking these strands are physically disrupted. Some of them reform but are of abnormal shape, with fragments and microspherocytes. Because the procoagulant factors are consumed, there is a strong bleeding tendency. Note the apparent paradox: DIC is primarily a hypercoagulable state presenting as a bleeding disorder (as well as a hemolytic state).*

There are numerous triggers that can activate intravascular coagulation. The most important are sepsis, necrotic tissue, malignant cells, and obstetric accidents.

4. **VASCULAR DEFECTS.**

Only two conditions need be mentioned: scurvy and hereditary hemorrhagic telangiectasia (the Rendu–Osler–Weber syndrome).

> **SCURVY.** The deficiency of vitamin C leads to poor collagen formation, including that in the vessel walls. This results in easy bleeding.
> **HEREDITARY HEMORRHAGIC TELANGIECTASIA** (the Rendu–Osler–Weber syndrome). This is a hereditary condition characterized by widespread telangiectatic lesions in the skin, the mucosae, and often in muscles. Large AV communications tend to form. These lesions tend to enlarge under the influence of estrogen.

Defects in Mechanisms Controlling Hemostasis

1. **CIRCULATING ANTICOAGULANTS.** At the general level, very little need be said. These patients will present with a bleeding tendency with little or no clinical features to alert one to the possibility. Here we are talking not of the natural anticoagulants, which are antithrombin, tissue factor pathway inhibitor and the protein C/thrombomodulin system; these act only on **ACTIVATED** coagulant factors (i.e., they are physiological). No conditions have been described where these are increased. Rather we talk here about acquired causes responsible for severe bleeding tendencies. These can arise in three situations:

   a. In multiply-transfused patients usually suffering from a congenital deficiency of a clotting factor.
   b. As an autoantibody.
   c. Of very great significance are the anticoagulants used therapeutically: heparin and the oral anticoagulants (this last also occasionally as a result of poisoning).

   The usual tests of the coagulation mechanism will be abnormal, but the identification of the nature of the problem must be left to the laboratory.

2. **INCREASED FIBRINOLYSIS.** Formation of fibrin is accompanied by the generation of plasmin, which breaks down fibrin and fibrinogen. Plasminogen from the liver is converted to plasmin by the action of tissue-plasminogen activator (t-PA) from the endothelium and/or by urokinase-type-plasminogen activator (u-PA) from the kinin system. These as well as plasmin are in turn controlled by various other factors. Investigation of abnormal fibrinolysis – even suspecting its presence – is generally a highly specialized task.

Pathological Thrombosis

To understand this properly, it is worthwhile to remember Virchow's triad. Rudolph Virchow, the great 19th century pathologist, identified three crucial factors in the pathogenesis of abnormal thrombosis:

1. Decreased blood flow (i.e., stasis)
2. Disease in or around the vessels
3. Alterations in the blood itself (in modern terms, abnormalities in the balance of coagulation, anticoagulation, and fibrinolytic processes).

These are still valid today; however, modern insights have tended to blur the clear distinctions between these in the role they play in thrombo-embolism, particularly with regard to endothelial damage and inflammation. Note that many of these causes are not primarily hematological. The condition is discussed in Chapter 22.

Summary

Hematology and hematology reports constitute a significant problem for clinicians and students. The reasons can partly be traced to the teaching of hematology and partly to a lack of understanding of the unusual nature of the system, its pathology and the nature of the tests used.

Heavy reliance is placed on a number of blood tests and the final approach is always an integrated activity involving both laboratory and clinical methodologies. Poor or misdirected teaching has been responsible for much of the traditional confusion that people experience. It has also resulted in a highly mechanistic approach to blood diseases.

Whilst the hematological system is unusual in many respects, it only requires some shifts in thinking, perspective, and approach for it to be entirely comprehensible. To be fully understood, the system should be seen firstly as integrated with the rest of the body systems, secondly as a dynamic system with several independent subsystems, and finally as a balanced system. This requires only a basic knowledge of

1. The possible pathological processes affecting the system. These comprise quantitative and qualitative disorders of production, disorders in the circulation, and disorders of the normal destruction of cells.
2. An understanding of the first-line tests – the FBC and the hemostatic screen. These form the basis of the investigation of the vast majority of suspected blood diseases. But their limitations and appropriate use must be understood.
3. A recognition that interpretation of these tests involves an understanding of the hematological system as

    a. A highly dynamic system.
    b. A balanced system, between production and disposal or utilization, and which is thus partially self-compensating. It is highly dependent on

normal nutrients and other stimulants. The most important nutrients are iron, folate, and vitamin B_{12}; their patho-physiology is best understood as being in a circulation, based on the red cell circulation itself.

    c. A system operating both in space and time.

4. Blood and its pathologies are intimately involved with all the body tissues and their pathologies. This contributes to an understanding of

    a. The signs and symptoms of blood disease
    b. The close interdependence between the pathology, the first-line tests, and the clinical features.

Hemostasis comprises several processes acting interdependently and concurrently: procoagulant activities rely on contact with foreign surfaces by platelets and certain clotting factors; natural anti-coagulants tightly control the extent of coagulation; and fibrinolytic processes remove the clot and restore circulation once the breach is healed.

> **The Basic Nature of the Diagnostic Process in Hematology** This is always an integrated activity involving both clinical and laboratory methodologies. But this implies that the tests are properly understood and interpreted, particularly the FBC.
>
> To stress: If the process as described is followed, the choice of tests in hematology will be made only after rational consideration. There is virtually no room for shotgun investigation.

> **A Final Word** The *bottom line* is that in hematology:
>
> 1. We cannot do without blood tests
> 2. Blood tests are not enough.

Exercise 2.1 A Quick Self-Test

Test your understanding of this chapter by answering true or false to the following statements. (Answers overleaf.)

True	False	Questions
		1. Lab tests in hematology are usually not critical for the complete diagnosis and management of blood diseases.
		2. The FBC is essentially a test for confirming clinical features.
		3. A morphological comment adds significant value (± one third) to a FBC report.
		4. The FBC is too expensive to use in clinical situations except as a last resort.
		5. The hematological system is a dynamic one with normally a balance between production and disposal.
		6. Increased bone marrow production is always called a myeloproliferative disorder.
		7. The role of the plasma is significant in the interpretation of the first-line tests.
		8. Band (stab, staff) cells are the developmental form immediately preceding the mature lymphocyte.
		9. The MCV is one of the most valuable indices in the FBC in the assessment of anemia.
		10. An acute destructive episode of the marrow will show decreasing counts of all three cell lines at the same time.
		11. Since the daily destruction of 6.4 g of hemoglobin per day releases 21 mg of iron, it follows that 21 mg of iron must be absorbed from the diet daily.
		12. Iron absorption is fixed at a maximum of 2 mg/day.
		13. Malabsorption of iron is the commonest cause of iron deficiency.
		14. In health the hematological system appears stable, with only minimal variation in its components from day to day. It follows that the system is based on standard fixed production and disposal of cells.
		15. Malabsorption is the commonest cause of vitamin B_{12} deficiency.
		16. Platelets play a subsidiary role in hemostasis and play no role in coagulation.
		17. Hemostasis is now recognized as occurring in distinct and separate phases.
		18. Hemostasis is normally set in operation by simultaneous activation of platelets and factor XI.
		19. An increase in the basophils in the blood is best referred to as *basophilia*.
		20. Erythrocytosis means an increase in the red cells or hematocrit only.

(continued)

True	False	Questions
		21. Polychromasia on a blood film means reticulocytosis.
		22. Diagnosis of a blood disease always requires a bone marrow examination.
		23. In adult males, the iron content of the body is 14.5–18 g.
		24. Neutrophils survive for about 120 days.

Exercise 2.2

Match the items in columns 1 and 2. (Answers overleaf).

Column 1	Column 2
A. Diagnosis of blood diseases	1. The commonest hereditary cause of a bleeding disorder.
B. Most abnormalities in the FBC in family practice	2. Can cause significant false results in the FBC
C. Most clinical diagnostic decisions in hematology	3. Based on the recognition of patterns
D. Disorders of plasma proteins	4. Iron
E. Neutrophils, monocytes, lymphocytes, eosinophils, and basophils	5. Antithrombin
F. Competent assessment of the blood morphology on stained films	6. Typically a combined laboratory and clinical activity
G. Bone marrow attempts at compensation	7. Has unique features because of the dynamic nature of the system
H. Breakdown product of red cells that is normally completely re-utilized	8. Adds ± one third of value to the FBC
I. Deficiency of the nutrient required for blood formation that is the easiest to develop	9. Folate
	10. Due to disease outside the hematological system
J. Coagulation	11. Leukocytes
K. Fibrinolysis	12. Recognized causes of hypercoagulability
L. Erythrocytosis	13. Is generated by the sequential activation in the form of a cascade of serine proteases
M. The major inactivator of thrombin	14. Measures factors I, II, V, VIII, IX, X, XI, and XII
N. The liver stores sufficient amounts for 4 years	15. The term given to the process causing the dissolution of thrombi
O. The pathology of the blood system	16. By increasing production
P. Defects in the mechanisms that control thrombin formation	17. The term used for increase in the hematocrit, not necessarily an increased red cell count
Q. von Willebrand disease	
R. Liver insufficiency	18. Vitamin B_{12}.
S. The partial thromboplastin time on its own	19. A common acquired cause of bleeding

Answers

Exercise 2.1

1: False. 2: False. 3: True. 4: False. 5: True. 6: False. 7: True. 8: False. 9: True. 10: False. 11: False. 12: False. 13: False. 14: False. 15: True. 16: False. 17: False. 18: False. 19: False. 20: True. 21: True. 22: False. 23: False. 24: False.

Exercise 2.2

A6; B10; C6; D2; E11; F8; G16; H4; I9; J13; K15; L17; M5; N18; O7; P12; Q1; R19; S14.

Further Reading

Lewis SM, Bain B, Bates I (2006). Dacie and Lewis Practical Haematology. 10th edn. London: Churchill Livingstone.

Ganong WF (2005). Review of Medical Physiology. 22nd edn. New York: McGraw Hill.

Hoffbrand AV, Pettit JE (2001). Essential Haematology. 4th edn. Oxford: Blackwell Science.

References

1. Neurath NJ, Joosten E, Riezler R, Stabler SP, Allen RH, Lindenbaurn J (1995). Effects of vitamin B_{12}, folate and vitamin B_6 supplementation in elderly people with normal serum vitamin concentrations. Lancet 345: 85–89.

Everything should be made as simple as possible, but not simpler.
(Albert Einstein)

Preview and Study Themes *Given that hematological diagnosis is so critically dependent on lab results, it is important that they be understood in terms of*

1. Their nature and value

   a. What they actually represent
   b. How they can vary and the reasons for this
   c. The resolution and limitations of the different tests, i.e., how clearly they can differentiate the normal from the abnormal

2. The degree of their reliability (i.e., of the actual measurements, assessments, and comments) as they emerge from the laboratory

Reaching a clinical decision on the basis of unreliable, misunderstood, or misinterpreted results can be worse than having no results at all.
Finally, some critical comments about algorithms and evidence-based medicine are made.

The Nature and Value of Laboratory Tests in Hematology

From the practical point of view, hematological tests can be classified very broadly into two major groups:

1. Numerical values (by far the majority) of measurements or counts of specific anatomical entities in (usually) the blood.
2. Morphological assessments of various anatomical structures and appearances. These assessments are commonly and pejoratively referred to as "subjective," but this label is misleading. A numerical result can be displayed or printed, appearing as evidently an absolute quantity, and is therefore granted the exalted status of "objective"; this does not automatically make the result cast in stone, as it were. The preconceived idea that a numerical result from a laboratory is necessarily an exact reflection of the truth must be demolished – **NUMERICAL VALUES FROM THE LABORATORY ALSO ARE ESTIMATES.** The criticism that "subjective" results are only in the mind of the observer is also a gross oversimplification – one has only to be involved in the prolonged training and constant cross-referencing that occurs in the education of a morphological hematologist or histopathologist to know that this is so. "Objective" results must be evaluated for validity as carefully as the "subjective" ones. They are simply different modalities of assessment, each with their weaknesses and strengths.

The results of all these tests are used to attempt to infer from them whether or not a disorder exists and what its nature is. To do this, values are correlated by clinical research workers with known, **CLINICALLY** identified, disease states, if possible relating the result to pathogenetic mechanisms of the relevant diseases. It is then decided to what extent an abnormal result predicts the

O.N. Beck, *Diagnostic Hematology*, DOI 10.1007/978-1-84800-295-1_3,
© Springer-Verlag London Limited 2009

existence, the nature, and/or the severity of a disease. If these predictions are found to be reliable, the tests are then assigned greater or lesser value in the clinical enterprise. These degrees of value depend primarily on what actions on the part of the clinician are triggered at different levels. The above constitute the major criteria for **CLINICAL ACCEPTABILITY** of a test.

To repeat, **ALL** laboratory testing procedures are really estimations, regardless of how carefully the tests are done and of the degree of sophistication of the equipment and personnel. The user should be aware of inherent limits that the laboratory operates within, no matter how good or even "certificated" or "accredited" it is, and should also know how clinical acceptability varies with different tests. The clinician cannot abdicate his responsibility in this regard and has therefore an obligation with regard to the taking and submission of specimens, and then deciding how to approach the results once received, for his clinical purposes.

It is as well to re-emphasize: the common preconception that not only are a laboratory's results "holy writ" but they are 100% reliable at all times **IS A FALLACY**. In addition, their predictive value varies enormously; this is discussed later in the chapter.

Before using a result for clinical purposes, one must decide the following:

1. Is the result normal or not? The answer to this depends in turn on the answer to some other questions, viz.
2. How certain can we be of the laboratory measurement? What can be the reasons for a result not reflecting the true value? What factors may have caused variation from the "true" value?
3. Are there inherent limitations to the test result/s? What are they?
4. How significant is the result from the clinical point of view?

   Each of these points is discussed in turn.

To exemplify our discussion, consider the simple result of a Hemoglobin (Hb) of 13.1 g/dl. After the presentation of the various problems and their causes that any result can be associated with, this result will be used as an example of the process of diagnosis, simplified here for didactic purposes.

TASK #1: IS IT NORMAL? This begs the question:

What is normal?

Up to now, we have used the meaning of the word "normal" with respect to results as being taken for granted. Clearly, one cannot decide anything about a possible abnormal result unless one knows what is normal; indeed, a large part of clinical training is the understanding and careful evaluation of any finding's normality. When is a patellar tendon reflex abnormally brisk? This can be very difficult in borderline cases.

It is generally accepted that there is an absolute true value for any analyte in any one patient (just as there presumably is an absolute normal intensity of patellar reflex in any one patient). This is referred to as the **HOMEOSTATIC SET POINT**. In other words, in any individual there would be say a hematocrit (Hct) that is exactly normal for him; any variation he would show in his Hct, **ASSUMING EXACT MEASUREMENT WERE POSSIBLE**, would be due to disease (or also in this case, a variant caused by the method of collection, or of the state of hydration). Thus, an "abnormal" result in most tests would (ideally) either indicate a specific disease process or be the result of environmental influences. (In **CHRONIC** environmental change, e.g., living at a very high altitude, the homeostatic set point may well be reset, but this is a complex and poorly researched matter). Consequently, the "normal" set point for a patient can also vary with **TIME** (it is likely that it therefore also varies with age). In the case of an abnormally brisk knee jerk, variation could be the result either of some form of upper motor neuron disorder or the effect of increased metabolic activity, such as hyperthyroidism, and so on. In the healthy person, we thus recognize one important set of causes for a given value to vary (even if it were true and accurate), and that is, environmental and physiological circumstances – commonly called "pre-analytic variation." This is discussed a little later.

However, homeostatic set points are potentially different in all individuals. We cannot possibly identify the set points of all tests in all persons (even a previous result of an analyte taken when the patient and his doctor claimed he was well, cannot without further ado be regarded as his set point). We are constrained therefore to look at values of **GROUPS OF PERSONS**. It follows that the results of an analyte tested in a **GROUP** of people will show a number (or **RANGE**) of results; the resultant range of values can reasonably be inferred as being "normal" – i.e., reflecting the **NORMAL POPULATION**; and we want to assess **WHETHER OUR PATIENT BELONGS IN THIS POPULATION**. Thus, testing an analyte in an individual necessarily will give a result, if he is healthy, that lies within **A RANGE OF VALUES**.

There is an important difference between the intensity of a reflex, for example, and a given hemoglobin estimation: it is very difficult to quantify a reflex (a reflex intensity has its own range within which it is **ADJUDGED** normal – or not), but the Hb level is already a quantity, with a measured range of what is taken to be normal – and is thus directly susceptible to statistical manipulation.

"Normal" and "Normal Ranges"

How can we be sure that everyone in the population that is surveyed to assess these "normal" ranges is truly healthy? How do we know that there is not an overlap with truly diseased values? These and other logical problems have caused the word "normal" to be replaced by "reference." These ranges are fairly arbitrarily defined in terms of the standard deviation (SD) (from the mean), or the coefficient of variation (CV), and mean that certain results near the limits are excluded, **POSSIBLY UNFAIRLY**, the idea being to exclude any sub-clinically abnormal results (which in fact may not be present). In Fig. 3.1, the range of reference values and their frequencies (i.e., how many subjects have a particular value) for Hb in apparently healthy adult males at an altitude of 5,000 ft, is depicted. In this case, the distribution is NORMAL (a confusing term, since here it means "bell shaped"). It will be seen that at both ends of the curve there are small tails of values that fall outside the ± 2SD range (defined by the two vertical black lines), statistically making them abnormal in possibly normal subjects.

A Hb of 13.1 at this altitude, by reference only to the distribution in the population, appears therefore to indicate anemia, but if and only if

1. The patient is a male – on looking at the range for females, we would see that the value would be perfectly normal.

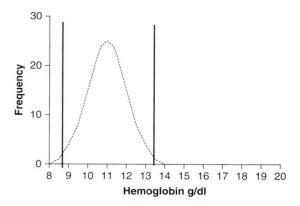

Fig. 3.2 Hemoglobin distribution in ACD at 5,000 ft

2. The patient is an adult. The value would be perfectly "normal" if he were 2 weeks old.
3. The patient is under around 65 years of age.

Nevertheless, apart from this and on looking further, even these conclusions seem questionable.

Observe that the range is large, and this holds considerable implications. First, equivalently large ranges also apply to sets of **ABNORMAL** results of the same analyte. In Fig. 3.2, one sees the range of values found in a group of male patients at the same altitude suffering from anemia of chronic disorders (ACD).

The curve is clearly to the left of that in Fig. 3.1, and it would seem that the populations are different and that a mild to moderate anemia is characteristic of ACD, and that therefore the Hb level would approach our ideal mentioned above, i.e., a test indicating a **DISTINCTLY DIFFERENT POPULATION**.

However, these "normal" and "abnormal" ranges are **NOT** entirely distinct, showing a degree of overlap, as can be seen in Fig. 3.3.

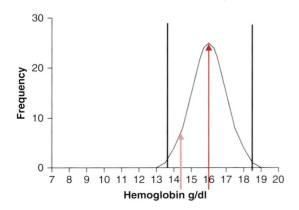

Fig. 3.1 The normal distribution of hemoglobin levels at 5,000 ft

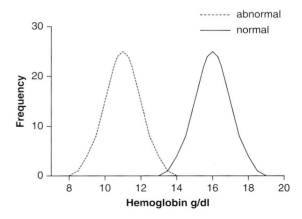

Fig. 3.3 Distribution of Hb in normal and in ACD at 5,000 ft

So, in this case the Hb of 13.1 does **NOT** identify with confidence a patient with anemia. What is one then to do in such a case? Very sophisticated statistical techniques have been developed for this, but in the end, the solution is still probabilistic. Usually in practice, other possibilities would be considered:

1. Is there any assistance from the rest of the FBC and related tests, such as the MCV, the WCC, and the ESR?
2. Has the patient until very recently lived at sea level, where the "normal" range of Hb values is lower?
3. There may be other clinical features that might explain the picture, independent of any cause of anemia, and so on.

These questions are all discussed in this and later chapters. Let us assume that none of the above-mentioned circumstances apply. In such doubtful cases, the use of language to facilitate your thinking may be of assistance. For instance, if our adult male patient appears otherwise fit, you should say to yourself "there is a possible anemia," and take it from there. You are at least now alerted to the possibility of disease and further clinical, and laboratory investigations can be undertaken if deemed important as a **CLINICAL** decision.

The second implication of the large range is as follows: even if his Hb were 14 (i.e., regarded as "normal"), his value a month before, had it been tested, could have been 18, and the Hb of 14 would represent a significant drop in Hb **FOR THAT PATIENT**, despite being within the reference range. This problem, with reference to occult bleeding, will be discussed later in the chapter; the principles would be the same regardless of the cause of the drop in Hb. The important conclusion therefore is that any measurement may be within the reference range and still be abnormal. These days, with laboratory tests being done extremely readily, often patients will know something about their previous results, or can get them. A general practice is ideal for this purpose, since it may be caring for a family for years or generations, with all the reports available. It should be clear therefore that the tendency for practices to dispose of "old" blood (and other) results is to be resisted if at all possible.

The third implication is more complex and has to do with the assessment of the **DEGREE** of a change in a value. Refer again to Fig. 3.1 and note the two arrows, one in pink pointing to a Hb of 14.4 and the other in red pointing to a Hb of 16. Both are "normal." Now assume both patients start consuming an inadequate diet with respect to iron. The "pink" patient will develop anemia (as defined by the reference range) far sooner than the "red" (other things being equal). So a Hb of 11 in patient "red" will reflect a far more severe anemia and state of

iron deficiency than patient "pink" at the same Hb. Imagine how much more severe the Hb of 11 would be had the patient's original Hb been 18. **THUS, AN HB OF 13.1 COULD REPRESENT SIGNIFICANT ANEMIA – IT CANNOT AUTOMATICALLY BE PASSED OVER AS INSIGNIFICANT.** This issue is very important, because of the common tendency to ignore very slight deviations from "normal" with many analytes as well as to slavishly follow published operating characteristics and ignore the specific circumstances of the patient.

> Therefore, the following point must be made: one cannot assess a value only by reference to the reference range, but also to what the value was before, preferably in a state of health. Without previous results, there should always therefore be reservations about the significance of a result – even an apparently normal result. The most sophisticated statistical techniques will not enable one to get around this problem.

We conclude that the patient with a Hb of 13.1 possibly has anemia, which may be more severe than the result suggests, and which therefore cannot be ignored. The next question now becomes very pertinent.

TASK #2: HOW VALID IS THE RESULT?

> How *certain* can we be of the laboratory measurement? Are there any obvious reasons for the result not to reflect the true value? What factors may have caused *variation* from the "true" value?

Variation, Uncertainty of Measurement, Reliability, and Quality Control

We return to our male patient with a Hb of 13.1 and assume we have decided that, **IF IT IS CORRECT**, then our patient **MAY** be anemic. But maybe the result was wrong in the first place. How do we proceed to decide whether the result is "correct"? A certain amount of knowledge and understanding is necessary here.

It is a mistake to assume that the laboratory bears all the responsibility for ensuring that the results are correct. Certainly, it bears a very heavy responsibility: all analytic procedures have an inherent variability – in the very nature of the analytical process. The various causes of this are collectively known as "**ANALYTIC**

VARIATION" and are entirely the laboratory's responsibility. It is unnecessary for the clinical user to be aware of the technical causes of laboratory variation; **WHAT HE HAS TO BE AWARE OF, HOWEVER, IS THAT THEY OCCUR, AND THAT THERE ARE CAUSES OF VARIATION FOR WHICH HE IS INDEED RESPONSIBLE.**

> It is necessary to have some insight into variation in results, both as a result of "natural" (pre-analytic) variation and that due to the inherent variability of measurement (analytic), else one can misinterpret results, to the disadvantage and sometimes unnecessary alarm to or unrealistic reassurance of the patient.

There are thus two broad causes of variation in results from the (unknown) homeostatic set point:

1. **PRE-ANALYTIC** (i.e., variations due to changes before the specimen reaches the laboratory) caused by

   a) Physiological and environmental conditions
   b) Circumstances surrounding the collection of the specimen

2. **ANALYTIC** (i.e., variations caused by and inherent in the actual process of analysis)

It is the laboratory's responsibility to ensure that its analytic variation is kept within acceptable standards, and to have the figures to prove this available for inspection. The laboratory also has a limited role in controlling pre-analytic variation, e.g., ensuring that certain specimens are or have been taken from a fasting patient, and so on; the laboratory will issue guidelines for this sort of thing.

Preventing most pre-analytic errors, however, is the responsibility of the clinician, and **A MAJOR SOURCE OF VARIATION LIES WITH THE PERSON COLLECTING THE SPECIMENS**. Too often, problems arise due to the condition of the specimen when it arrives in the laboratory. Specimen management is one of the prime responsibilities of the collector – bear in mind that serious, avoidable, even life-threatening errors can be made with a substandard specimen, through **NO** fault of the laboratory.

> Preventing certain laboratory errors is the responsibility of the clinician, and can interfere with the interpretation of the tests. They are to do with: *how you handle your specimens*, and *the recognition that different physiological and environmental states can affect the results.*

Specimen Management

1. **CARE MUST BE TAKEN WHEN TAKING BLOOD FOR YOUR TESTS**. If using a syringe, do not apply too much suction. Get the blood into the relevant tubes promptly.
2. Make sure you use the correct tubes. In particular, do not use a heparinized tube for the FBC. Significant platelet clumping occurs very rapidly, giving a falsely low platelet count. Also, stained smears made from this blood are unsatisfactory.
3. If, having taken the blood with a syringe, you are putting the blood into an evacuated tube (containing the relevant anticoagulant) through the needle, do not apply pressure – let the vacuum do the work for you. However, you must make sure that the tube has filled optimally (see point 5 – sometimes tubes get old and the vacuum decreases, particularly if they have been left in the sun).
4. If you are putting the blood into an ordinary, non-evacuated tube containing the relevant anticoagulant, remove the cap and the needle and **GENTLY** push the blood into the tube.
5. The ratio between anticoagulant and blood is very important.

   a) With respect to the FBC, 3–4 ml of blood should be added to the EDTA tube. The effects of adding too little blood to the EDTA tube are serious. Adequate anticoagulation for the FBC requires about 1.2 mg EDTA per milliliter of whole blood. The usual evacuated tube is engineered to draw in about 4 ml of blood, and thus the tube contains ±5 mg. of EDTA salt. Inadequate filling, if severe enough to produce a concentration of 2 mg EDTA/ml of blood (i.e., 1.7 ml of added blood), will cause shrinkage with a falsely decreased MCV and thus Hct, and degenerative changes particularly in the white cells and platelets. Thus

      - Decreased Hct
      - Increased MCHC
      - Degenerative changes in leukocytes, observable morphologically
      - Disintegration of platelets, causing a falsely raised platelet count

   b) With respect to coagulation studies, as accurately as possible, 4.5 ml of blood should be added to the citrate-containing tube. The effects of adding the wrong amounts of blood to the tube are possibly even more serious than with the FBC. This requires explanation: the reason the blood in these tubes does not clot is the citrate binds the Ca^{2+} in the plasma, and Ca^{2+} is required for most of the steps in the hemostatic process. In the tests, a standard amount of Ca^{2+} is added, and the final concentration is critical for reproducible results. Therefore, the ratio of blood to anticoagulant will affect this final concentration. Overfilling (or more usually underfilling) the tube will therefore be seen to be serious sources of erroneous results. However, the extent of the resultant errors and consequently the negative influence of underfilling vary with whether the patient is receiving anticoagulant therapy: normal subjects will have accurate results in tubes filled to $\geq 65\%$ of optimum; in patients on anticoagulant therapy, tubes filled to $\leq 80\%$ of optimum are not accurate. Note that a very high hematocrit (>55 l/l) by the same reasoning will lead to incorrect results. The laboratory should be consulted, and asked to provide tubes with different amounts of citrate depending on the hematocrit. (Incidentally, a **LOW** hematocrit requires no adaptation.)

6. Tests of coagulation are attempts to mimic in vivo processes. Blood anticoagulated with citrate does not clot (spontaneously), but this does not mean that there has not been a tendency to partial activation of the coagulation cascades and the platelets; this tendency will only be aggravated by increased levels of certain factors. Consequently, every effort should be made to minimize these potential activators:

   a) Capillary samples (e.g., finger-pricks) should be avoided – endothelial and tissue injury can easily be responsible for thromboplastic activation.
   b) Stress and exercise should be avoided prior to the collection, since these increase factor VIII, von Willebrand factor, and fibrinolysis.
   c) Venous occlusion to facilitate drawing of blood causes hemo-concentration, increased fibrinolytic activity, platelet activation, and activation of some clotting factors. Thus, occlusion should be applied for less than a minute. Even then, the first tube filled should not be used for coagulation studies.
   d) Good-quality plastic syringes and tubes should be used. If glass is used, the containers should be properly siliconized.

7. Most laboratories make their own smears from the EDTA tube. However, if you make your own smears, try to make them from non-anticoagulated blood, from either the syringe or the last drop in the needle. Make a good tapering bullet-shaped smear and let it dry **NATURALLY**; do not wave it about or put it on the radiator or in the sun to dry. There is an advantage

in using fresh blood: normally in fresh blood, platelets tend to form little aggregates; if this does not happen in fresh blood, one has suggestive evidence for a platelet function defect (the poor man's platelet function test).
8. Correct labeling of the specimens is obviously critical.
9. The specimens must reach the laboratory promptly, generally speaking within an hour or two. There are numerous effects if there is delay. Logistic problems often occur, however, and you should be aware of the effects of delay, and indeed if you can spot the pattern of changes, a lot of grief can be avoided.

   a. Changes occur with all anticoagulants, the worst being with EDTA (i.e., the one used for the FBC).
   b. The red cells swell, raising the MCV and thus the Hct.
   c. The effect on morphology is serious. Changes can be seen at 3 h and at 12–18 h they are striking.

10. Specimens for certain tests need to be submitted in very special ways. For example, most laboratories require specimens for tests of fibrinolysis to be submitted on a bed of crushed ice. Your laboratory will have available clear guidelines on these special requirements for submission of specimens.
11. Since the interpretation of these tests is so clinical in nature, the more clinical information you give the laboratory the better. However, this can lead to overkill. Hospital patients particularly have complex clinical problems. Judgment (and therefore insightful knowledge) must be used in what data to give the lab. The same thing applies to drugs – not all drugs can have hematological complications. Supply the names and duration of use only of those that have. See Appendix A for lists of drugs relevant here.

    By the same token, certain clinical diagnoses are more relevant to the lab than others. A submitted diagnosis of "myxedema" with a FBC will considerably assist the laboratory in understanding the reason for a macrocytic anemia; on the other hand, a submitted diagnosis of "panic disorder" is unlikely to be of any assistance to the laboratory hematologist.
12. Early or emergency treatment can have an effect on interpretation of specimens collected later. Many anemias are difficult to diagnose on the basis of the clinical examination and the FBC; commonly it is necessary to proceed to further tests, notably bone marrow aspiration. Certain forms of emergency or early treatment can seriously interfere with many of these further tests, particularly including the bone marrow cytology. The treatment can also alter the FBC, and since the interpretation of the marrow cytology is very much facilitated by a FBC taken at roughly the same time so that the dynamic relationships between production and disposal can be assessed, the marrow cytology may

be rendered quite unrepresentative of the underlying state of affairs. Common scenarios are the following:

a. The patient is admitted with a severe anemia, perhaps with angina or cardiac failure. Urgent blood transfusion is frequently necessary in these circumstances, before time can be spent in investigating the nature of the anemia. But transfusing several units of packed cells can seriously interfere with subsequent investigations, especially with nutritional anemias (and the FBC can by no means always be relied upon to identify these). Packed cells contain relatively large amounts of nutrients, particularly iron and folate. Interpretation of a subsequent bone marrow as well as many other confirmatory tests can be considerably modified by their effect. In this sort of case, it is strongly recommended that a bone marrow aspirate be done as an urgent procedure and extra blood be taken and kept.

b. The patient is admitted with a moderate anemia. Such symptoms as were present before have lessened (all experienced clinicians will be aware of the phenomenon of the symptoms of truly ill patients ameliorating considerably once admitted to hospital). And thus, for various reasons, a few days elapse before the nature of the anemia is found to be a conundrum, and a marrow aspirate is done. In the meantime, the patient has been on a ward diet, which may be sufficient to have stimulated erythropoiesis, and obscure many of the original diagnostic morphological changes.

c. A patient is admitted with a serious pulmonary embolism. For one of various reasons, e.g., age, he cannot be given thrombolytic therapy, and it is decided to urgently anticoagulate the patient. The patient is very ill and a decent history cannot be obtained. Only on the following day are a strong family history and a history of previous emboli obtained. It is now too late to do most of the studies to look for thrombophilia. Blood for these tests should have been drawn before commencing anticoagulation.

We recommend that, apart from the marrow aspirate, the following tubes of blood be taken before urgent transfusion or anticoagulation therapy is instituted (if no immediate tests are contemplated, ask the laboratory to keep the tubes):

1. Two FBC tubes plus six smears made from FRESH blood
2. Two or three citrate tubes
3. 10 ml clotted blood
4. Possibly emergency bone marrow aspiration

Environmental and Physiological Causes of Pre-analytic Variation

There are a number of environmental and constitutional causes of physiological variation in all measured elements. Naturally, this applies also to the various components of the FBC and hemostatic screen, and this will impact on your interpretation in several ways. It is essential that the laboratory be informed of these environmental and physiological circumstances.

See Table 3.1 for a list of the most important causes of this type of variation in the FBC and Table 3.2 for causes of this type of variation in the hemostatic screen.

Notes with respect to the data in Table 3.1:

Table 3.1 Physiological causes of variation

Component	Value	Causes	Remarks
Hemoglobin, hematocrit, red cell count	Decreased	Pregnancy[1]	Mild true increase masked by plasma expansion
		Old age[2] (men) Recumbency[3] Severe exercise	Changes in plasma volume
	Increased	Standing from recumbency	Release from spleen. The effect may be enhanced by fluid loss
		Altitude[4] Mornings[5] Smokers[6]	Changes in plasma volume / Mediated by hypoxia
Total WCC	Lowest	Mornings at rest	Diurnal variation
	Highest	Afternoons	
Neutrophils	Decreased	Loss of antigen Race	Constitutionally lower in Blacks
	Increased	Menstruation Extreme environmental temperature Eating. Heavy smokers Exercise especially if unfit	Decreased marginal pool[7] See note 8
	Left shift	Pregnancy[9] Pregnancy[9]	
Eosinophils	Decreased	Increased	Morning Evening Menstruation
Diurnal variation, inverse relation to plasma cortisol			
Basophils	Decreased	Stress Ovulation	
Platelets[10]	Decreased	Menses	
	Increased	Ovulation. Sudden prolonged exercise[8]	
ESR	Increased	Pregnancy. Age	

1. The RCC, Hb, and Hct return to normal about 1 week after delivery. Ferritin falls in early pregnancy and remains low throughout, even if supplementary iron is given.

2. In old age, the Hb falls progressively, about 5–10% per decade from 65 years on in men, but much less in women (indeed, in some women the Hb actually rises a bit). The effect is that women tend to catch up with men with time. There is also an increase in serum iron. Ferritin levels remain higher in men than in women.

3. The increase in Hb and Hct of about 5% from lying to sitting particularly occurs in women. The drop from walking about to lying down is by 5–10% and occurs within 20 min, and then is stable. The position of the arm during venesection also is important: the Hct is 2–4% lower when the arm is held at atrial level than when hanging down.

4. The effect of altitude depends on the partial pressure of oxygen at that height. At an altitude of 6,000 ft (with a P_{O_2} of 640 mm), the increase in Hb is about 1 g/dl; at 10,000 ft it is about 2 g/dl.

5. The difference is about 8%. This is important particularly where serial measurements are made; it is a good idea to have the blood drawn at more or less the same time of the day.

6. The mechanism in smokers is complex and not fully understood. Carboxyhemoglobin formation (from CO in tobacco smoke, especially cigars) does play a role, but reduction in plasma volume, probably due to redistribution in the lungs, plays the greater part. Of course, this may be aggravated by chronic chest disease brought on by smoking.

7. All causes of decreased marginal pool are due to release of catecholamines.

8. There are several factors operating to cause a neutrophilia (as well as a monocytosis and lymphocytosis) in severe exercise:
   a. Decreased splenic blood flow (through the red pulp), with less sequestering
   b. Release from the spleen and previously shut down capillaries

9. A moderate neutrophilia is common in pregnancy and reaches its maximum about 8 weeks before birth. A left shift also is very common, with a significant increase in band forms.

10. Some authors have reported that the platelet count is about 20% higher in women than in men.

There are far fewer causes of pre-analytic variation in the tests for hemostasis; they are, however, extremely important. See Table 3.2.

Table 3.2 Physiological causes of variation

Component	Value	Causes	Remarks
Coagulation times	Prolonged	Hematocrit >55	Over-citration
Factor VIII	Raised	Stress, exercise	
Von Willebrand factor	Raised	Stress, exercise	
Fibrinolytic tests	Raised	Stress, exercise	
Factors I, VIII	Raised	General, subacute or chronic disease	Acute phase reactants
Platelets, fibrinolysis, clotting factors	Activated	Prolonged venous occlusion (>1 min)	Causes local hemo-concentration

Analytic (Laboratory) Variation

As said earlier, all laboratory measurements are in fact estimates, by the very nature of things. There are many causes for this, some to do with inherent variables in the process of measurement, and others to do with "peripherals" such as how pipettes are calibrated and washed. With two exceptions, all you need to know here is that there are many technical causes for a test done in a laboratory to show variation in results. The exceptions are to do with **PRECISION AND ACCURACY**, since an insight into these concepts will assist with gaining clarity with respect to the validity of your results and their interpretation.

If any estimation is done numerous times, with respect to

1. The **SAME** test on the **SAME** sample from the **SAME** patient one after the other (i.e., sequentially and called within-run variance),
2. The **SAME** tests on the **SAME** sample from the same patient at **DIFFERENT TIMES** (without-run variance),
3. The **SAME** test on **DIFFERENT** samples from the **SAME** patient at **DIFFERENT TIMES** (serial variance),

then in good hands the results will be in clusters, more or less closely about the assumed "true" value. The within-run variance will show the closest clustering, followed by without-run variance, and then serial variance. These are expressed as coefficients of variation (CV).

This degree to which results cluster is referred to as **PRECISION OR REPRODUCIBILITY**. The "true"

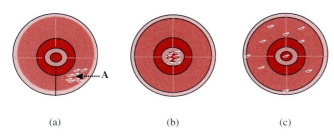

(a)   (b)   (c)

Fig. 3.4

value strictly speaking is unknown, since that is the whole point of doing the test. **ACCURACY** refers to how closely a result is to the theoretical true value.

To make clear the critical difference between precision and accuracy, see Fig. 3.4.

Figure 3.4 represents a primitive dartboard. Imagine that you throw 10 darts (illustrated by the white wedges) at the board, and they all miss the bull but cluster closely together around a point (**A**), as demonstrated in Fig. 3.4a. This clustering represents good precision, i.e., the "results" are all close together, although they are not accurate. That is, you habitually tend to throw all your darts off-center to more or less the same degree, i.e., quite **PRECISELY**. In Fig. 3.4b, the same precision is achieved, but they all cluster around the bull, indicating both accuracy and precision. Figure 3.4c shows very little precision (at least all the darts are on the board!).

It should be clear that without precision, accuracy is meaningless. A laboratory producing results as depicted in Fig. 3.4a is at least consistent – repeated results (e.g., follow-up tests on a patient) will reliably show changes varying with the course of the disease, and are thus clinically useful. A lab producing results as in Fig. 3.4c is totally unreliable – the value of the occasional accurate result is completely outweighed by the others. The ideal laboratory first achieves good precision, and then gradually moves the whole cluster as close as possible to the bull.

Note that the above types of result can obtain in any laboratory even if the analytical techniques used are extremely sensitive and the tests are performed meticulously. The laboratory bears the major responsibility to ensure that the results it produces are clinically acceptable, and to achieve this it implements certain quality control (QC) programs. It is important that the user acquaint oneself with the results of the quality program of a laboratory that one intends to use, at least in very general terms, and particularly with respect to precision and Accuracy. Any laboratory should be able to provide documentary evidence of its performance in these areas – if it cannot, one should find another one – one's patient's well-being may depend on it.

For practical purposes, the pre-analytic and analytic causes of variation can be aggregated into one percentage,

the "total allowable error." In the examples used in this book, you will see two extra columns in many of the reports, entitled "Possible Range," which in fact means "total allowable error" (TAE) but expressed as a range. They are not included in routine reports, and one could argue that they should be. Bear in mind that your laboratory might have slightly different values for TAE; these you should get from them.

To repeat, it is the **LABORATORY'S RESPONSIBILITY** to ensure that the results sent out are acceptable from the quality control point of view within predefined limits. It is the **USER'S RESPONSIBILITY** to find out what standards are being maintained in the laboratory he uses. (For those interested, these TAEs are also referred to as the "Uncertainty of Measurement" (or MU), which is defined as "A parameter associated with the result of a measurement, which characterizes the dispersion of the values that could reasonably be attributed to the measurand.")

The use of TAEs in this book will get you used to the concept. Of great importance is that it permits the clinician to understand when SERIAL results show a significant change or not. This turns out to be a major problem, and one that is responsible for large numbers of diagnostic, management, and prognostic errors. To state the problem: how is one to know whether sequential results on a patient represent significant change? Again there are sophisticated statistical methods to assess this; however, these require extensive computer power as well as access to the raw QC data of the laboratory. Some modern laboratory management computer programs can do this. In brief, the technology requires calculation and statistical manipulation of within-run and without-run CVs of the relevant tests **DONE ON THE DAYS IN QUESTION**. It is surprising how large the gap between results must be for significance. Clearly, this depends on the laboratory and on the test, but generally **ONE CANNOT INFER THAT SERIAL RESULTS MEAN ANYTHING UNLESS THEY ARE, IN MOST CASES, AT LEAST 10–15% APART – SOMETIMES UP TO 20% APART.**

To summarize: the departure from "normal" in any result must thus, in the first instance, be evaluated in terms of this natural variation **AND** of your own assessment of how good your laboratory is.

Variation works for apparently normal as well as abnormal results: just as a truly normal result may spuriously be in the abnormal range, **SO CAN A TRULY ABNORMAL RESULT BE IN THE NORMAL RANGE**. It is commonly taught that all abnormal results should be checked, and there is much to be said for this. However, using the same logic, one should check all normal results as well, but this becomes a serious financial

There is a tendency among some laboratories to report serial results in dated columns. This is very convenient for easily seeing changes in time. However, this practice cannot unconditionally be endorsed:

1. The columnar results do not show the possible allowable ranges and often the reference ranges are also not given.
2. Therefore, a change in a value with time may be misconstrued as being significant, when in fact it is within the possible range.
3. A blanket permitted allowable error can only be given in terms of percentages. This would mean that the clinician himself would have to work out the possible ranges of every result himself.
4. It is all very well saying that spotting a trend over a long period would be very useful, and that in this case the possible ranges are not significant. A Hb level falling from 11 to 7 in a week is undoubtedly significant, but it is an unusual situation where a clinical decision to intervene has not had to be made *before* the week was over, on the basis of clinical and other manifestations.
5. In practice, we believe this practice is only really useful and justifiable in the ICU and High Care Unit, and in certain chronic diseases being followed up *regularly and frequently*, especially with reference to the Hct, MCV, MCH, white cells, band cells, platelets, and activity tests.

problem. Once again the importance of the clinical features is emphasized – one should probably check ALL results that contradict your clinical findings (and if the re-test checks out, you must check your clinical findings and conclusions – clinical certainty is fraught with difficulty). Even so, this is not the whole answer. By all means consult with the laboratory and your senior colleagues: you do not want to miss anything and you do not want to waste money. The important point is that blind faith in a laboratory report is indeed an abdication of one's clinical responsibility to **THINK**.

By now it should be clear that a first-stage diagnosis might falsely be made if the various causes of variation are not considered, and where necessary, discounted. A relevant history and examination should be undertaken before interpreting the FBC – and unless you inform the

laboratory of your findings, they will be able to make only very general comments in most cases – remember, the laboratory **WANTS** to help.

A demonstration of the practical importance of variation: assume that an ill-informed colleague, perhaps a junior, decides to see the effect of oral iron therapy in our patient with the Hb of 13.1 (he is ill informed because there is **NOTHING** to suggest iron deficiency. He may have been seduced by a bureaucratic approach that said "If the anemia requires treatment, then, since iron deficiency is by far the commonest cause of anemia, iron therapy is, in the first instance, appropriate"). A week later the Hb is 13.7 g/dl. He tells you that this proves that the mild anemia was due to iron deficiency. Since you are aware that the possible range for the original hemoglobin was 12.7–13.7 g/dl, you can confidently inform him that there is no evidence that the patient has shown a response to therapy. Giving iron to such a patient may result in serious harm.

> **Variation in a Result** *A hemoglobin result of 13.1 g/dl means that the actual result can lie anywhere between say 12.7 and 13.7, depending on the type (level) of laboratory.*

So far, we have considered the lab result only in terms of its technical reliability. But what of the test itself? How useful is the Hb test in diagnosing anemia in the first place, even assuming that the result is acceptable? This issue must be addressed.

TASK #3: WHAT ARE THE LIMITATIONS OF A TEST IN TERMS OF ITS PURPOSE?

> For us to be able to use our tests, we first must be aware of their limitations. *No test is perfect in this regard.*

Limitations of Tests: Clinical Epidemiology

None of our techniques and tests is perfect in terms of what they mean, and it is essential that we understand the principles underlying these limitations. It should be understood that modern medicine is moving very rapidly in this, the epidemiological, direction. The topic is simplified as much as possible. There are two broad aspects to the understanding of the limitations of tests:

1. **THE RELATIONSHIP BETWEEN GIVEN RESULTS AND ABNORMALITY**. In other words,

   a. Whether results outside the given reference ranges always mean an abnormality and
   b. Whether results within the given reference ranges always mean the absence of abnormality

To discuss these issues, it is valuable to look at how most tests originate. Generally, for one of several possible reasons (theory, serendipity, tradition, etc.), a test is thought to reflect the presence of disease A. Large numbers of patients with this disease are selected, primarily on the basis of definable clinical features, and the diagnosis confirmed where possible with a so-called gold-standard test. They are then submitted for testing with the new test under consideration. Assuming a large enough (significant) proportion show positive results, the data is then manipulated to decide which is the most valuable level to use (the statistical techniques here are very complex). **BEAR IN MIND THAT THE ORIGINAL GROUP WAS HIGHLY SELECTED.**

The test is now introduced as a routine diagnostic test on patients who do not have all (or perhaps any) of the clinical features of the disease, and it is found, after considerable investigation, that the test does not live up to its promise: usually it picks up too many false positives. Consider, for example, the ANA test for SLE: this test is very sensitive in confirming the diagnosis **IN PATIENTS WITH KNOWN CLINICAL MANIFESTATIONS OF SLE**, but is pretty useless in a shotgun approach to the diagnosis. (This type of statement serves to underscore the vital role that clinical evaluation – and justification for testing – plays in diagnosis.) Issues such as false and true positives are given by the operating characteristics.

2. **THE OPERATING CHARACTERISTICS OF THE TESTS**

It is extremely important to know just how the test/s you are looking at reflect actual pathology. This data is given by the operating characteristics of the tests, but with several caveats. These characteristics are inherent in Evidence-Based Medicine (see later). These data are very valuable in their application to confirmatory tests, but much less so with reference to the first-line tests. However, this is a very topical issue in medicine, and something must be known about it.

The Operating Characteristics of Tests

Assuming all the previous issues have been taken into account, we still have to decide how reliably a test result is going to reflect actual disease. A test only has value if it can trigger an appropriate clinical reaction, and to do this it needs to distinguish between populations with and without a specific disease, and preferably without overlap. There are indeed tests that do this, but frequently there is overlap, as in our example Hb of 13.1 (with respect to the ranges in "normals" and ACD).

We attempt to evaluate tests in this regard by understanding their operating characteristics, that is, attempting to measure the information they provide as accurately as possible. These terms are frequently mentioned and can be the cause of some confusion. To introduce the concepts as gently as possible, let us start with the following definitions:

1. **SENSITIVITY.** This is the probability that a test will be positive when disease is present, i.e., $p(T^+|D^+)$. This group of results comprises the true positives (TP).
2. **SPECIFICITY.** This is the probability that a test will be negative when disease is absent, i.e., $p(T^-|D^-)$. This group of results comprises the true negatives (TN).
3. **FALSE-POSITIVE RATE.** This is the probability that a test will be positive when disease is not present. This group of results comprises the false positives (FP).
4. **FALSE-NEGATIVE RATE.** This is the probability that the test will be negative when disease is present. This group of results comprises the false negatives (FN).

CALCULATING SENSITIVITY AND SPECIFICITY requires knowing the false-positive and false-negative rates for that test. Thus,

$$Sensitivity = (TP/(TP + FN))$$

In other words, sensitivity is what is left after the number of true positives in a sample or population is divided by the number of true positives plus the number of false negatives. This will clearly be ≤ 1. In the same way,

$$Specificity = (TN/(TN + FP))$$

In other words, specificity is what is left after the number of true negatives in a sample or population is divided by the number of true negatives plus the number of false positives. This will also be ≤ 1.

Sensitivity and specificity are actually difficult concepts, since their meanings are somewhat counterintuitive. Examine the following examples:

1. You suspect anemia in a patient at sea level: a Hb < 18 g/dl has a sensitivity of 1 (**FOR THE DIAGNOSIS OF ANEMIA**); this means that 100% of patients with anemia will have a Hb of < 18. So, at the Hb level of 18, the test is extremely sensitive **FOR ANEMIA**, but is not much good in practice, for example, as a screening test – you are going to end up with no patients at all. The same test has a specificity of 0.2: this means that in 20% of patients with anemia the Hb will not be < 18 – again, it is difficult to see the value to the clinician. The major point to be made here is that the sensitivity and specificity of the test for any analyte vary with

   a. The level of the analyte under consideration
   b. What condition or state is being considered

2. You suspect anemia in a male patient at 5,000 ft: a Hb of 14.0 has a sensitivity of 0.48; this means that 48% of patients with anemia will have a Hb of <14.0. The specificity at this level is (around) 0.75; this means that in 75% of patients the Hb will be <14 if they are anemic.

3. In the same patient, a Hb of 4 g/dl has a specificity of say 0.01.

The ideal test would have both sensitivity and specificity of 1. However, in practice, sensitivity and specificity tend to counteract each other, and therefore the choice of a test depends rather on what you want to do with it:

1. When you want to **EXCLUDE DISEASE** in the clinical situation, you use a very sensitive test.
2. When you want to confirm a diagnostic possibility in the clinical situation, you use a very specific test.

   To restate the above,

1. Tests with a low sensitivity but a high specificity are helpful only if positive.
2. Tests with a low specificity are only requested with a strong clinical suspicion.

This re-emphasizes the point that it all depends what disease you are considering, what level you are testing at, and what you want to do with the test, i.e., confirm or exclude a diagnosis.

There are four further important points to realize with sensitivity and specificity of a test:

1. They are the same wherever the test is done, but the predictive value changes with the prevalence of the disease in the population.
2. It can be seen that at the outer limits of results the sensitivity and specificity are easier to understand;

however, it is when one is dealing with borderline values that things get difficult, for example, in our example patient with a Hb of 13.1 (in an adult male at 5,000 ft). The sensitivity at this level drops to about 0.25 and the specificity has risen to say 0.90. One could argue that, since the test has a high specificity, a Hb of > 13.1 g/dl would tend to exclude disease; we shall see later that this is not necessarily so.

3. Regardless of the sensitivity and specificity of a test, its result does not tell you whether the disease tested for is present. All they do is modify your pre-test hypothesis upwards or downwards. (Remember that your pre-test hypothesis is essentially your provisional, starting diagnosis).

4. The pre-test hypothesis exerts a profound effect on the diagnostic process, and this reinforces the idea that the clinical assessment, used for the pre-test diagnosis, is enormously significant, and not the test result per se. Pre-test is an assessed probability of a disease being present and is derived from three sources:

   a. The history
   b. The clinical examination
   c. The knowledge of the prevalence of the disease in the community

This is **BEFORE** any special investigations are done.

> Tests are only ordered with a clinical suspicion. Conversely, if a test suggests abnormality and the patient features do not support this, the test should be re-evaluated.

Sensitivity and specificity have (some) predictive value. However, the probability that a test will be positive when the patient has the disease (i.e., $p(T^+|D^+)$) is **NOT** what the patient or the doctor actually wants to know – they both want to know what the chances of having the disease are if the test is positive ($p(D^+|T^+)$)! How do we achieve this? It turns out that the answer very much depends on the prevalence of the suspected disease in the community; this enables us to arrive at positive and negative predictive values.

To place the problem in perspective, consider the following situation. Let us assume that a new blood test has been developed for the diagnosis of schistosomiasis. (When we consider that schistosomiasis is the largest single cause of splenomegaly and probably therefore of hypersplenism in the world, it would be extremely valuable to have a reliable screening test to identify early disease.) We assume that extensive evaluation has shown that this test is 99.9% **SENSITIVE** and 99.9%

SPECIFIC (extremely unlikely in practice), and thus appears, on the face of it, to be an outstanding test. We further assume that we are currently in Egypt where the prevalence of schistosomiasis is 1% (in fact it is higher, but let us simplify our calculations). We apply this test to 1,000,000 people; of these 10,000 would be infected with the schistosoma. With a sensitivity of 99.9%, our new test will

1. Find 9,990 cases who are actually infected; these are true positives (TP)
2. Miss 10 such cases; these are the false negatives (FN)

On the face of it, this is a very good test. However, we think a bit further and realize that of our 1,000,000 patients, 990,000 are not infected. Looking at our test results again, our test shows that

1. 989,010 are found to be clear of the infection; these are true negatives (TN).
2. **990** uninfected patients are found to be positive; these are false positives (FP). It would be poor medicine to treat these patients for schistosomiasis, and therefore further confirmatory tests would have to be undertaken.

Now consider that we apply the same test in the United Kingdom, where the prevalence is say 0.1%, i.e., 1,000 patients will have the disease (in this case an **OVER** estimate). Our test results will find 999 cases who are actually infected, with only one patient wrongly identified; and of the 999,000 patients who are not infected the test would label 990,009 patients negative for infection **BUT WOULD IDENTIFY 9,991 NON-INFECTED PATIENTS AS INFECTED.** The effect of prevalence is dramatically illustrated. And even with a test with these incredible operating characteristics, the dangers of relying on them at the expense of common sense are explicit.

Positive and Negative Predictive Values and Likelihoods

The probability that the patient has the disease (under consideration) if the test (under consideration) is positive is given by the **POSITIVE PREDICTIVE VALUE**. Conversely, the **NEGATIVE PREDICTIVE VALUE** of the test is the probability that the patient does not have the disease if the test is negative. Formally

POSITIVE PREDICTIVE VALUE (PPV) is the **PROPORTION** of patients with a positive test who in fact have the disease; or

$$p(D^+|T^+) = \frac{\text{The number of True Positives}}{\text{True Positives + False Positives}}$$

NEGATIVE PREDICTIVE VALUE (NPV) is the **PROPORTION** of patients with a negative test who in fact do not have the disease; or

$$p(D^-|T^-) = \frac{\text{The number of True Negatives}}{\text{True Negatives + False Negatives}}$$

In our patient (i.e., with a Hb of 13.1), the PPV [$p(D^+|T^+)$] is about 0.35, i.e., there is a reasonable chance that the patient is in fact anemic.

This however is not good enough: the PPV and NPV of a test change with the prevalence of the disease in a community. For example, the antigen test for **PLASMODIUM FALCIPARUM**, which has an excellent specificity and pretty good sensitivity, will give a low PPV in the Antarctic. Anemia, however, is very common worldwide, and tests for anemia thus will have a higher PPV and NPV.

Therefore, to interpret the PPV and NPV properly you must know the prevalence of that disease in your community, i.e., what percentage of people at one time have the disease. So, we want to know how much more likely is a test positive among those with the disease as opposed to those without disease.

It has been found that the most convenient way of using sensitivities, specificities, and predictive values in practice is by means of the Likelihood Ratios, which consolidate these concepts.

LIKELIHOOD RATIOS (LR). These express the likelihood of a disease being present if a relevant test is positive, and the likelihood of the disease being absent if the test is negative. They are expressed as follows:

1. A single figure for a positive test
2. A single figure for a negative test

$$\textbf{Positive LR} = \frac{p(T^+ \text{ if diseased})}{p(T^+ \text{ if not diseased})}$$
$$= \frac{\text{Sensitivity}}{1 - \text{Specificity}}$$

$$\textbf{Negative LR} = \frac{p(T^- \text{ if diseased})}{p(T^- \text{ if not diseased})}$$
$$= \frac{\text{Specificity}}{1 - \text{Sensitivity}}$$

The LR does not directly achieve what we want – i.e., the probability that the patient has the disease if the test is positive. What it does is indicate by how much the test will alter the **PRE-TEST PROBABILITY** of the patient having the disease. Formally, the pre-test probability of a diagnosis multiplied by the LR of a particular test equals the post-test probability (this reflects Bayes' theorem – see Chapter 5).

How to Interpret the LR

If LR = 1 then pre-test probability = post-test probability, i.e., you are back where you started.

If LR > 1 then the probability that the disease is present is increased (by that amount).

If LR < 1 then the probability that the disease is present is decreased (by that amount).

In practice, we like to see a LR+ of over 5 before we feel convinced as to the usefulness of the test.

From here it is an easy step to get to the post-test probability, by using the famous Fagan nomogram. This, with instructions, is shown in Appendix B.

Note however that the process is still not over: once special investigations are done, a further assessment is done, based on the knowledge of the likelihood of a disease suggested by a positive test actually being present. For example, a prolonged PTT in a healthy 40-year-old man gives only a 0.15% chance that the patient in fact has a bleeding disorder.

The Choice of Tests in a Particular Clinical Situation

It should be clear that LR can and should be used to list in order of priority the tests to be used in a clinical situation, as long as some flexibility is used – in one sense, every single clinical situation is unique.

"GOLD-STANDARD" TESTS. In essence, the gold standard defines the disease in question, and its major use is to compare the efficacy of a new test. This implies that a test to be regarded as the gold-standard test must be extremely specific and sensitive. Some characteristics of a gold standard are given:

1. It is usually expensive and/or invasive.
2. It is assumed to be "correct."

Frequently, these tests are not easily available routinely; however, other tests for the disease can be compared, in a research project, to the gold standard and their operating characteristics quantified for routine work.

As far as our patient with the Hb of 13.1 is concerned, we have no indication which gold-standard test to use, and we wish if possible to avoid a shotgun approach. This discussion is continued in the next section.

THE ABOVE NOTES ON THE LIMITATIONS OF OUR TESTS ARE FAIRLY BASIC. In Chapter 5, an example is presented to illustrate the data given. At the general level, there is no need to memorize these notes since the data for the bulk of hematological tests are not yet properly defined. However, research is continuing and eventually it will be necessary to use these data as they become available in your interpretations. It was considered useful to include this section at this stage, to prepare for the future. A general grasp of the issues is all that is required at present. The good news is that, as will be seen, a systematic clinical approach to our reports will generate conclusions not significantly different from any calculations.

TASK #4: HOW SIGNIFICANT IS THE RESULT FROM THE CLINICAL POINT OF VIEW? SPECIFICALLY: HOW ABNORMAL MUST A RESULT BE TO TRIGGER INTERVENTION? This is a hugely difficult problem and there are several approaches, but to name just two:

1. Consensus conferences and documents
2. Individual clinical judgment, considering the patient as a whole, including his support structure

Clearly, having a set of tests of high quality is not going to be of much use unless you know their clinical relevance. The most important question is, what, if anything, does the test do to the diagnostic process? To the decision to institute therapy?

Up to this point we have spoken about our tests purely in statistical terms. Experience over the last few decades has shown that this approach is incomplete. Most test results are used in clinical monitoring. Many models have been proposed to decide which changes are clinically relevant and what levels of probability should be adopted. None of these models have provided the full answer. A number of challenges therefore face the practising doctor:

1. How abnormal must a test be to generate action (i.e., what are the decision levels)? Alternatively, how large should a change in value be to trigger a response? Note that ideally this must take into account the various issues already discussed:

   a. The width of the known reference range
   b. Any previous results
   c. The known efficacy of the laboratory

2. Does any abnormal result necessarily require action? If not, how can this be, and what then are the criteria with which to decide?

3. How can we be sure that the results within the normal range are in fact normal?

It should be realized that these questions go to the heart of modern clinical medicine – no practitioner, even at the most general level, can afford not to understand the implications of these points. The answer to these questions rests on many legs:

1. **TEST RESULTS ARE USED IN MANY DIFFERENT CLINICAL SITUATIONS**. It is probably impossible to try to define a single set of performance characteristics for a test to be used in all circumstances. For example, a platelet count of $120 \times 10^{12}/l$ in a healthy pregnant woman, without any other abnormality in the FBC, etc., will not require any intervention at all.

2. **EXTENSIVE CLINICAL STUDIES** have suggested that decision levels about certain tests are very different from the usual coefficient of variation approach: the prime example here would be cholesterol levels; there is suggestive evidence that Hb levels nearer the lower limit of "normal" prior to routine major surgery may stand the patient in good stead; there is some evidence that a high "normal" hematocrit is an independent risk factor for myocardial infarction; and in septic shock in the ICU, lower Hb levels are unquestionably associated with better survival. These considerations apply to certain clinical features as well, the most prominent of which currently is the level of blood pressure control.

3. **THERE ARE MANY SOMEWHAT CONFLICTING IDEAS** about what constitutes desirable practice, suggesting that nobody currently has the complete answer.

4. There are performance characteristics of tests other than precision, accuracy, sensitivity, specificity, and other characteristics derived from these, such as specimen volumes, perhaps undue invasiveness, personnel abilities, and capital and cost aspects.

There has thus been, in recent years, a significant tendency to ask clinicians for and to respect their opinions of their views on these issues.[9,10] As mentioned earlier, no test is worth doing in routine practice unless it is going to trigger a therapeutic (in the broadest sense) response, or potentially require a response, pending a clinical decision.

So, once we have evaluated the result obtained as reliable (tasks #1 and #2), we need to assess whether the test result requires intervention or not.

1. **THIS CAN BE STRAIGHTFORWARD**: a Hb level of 4 or 21 in an adult, as examples, unquestionably requires some sort of response. These are assessed and followed up as described in Chapter 4.

2. **THE BORDERLINE CASES ARE THE REAL PROBLEMS**. There are many ways of handling these:

   a) Make a search for previous results and see if there has been a significant change. Life insurance companies are particularly keen on this approach, indicating its usefulness.

   b) Look more globally at other investigations and clinical features.

   c) Wait and see. Repeating the results after a time is a common strategy.

   d) Investigate fully – this is usually **NOT** advisable.

   e) Be guided by best clinical practice. Many case examples in this book will show what we consider to be best practice.

Every such case must be handled individually, using all one's clinical acumen and personal experience in making the decision; this includes strong involvement of the patient in the decision. There are serious questions about the evidence-based medicine approach with its algorithms as a solution. Indeed, algorithms are questionable and dangerous in borderline cases. This is discussed later. We shall now discuss possible approaches in greater detail from a primarily clinical point of view.

Deciding on the "Normality"/"Abnormality" of a Result

There are five common scenarios to consider:

1. The single (i.e., only one test was done), isolated "abnormal" result
2. The single, isolated "normal" result
3. One "abnormal" result in a set of tests done (more or less) at the same time
4. More than one "abnormal" result in a set of tests done (more or less) at the same time
5. "Normal" and "abnormal" results of an analyte at different times

It will be seen that handling these problems will require a combination of clinical skill ("sense") as well as a clear understanding of the nature of laboratory tests. The approaches suggested are merely possibilities.

The Single Isolated "Abnormal" Result

The following approach is suggested: we assume only a single test, e.g., Hb, is requested (no previous results are to hand). It is decreased. This can have very important consequences, e.g., an operation may have to be postponed. It can readily be seen that the any decisions based on this finding are primarily clinical, i.e., using clinical thinking:

1. Probably the most important consideration is the Hb level itself: a very low Hb would clearly require urgent attention – repeating the test but as part of a FBC, and proceeding as outlined in Chapter 5.
2. With a borderline result, the reason for requesting the Hb in the first place would be important. On the one hand, the patient may obviously be pale, and the lowish Hb would necessarily require full investigation. Otherwise, this may have been a routine "pre-op" or routine pre- or post-natal in an otherwise evidently healthy young person, and where typically, further clinical examination would reveal no suggestion of a cause for anemia. Consider the case of a healthy young woman who is 30 weeks pregnant, and her Hb is 11.8 g/dl: the pre-test probability of disease is very low, and no further action is contemplated. One approach here would be to repeat the test but as part of a FBC: if the low Hb persists and the rest of the count is normal, the patient's problem could be approached as a normocytic anemia (see Chapter 10), or a wait-and-see approach could be adopted; if, instead, the Hb is now normal in this normal FBC, one is probably justified in regarding the first test as a laboratory error (remember, statistically, 1 in 20 to 1 in 40 Hb results will show spurious abnormality, through no fault of the laboratory).
3. A seriously low Hb would clearly have to be followed up – re-test with a FBC, and take it from there.
4. The clinical features may indicate a possible pathological reason for the change, in which case it would have to followed up in the traditional way.

The Single Isolated "Normal" Result

We are all more or less conditioned to focus on abnormal results and to more or less ignore the normal ones. This can lead to serious errors (for example, with the MCV as discussed above). So, what specifically does a negative or "normal" result of a single investigation mean? (We are not now discussing the issue of variation causing spurious "normal" and "abnormal" results, as discussed previously.)

As stated before, statistically 1 in 20 results of a group of tests on the same patient at one time will significantly vary from what it should have been. This variation however may not be enough for the result to fall out of the reference range for that analyte. So here we have two possibilities:

1. **ANY RESULT WITHIN THE REFERENCE RANGE COULD ACTUALLY LIE OUTSIDE THE "NORMAL" RANGE.** Generally speaking, this is an impossible situation to handle, unless

a) There are strong clinical reasons to suspect this.
b) The result does not "fit in" with an otherwise comprehensible pattern.
c) Previous results raise strong suspicions.

2. **ANY RESULT WITHIN THE REFERENCE RANGE INDEED BELONGS IN THIS RANGE, BUT IS INACCURATE.** This similarly is an impossible situation unless one is alerted to the possibility by a different previous result.

> *Negative or "Normal" findings have positive value.* **!**

A negative or "normal" finding should never be ignored. It is incorrect to suggest that such a value implies the absence of information; a "normal" finding is just as informative as an "abnormal" one. Nor should information given by negative results be considered insignificant – some "positive" (i.e., "abnormal") results are also sometimes viewed as insignificant: how often have you not concluded that a WCC of 11.3×10^9/l as an isolated finding, in a patient without any suggestion of infection, is clinically insignificant?

A number of questions should be asked about "normal" results:

1. **COULD THE SO-CALLED "NORMAL" RESULT IN FACT REPRESENT A CHANGE FROM BEFORE**, yet lie within the "normal" range (and this is especially important where the "normal" range is very wide)? Previous reports are invaluable here.
2. **HOW GOOD WAS THE CLINICAL INFORMATION** that led to the test being requested in the first place?
3. **WOULD THE NEGATIVE RESULT IN ANY WAY INFLUENCE YOUR DIAGNOSIS OR MANAGEMENT**?
4. **DOES THE PATIENT NOT FALL INTO A "NORMAL TAIL"** on the distribution curve of that test? For example, as in Fig. 3.2, a patient with established active rheumatoid arthritis, typically associated with ACD, can have a Hb of 13.7 – apparently "normal."
5. **WAS THE SPECIMEN COLLECTED AND HANDLED IN THE PROPER MANNER**?
6. **IF THE TEST OUGHT TO BE POSITIVE**, as suggested by strong clinical evidence, can this evidence not perhaps be interpreted differently? Or have you missed something? Or are you perhaps dealing with something new?

Negative (or "normal") values can also have advantages in different situations:

1. **THE EFFECT ON THE PATIENT**. Either he is very relieved and goes home, or gets very upset and asks "What then is the matter with me?" Perhaps he has been told that he looks pale and must be anemic. He has talked himself into believing that anemia is the cause of his tiredness and pallor. Now his Hb is found to be 15 g/l and his coronary artery disease has yet to be thought of!

2. **THEY ARE VERY VALUABLE IN THE FOLLOW-UP** of chronic patients, particularly since their previous values are known.

3. **WHEN A TEST IS VIRTUALLY INVARIABLY POSITIVE IN A PARTICULAR CONDITION** that is diagnosed in the patient: here it can be extremely useful for reviewing one's diagnosis.

"The long silent period before the onset of symptoms[4]" also has a close relationship to negative or "normal" results. In modern practice we attempt to detect the earliest signs of disease, before the stage of significant tissue damage. Much care and clinical judgment is necessary in this type of situation.

One "Abnormal" Result in a Set of Tests Done at (More or Less) the Same Time

For example, let us say that, in a FBC, all the results fall within the reference ranges except for the Hb, which is decreased. With a FBC, one is fortunate because of the functional interrelationships of many of the elements. Thus, the "normal" MCV would immediately suggest that **IF THERE IS INDEED AN ANEMIA**, then it should be investigated as a normocytic anemia. The problem, however, is to decide whether the result is significant, and this would essentially be what has been discussed.

Certainly, a search for previous FBCs would be justified. Failing this, and in the absence of positive or suggestive clinical findings, a repeat would be justified. Only then would an approach to a normocytic anemia be warranted.

More Than One "Abnormal" Result in a Set of Tests

The major task here is to look for a known pattern, and go on from there. On the other hand, the results could appear to be contradictory, e.g., in a level 1 laboratory (where the

level of expertise is perhaps wanting), the Hb could be low with a normal Hct – this would strongly suggest a laboratory error.

"Normal" and "Abnormal" Results of Analytes at Different Times

This is where things can get very involved. The approach depends on whether a clinical pattern has been identified in the results, plus an understanding of how they can change in different clinical situations. The clinical patterns are discussed in Chapter 4.

> We have reached the end of our general discussion of the first-line tests, their value and their significance. We have covered the nature and basic pathology of the system, the system as in space and time, the nature of the first-line tests in accessing the system, and how to evaluate the quality of the tests received.
>
> Thus, by now you should have a clear idea as to whether a reported abnormal result is truly pathological and what its relevance is.

We have to complete the process of making the result **CLINICALLY RELEVANT** (vis-à-vis the patient) by integrating the best available information with what we have already learned so as to be as sure as possible about what the results mean and how they fit into the total evaluation of the patient, and with what degree of certainty. There are two general problems:

1. **HOW TO USE SUCH DATA AS WE HAVE TO MAKE A DIAGNOSIS**. Here there are two general approaches:

   a. Reducing the problem to a mechanical process, primarily using **ALGORITHMS**.

   b. **USING AN INTELLECTUAL PROCESS** based on all available results, knowledge of basic pathogenetic processes and pathology, and rigorous logic, to infer the likelihoods. There are several legitimate methods here, starting with pattern matching (see later).

2. **HOW TO EVALUATE THE SIGNIFICANCE AND VALUE OF OUR RESULTS**. Again there are two approaches:

   a. **GOING STRICTLY ACCORDING TO THE STATISTICS** of published results and research, again in a somewhat mechanical fashion.

b. **USING EXISTING RESULTS** where they are applicable (and available), but evaluating them with reference to the individual patient. This approach is a logical intellectual process and an integral part of the clinical enterprise.

Algorithms

ALGORITHMS ARE NOT THE MAGIC ANSWER TO INTERPRETATION. Because of the problems attendant upon interpretation, particularly with the FBC with its potential complexity, there is a tendency to reduce the subject to a series of algorithms. These are very useful in a restricted group of common conditions, primarily of single abnormalities. But there are a number of limitations.

1. The definition of an algorithm is "A procedure that guarantees a solution to a problem." We all know that in medicine there is too often not a guaranteed answer available. In a significant minority of cases, even the experts struggle to reach agreement.
2. They are very mechanistic in their approach and demand very little insight. The author suspects that often the patient's problem is forcibly made to fit the algorithm. He finds algorithms frustrating to follow, and makes him feel reduced to a technician. Actually, hematology is not difficult if a number of essentials are understood.
3. They often oversimplify the problem. In one text the author reviewed he saw, in a chapter about the red cell disorders, an algorithm portraying the approach to suspected anemia. The very first instruction was to measure the hemoglobin and if this was within the normal range, to stop the process. This is clearly nonsensical. Should a patient's (truly) normal hemoglobin be 16.5 and he were to lose a liter of blood fairly rapidly, his hemoglobin after a day or so would have come down to say 15 g/dl – still well within the "normal" range, but he, the patient, is undoubtedly anemic! He is very likely to show other changes in the blood count from which a recent bleed could be inferred or suspected, and which, were the above algorithm followed, would not be looked at **OR EVEN LOOKED FOR**. Imagine trying to convince a third-party funder to finance the further investigation of such a patient when according to their criteria he is not even anemic! Even the WHO commits this error: it calls males anemic if the hematocrit is < 0.39 l/l, and females if the hematocrit is < 0.36 l/l. Since the recommendations for treatment are also based on levels, this has serious consequences. Again, the functional (indeed clinical) approach is emphasized.

Thus, oversimplifying the problem really does the patient a disservice. To repeat, "Everything should be made as simple as possible, **BUT NOT SIMPLER.**"

4. They are unsuitable for patients with multiple problems that in hematology are an all too common occurrence.
5. In an attempt to cater for all the variants they usually become so complicated as to be self-defeating. There are authors who seem to take a perverse delight in constructing horribly complicated algorithms.
6. The very fact that health-care funders love them should make them suspect. A large part of the answer to rising costs lies in sensible, patient-oriented approaches. However, there are some outstanding exceptions in the philosophy and practice of health-care funders: some explicitly state that their algorithms must be used only as a guide, and that clinical, **PERSONALIZED** assessment is crucial. In addition, the research that has gone into producing many of the algorithms is frequently extensive and of a high order (e.g., "The Medical Algorithms Project"[5]).
7. Part and parcel of the use of algorithms is the tendency to rely too heavily on measurable entities, particularly biochemical entities, glossing over the fact that these measurements can be wrong, or are not satisfactory on their own for making decisions. It is more or less standard these days to assume that all disease processes can be reduced to changes in chemical constituents; this reductionism is not logically sustainable. One only has to look at the (poor) value of folate levels in the diagnosis of macrocytosis for this point to be valid. Nothing can supplant a thorough examination and the cultivation of **PERSPECTIVE** in evaluating any results. There is also a lingering suspicion: that of the desire to minimize patient contact, and reduce all problems to specialized testing.

Studying one or two typical algorithms will be of much benefit, to enable the gaining of the necessary perspective. There are any number of algorithms available, particularly for anemia; this is itself significant – if it were so simple, a standard algorithm would long ago have been agreed upon. There appear to be three common characteristics of published algorithms in hematology:

1. All the algorithms minimize, sometimes to the point of disappearance, a clinical approach to the patient himself. This is strange, especially when one considers that a proper clinical assessment goes a long way in solving the diagnostic problem.
2. They also all minimize the importance of morphology. The motivation for this is obscure. In part, probably, it

lies in a manpower problem – as stated before, hematologists are expensive; in addition, however, there seems to be an awed obsession with mechanization, with machine-produced results.

3. They all emphasize a sequential list of tests. Each test takes time; depending on the result there is another test that must be done, and so on. If the blood for all the possible tests are taken in one go (thus minimizing repeated assaults on the patient), one is likely to find a lot of blood being discarded. In any case, the process is economically self-defeating: hospital stay is extremely expensive, and it seems that following algorithms wastes time.

The following algorithm for the diagnosis of anemia was constructed as an exercise by a resident in the department (Fig. 3.5). He was told to restrict his algorithm to the red cells only.

Discussion of Fig. 3.5 with Critical Comments

1. The issue of anemia in the presence of a "normal" Hb has already been discussed before.

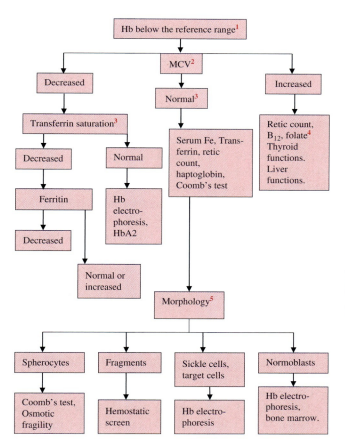

Fig. 3.5

2. A similar argument applies to the MCV: assume a person's MCV normally is say 85 fl; she is in the process of developing hypothyroidism, and her MCV starts to rise; by the time she presents to her doctor her Hb is 11.9 and the MCV is 98 fl – still in the published "normal" range but for her, the picture is macrocytic.

3. Serum iron particularly is susceptible to technical problems, and spuriously raised or decreased levels can occur, which can put one very much on the wrong track. Nor is there any mention in the algorithm of what to do with raised serum iron levels, as can occur in a number of conditions.

4. Folate in particular is unreliable as a **DIAGNOSTIC** measurement. But many other elements demonstrate the same problem.

5. Morphology comes late in the process. Had it been done earlier, many of the steps could have been short-circuited. The presence of round hypochromic macrocytes (assuming that no clinical evidence for hypothyroidism was seen) could have avoided the expensive vitamin B_{12} and folate tests. The diagnoses listed under morphology are very limited – what about elliptocytosis, for instance?

6. The clinical assessment hardly appears at all. It could have short-circuited many steps.

All in all, this exercise, while actually very revealing, was considered a waste of time.

Consider another algorithm (in fact only part of one, since the complete algorithm occupies a full A4 page, contains 36 decision blocks, and 44 possible directions to move in!). To arrive at a diagnosis of renal anemia, the following parameters must have been measured or taken note of **IN SEQUENCE**: MCV and RDW; reticulocyte count; haptoglobin and LDH isoenzyme; and only then, investigation for possible renal disease as part of a long list of possibilities: infectious and inflammatory disease, liver disease, kidney disease, endocrine disease, and alcoholism (no mention of morphology whatsoever!). **THE REAL CLINICAL WORLD SIMPLY DOES NOT WORK THIS WAY – ASK ANY COMPETENT, EXPERIENCED, AND SENSIBLE PHYSICIAN!** Kidney disease in most cases would be suspected **BEFORE** the anemia was investigated (hypertension, sallow facies, history of perhaps frequent urinary tract infections, easy bruising, and bleeding, routine urinalytic abnormalities); morphological examination of the film would in most cases have shown the typical normochromic anemia, perhaps with burr cells, the right shift of the neutrophils. Biochemical tests would easily have proven the diagnosis.

The Logical Generation of the Provisional Diagnosis

First some general conceptual issues are briefly considered. The psychological process known as the clinical approach is engrossingly complex, and despite all attempts cannot be simplified (certainly given the current state of technology).

This applies also to laboratory tests and their interpretation.

> All laboratory reports require some element of clinical thinking, but it is really only in hematology that this is critical, because of
>
> 1. The peculiar nature of the blood system itself
> 2. The peculiar nature of the first-line tests, particularly the FBC

The essence of clinical medicine is the making of decisions, often in the face of insufficient data (a major drawback about algorithms). We try to **INFER** the nature of an abnormal internal process from subjective data reported by the patient (always a process requiring considerable judgment) and from external alterations, either anatomical or functional, or both. After integrating these findings, we try to come up with a set of possibilities, which we then proceed to confirm of exclude by further clinical tests and by special investigations. As we proceed along this process, we are constantly asking ourselves questions, notably (and repeatedly)

1. "Does the patient or any particular symptom or sign, or one or more features in the FBC, deviate sufficiently from 'normal' (however this is defined) for him (or the finding) to be regarded as diseased or indicative of disease?"
2. "What are the probable nature, cause and severity of the disease or deviation?"
3. "What further investigations need be done to narrow the possibilities?"
4. "What is the optimal form of therapy and or management for this patient in these circumstances?"

The answer to each of these questions is generally a major intellectual undertaking that, with increasing experience, we tend to take for granted, and requires high intelligence and the long training we undergo. All problem solving is essentially an **INFERENTIAL PROCESS** leading to the generation of a set of hypotheses regarding the nature of the problem. Because it is inferential, it is also **PROBABILISTIC**. Indeed, whichever method of reaching decisions is used, we can never be completely certain of our diagnosis (or treatment regime – arrogance has no place in medicine!). In our thinking we form hypotheses (in the form of **DIFFERENTIAL DIAGNOSES**) that describe a context (or "**PROBLEM SPACE**") within which further investigations take place, either clinical, laboratory, radiological, etc., that then validate and strengthen one or more of the hypotheses, and require the discarding of others – with the proviso that one understands that this is always done with a degree of probability.

Probability and Inference

Thus far we have taken the existence of the provisional or pre-test diagnosis as a given. However, the generation of this diagnosis is one of the most crucial parts of the whole exercise (and one of the most difficult): if this is wrong, all the subsequent activities will be wrong. And this comment is particularly relevant to the first-line tests especially the FBC, where there is a marked tendency to simplistic and slapdash thinking.

The probabilistic aspects of our thinking have been overemphasized, whereas the inferential part of the process should receive more attention. Unfortunately, over the years, the author has seen countless examples of sloppy thinking, jumping to conclusions, using preconceived ideas of what the problem is, taking results and clinical features out of context, and other forms of laziness, resulting only in wrong diagnoses and detriment to the patient. It has thus been adjudged necessary to discuss, as simply as possible, some basic intellectual approaches to problem solving, especially in hematology.

It is true that some forms of advanced thinking are extremely difficult if not impossible to map, involving as it does such elements as logical leaps; the sudden, almost eidetic grasp of the whole picture at once; strange "hunches"; and so on. However, in most cases and when faced with **ANY** practical problem, whether a FBC, a clinical problem, a sudden electrical outage in the home, or a noise that goes bump in the night, most of us seem to work according to a fairly typical pattern (at least in the first instance):

1. To look for features of the problem presented that one can recognize.
2. Search one's memory for a possible answer and any remembered associated features.
3. Make an assumption (working hypothesis) that this answer is the correct one.
4. Use the assumption as the **BASIS OF A LOGICAL ARGUMENT**, and examine the rest of the features of the problem, and if necessary make further investigations to find other features, and see if they fit – i.e., are logical.

5. If they do, we tend to conclude that the assumption states the facts of the case correctly.

6. Alternatively, as soon as one comes across a contradictory feature, the assumption is reconsidered.

This approach is potentially extremely successful, the degree of success depending on a number of variables:

1. One must know enough about the general type of problem to be able to recognize an abnormality. This can be easy – anyone can recognize an electrical outage; or it can be very difficult – an intermediate year student is probably going to be hard-pressed to recognize a mild sixth nerve palsy or a mild macrocytosis. Thus, a certain amount of essential knowledge is necessary even at this early stage. If one cannot recognize the abnormality at this stage, it is pointless going further.

2. The second stage too involves a certain amount of knowledge. A child of 5 years is very unlikely indeed to be able to suggest possible causes of a power outage; a properly educated student will recognize immediately that a Hb of 9 g/dl is abnormal, and will immediately be able to think of several possible general causes. He will know where next and for which associated features to look.

3. In most cases, the above leads directly to the making of an assumption, which enables action. In the case of a power outage, one could generate (say) one of two assumptions:

   a. That it is due to a central or regional power failure; this would lead to the action of (say) checking with the neighbors that this seems to be the case, and then phoning the power company to complain.

   b. That it is due to a domestic problem, perhaps from an overloaded circuit; this would lead to checking the home's distribution board and if found to the cause, to take further appropriate steps.

   Whatever assumption is made first, if action indicates it to be false, the other one would then be used.

   Similarly, in the case of an anemia (with a normal WCC and PC), he would examine the MCV. If this were decreased, he would almost certainly generate an assumption that the patient was iron deficient; this would lead to the further action of studying the rest of the count to see if there was anything contradictory (e.g., a raised ESR, a raised RCC), in which case he would generate a new assumption and go on from there.

   It is obvious that the assumptions he generates (and their quality and applicability) and how he follows them through depend very much on his knowledge, thoroughness, and intellectual integrity.

4. The next point is great significance: if no contradiction is found to an assumption, the tendency is to deem the assumption proven. This is a fallacy, both logical and medical. The great philosopher of science, Karl Popper, has shown quite clearly that **ONE CANNOT PROVE THE TRUTH OF AN ASSUMPTION** (hypothesis); one can, however, **DISPROVE** ("falsify") it. This has the very powerful implication that we must keep an open mind; as we act on our hypothesis we must assess very carefully how strong our evidence is, and watch the results of intervention very critically.

5. The above logical sequence cannot in most cases be bypassed without the danger of serious errors.

As stated before, the FBC can simply be a confirmatory (of a clinical diagnosis) test or one that is actually required to make the diagnosis in the first place. In the more typical type of clinical presentation such as in a patient with a swollen joint or one in whom we find a cardiac murmur, the above approach is, with training and experience, usually straightforward, and **PRIMARILY CLINICAL**. Such tests that are done in this sort of case are primarily **CONFIRMATORY**. The confirmatory tests are often hematological.

Consider a very simple example: a young woman of 19 years (revisiting our example briefly introduced in Chapter 2) complains of central abdominal pain for 1 day, which then moved to the right iliac fossa, anorexia, mild dysuria, and an episode of vomiting. On examination, she is mildly pyrexial with considerable tenderness over McBurney's point. A provisional diagnosis of acute appendicitis is confidently made; the only important consideration is to exclude an atypical urinary tract infection or mesenteric adenitis as the cause. A urinalysis reveals only small numbers of inflammatory cells, and the (abbreviated) FBC is shown in Table 3.3. It will be seen that the role of the FBC is entirely confirmatory (of the clinical diagnosis).

CASE #2

Table 3.3

	Value	Units	Reference range Low	Reference range High
Hemoglobin (Hb)	12.1	g/dl	12	15
White cell count	**11.89**	$\times 10^9/l$	4	10
Neutrophils	83.4	%		
Band cells	3.0	%		
Lymphocytes	10.0	%		
Monocytes	3.4	%		
Eosinophils	0.1	%		
Basophils	0.1	%		
Neutrophils abs.	**9.92**	$\times 10^9/l$	2	7
Band cells abs.	**0.36**	$\times 10^9/l$	0	0
Lymphocytes abs.	1.19	$\times 10^9/l$	1	3
Monocytes abs.	0.40	$\times 10^9/l$	0.2	1
Eosinophils abs.	**0.01**	$\times 10^9/l$	0.02	0.5
Basophils abs.	**0.01**	$\times 10^9/l$	0.02	0.1
Platelet count	**441.0**	$\times 10^9/l$	150	400
Sedimentation	**27**	mm/h	0	20

In summary, this blood count shows

1. A leukocytosis because of a mild neutrophilia
2. A left shift in the neutrophils (Band cells)
3. A mild increase in platelet count and sedimentation

The features are very much against a urinary tract infection or mesenteric adenitis and very much **SUPPORTIVE OF THE CLINICAL IMPRESSION** of appendicitis.

1. The diagnostic approach was essentially clinical (in the traditional sense). No test by itself could give or even suggest the diagnosis (except rarely sonography).
2. The clinical features were obvious, and followed the pattern found in the majority of cases of acute appendicitis.
3. The laboratory tests were only of confirmatory value.
4. Note that the FBC was evaluated with respect to the clinical features but that the evaluation was not particularly clinical – in fact, it was essentially **PATTERN RECOGNITION**, in the clinical context: the presence of a mild neutrophilia, the absence of a lymphocytosis and of any other abnormalities.
5. However, we all know that appendicitis can occur without a neutrophilia. The absence of a neutrophilia does not falsify our clinical diagnosis, it can only make us more careful. So, neutrophilia does not prove the diagnosis of appendicitis (indeed, the word "confirmatory" is misleading), nor does its absence negate it; its role here is to provide **SUPPORT**.

Very often, however, the FBC plays a far more fundamental diagnostic role – the identification of the nature of the disease process itself. Such cases are presented throughout the book.

Common Methods of Generating Pre-test Hypotheses

By far the most commonly used techniques for generating pre-test hypotheses are what are known as heuristics. This is the fancy name for mental shortcuts we use all the time in our daily lives. The only difference in professional work is that their use there is supported by wide knowledge and experience, as well as a keen appreciation of their potential shortcomings. At the general level, we will discuss (very largely) only the use of heuristics in approaching our first-line tests. Very complex problems will require a much more involved thinking process and will almost certainly require referral to a competent specialist (and the implication that the specialist will be able to think at this level is true – this is what is expected of him).

The Use of Heuristics in Generating Pre-test Hypotheses

At the general level, heuristics are the most commonly used mental methodologies in our interpretation of our tests. It is critical to understand a number of issues:

1. The limitations and proper usage of these heuristics
2. How to assess whether they have succeeded or not
3. What to do if they have indeed failed

Pattern recognition is one of the **HEURISTIC** (mental shortcut) methods; in this book, only two **HEURISTIC** methods will be discussed.

THE AVAILABILITY HEURISTIC. This is a very common strategy – the solution that most easily comes to mind is the one that is adopted; and the reason it most easily comes to mind is that it has been recently and/or commonly seen. This heuristic is particularly useful in an epidemic. It is commonly correct. Unfortunately, it is also the one that is most open to abuse: the probabilistic nature of our inferences can be exaggerated and distorted to cause marked oversimplification of the issue. The principle, commonly and inappropriately called the probabilistic approach to diagnosis, is that the disease fitting the findings that is most prevalent in the community **IS THEN USED FOR THE FINAL DIAGNOSIS**; only when treatment fails is the diagnosis reviewed. In the process, a great deal of anxiety can be avoided by a bit of thought and care (Examine Table 3.4).

Here, no morphological comment was provided. The patient was told by the nurse (an algorithm presumably having been consulted) that the commonest cause of a low platelet count was ITP, and that this was probably precipitated by a recent viral infection (in view of the "lymphocytosis"). She was placed on high tapering doses of prednisone and told to come back in 6 months, and if not improved a bone marrow examination would be done. She experienced no clinical improvement. After 4 months she went overseas to visit family. While there she deteriorated and was seen at the hematology clinic of a teaching hospital. A bone marrow examination revealed a myelodysplastic syndrome that was already transforming into an acute leukemia. There are numerous instructive comments that can be made:

a. A number of subtle clues in the FBC were present: the very high RDW and the relatively prominent monocytes.

CASE #3

Table 3.4

Patient: Miss E J	Age: 32	Sex: F	Race: W	Altitude: sea level
The patient complained to the nurse at the HMO of tiredness, weakness, epistaxis, bleeding gums, and cold sweats. She was found to be slightly pale and a tip of spleen was palpable. She was referred for a blood count.				

	Value	Units	Reference range Low	High
Red cell count	**3.78**	$\times 10^{12}/$ l	3.8	4.8
Hemoglobin (Hb)	12.1	g/dl	12	15
Hematocrit (Hct)	0.36	l/l	0.36	0.46
Mean cell volume	89	Fl	80	99
Mean cell Hb	**32.0**	pg	27	31.5
Mean cell Hb conc.	33.6	g/dl	31.5	34.5
Red cell dist. width	**19.2**	%	11.6	14
White cell count	4.1	$\times 10^9/l$	4	10
Monocytes	**16.0**	%		
Neutrophils abs.	2.00	$\times 10^9/l$	2	7
Lymphocytes abs.	1.39	$\times 10^9/l$	1	3
Monocytes abs.	0.66	$\times 10^9/l$	0.2	1
Eosinophils abs.	0.05	$\times 10^9/l$	0.02	0.5
Basophils abs.	0.00	$\times 10^9/l$	0.02	0.1
Platelet count	**7.1**	$\times 10^9/l$	150	400

b. The smear was evidently not examined. It is almost certain that the dysplastic changes in the neutrophils would have been noticed. There even may have been one or two blasts.

c. Some of the clinical features should have alerted whoever was responsible to look deeper.

　　The concept of likelihood was misdirected. It was being used by the HMO purely as a device to minimize costs; a pre-test "diagnosis" of ITP was made on the basis of insufficient data. The prevalence of a disease is only a pointer to the direction in which further **THINKING** should be done. **"THE LR DOES NOT DIRECTLY ACHIEVE WHAT WE WANT – I.E., THE PROBABILITY THAT THE PATIENT HAS THE DISEASE IF THE TEST IS POSITIVE. WHAT IT DOES DO IS INDICATE BY HOW MUCH THE TEST WILL ALTER THE PRE-TEST PROBABILITY OF THE PATIENT HAVING THE DISEASE."** Indeed, the whole concept of probability was abused at the expense of logical inference (and good patient care).

d. One of the core principles of decision analysis was ignored: it is true that additional testing should (only) be done if subsequent management will differ as a result of the new information – but then it **MUST** be done.

e. This is the sort of thing that can happen when bean counters take control of the medical profession. The fact that the above HMO approach would be successful in say 80% of cases is not the point, not if your patient's well-being is your primary concern.

THE REPRESENTATIVE HEURISTIC: THIS IS THE MOST USEFUL, PRACTICAL AND WIDELY USED OF ALL METHODS. The diagnostic possibilities are triggered by the resemblance of the current clinical picture to that of a well-known pattern (i.e., pattern recognition – the syndromic approach). And this is particularly relevant with the FBC, because certain patterns in the FBC are very suggestive and can thus trigger a hypothesis very rapidly. The proviso of course is that

a. The various patterns are known.

b. Common exceptions to the patterns are known.

c. When a pattern does not "fit" with anything known, one must be prepared to think at a more fundamental level – and this requires a certain amount of basic pathophysiological knowledge.

Thus, at the general level (i.e., for most readers), the emphasis is on the **REPRESENTATIVE HEURISTIC** – i.e., the **RECOGNITION OF PATTERNS** understood as representative of a typical diagnostic or suggestive picture. These patterns are built up gradually throughout the book, such that toward the end, the general reader will be competent to handle quite complex pictures. This is not to say that the basic knowledge required for their understanding will be neglected – patterns are difficult to remember without understanding their basis. At the advanced level, the **CATEGORICAL REASONING APPROACH** is often necessary and requires specialist knowledge and understanding (but there is nothing stopping the concerned generalist from becoming acquainted with the approach).

In practice, probably the major problem with the representative heuristic is the danger of forcing your interpretation of a report into a known pattern when in fact there are contradictory features – the Crime of Procrustes! Procrustes was a mythical innkeeper in ancient Greece. His inn was on a country highway. When a traveler sought accommodation for the night, Procrustes would take him to a bed; if the traveler was too long for the bed, he would saw off enough of his legs **TO MAKE HIM FIT THE BED**; conversely, if he was too short, he would stretch him. This is a very seductive error and very common, to be avoided at all costs.

The point is that if the report does not have a recognizable pattern, or worse, if features in a report contradict one's first impression, one **MUST** abandon pattern matching for something more fundamental: **CATEGO-RICAL REASONING**.

Categorical reasoning (or causal inference) requires a good and systematic knowledge of on the one side the pathophysiology of the hematological system and how it integrates with other systems and on the other of the multitude of clinical correlates that are gained from experience. These are usually expected of specialists, but there is nothing to prevent a generalist from acquiring and using these. However, it is not practicable to teach these formally – instead they will be demonstrated in our discussions of cases later in the book. Note there are other reasoning techniques often used.

Please note, however, the following:

1. All methods embrace the concept of validation of any hypotheses generated. The **VALIDATION** of any one hypothesis can be very difficult and requires a judicious choice of further tests as well as, very often, very judicious reasoning.
2. Subconscious biases. These usually relate to

   a. **CONTENT** and **BELIEVABILITY.** If it seems to be true, one tends to believe in its validity.
   b. **CONFIRMATION BIAS**. This is the tendency to seek evidence confirming the theory rather than that tending to disconfirm it.
   c. We tend to pay less **ATTENTION TO THE PREMISES OF OUR ARGUMENT** and more to the conclusion. If explicit attention is paid to the premises, the conclusion is more likely to be valid.

3. An overriding concern is the **RATIO BETWEEN BENEFIT AND RISK**: this is often an estimate based on clinical experience, judgment, and so on. The point is, the lower the benefit:risk ratio the more certain one must be of the diagnosis – i.e., this situation would have a **HIGH TREATMENT THRESHOLD** (in the Bayesian paradigm).
4. All methods – clinical and laboratory – have limitations, and we wish to be able to measure the information they provide as exactly as possible. This is done by understanding the **TEST OPERATING CHARACTERISTICS**.
5. Once a provisional diagnosis has been reached, the next phase is entered.

It is abundantly clear that the use of heuristics can lead to serious errors, and while their use is common and very useful, it is worthwhile to consider just what it is that one does with heuristics and indeed most forms of thinking.

The Final Diagnosis

THE ELEMENTS OF THE DIAGNOSTIC PROCESS DESCRIBED UP TO THIS POINT ARE FAIRLY INVOLVED. THE FINAL ASSESSMENT IS ALWAYS CLINICAL – I.E., ETIOLOGY, COMPLICATIONS, PROGNOSIS, MANAGEMENT, AND MONITORING PARAMETERS. THE ISSUE IS DISCUSSED IN THE DIFFERENT CHAPTERS.

No matter how good the laboratory is, it cannot perform **YOUR** essential duty – integrating the results with the clinical picture. And before you can do this you need to have some insight into the type and quality of laboratory you are using.

However, we still have to complete the process of making the result **CLINICALLY RELEVANT** by integrating what we have already learned so as to be as sure as possible about what the results mean and how they fit into the total evaluation of the patient, and with what degree of certainty. This we do after considering the process of diagnosis in hematology, which has many unusual features.

For two reasons, it is necessary to spend some time on the actual diagnostic process. This is done in the Chapter 5.

1. In our experience, most students and most practitioners do not have a firm grasp of how to take an effective history from or to perform a sensible clinical examination on a patient with respect to the hematological system. Ironically, this is also essential for the proper evaluation of the first-line tests.
2. The process in hematology is unusual. It will be shown that the clinical contribution to diagnosis in blood diseases is as essential, albeit different, as it is in neurology or cardiology.

Evidence-Based Medicine (EBM)

In the words of David Sackett, of the Center for Evidence-based Medicine, EBM is "the conscientious, explicit and judicious use of current best evidence in making decisions about the care of individual patients.[2]"

Advances in diagnostic technology have clearly demonstrated that traditional clinical diagnoses were very often wrong. Forty-odd years ago, in a series of routine autopsies, in at least half of the autopsies performed either the main clinical diagnosis was wrong or a major complication was missed. Fifty and more years ago, heavy reliance was placed on personal clinical experience even with specialist consultations. However, it did not, in many cases, matter too much if the clinical diagnoses were wrong. Clinicians could learnedly discuss (or pontificate about) the nature of a cardiac murmur, and since very few specific therapeutic modalities were available, it did not matter much anyway (except of course to the patient, who at least wanted a diagnosis). The amount of published knowledge was not huge, and reading a few reputable journals regularly was sufficient to keep in touch. Also, the articles tended not to have little or no statistical analysis of their data.

(It should not be forgotten, however, that the doctors at the time were superb clinicians and extremely patient orientated. They worked almost exclusively from their own experience, without any formal peer review but with considerable informal sharing of ideas and problems; it was often based on very insubstantial biochemistry and pharmacology.)

Today, the circumstances have changed dramatically. There are massive amounts of material available – it is quite impossible for any individual to keep abreast of all new diseases and technologies, which are being discovered regularly. Statistical methods are an integral part of today's article, and one needs specialized knowledge to understand them. Third-party health funders are demanding solid evidence for the need for a diagnostic or therapeutic regime, which has in the meantime become enormously expensive.

In 1972, Archie Cochrane recognized the problems, and started the huge collaborative effort that bears his name. Data, good, bad, and indifferent, is available on huge numbers of diseases, procedures, and therapies, with outstanding (and some not so outstanding) interpretive assessments. These trends are in line with the scientific method applied to medicine.

Many reservations about EBM have however been expressed. For example, Charlton[3] has expressed many of these in the form of a set of questions: are the proponents of EBM suggesting, he asks,

1. That previous medical practice was based on the **WORST** evidence, without reference to data from patients and their communities?
2. That previously doctors' decisions were dictated by habit and thoughtless following of medical traditions?
3. That statistical data had no place in their practice?
4. That if they derived relevant therapeutic and prognostic conclusions from their clinical experience, this data was not ever used in modifying their practice?
5. That, by following EBM guidelines, doctors have no need to check their own performance?

Walker and Labadarios[6] have raised disturbing questions about the powerful effects of the unquantifiable factors that are part and parcel of therapy – emotional factors, religious faith, the surroundings, a wife's love, and so on.

Aveyard[7] stated that "... the contribution of nursing, physiotherapy, and other specialties to the healing process is often unknown.... In the effort to make clinical practice evidence-based, we must not neglect to find and use those beneficial aspects of care that cannot be prescribed."

There are a number of points that further can be raised:

1. While it is true that the proponents of EBM acknowledge that many aspects of patient care are only partly subject to scientific methods, and strictly speaking EBM tries to quantify only those aspects that are essentially subject to scientific methodology, the effect, albeit subtle, has been to reduce the relevance of individual judgment and experience. In particular, the message being sent to students tends to be misinterpreted – "refer to (and quote) published results and/or statistics and it is no longer necessary to think critically." This has developed to the point that programs are available for palmtop computers to retrieve and calculate the significance of results of tests and therapeutic modalities, further making individual thought irrelevant. "The patient is pale – what can this mean and what do I do? Let's look up the relevant tests and their value in this case!" One effect is the evident decreasing ability among students to see often complex clinical situations in perspective. There are various levels of quality of evidence, and the opinion of the individual expert in the field is now held to be the least relevant! These effects are not the fault of EBM per se, but of humanity's chronic predisposition to intellectual laziness.
2. All research in the field is based on population studies, usually in one part of the world, and in one area. It is simply not acceptable to assume that results of a survey in say Japan, no matter how well done, can without consideration be applied to patients in Edinburgh. Also, these figures usually represent big pools of data, and this makes it very difficult always to apply the results of the study to your individual patient. Such pooling of data ignores other diseases or physiological states the individual patients comprising the pool showed.
3. These studies are also usually done on a highly selected population, either positive or negative for a well-defined condition. They tend thus to be intended for patients with a high pre-test probability of a disease and are therefore not necessarily very helpful in a routine setting. The example quoted earlier of the value of the ANA test for SLE is apposite.
4. Sensitivity and specificity studies on the same test done by different researchers do not always (in fact seldom) correspond. They must always only be used as a guideline and interpreted with circumspection and perspective.

5. There is a tendency to a gross oversimplification of the complexities of clinical diagnosis and therapy. The diagnostic emphasis is on tests and not clinical methods, which tend to be regarded contemptuously (forgetting that in the end, the patient's status as an individual is the overriding consideration).

6. EBM has become politically loaded. Bureaucrats and funders have seized upon some of the principles of EBM. The door to bureaucratic control of medical practice has been opened, in the process changing it out of all (humane) recognition.

7. As far as hematology is concerned, the research on the operating characteristics of the various tests has been of varying quality and usefulness. Current practice is to approach hematological results on the basis of the primary changes (for example, microcytosis), as revealed in the first-line tests. Each of these changes however has a number of possible causes, and the operating characteristics of the primary measurement used for differentiation do not usually effectively discriminate between the various **SPECIFIC** causes (e.g., differentiating between iron deficiency and anemia of chronic disorders). These changes require a different approach, which is described in this book. As far as confirmatory tests are concerned, however, their operating characteristics do indeed have great value, e.g., the sensitivity of a decreased ferritin in diagnosing iron deficiency.

There are many aspects to EBM, such as the evaluation of clinical trials, decisions to treat, and evaluation of journal articles. In this book we are concerned only with one aspect – **THE EVALUATION OF DIAGNOSTIC TESTS, IN TERMS OF TWO ISSUES:**

1. **THEIR VALIDITY AS DIAGNOSTIC AIDS.** The major consideration is to attempt to quantify the added contribution a test result would make in changing our pre-test hypothesis. This in turn requires an assessment of what the different tests can be used for. With respect to our first-line tests, different expectations would obtain

   a. **THE HEMOSTATIC SCREEN.** Since this is never done without a clinical indication, its usefulness in such a patient is high – a positive finding in the screen in a patient with a bleeding disorder is of the order of 95% or more.

   b. **THE FBC.** Here the situation is very different, since the FBC is often used in an attempt to find a disease, often as a last resort. So its yield depends very much on the clinical presentation. Thus, in a pale patient the FBC should yield a usable result in at least 90% of cases, while in a patient with say chronic fatigue

without any suggestive clinical features, its yield is going to be low.

2. **THEIR APPROPRIATENESS.**[8] This issue applies not only to the first-line tests but (perhaps more particularly) also to the many confirmatory tests that are available. It is important that these tests be used appropriately. Some specific questions must be answered before one should use them and before one can apply valid evidence about them:

   a. Is the test easily available, affordable, accurate, and precise enough for your purposes?

   b. Can you generate a clinically sensible estimate of the patient's pre-test probability?

   c. Will the resulting post-test probabilities affect your management in a positive sense? Would your patient be willing to carry out the management suggestions?

   d. Would the consequences of the test help your patient? It is important to try to quantify the potential benefit to the patient.

Our approach to these topics is cautious. It is necessary that students know the principles, and these are discussed in various chapters, but with due perspective and critical judgment. This is particularly relevant to hematology, since laboratory tests play such a large part in our practice – and the danger is that the integrated methodology that we are striving for will be abandoned, to the detriment of good patient care. There is undoubtedly an element among some students and doctors to decide on a test only on the basis of its operating characteristics: for example, a patient may present with a history of repeated hematemesis; the FBC shows an MCV of 84 fl. The doctor decides that the sensitivity of the MCV for iron deficiency is high only at a level of < 80 fl and thus that the patient (most likely) does not have iron deficiency and therefore does not need iron studies; in the meantime, his underlying liver disease has not been taken into account (responsible for a rise in MCV). If he had looked critically at the rest of the FBC – which this book intends to teach him – he would not have fallen into this reductionist trap.

We strongly contend that EBM cannot supplant clinical judgment.

Summary

1. Laboratory tests have a central role in hematological practice. Results are of two kinds, each having their strengths and weaknesses:

   a. Numerical, commonly and misleadingly referred to a "objective." They are always **ESTIMATES**.

b. Morphological, commonly and misleadingly referred to as "subjective." Their importance is underestimated.

2. Using a lab result sensibly requires the answers to a number of essential questions:

a. Is it normal? This begs the question – what is normal? Statistical analyses are very helpful but cannot answer all the problems, especially in cases of overlap between "normal" and "abnormal." The "normality" of a result is assessed in the first instance by reference to a reference range. This is often broad and reflects a population, not the individual. To attempt to gain an idea of the patient's "true" normal value (for any analyte), previous results should be consulted.

b. How valid is the result? There are many causes of a result not reflecting the "true" value:

   i. The inherent variability of the testing process
   ii. Variations due to incorrect methods of obtaining and handling the specimen
   iii. The physiological causes of variation

c. With reference to the range of reference results, by how much does the patient's result differ? Then, within this range, if there is information as to previous results in a state of apparent health, by how much does the new result differ?

d. What associated features, clinical and laboratory, throw light on the pathogenesis of an abnormal result?

e. What are the limitations of the test/s? This data is provided by the operating characteristics of the test, in terms of

   i. Sensitivity. This parameter reflects the degree to which a test is positive if disease is present. A test of high sensitivity is used to **CONFIRM** a diagnosis. The degree to which the test is positive if disease is absent is known as the false positive rate.

   ii. Specificity. This parameter reflects the degree to which a test is negative if disease is absent. A test of high specificity is used to **EXCLUDE** a diagnosis. The degree to which the test is negative if disease is present is known as the false negative rate.

   iii. Sensitivity and specificity do not answer directly the clinical questions raised. The answers come from the positive and negative predictive values and the likelihood ratios, derived from sensitivities and specificities in relation to prevalences of the disease in the relevant community.

f. At what level does a particular result of a particular analyte require clinical action? This is sometimes a complex and difficult issue.

3. Algorithms are shown not to be the final answer in handling hematological problems.

4. The concept and use of evidence-based medicine is examined and its pros and cons discussed.

We believe that the optimal approach to diagnosis is professional, informed and experienced assessment of the facts in the case, and using one's best logic to infer the nature of the problem, often in the face of insufficient evidence.

This is the subject matter of our next three chapters: how to reliably obtain the data we need and then how to use it to get to a diagnosis, and a survey of some of the essential knowledge required for this process.

The two outstanding characteristics of a good physician are

Perspective & Thoroughness

It is strongly recommended that these two qualities be nurtured. One can always find the necessary knowledge elsewhere.

Exercise 2.1

A quick self-test (Answers on page 79)

True	False	Questions
		1. Laboratory reports cannot always be trusted
		2. Heuristics are a fundamentally unreliable approach to making a diagnosis
		3. Since algorithms by definition guarantee a correct result, their use in hematology is restricted
		4. The "reference range" refers to the same concept as "clinical acceptability"
		5. Pregnancy causes significant physiological changes in the FBC
		6. Severe anemia results in systolic and diastolic hypertension
		7. Anticoagulants are a known possible cause of spurious abnormalities in the FBC
		8. The laboratory is always at fault if results are incorrect
		9. A laboratory result can always be relied upon to give the exact and true measurement of any constituent
		10. Great care must be taken when doing venesection for obtaining specimens for analysis
		11. Blood in an EDTA tube remains fully usable for the FBC for up to a week
		12. All diagnoses are in fact hypotheses and their value should be assessed in terms of probability
		13. Physiological variation is a significant potential cause for confusion in the interpretation of lab results
		14. The race of the patient has no effect on any of the elements of the FBC
		15. The sensitivity and specificity of tests are all that are required to use the tests for confident diagnosis
		16. The pre-test stage of diagnosis is an attempt to evaluate the likely possible causes in terms of prevalence, by using the history and clinical examination
		17. Anemia developing in a particular patient does not progress along a standard or set course
		18. Negative or "normal" results are just as informative as "abnormal" or positive results
		19. A laboratory's results are always 100% accurate
		20. The homeostatic set point for the value of Hb in an adult male at sea level is fixed at 14.9 g/dl
		21. An isolated Hb result in a patient is of no clinical value

True	False	Questions
		22. The proportion of citrate anticoagulant to blood in a tube for coagulation studies is critically important
		23. If an algorithm is properly constructed, applying it to a hematological problem will always lead to the correct answer
		24. Using EBM guidelines is always demeaning to a professional
		25. Clinical judgment plays a minimal role in diagnosis when compared with the contribution made by the operating characteristics

Exercise 2.2

Match the items in columns 1 and 2 (Answers on page 79)

Column 1	Column 2
1. Numerical laboratory results	A. May or may not reflect disease
2. The homeostatic set point	B. While of value in simpler presentations, they can be very unpractical in many situations
3. 'Normal' and 'abnormal' ranges for an analyte	C. May be a false result due to the age of the specimen
4. Analytical variation	D. Are not inherently more reliable than morphological assessment of anatomical elements
5. A result within the given 'normal' or reference range	E. Potentially causes multiple abnormalities in the blood and the first-line tests
6. Common causes of pre-analytical variations in results	F. This refers to the true individual normal value for any test in a particular person
7. The operating characteristics of tests	G. Are totally unreliable
8. A value for an analyte just outside the reference range	H. Is not sufficient for proper evaluation of a test's utility
9. Knowing the sensitivity and specificity of a test	I. Does not imply that the result is necessarily normal for that patient
10. The most useful practical operating characteristic of a test	J. Are due to poor specimen management on the part of the referring clinician
11. Algorithms	K. Are critically important in evaluating their utility
12. Final (complete) diagnosis in hematology as in general medicine	L. Is mainly the responsibility of the laboratory but the clinician can contribute to this
13. The data provided by articles on Evidence-Based Medicine	M. The likelihood ratios
14. Smoking	N. Is ultimately a clinical decision

Column 1	Column 2
15. Laboratory results that are accurate but without precision	O. Are invaluable to the practitioner but do not supplant individual judgment
	P. Can cause numerous hematological abnormalities and changes in the FBC
	Q. Reflect the range of results found in a population

ANSWERS
EXERCISE 2.1

1: True; 2: False; 3: False; 4: False; 5: True; 6: False; 7: True; 8: False; 9: False; 10: True; 11: False; 12: True; 13: True; 14: False; 15: False; 16: True; 17: True; 18: True; 19: False; 20: False; 21: False; 22: True; 23: True; 24: False; 25: False

EXERCISE 2.2

1D; 2F; 3Q; 4L; 5I; 6 J; 7 K; 8A; 9H; 10 M; 11B; 12 N; 13O; 14P; 15G.

References

1. Lewis, SM, Bain, B, Bates, I (2006). Dacie and Lewis Practical Haematology. 10th edn. Philadelphia, Churchill Livingstone.
2. Sackett, DL. Evidence-based medicine. Lancet (1995) 346: 840.
3. Charlton, B (1996). The Limits of Evidence-Based Medicine (Editorial), Hospital Update, September.
4. Seegal, D. J. Chron. Dis. (1963) 16: 195.
5. www.medalreg.com.
6. Walker, ARP, Labadarios, D Evidence-based medicine – how much does it explain? S. Afr. Med. J. (1996) 86: 939.
7. Aveyard, P. Evidence-based medicine. Lancet (1995) 346: 840.
8. From EBM Syllabi; manuals are available from Radcliffe Medical, 18 Marcham Rd, Abingdon, Oxfordshire, UK.
9. Barnett, AE et al. A clinical view of analytical goals in clinical biochemistry. J. Clin. Pathol. (1979) 32: 893–896.
10. Campbell, DG et al. The physician's view of laboratory performance. Aust. Ann. Med. (1969) 18: 4–6.

Further Reading

Lewis, SM, Bain, B, Bates, I (2006). Dacie and Lewis Practical Haematology. 10th edn. London, Churchill Livingstone.

Clinical Interactions Between the Blood and the Other Systems

4

There are no lengths to which men will not go to avoid the labor of thinking.

(Thomas Edison)

Preview *In the first section of this chapter, a number of general pathophysiological processes or states, secondary to changes in other systems, are discussed; their relevance is that the changes they can cause in the FBC can mimic more serious diseases and are often the source of considerable difficulty in the interpretation of the FBC.*

In the second section, disease processes in other systems as they are reflected in the first-line tests are discussed at greater length. As previously stated, the blood itself is not accessible for clinical examination; since it flows through all the other tissues, both affecting them and being affected by them, changes in the rest of the body can, and do, reflect changes in the blood, facilitating clinical diagnosis and evaluation of blood and test abnormalities. At the same time, specialists in different fields (e.g., rheumatology or neurology) are able to see the hematological associations of the diseases in their purview.

These associations are a necessary introduction to the description of the clinical examination in Chapter 5. The discussions also conveniently facilitate an overview of diseases in other systems.

General Pathophysiological Processes or States Affecting the Interpretation of the FBC

The following are discussed:

1. The physiological response to acute hemorrhage
2. The physiological response to hypoxia
3. The raised hematocrit
4. Splenectomy and Hyposplenism

In these, you will be able to understand

1. How the FBC changes after an acute hemorrhage may significantly resemble certain disease states and can be the cause of significant confusion and misdiagnosis
2. The different ways in which chronic hypoxia affects the blood, and especially the FBC
3. That the raised hematocrit is the end-result of a number of completely different pathophysiological processes and each must be understood

before this common presentation can be approached successfully
4. Splenectomy and hyposplenism, of which there are many causes, has specific effects on the blood and are causes of potential confusion

The Physiological Response to Acute Hemorrhage and the Effects on the FBC

One of the most dynamic and rapidly changing FBC findings occurs after an acute hemorrhage. A lot depends on when the blood is drawn after the episode. As you read the following description, imagine that each count presented is the first FBC you see – you can get a very disturbing and misleading picture. This is particularly so where the bleed is occult.

O.N. Beck, *Diagnostic Hematology*, DOI 10.1007/978-1-84800-295-1_4,
© Springer-Verlag London Limited 2009

Table 4.1

	Value	Units	Reference range Low	Reference range High	Possible range Low	Possible range High
Red cell count	5.27	$\times 10^{12}$/l	4.77	5.83	4.61	5.93
Hemoglobin (Hb)	15.5	g/dl	13.8	18.0	15.0	16.0
Hematocrit (Hct)	0.47	l/l	0.42	0.53	0.46	0.48
Mean cell volume	87	fl	80	99	77.9	96.1
Mean cell Hb	29.4	pg	27	31.5	26.3	32.5
Mean cell Hb conc.	33.0	g/dl	31.5	34.5	32.3	33.6
Red cell dist. width	12	%	11.6	14	11.1	12.9
Retic. count	0.5	%	0.27	0.80	0.5	0.5
Retic. absolute (abs.)	26.4	$\times 10^9$/l	26	100	23.7	29.0
White cell count	6.5	$\times 10^9$/l	4	10	5.85	7.15
Neutrophils abs.	3.97	$\times 10^9$/l	2	7	3.57	4.36
Lymphocytes abs.	2.28	$\times 10^9$/l	1	3	2.05	2.50
Monocytes abs.	0.20	$\times 10^9$/l	0.2	1	0.18	0.21
Eosinophils abs.	0.07	$\times 10^9$/l	0.02	0.5	0.06	0.07
Basophils abs.	0.00	$\times 10^9$/l	0.02	0.1	0.00	0.00
Platelet count	195.0	$\times 10^9$/l	150	400	170.6	219.4

Table 4.2

	Value	Units	Reference range Low	Reference range High	Possible range Low	Possible range High
Red cell count	5.25	$\times 10^{12}$/l	4.77	5.83	4.59	5.91
Hemoglobin (Hb)	15.6	g/dl	13.8	18.0	15.1	16.1
Hematocrit (Hct)	0.48	l/l	0.42	0.53	0.47	0.49
Mean cell volume	88	fl	80	99	78.8	97.2
Mean cell Hb	29.7	pg	27	31.5	26.6	32.8
Mean cell Hb conc.	33.0	g/dl	31.5	34.5	32.3	33.7
Red cell dist. width	13.1	%	11.6	14	12.1	14.1
Retic. count	0.41	%	0.27	0.80	0.4	0.4
Retic. absolute	21.5	$\times 10^9$/l	26	100	19.4	23.7
White cell count	10.7	$\times 10^9$/l	4	10	9.63	11.77
Neutrophils abs.	6.42	$\times 10^9$/l	2	7	7.14	8.72
Lymphocytes abs.	2.40	$\times 10^9$/l	1	3	2.02	2.47
Monocytes abs.	0.32	$\times 10^9$/l	0.2	1	0.29	0.35
Eosinophils abs.	0.11	$\times 10^9$/l	0.02	0.5	0.10	0.12
Basophils abs.	0.00	$\times 10^9$/l	0.02	0.1	0.00	0.00
Platelet count	**927.0**	$\times 10^9$/l	150	400	811.1	1042.9

Briefly, the sequence of changes after an acute hemorrhage (of sufficient degree) is as follows:

1. **THROMBOCYTOSIS.**
2. **NEUTROPHILIA**. Neutrophilia can occur first.
3. **ANEMIA**.
4. **RETICULOCYTOSIS**.

To illustrate, we shall use blood of an adult male. He suffered a large sudden duodenal bleed without hematemesis; that is, he had no idea at the time that he had suffered a bleed. His only symptoms were suddenly feeling peculiar, a feeling of weakness, some palpitations, and a dull pain low down in the chest (raising the suspicion of an infarct or angina); but there was nothing clinical (yet) to indicate to him or to his doctor that he in fact had a bleed. Table 4.1 displays his pre-incident FBC.

Thrombocytosis

An increase in the platelet count is almost invariable and usually the first response to a significant bleed.

Thrombocytosis usually occurs within 1–2 h. (See Table 4.2.) Note that until thrombocytosis (or neutrophilia) occurs, there are **NO** changes in the FBC.

NOTES:

1. If the first FBC were drawn now and assuming that bleeding had not been recognized, the picture would be puzzling and indeed very alarming.

2. The thrombocytosis can be profound, even up to 1 million per mm^3, and one may be misled into thinking of a myeloproliferative condition. The thrombocytosis persists for a few days, **SHOWING THE IMPORTANCE OF INTEGRATING THE CLINICAL ASSESSMENT OF THE PATIENT WITH THE INTERPRETATION OF THE FBC.**

Neutrophilia

Neutrophilia is a frequent reaction to a significant bleed and sometimes can be the first change, even before the thrombocytosis.

Neutrophilia does not always occur after an acute bleed. It can be the earliest change, within an hour or two. Usually, however, it occurs a little later, after the platelets start rising. Assume that the first FBC is drawn 2 h after the incident and he does develop a neutrophilia. Look at the FBC (Table 4.3), drawn 1 h after the incident. Your first thought could well be an acute infection.

Note the following points about this FBC:

1. The variation from the pre-incident FBC in the red cell parameters and the platelets can be entirely due to "natural" variation. If you look at the "possible ranges", you will see that the varying results are all within these limits.

2. The total leukocyte count is within "normal" limits. Only when you look at the neutrophil count, particularly the absolute count, is the neutrophilia noticed.

Table 4.3

	Value	Units	Reference range Low	Reference range High	Possible range Low	Possible range High
Red cell count	5.29	$\times 10^{12}/l$	4.77	5.83	4.63	5.95
Hemoglobin (Hb)	15.2	g/dl	13.8	18.0	14.7	15.7
Hematocrit (Hct)	0.46	l/l	0.42	0.53	0.45	0.47
Mean cell volume	88	fl	80	99	78.8	97.2
Mean cell Hb	28.7	pg	27	31.5	25.7	31.8
Mean cell Hb conc.	33.0	g/dl	31.5	34.5	32.4	33.7
Red cell dist. width	12.5	%	11.6	14	11.6	13.4
Retic. count	0.45	%	0.27	0.80	0.4	0.5
Retic. absolute	23.8	$\times 10^9/l$	26	100	21.4	26.2
White cell count	10.3	$\times 10^9/l$	4	10	9.27	11.33
Neutrophils	74.0	%				
Band cells	3	%				
Lymphocytes	21.0	%				
Monocytes	2.0	%				
Eosinophils	0.0	%				
Basophils	0.0	%				
Neutrophils abs.	**7.93**	$\times 10^9/l$	2	7	7.14	8.72
Lymphocytes abs.	2.16	$\times 10^9/l$	1	3	1.95	2.38
Monocytes abs.	0.21	$\times 10^9/l$	0.2	1	0.19	0.23
Eosinophils abs.	0.00	$\times 10^9/l$	0.02	0.5	0.00	0.00
Basophils abs.	0.00	$\times 10^9/l$	0.02	0.1	0.00	0.00
Band cells	3	%	0	0		
Platelet count	209.0	$\times 10^9/l$	150	400	182.9	235.1

Table 4.4

	Value	Units	Reference range Low	Reference range High	Possible range Low	Possible range High
Red cell count	4.95	$\times 10^{12}/l$	4.77	5.83	4.33	5.57
Hemoglobin (Hb)	14.4	g/dl	13.8	18.0	13.9	14.9
Hematocrit (Hct)	0.41	l/l	0.42	0.53	0.40	0.42
Mean cell volume	91	fl	80	99	81.4	100.6
Mean cell Hb	29.1	pg	27	31.5	26.0	32.1
Mean cell Hb conc.	33.0	g/dl	31.5	34.5	32.3	33.7
Red cell dist. width	13.1	%	11.6	14	12.1	14.1
Retic. count	0.53	%	0.27	0.80	0.5	0.6
Retic. absolute	26.2	$\times 10^9/l$	30	100	23.6	28.9
White cell count	7.21	$\times 10^9/l$	4	10	6.49	7.93
Neutrophils	72.0	%				
Lymphocytes	23.0	%				
Monocytes	3.0	%				
Eosinophils	1.0	%				
Basophils	1.0	%				
Neutrophils abs.	5.19	$\times 10^9/l$	2	7	4.67	5.71
Lymphocytes abs.	1.66	$\times 10^9/l$	1	3	1.49	1.82
Monocytes abs.	0.22	$\times 10^9/l$	0.2	1	0.19	0.24
Eosinophils abs.	0.07	$\times 10^9/l$	0.02	0.5	0.06	0.08
Basophils abs.	0.07	$\times 10^9/l$	0.02	0.1	0.06	0.08
Platelet count	**1011.0**	$\times 10^9/l$	150	400	884.6	1137.4

3. Notice that there is a small percentage of band cells, i.e., slightly earlier forms of neutrophil than normal. This suggests a left shift. However, the criteria for a left shift are fairly stringent and will be discussed in Chapter 6. The point to be made is that these band cells NEED NOT, other things being equal, necessarily mean a left shift in the clinically significant sense (being in this case due only to stress). Also note that no absolute numbers are given for the band cells. Usage in this regard varies in different hands. In the author's view, it is only in the critical care unit that an absolute band cell count is necessary, particularly for monitoring progress.

4. The neutrophil count seldom rises by more than 50% and usually subsides within hours.

Anemia

ANEMIA IS THE MOST LOGICAL RESPONSE TO ANEMIA, YET IT DOES NOT OCCUR IMMEDIATELY.

Students are often surprised that a large bleed does not immediately lead to anemia – just remember that not only red cells are lost, also plasma. **ANEMIA ONLY DEVELOPS WHEN THE PATIENT'S BLOOD VOLUME IS RESTORED WITH CRYSTALLOID OR HE WITHDRAWS FLUID FROM HIS TISSUES TO THIS END.**

The latter process takes anything up to 24 h for completion. Table 4.4 shows the FBC drawn after 24 h.

Were this the first FBC drawn, the picture would be as worrying. Note, however, that there is still no reticulocytosis, and indeed the Hb is within the "normal" range. Only the thrombocytosis should alert you to the possibility that there has been an occult bleed.

Reticulocytosis

The expected reticulocytosis occurs from the 4th day, rising by the 10th day to a level proportionate to the anemia, **IF THE BONE MARROW IS FUNCTIONALLY ADEQUATE.** (See Response of the Bone Marrow to Anemia in Chapter 7.)

The Physiological Response to Hypoxia and the Effects on the Full Blood Count

FIRST WE MUST SPECIFY WHAT WE MEAN BY HYPOXIA. The four traditional classes are hypoxemic, stagnant, anemic, and histotoxic. However, from the functional point of view there are two broad groups:

1. **HYPOBARIC.** This refers to hypoxia in the presence of a blood supply with a decreased Po_2. This is **HYPOXEMIC HYPOXIA** and is always due to defective

oxygenation of venous blood in the lungs (apart from the case of a large AV fistula or connection).

2. **NORMOBARIC.** This means hypoxia in the presence of a blood supply to the tissues with a normal Po_2. This is found in hypoxia due to anemia and tissue toxicity.

This distinction is valuable for a number of reasons:

1. **THE EPO RESPONSE (AND THEREFORE THE RETIC. RESPONSE) IS DIFFERENT,** particularly when one contrasts anemic with hypobaric hypoxia. **IN ANEMIC HYPOXIA, EPO SECRETION, AND THEREFORE RETICULOCYTOSIS, IS CONSTANT AND DIMINISHES ONLY AS THE HB IMPROVES, WHEREAS IN HYPOBARIC HYPOXIA, EPO SECRETION (AND RETICULOCYTOSIS) IS INTERMITTENT AND SOMETIMES APPEARS NOT TO OCCUR AT ALL.** Thus in, e.g., chronic chest disease, reticulocytosis is not always present – the important point is that the absence of a reticulocytosis does not rule out hypoxia. Nevertheless, in most cases the Hb tends to increase, other things being equal, whether or not a reticulocytosis is noted. Very roughly, **THE INCREASE IN HB (ASSUMING STRUCTURALLY NORMAL HB AND RED CELLS) WILL PARALLEL THE DEGREE OF CHRONIC HYPOXIA AVERAGED OVER A PERIOD OF TIME.**

2. **PATIENTS WITH HEMOGLOBINS SHOWING INCREASED OXYGEN AFFINITY CAN HAVE NORMAL HB LEVELS AND YET THE PATIENT CAN BE HYPOXIC.** These hemoglobins are either inherited or acquired. There are over 50 inherited types, the best known probably being Hb Chesapeake and Kansas. **NOTE THAT ONLY ABOUT TWO THIRDS OF THESE HAVE ABNORMAL ELECTROPHORETIC PATTERNS; THE REST RUN AS HBA.** The inherited forms all show compensatory erythrocytosis. The acquired forms are methemoglobin, sulfhemoglobin, and carboxyhemoglobin (there are also hereditary forms of methemoglobinemia). **CARBOXYHEMOGLOBINEMIA WHEN CHRONIC IS TYPICALLY ASSOCIATED WITH ERYTHROCYTOSIS, BUT THIS IS UNUSUAL IN THE OTHER TWO.** (Note that there also exist hemoglobins with **DECREASED** affinity – these patients have normal oxygenation (usually) at a lower Po_2 and consequently a mild anemia without tissue symptoms.)

The Raised Hematocrit

A raised Hct and/or Hb and/or RCC is often the first abnormality in a FBC that hits the eye, so to speak. The functional interrelationship between these three measurements is very important to understand. The prime considerations when one sees a raised hematocrit are **POLYCYTHEMIA** and **ERYTHROCYTOSIS**, and it may well be asked why the RCC does not have primacy as a diagnostic presentation.

It is true that, strictly speaking, erythrocytosis refers to a raised RCC; the problem, however, is that, from the functional point of view, the viscosity of blood is more important biologically than the number of circulating red cells – and the Hct is the largest single determinant of whole blood viscosity. The significance of the viscosity is that it plays a profound role in the efficacy of tissue perfusion and hence tissue oxygenation (apart from issues like stagnation and tendency to thrombosis in the presence of high viscosity, as well as aspects of endothelial function). Thus the whole blood viscosity can be normal with a very high RCC if the Hb is low enough to result in a normal Hct (as, for example, in thalassemia or venesected erythrocytosis). In these cases the Hb is low because the red cells are smaller than normal (i.e., are microcytic).

Therefore from the practical point of view, the Hct is the preferred measurement to take note of. Of course, if the red cells are normal in size, the Hb and RCC will parallel the Hct, but they can never be relied upon – the physiological factors determining the average red cell **SIZE** are largely independent of those determining the **NUMBER** of red cells.

Note that the above arguments apply also to a decreased RCC: for example, if the red cells are macrocytic in an anemic patient, the RCC will be disproportionately lower than the Hb and Hct would suggest.

(The above discussion is another argument why measuring the Hb as an isolated test is fraught with danger.)

The other major point in this regard is that the Hct is a concentration (a ratio between a given mass of red cells suspended in a volume of plasma). Bearing in mind that ~93% of the plasma is water, it is easy to see that loss of plasma water can significantly affect the Hct. Loss of plasma water leading to hemo-concentration and thus **APPARENT** increase in cell concentrations usually results only in erythrocytosis (red cells account (normally) for over 99% of circulating blood cells) but a short-lived generalized increase can occur acutely – presumably because the natural life span of the WBC and PLT are very brief compared with that of the RBC, the spurious increase is adjusted as new cells emerge from the marrow, but in fact the mechanism is not known.

From our point of view, either the Hct alone is affected or, in addition (and only occasionally), the WCC and PC are affected by dehydration. Obviously therefore when faced with either polycythemia or erythrocytosis (see the introductory section for definitions), **DEHYDRATION MUST ALWAYS BE CONSIDERED FIRST AS A CAUSE.**

Dehydration May Be Either Hyponatremic or Hypernatremic Extensive discussion of these is beyond the scope of this book and hence discussed in brief here.

Hyponatremic dehydration (serum $Na^{1+} <$ 130 mmol/l by definition) is found in losses from the GIT, the skin, the lungs, and the kidneys due to diuretics, renal damage, and partial outflow obstruction. Characteristics are

1. Decreased osmolality with a **low** Na^{1+}
2. Increased blood urea, creatinine, and urate levels
3. Urinary osmolality and Na^{1+} are variable, depending on the cause.

Hypernatremic dehydration (serum $Na^{1+} >$ 150 mmol/l by definition) is found wherever loss of water is greater than the loss of Na^{1+}, including in the causes mentioned above where water replacement is sub-optimal or the thirst mechanism is inoperative, and particularly in renal causes, glycosuria, and adrenal deficiency syndromes. Characteristics are

1. Increased osmolality with a **high** Na^{1+}.
2. Increased blood urea and creatinine levels
3. Urinary osmolality and Na^{1+} are again variable.

It can be seen that Na^{1+}, osmolality, blood glucose, urea, creatinine, and urate levels are the most valuable in assessing dehydration.

Losses into extravascular spaces: These can be dramatic and rapid, such as acute pancreatitis with peritonitis and effusion and some other causes of ascites.

Third-space losses: A common occurrence in the critically ill with multiple system failure is the edematous patient who nevertheless requires fluid replacement to maintain the circulation. The mechanism is still uncertain but it is probable that part of the pathogenesis is decreased tissue perfusion (whether due to prolonged hypotension, hyperviscosity, or micro-vascular damage due to endothelial swelling) resulting in more fluid being returned to the circulation from the interstitium than is entering it; decreased interstitial fluid results in reduction in tissue nutrition and oxygen

supply with damage to the sodium pump; hence intracellular water accumulates, the cells swell even further, and large volumes of water are effectively cut off from the circulation. A particular problem with third-space losses is that the extent of dehydration is commonly underestimated, and the electrolytes and osmolality are frequently ambiguous.

NOTE: The acute/subacute dehydration discussed above must be distinguished from chronic decrease in plasma water found in another condition, Gaisbock syndrome, discussed in Chapters 6 and 17.

Splenectomy and Hyposplenism

Splenectomy is performed for many reasons. Hyposplenism is an unusual condition and is found in association with a few diseases, to be discussed shortly. There are characteristic FBC features that are found, regardless of why the splenectomy was done or the cause of hyposplenism.

1. **ANISOCYTOSIS** with a rise in RDW, because the culling function of the spleen, which is very efficient at removing deformed, abnormal, or aged cells, is now absent (clearing the blood of these cells is now the function mainly of the rest of the reticulo-endothelial system, which is not nearly as efficient).
2. Thus **ABNORMAL CELLS ARE FOUND**, classically target cells, crenated cells, Howell–Jolly bodies, and so on.
3. **PLATELETS CHARACTERISTICALLY ARE INCREASED**, except in some cases where the splenectomy was done for thrombocytopenia. The platelet count (PC) can exceed 1000×10^{12}/l. In most cases the PC returns to normal, over a period usually of weeks but sometimes months or years; occasionally the PC is permanently raised. Giant platelets are sometimes seen.
4. Note that if the splenectomy was performed for a hematological disorder, the features of that disorder will in addition be visible.

Hyposplenism

This is found in association with a number of other conditions:

1. **SICKLE ANEMIA**. The splenic pulp becomes destroyed by the micro-vascular complication of sickle disease. Note one very important fact in this regard:

while the spleen eventually becomes non-functional (usually by the age of 18–24 months), it is not necessarily small – it can be palpable and is often the site of calcification, which can be seen on straight X-ray.

2. **CELIAC DISEASE.**
3. **INFLAMMATORY BOWEL DISEASE,** especially ulcerative colitis.
4. **OCCASIONALLY IN COLLAGEN VASCULAR DISEASE AND OLD AGE.**

Note that patients without functional spleens are very prone to pneumococcal and hemophilus infections and are in great danger when getting malaria.

Clinical Interactions with Other Systems

In the following sections we study relevant abnormalities in other systems, primarily their general features and pathogenesis. There is considerable interaction with the blood, often of great value in the diagnosis of blood disease and blood changes. Our major emphasis is on disorders of the blood that are reactive and secondary to changes in other systems. Students are advised that this section need be used only for reference, after a careful and comprehensive reading. Note that the clinical features per se are discussed in Chapter 5.

With each of the systems discussed, however, it should be understood just how the pathological changes described affect the blood, and thus how to infer the nature of the effects on the blood and the blood tests.

Bear in mind that the converse also is true – primary, secondary, and sometimes even reactive blood diseases can affect the tissues. However, these are not the primary concern of this book.

CLINICAL SUSPICION AND ASSESSMENT OF BLOOD DISORDERS IS PRIMARILY BY REFERENCE TO FINDINGS IN OTHER SYSTEMS, VIZ.,

1. The immune system, infections, and blood diseases
2. The cardiovascular system and blood diseases
3. The gastro-intestinal tract and blood diseases
4. The skin and blood diseases
5. The genito-urinary system and blood diseases
6. Pregnancy and changes in the blood
7. The musculo-skeletal system and blood diseases
8. The nervous system and blood diseases
9. The endocrine system and blood diseases
10. The lungs and blood diseases
11. The hematology of malignant disease

The Immune System, Infections, and Blood Diseases

Disorders of the immune system may be primary or secondary and may affect the cellular elements (neutrophils, eosinophils, monocytes, and lymphocytes) or the protein elements (mainly complement and immune globulins) or sometimes both.

Disorders of the cellular elements may be due to decrease in their concentration or an abnormality in their functions, and a large number of conditions have been described. Disorders of the protein elements may be due to deficiencies or molecular abnormalities; the important disorders are discussed in Chapters 12 and 22.

An introduction to the types of immune response is relevant at this point, since many other diseases that we will be discussing are due to their abnormalities:

1. **TYPE I (OR "IMMEDIATE" REACTIONS).** These are IgE-mediated leading to eosinophil chemotaxis and frequently accompanied by **EOSINOPHILIA.** Allergies are a prominent example.
2. **TYPE II REACTIONS.** These are characterized by the assembly on membranes of antigen–antibody complexes, with **ACTIVATION OF NEUTROPHILS AND COMPLEMENT.** There are two fundamental-pathogenetic mechanisms, both mediated by IgM/IgG:

   a. **CYTOTOXICITY** (cell lysis), with complement activation. Examples are **TRANSFUSION REACTIONS, AUTOIMMUNE HEMOLYSIS,** effects of **METHYLDOPA (SOMETIMES ASSOCIATED WITH AN INDUCED AUTOIMMUNE HEMOLYSIS),** and **GOLD** (used in rheumatoid arthritis and frequently associated with **NEUTROPENIA**). **ITP** is regarded as type II reaction.
   b. **RECEPTOR BLOCKAGE,** such as in **PERNICIOUS ANEMIA.**

3. **TYPE III REACTIONS.** These are characterized by circulating immune complexes. When these are deposited in various organs, various syndromes develop. Again, there are two fundamental pathogenetic mechanisms, both mediated by IgA/IgG:

   c. **ANTIBODY EXCESS** (Arthus-type reaction): An important example is bronchopulmonary aspergillosis, which characteristically is accompanied by **SEVERE EOSINOPHILIA.**

d. **ANTIGEN EXCESS** (serum sickness type): An important example is **HENOCH–SCHöNLEIN "PURPURA"** (vasculitis).

4. **TYPE IV REACTIONS** (or "delayed hypersensitivity"). These reactions are T-cell mediated, resulting in the accumulation of monocytes and lymphocytes. An important example is the **GRAFT-VERSUS-HOST REACTION**, as in complications of bone marrow transplants and blood transfusion.

Immunohematology

Traditionally, this term has a restricted meaning: it refers mainly to antigen–antibody interactions with blood cells and as such encompasses transfusion as well. Transfusion is covered in Chapter 19, and here we present only a discussion of the relevant antigens and antibodies and their interactions.

The major clinical relevance apart from transfusion reactions is of course other immune destruction of red cells (i.e., hemolysis), white cells, and platelets. Our major interest at this stage is in the pathogenesis of immune **HEMOLYSIS**.

An understanding of immune hemolysis is very difficult without some insight into the basic pathogenetic processes. With respect to immune hemolysis, a number of factors are relevant:

1. The type of antibody. The antibodies are of two broad types, IgG and IgM. IgA is rarely implicated.
2. The ease with which complement can be bound and activated.
3. Interaction with phagocyte receptors.

The Antigens and Antibodies Associated with Red Cells

The red cells, like all other cells, contain on their surface a vast number of receptors and other functional molecules that can act as antigens. In many conditions antibodies to these antigens are found. Antibodies may be

1. **ALLOANTIBODIES**. These may be

   a. **PRODUCED BY THE PATIENT** against foreign antigens as in blood transfusion or pregnancy.
   b. **SECONDARILY ACQUIRED** as in drug-induced hemolysis.

2. **AUTOANTIBODIES**. These are produced by the patient and are directed against the patient's own antigens. Autoantibodies are of two types:

a. **WARM TYPE**. These are most active at 37°C. They are mostly IgG and are polyclonal. The red cells are coated with IgG and sometimes complement. These are usually "incomplete" antibodies – i.e., they cannot agglutinate red cells in saline. Hemolysis is due to splenic phagocytosis: the spleen recognizes the coated red cells as abnormal (the splenic macrophages have receptors for these antibodies as well as for complement).

b. **COLD TYPE**. These are either monoclonal, as is found in the cold hemagglutination syndrome or associated with lymphoproliferative disease, or polyclonal as is found after some infections, notably due to mycoplasma and EB virus. They are mostly IgM and are "complete"; thus they are capable of binding neighboring red cells, causing agglutination, particularly in the cold. These antibodies attach to the red cell in the periphery, where the temperature is lower. When the blood reaches the core, the antibody is released; however, if complement has been bound, the cell is prone to being phagocytosed, mainly in the liver (see below). Sometimes, however, true intravascular lysis occurs.

The essential and critical point to understand is that, for an antibody to activate the C1 component of complement, it must bridge at least two antigenic sites (of the same type).

Figure 4.1 shows a part of a red cell membrane with several antigens (in pink) and two IgG molecules (in red and **NOT** drawn to scale).

In Fig. 4.1, it can be seen that the upper IgG molecule cannot span the two neighboring antigens. In this case, even if the Fc fragment were to be attached to a receptor on a macrophage, no complement would be activated. The lower IgG molecule does indeed span two antigens; were the Fc fragment now to become attached to a macrophage, phagocytosis would in principle be activated. Note that, while it is possible for an IgG molecule to bridge antigens on two neighboring red cells, this is most unlikely since the red cells tend to repel each other because of surface negative charges. The IgG molecule is smaller than the average distance this repulsive force maintains

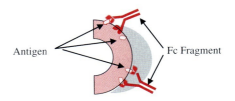

Antigen   Fc Fragment

Fig. 4.1

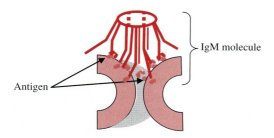

Fig. 4.2

(18 nm). Therefore the formation of agglutinates in the blood is very unusual in IgG-mediated hemolysis.

Figure 4.2 shows a part of two red cell membranes with several antigens (in pink) and an IgM molecule (in red and **NOT** drawn to scale). It will be remembered that the IgM molecule is a pentamer and is very large; potentially each IgM molecule can bind many antigens and, being so large, has a much greater "span". IgM is also very avid and can bind neighboring red cells, thus tending to form agglutinates.

In Fig. 4.2, it can be seen that the IgM molecule spans more than two neighboring antigens, including those on different cells. There is a strong tendency for complement to be activated (the classical pathway). If the Fc fragment were to be attached to a receptor on a macrophage, lysis could occur. However, what happens at this stage is variable. In most cases, activation of the complement pathway halts at the C3 stage; C3 is altered by the membrane to an inactive form, and thus the MAC is not generated, and lysis does not occur. In a minority of cases, complement activation proceeds to completion, resulting in lysis. The exact reasons why this should happen are not clear.

The Basis of the Antiglobulin Test (Coombs)

When any form of immune hemolysis is suspected, it is necessary to prove its existence. This is done by the Coombs test: antibodies against human IgG are raised in animals; adding these antibodies to human red cells that are coated with IgG will cause the cells to agglutinate, proving their presence. Antibodies to C3 would in turn detect the presence of complement (and by extension, IgM).

The Autoimmune Hemolytic Anemias (AIHA)

There are two broad groups of autoimmune hemolytic anemias:

1. **THE PRIMARY OR IDIOPATHIC TYPE.**
2. **SECONDARY AIHA.** These in turn are mainly associated with four groups of conditions or circumstances:

   a. **LYMPHOMAS** and related disorders – see Chapter 22.
   b. **OTHER AUTOIMMUNE DISEASE**, notably SLE.
   c. **CERTAIN INFECTIONS**, notably mycoplasma and many viral infections.
   d. **CERTAIN DRUGS**, notably methyldopa.

The clinical features depend to an extent on whether the responsible antibody is cold or warm, how much antibody is present, and to what extent complement is bound. The clinical presentations are discussed in Chapter 5.

Drug-Induced Hemolytic Disease

Drug-induced hemolysis is by one of three mechanisms:

1. **ANTIBODIES DEVELOPED AGAINST A DRUG** that has been complexed with the red cell membrane. This is mostly found with the penicillins and cephalosporins. It only develops after prolonged, especially high-dosage therapy. The antibody is an IgG and the Coombs is only positive in the presence of the offending drug; the anti-C3 is negative.
2. **DEPOSITION OF IMMUNE COMPLEXES** on the red cell membrane, with activation of complement. This is found classically with quinine and quinidine. Hemolysis only occurs on the second or third exposure to the drug. It is an IgG or IgM antibody and causes intravascular hemolysis. Thus the anti-IgG and the anti-C3 are both positive.
3. **AN AUTOIMMUNE MECHANISM** (as described above). This is a mild extravascular hemolysis. The Coombs test is positive without the drug being present and can remain positive for years.

Autoimmune Diseases and the Blood: Other Aspects

Why the organism should produce antibodies against its own tissues is still imperfectly understood. There are at least two valuable clues:

1. It is known that certain viruses, apart from themselves being antigenic, can attach to cell membranes and induce the formation of antibodies with specificity to that cell type (and perhaps to related cell types). Many of the cytopenias, for example virus-associated

neutropenia, are the result of antibodies raised against the relevant cell type by viral induction.

2. The differing gender prevalences and the possible effect of pregnancy. In the Western world, ± 75% of patients who suffer from autoimmune disease are female. The following factors are known to, or are strongly suspected to, play a role in the pathogenesis:

a. The effect of sex hormones and hormone-related genes. There is good evidence that corticosteroids and progesterone, produced in high quantities during pregnancy, are suppressive of cellular and humoral immunity, by shifting the cytokine balance. There are differing immune environments in males and females, as well as in pregnancy and the non-pregnant state. This is particularly notable in the patterns of cytokine production, especially by the CD4 lymphocytes in response to an infection: males and non-pregnant females are more likely to develop a T_H1 response (dominated by IL-1, IFN-γ, and lymphotoxin) whereas in pregnant females a T_H2 response is predominant (characterized by IL-4, IL-5, IL-6, IL-10, and TGF-β).

b. To some extent overlapping with the above, there is also strong evidence that maternal immune responses during pregnancy are shifted toward antibody-mediated responses and away from cell-mediated responses.

c. There is a strong tendency for women who have complicated pregnancies to produce autoantibodies (not the case in uncomplicated pregnancies). Whether these are due to exacerbation of previously undiagnosed autoimmune disease or to an unknown immune response is not known.

The suggestion thus is that pregnancy, particularly complicated pregnancy, plays a role in facilitating the development of autoantibodies and autoimmune disease. The relation of autoimmune diseases to pregnancy is further discussed later in the chapter in "Pregnancy and Changes in the Blood".

HIV/AIDS, Primarily from the Hematological Perspective

Hematological complications are among the most common features of HIV infection. The blood count almost always shows changes, and just about any abnormality can be found. The hemostatic system is less dramatically involved. There are two basic variants of the HIV virus affecting humans: HIV-1 is prevalent throughout the world and is characterized by slow, progressive deterioration and, without treatment, is almost uniformly fatal; HIV-2 virus is found primarily in West Africa and is characterized by a more benign course.

The **PRIMARY** pathway of HIV infection is the T helper (CD4) cell. This lymphocyte orchestrates the immune responses to infectious organisms as well as to tumor cells. The $CD4^+$ glycoprotein is the receptor for the HIV-1 virus. The CD4 cells are normally long-lived, but once infected their half-life is 1.6 days, with up to 5% of total CD4 cells being destroyed each day. As the CD4 cells decrease, there is not necessarily a lymphopenia until fairly late, since CD8 cells tend to increase.

Of great importance, it should be realized that the rate of progression to AIDS varies: 80% of HIV-infected persons progress within 10 years (the **TYPICAL PROGRESSORS**); 20% develop AIDS within 5 years (the **RAPID PROGRESSORS**; and 2% remain asymptomatic for 12–15 years (the **LONG-TERM NON-PROGRESSORS**).

As the virus multiplies eventually the CD4 cells become depleted, resulting in the gradual development of immune deficiency, and hence with the development of infections and malignancies, as well as damage to several organs. The infections can of course be any, but there is a strong tendency to infection with opportunistic organisms that do not normally cause disease. Similarly the malignancies that often develop are frequently very unusual and are rare in normal people, except for the lymphomas.

There seem also to be **SECONDARY** pathways of infection, notably marrow cells and brain cells. It is thought that the primary effect on the marrow is on the stromal cells and less on hemopoietic precursors, and that the major effect on hemopoiesis is thus most likely to be by interference with cytokine production (by the stromal cells). However, there are numerous other effects on the marrow.

The pathogenesis of hematological changes in HIV is often obscure. Some important factors appear to be

1. **CD34 CELLS** (the stem cells, from which all hematopoietic cells originate, express low levels of CD4, suggesting direct infection by HIV).

2. **MONOCYTES** infected by HIV produce various cytokines that suppress hematopoiesis.

3. **THE ERYTHROPOIETIN RESPONSE** is blunted for the level of anemia. This is a feature of the anemia of chronic disorders. See Chapter 8.

4. **INFECTIONS**, particularly CMV, parvovirus, mycobacteria, and histoplasma.

5. **MARROW INFILTRATION** (by lymphoma, fibrosis, etc.).

6. **HEMOPHAGOCYTOSIS**. This condition will be further discussed in Chapter 13. In brief, increased

numbers of marrow histiocytes are seen to phagocytose precursors, causing cytopenias.

7. **DRUGS**, notably AZT, co-trimoxazole, amphotericin B, and gancyclovir. Drugs are particularly important in the pathogenesis of **ANEMIA**:

    a. **AZT** has pronounced effects:

        i. It inhibits the development of precursor colonies.

        ii. Severe anemia develops in 25% of patients taking 1500 mg/day.

        iii. Macrocytosis develops within weeks of starting AZT; this appears to be due to impaired red cell maturation – it is not corrected by vitamin B_{12} or folate administration. (Note that macrocytosis is a good marker for patient compliance.)

    b. **AMPHOTERICIN B** suppresses EPO production.

    c. **TRIMETHOPRIM** interferes with folate metabolism.

8. **VITAMIN B_{12} DEFICIENCY**. This is found in ± ¼ of cases, even in early asymptomatic disease. It is considered to be due to malabsorption, of uncertain mechanism.

9. **GASTRO-INTESTINAL (GIT) BLEEDING** can occur with involvement of the GIT by Kaposi sarcoma and MALT lymphoma.

10. **MALNUTRITION, NEGLECT, AND CONCURRENT CHRONIC INFECTION**. Folate and iron deficiency contribute to anemia.

The Incidence, Significance, and Pathogenesis of Certain Hematological Findings in AIDS

ANEMIA. Roughly 80% of patients develop anemia, at all stages of the disease:

1. ± 20% of asymptomatic patients are anemic; 5% of patients with a CD4 count of > 700/mm^3 are anemic.
2. 50% of early symptomatic patients are anemic.
3. 75% of later symptomatic patients are anemic.

Note that anemia is an independent risk factor for death, and recovery from anemia is associated with an improved prognosis. The degree of anemia tends to parallel progression of the disease, independent of other factors, such as therapy. There are numerous causes, but not all the mechanisms are known completely.

NEUTROPENIA. The **INCIDENCE** of neutropenia increases with progression of the disease. Bone marrow dysfunction is the major cause. Of interest and clinical importance is that the neutropenia responds well to growth factors (such as GM-CSF).

THROMBOCYTOPENIA. This is very common and may be the presenting feature. The pathogenesis in most cases appears to be immune in origin.

LUPUS ANTICOAGULANT. This is an antibody to the prothrombin complex formed during coagulation. It prolongs the PTT but paradoxically causes thrombosis. See Chapter 21.

LYMPHOMA. The incidence of non-Hodgkin lymphoma is very high and most of these are high-grade B-cell malignancies.

IMMUNOLOGICAL CHANGES. The CD4 count decreases by 40–80 cells/μl per year. The CD8 count increases.

Other Infectious Diseases and the Blood

From the point of view of infectious disease, a very large association with the blood can be predicted. Only a brief overview can be given. Clearly the relationship of blood to infectious process can work in either direction – the blood may show a (part of the) reaction to the infection, and infection can cause damage to the blood and marrow.

Of major clinical and epidemiological significance is hemolytic anemia caused by **INFECTIONS**, and it is necessary to put hemolysis into perspective. A great deal (possibly too much) emphasis is placed on immune causes of hemolysis. **IN FACT, MALARIAL INFECTIONS ARE THE GREATEST CAUSE OF HEMOLYSIS IN THE WORLD.** Many organisms invade the red cell and destroy or damage the red cell membrane. The resultant hemolytic states can vary clinically from the extremely acute and severe to chronic hemolysis (sometimes lasting for years).

In general, infections cause hemolysis by a variety of mechanisms:

1. Direct damage to circulating reticulocytes and/or mature red cells.
2. Some organisms evidently act by inducing antibodies to red cells.
3. Some organisms act by activating the coagulation mechanism, causing DIC; the resultant intravascular fibrin strands directly damage the red cells.

Viruses

There are several hematological conditions or presentations that are associated with viruses. These can present as (more or less in order of frequency)

1. **LYMPHOCYTOSIS**. The most common viruses causing lymphocytosis are

   a. **EPSTEIN–BARR VIRUS** (EBV). Classically this causes infectious mononucleosis and is accompanied by very specific morphologically identifiable atypical lymphocytes. However, it can cause a more non-specific lymphocytosis.
   b. **CYTOMEGALOVIRUS** (CMV).
   c. **HERPES SIMPLEX VIRUS** (HSV).
   d. **VARICELLA–ZOSTER VIRUS** (VZV).
   e. **RUBELLA**. Rubella tends to be forgotten as a cause of changes in the white cells, partly because it is a very mild disease clinically, and the typical rash is often evanescent or even absent.
   f. **HUMAN T-CELL LYMPHOTROPIC VIRUS 1** (HTLV-1).
   g. **ADENOVIRUS**.
   h. Any of the **HEPATITIS VIRUSES**.
   i. In the early stages of **HIV INFECTION** lymphocytosis is frequently observed due to increase in CD8 + cells, despite decrease in CD4 + cells.

   Note that all viral infections tend to cause "atypical" lymphocytes to appear; there may indeed not be an absolute lymphocytosis with viral infections, but a reversal of the neutrophil:lymphocyte ratio is very common indeed.

2. **THROMBOCYTOPENIA**. Acute thrombocytopenia due to viruses is very common in childhood but less common in adults. A large number of common viruses have been implicated. The most common ones appear to be EBV, Rubella, and CMV. Viruses may induce thrombocytopenia in several ways:

   a. Early in the infection, viruses can invade megakaryocytes and thence interfere with platelet production.
   b. Viruses can attach to platelets and cause thrombocytopenia either by promoting intravascular aggregation or by precipitating clearance by the spleen.
   c. Viruses may have a direct toxic effect on platelets.
   d. Virus-induced vasculitis may lead to microangiopathy with platelet adherence.
   e. Occasionally, some viruses may cause a DIC-like picture, with consumption of platelets, etc.

3. **NEUTROPENIA**. Many viruses have been implicated in the pathogenesis of neutropenia, such as respiratory syncytial virus (RSV), EBV, influenza, CMV, HIV, hepatitis, rubella, adenovirus, coxsackie viruses and parvovirus. The mechanisms are generally uncertain; some, such as parvovirus and HIV, are thought to act via virus-induced antineutrophil antibodies.

4. **LYMPHOPENIA**. Many viruses have been implicated in transient lymphopenia. HIV, of course, is the classic cause of a permanent lymphopenia.

5. **PANCYTOPENIA**. The biggest culprit here is parvovirus B19, which, while it can cause conditions in other systems like erythema infectiosum ("slapped cheek" syndrome or fifth disease) and polyarthropathy, has a major impact on the blood system, where it can cause aplastic anemia, especially in patients with a previously **COMPENSATORY** hypercellular marrow (as in hereditary spherocytosis).

6. **BLEEDING DISORDERS**. Viruses may be associated with a bleeding tendency in several ways:

   a. **THROMBOCYTOPENIA**.
   b. **DIC**, particularly arboviruses. (With viruses, DIC tends to take a somewhat more chronic and in many ways an atypical form, especially arboviruses.)
   c. The **VIRAL HEMORRHAGIC FEVERS**. A large number of viruses are associated with generally extremely serious bleeding disorders with fever and a very poor prognosis.
   d. Some viruses are known to be associated with the development of **ACQUIRED INHIBITORS OF COAGULATION FACTORS**, notably factor VIII. The bleeding from this acquired hemophilia can be very serious.

Bacteria

Again there is a typical and non-specific reaction to bacterial infections – neutrophilia, characteristically associated with a left shift and toxic granulation (see Chapter 15). The organisms attacking immuno-compromised subjects are often unusual.

Protozoa

A few organisms are significant in blood disease: plasmodia (malaria), toxoplasma, filariae, and trypanosomes.

1. **MALARIA**. This is one of the single biggest killers in the world. The specific organismal type varies:

   a. **PLASMODIUM FALCIPARUM**. This form of malaria is the commonest in Africa, but it also occurs in Asia, Central and South America, and the Middle East. It commonly presents with high fever, anemia, jaundice, mental confusion, and renal failure. Overt DIC may develop. Hemoglobinuria ("blackwater fever") may occur.
   b. **PLASMODIUM OVALE** occurs only in Africa.
   c. **PLASMODIUM VIVAX** is the commonest form in Asia but otherwise has a similar distribution as falciparum. It is said not to be common in Africa – this is

incorrect; indeed double infections with falciparum and vivax occur quite regularly in certain regions.

d. **PLASMODIUM MALARIAE** is uncommon and occurs in all malarial areas.

2. **FILARIASIS**. Two species of filaria are relevant to hematology. These are often associated with marked eosinophilia:

a. **WUCHERERIA BANCROFTI**. This is especially common in Asia, but also found in Africa and the Pacific Islands.

b. **BRUGIA MALAYI**. This is found in China, Indo-China, Thailand, Malaysia, Philippines, and southeast India.

3. **TRYPANOSOMIASIS** (sleeping sickness).

a. **TRYPANOSOMA BRUCEI RHODESIENSE** is endemic to East Africa.

b. **TRYPANOSOMA BRUCEI GAMBIENSE** is endemic to West and Central Africa.

4. **TOXOPLASMA GONDII**. Its only hematological association is as a cause of the infectious mononucleosis syndrome – see below – and in the differential diagnosis of cervical lymphadenopathy.

Nematodes and Trematodes

The effect on the blood is primarily an eosinophilia. This is discussed in Chapter 15. **SCHISTOSOMIASIS** deserves a special mention. It is the most common cause of hepatosplenomegaly in the world and frequently leads to portal ("pipe-stem") fibrosis, portal hypertension with bleeding varices, and hypersplenism (with anemia and/or leukopenia and/or thrombocytopenia).

The Infectious Mononucleosis (IM) Syndromes

The classic IM syndrome is caused by the EB virus. There are four other organisms that can produce a very similar clinical syndrome: cytomegalovirus, HHV-6 (human herpesvirus-6), HIV, and toxoplasmosis. Their distinction as well as the clinical features of IM are discussed in Chapter 15.

The Cardiovascular System and Blood Diseases

The cardiovascular system (CVS) is relevant to hematology in five groups of conditions or states:

1. **THE REACTION OF THE CVS TO ANEMIA**. This is discussed earlier in this chapter.

2. **MISDIAGNOSIS**.

a. **SEVERE CORONARY ARTERY DISEASE** as well as chronic cardiac failure, especially left ventricular failure, tends to cause, in many patients, considerable pallor, which may be misconstrued as anemia.

b. **CONGESTIVE CARDIAC FAILURE** may be misdiagnosed in the superior vena cava syndrome, where the JVP is very high but is not pulsatile and without hepatojugular reflux. The patient appears plethoric but in fact is anemic.

c. **THE SUBCLAVIAN STEAL SYNDROME** (obstruction of the subclavian artery, usually on the left side) may cause plethora of the head.

d. Finally, **SEVERE CORONARY ARTERY DISEASE** might be diagnosed in a patient presenting with angina and even submitted to catherization if the severe anemia were not noticed. The majority of patients over the age of 50 with severe anemia **PRESENT** with angina; this is not to say that the patients do not have coronary artery disease – it merely means that its severity is overestimated; the anemia needs to be corrected first and urgently.

3. The coronary arteries may be involved in various **VASCULITIC SYNDROMES**.

4. **PULMONARY ARTERIAL HYPERTENSION** can complicate a number of hematological conditions, and the mechanisms are frequently obscure:

a. Chronic myeloproliferative disorders,
b. Thalassemia major (see Chapter 8) and sickle disease (see Chapter 10),
c. Some chronic hemolytic anemias including paroxysmal nocturnal hemoglobinuria.

5. **MICRO-VASCULAR DISEASE** with endothelial swelling and dysfunction, typically associated with disturbances of coagulation, is a pathogenetic mechanism that is achieving greater and greater prominence, particularly in the complications of diabetes and the pathogenesis of septic shock, multiple organ dysfunction and inflammatory bowel disease.

The Gastro-intestinal Tract (GIT) and Blood Disease

The relationship of the blood to the gut is especially important. Many blood diseases (of the reactive and secondary types) are caused by pathology in the GIT;

conversely, some blood diseases have secondary effects on the GIT, often of importance as diagnostic clues. Thus, in developed countries, the commonest source of iron deficiency is bleeding from the GIT and is sometimes very difficult to find. Many of these bleeding lesions produce lesions in other systems, enabling at least a suspicion of what the underlying pathology is.

Generally, however, there are several pathological processes of relevance to the blood. Some of these processes will be local to a site, but others can span many (or all) of the different parts of the tract. An overview of these basic clinico-pathological presentations is as follows:

1. **BLEEDING**. Bleeding can occur from any site along the length of the tract. If acute, it can result in **HEMORRHAGIC SHOCK AND LATER ANEMIA**; if chronic it may present with **IRON DEFICIENCY**. GIT bleeding can be divided into local causes and general (systemic) causes:

    a. **LOCAL CAUSES**.

        i. **BENIGN CONDITIONS**, such as polyps.
        ii. **MALIGNANT EROSIVE CONDITIONS**. The most important conditions here are carcinoma and lymphoma.
        iii. **CHRONIC INFLAMMATORY CONDITIONS** ⎱ These can
        iv. **VASCULAR ABNORMALITIES** ⎰ be fairly general.

    b. **SYSTEMIC (USUALLY GENERAL) CONDITIONS**.

        i. **POLYCYTHEMIA VERA**.
        ii. **ESSENTIAL THROMBOCYTHEMIA**.
        iii. **PORTAL HYPERTENSION**.
        iv. **PEUTZ–JEGHERS SYNDROME**.
        v. **POLYARTERITIS NODOSA**.
        vi. **HENOCH–SCHöNLEIN VASCULITIS**.
        vii. **AMYLOIDOSIS**.
        viii. **TYPE IV EHLERS–DANLOS SYNDROME**.

2. **DIVERTICULAR DISEASE**,
3. **COMPLICATIONS OF GASTRO-INTESTINAL SURGERY**.
4. **FUNCTIONAL DEFICIENCIES**.

    a. **ACHLORHYDRIA**.
    b. **LOSS OF TEETH, ILL-FITTING DENTURES, DISORDERS INTERFERING WITH CHEWING ABILITY**.
    c. **RAPID TRANSIT SYNDROMES**.

5. **LIVER, BILIARY, AND PANCREATIC DISEASE**.

    a. **ACUTE** and **CHRONIC HEPATITIS**.

    b. **BILIARY DISEASE**.
    c. **PANCREATIC DISEASE**.

6. **MALABSORPTION**.
7. **MISCELLANEOUS CONDITIONS**.

Bleeding

The clinical features of gastro-intestinal bleeding should be well known to you. It is a very common cause of iron deficiency and may be occult.

1. **BENIGN CONDITIONS**.

    a. **PEPTIC ULCERATION** should require no special discussion, except that it can occur in some atypical areas: the esophagus, in a hiatal hernia, and in a Meckel's diverticulum. The latter two especially may be very difficult to suspect.
    b. **IRRITANTS**, especially to the gastric mucosa, such as very spicy food, alcohol, aspirin, NSAIDS.
    c. Bleeding may occur as a complication of

        i. **DIVERTICULOSIS**. Diverticular disease mainly affects the colon, but can affect the small bowel as well. Apart from perforation and peritonitis, a major complication is infection and bleeding.
        ii. **POLYPS**.
        iii. **ISCHEMIC COLITIS** (in the elderly).

2. **MALIGNANT EROSIVE CONDITIONS. CARCINOMA** of the stomach is far less common than previously, but carcinoma of the colon is a major health problem. However, advances in diagnosis, surgical techniques, and other therapy have significantly reduced their impact. Surgical intervention has several potential hematological sequelae, and these are discussed below.

    LYMPHOMA OF THE STOMACH is not rare, especially of the MALT-type. This appears to be associated with **HELICOBACTER PYLORI** infection and this can cause chronic bleeding apart from the effects of the lymphoma itself.

3. **CHRONIC INFLAMMATORY CONDITIONS**. Bleeding frequently occurs as a complication of inflammatory bowel disease, diverticulitis, and dysentery.

4. **VASCULAR ABNORMALITIES**. Because of their propensity to bleed, vascular malformations are important, especially as causes of occult and obscure bleeding (these two terms will be defined in Chapter 5). Also, they tend generally not to be thought of. There are a great many types of these lesions:

a. **HEREDITARY**. These are generally rare except for the Rendu–Osler–Weber syndrome (hereditary hemorrhagic telangiectasia or HHT).

HEREDITARY HEMORRHAGIC TELANGIECTASIA.

This condition is inherited in an autosomal dominant fashion with an equal incidence in all racial groups and both sexes. It is characterized by

i. Telangiectases that blanch under pressure and are found in the skin, mucosa, and soft tissues. These can be responsible for occult and obscure bleeding. Epistaxis is the commonest feature.

ii. AV malformations. These can be found anywhere, but can be responsible for severe morbidity when in the lungs: there is a tendency for coagulation to be initiated in these fistulae; the resultant thrombi tend to cause paradoxical emboli to the brain, with potentially disastrous results.

The diagnosis is made by using the Curaçao criteria (see Chapters 6 and 8).

THE PEUTZ–JEGHER SYNDROME.

This syndrome is characterized by freckling of the lips and palms and associated with multiple hamartomatous malformations throughout the gut, which tend to bleed, since they generally are very vascular.

b. **ACQUIRED**. These include radiation-induced ectasias and vascular tumors, but by far the most important is angiodysplasia.

ANGIODYSPLASIA can affect any part of the GIT and can be widespread. It is found in 2% of autopsies. While it is far more common in patients over 60 years, it has been found in persons in the age group of 20 to 30. The etiology is uncertain. These abnormalities are usually quite small with a stellate pattern and are thin-walled, often consisting only of endothelium. They tend to bulge into the lumen and bleed readily. The risk of bleeding is increased in bleeding disorders, particularly von Willebrand disease. These lesions have been associated with other conditions, most prominently aortic stenosis (Heyde syndrome): in this condition von Willebrand factor is used up because of the high shear stress across the valve; this deficiency then appears to promote bleeding from the angiodysplastic lesions. Diagnosis can sometimes be made by scintigraphy, but usually requires endoscopy. Of particular difficulty in this regard is angiodysplasia of the small bowel, since enteroscopy is not widely available.

5. **SYSTEMIC CONDITIONS** (as listed above). These are rare.

Diverticular Disease

Congenital diverticulae can be found in any portion of the GIT – indeed 15% of normal people have a few. The pathogenesis of acquired diverticulae is uncertain, and possible causes vary with the site.

1. **COLONIC DIVERTICULAE** are most common in the sigmoid. They are very common in the West and rare in, for example, Africa. Their prevalence parallels the increase in consumption of refined carbohydrates and decrease in the consumption of fiber. The resultant tendency to constipation will tend to increase the intraluminal pressures, acting on areas of natural weakness, such as the entrance of vascular loops. The complications are infection and bleeding, which can be severe.

2. **JEJUNAL DIVERTICULAE**. The cause is unknown; some patients probably have either a localized form of systemic sclerosis, autonomic neuropathy, or myenteric plexus abnormality. Only about a quarter of patients are symptomatic, and the symptoms are suggestive of chronic intestinal obstruction. Bleeding is rare.

3. **MECKEL'S DIVERTICULUM**. It is found in the ileum "**2** ft from the ileo-cecal valve, in **2**% of people, and is **2 INCHES** long". It is usually asymptomatic. Some develop ectopic gastric mucosa with the production of acid and consequent peptic ulceration and bleeding. Diagnosis is very difficult.

Gastro-intestinal Surgery and Its Complications

Gastric Surgery

The important hematological sequelae are iron deficiency from blood loss, malabsorption, and decreased intake; vitamin B_{12} deficiency from malabsorption; folate deficiency; and occasionally vitamin K deficiency.

1. **TOTAL GASTRECTOMY** is usually performed for carcinoma. One can predict that vitamin B_{12} deficiency (due to lack of intrinsic factor from the proximal

stomach) would supervene after 4 years. Previously, survival after surgery was poor, with insufficient time for vitamin B_{12} deficiency to develop. Earlier diagnosis, however, is leading to progressively improved survival and thus the development of megaloblastic anemia. Note that, in contrast, iron deficiency can, depending on the state of the stores and complications of surgery, develop quite rapidly.

2. **PARTIAL GASTRECTOMY.** With the development of triple therapy for **H. PYLORI** infections, this operation is done very infrequently. But there are still many patients on whom the operation was done in the past. On most of them it would have been vagotomy plus some sort of drainage procedure, such as gastrojejunostomy. However, among the elderly, one still occasionally comes across Billroth II and even Billroth I types. Possible hematological effects are as follows:

   a. Since vagotomy was done more or less as a routine, the effects of **HYPO- OR ACHLORHYDRIA** may be seen – essentially on iron absorption (see Chapter 2). More recent techniques have permitted far more selective vagotomy, which reduces this complication.

   b. **SECONDARY MUCOSAL ATROPHY** (10–15% incidence) may eventually result in intrinsic factor and therefore vitamin B_{12} deficiency.

   c. **BLIND LOOPS** may occur as a result either of the types of surgery (Billroth II) or due to post-operative adhesions. Overgrowth of bacteria in these loops can lead to consumption of vitamin B_{12} and hence megaloblastic anemia. (See later under Bacterial Overgrowth Syndromes.)

   d. **STOMAL ULCERATION** may result in chronic or acute bleeding.

   e. **MALABSORPTION** may result from the dumping syndrome or steatorrhea (after Billroth II); this can be aggravated by a blind loop. Malabsorption of heme iron (i.e., in red meat) is common after **SUBTOTAL GASTRECTOMY** (interestingly, medicinal iron is usually well absorbed).

Anemia After Gastric Surgery: A Summary The commonest causes are due to iron, vitamin B_{12}, and/or folate deficiencies. There are several mechanisms:

1. Food intake is often diminished after gastric surgery, although this is rarely the main cause of an anemia.
2. Vitamin B_{12} deficiency may develop as a result of lack of intrinsic factor (gastric atrophy) or be

due to bacterial overgrowth, with bacterial consumption of the vitamin.
3. Iron deficiency can result from chronic bleeding (stomal ulcers, etc.) or malabsorption (notably after Billroth II operations).
4. Folate deficiency may result from any cause of intestinal hurry (e.g., dumping syndrome) or steatorrhea.

Intestinal Surgery

In discussing the hematological sequelae of intestinal surgery, much depends on what parts of the bowel are resected.

RESECTION OF UP TO 50% of the middle parts of the small intestine is well tolerated. However, **RESECTION OF 70–80%** results in catastrophic malabsorption. The effects are aggravated by the frequent development of hyperchlorhydria, as well as by increased colonic secretions due to hydroxy fatty acids (from bacterial hydroxylation of unabsorbed fat).

RESECTION OF THE DUODENUM OR DISTAL ILEUM results in symptoms associated with malabsorption in, respectively, the most proximal regions (iron, calcium, and folate) and of the most distal (vitamin B_{12}, and of bile salts which have an effect on vitamin K absorption).

Functional Deficiencies

1. **ACHLORHYDRIA.** This is quite a common condition. It may have specific causes, such as gastric mucosal atrophy, or may be found in general conditions such as cachexia, severe debility, etc.
2. **RAPID TRANSIT SYNDROMES**. These vary from anatomical disruptions caused by certain types of gastric surgery to post-gastrectomy dumping syndrome to infections to certain hormonal abnormalities.

Liver and Biliary Disease

Liver disease is a major cause of hematological abnormalities in practice; practically all the different FBC and hemostatic test appearances can be found.

JAUNDICE is a cardinal feature suggesting liver disease. Any of the three types of jaundice – hemolytic, hepatocellular, and obstructive – may have implications for blood disease.

1. **HEMOLYTIC JAUNDICE.** The blood will almost always show a reticulocytosis, and the smear may show clearly what the likely cause is. Hemolytic anemias are discussed extensively in Chapter 2 and in this chapter.
2. **OBSTRUCTIVE JAUNDICE.** Hematological findings are discussed below.
3. **HEPATOCELLULAR JAUNDICE.** Findings here are also discussed below.

HEPATOMEGALY may reflect disease (such as cirrhosis) that can cause blood changes or coagulation defects or it may be the result of blood disease, such as infiltration by leukemia, lymphoma, or amyloidosis.

Hemostatic Changes

THROMBOCYTOPENIA is common. There are several mechanisms:

1. **ADHERENCE OF PLATELETS** to activated endothelium within the sinusoids. This activation in found especially in cirrhosis, where the nodules stretch the sinusoids.
2. Due to **HYPERSPLENISM** complicating portal hypertension.
3. **ASSOCIATED WITH DIC** complicating hepatic insufficiency.
4. **BONE MARROW DISEASE** due to alcohol and/or folate deficiency.

COAGULATION DEFICIENCY AND FIBRINO-LYTIC ABNORMALITIES too are common. The mechanisms are as follows:

1. **THE LIVER MANUFACTURES AND CONTROLS** the plasma levels of most of the factors of the coagulation and fibrinolytic system (the exceptions being von Willebrand factor and plasminogen activators). Normally it maintains the plasma levels within narrow limits.
2. **THE LIVER CATABOLIZES** many of the factors.
3. **THE LIVER PERFORMS A VITAL MOLECULAR MODIFICATION** of factors II, VII, IX, and X, as discussed in Chapter 2.
4. **THE RETICULO-ENDOTHELIAL SYSTEM** in the liver is one of the prime tissues responsible for the clearance of activated clotting and fibrinolytic factors, activation complexes, and end-products of fibrin formation from fibrinogen.

Thus in summary, **LIVER DISEASE MAY LEAD TO IMPAIRED COAGULATION DUE TO**

a. **DECREASED PRODUCTION OF CLOTTING FACTORS** (synthesis)
b. **PRODUCTION OF FUNCTIONALLY DEFEC-TIVE COAGULATION FACTORS** (vitamin K deficiency)
c. **INCREASED CONSUMPTION** of coagulation factors
d. **DISTURBED CLEARANCE** of circulating activation components

From the clinical point of view, it is worthwhile to look at the hemostatic changes in different types of liver disease.

ACUTE AND NON-CIRRHOTIC CHRONIC HEPATOCELLULAR DISEASE. In acute mild hepatitis and acute alcoholism there may be no changes. However, mild decreases in the vitamin K-dependent factors, particularly factor VII, tend to occur early. The prothrombin time (PT) may thus be slightly prolonged. The PT is probably the best liver function test in acute liver disease. With progressive or more serious disease, other factors may be diminished, thus producing a prolonged partial thromboplastin time (PTT), with the exception frequently of factor VIII, which may be markedly elevated, and of fibrinogen which may also be increased.

SEVERE OR FULMINANT LIVER DISEASE shows a number of changes: more severe prolongation of the PT and PTT and a sharp drop in fibrinogen levels. The latter may only be obvious with functional assays of fibrinogen, since dysfunctional fibrinogen molecules are frequently found. In addition: other features of DIC may be present; increased fibrinolytic activity may be found; and thrombocytopenia, usually mild, is common.

CIRRHOSIS. Once again, hemostatic defects tend to mirror the degree of the disease. The defects are in the procoagulant factors, the liver-dependent anticoagulant and fibrinolytic factors, and defects in platelet function and sometimes platelet numbers. Different aspects of the hemostatic mechanism are affected at different stages. Thrombocytopenia and platelet dysfunction are common.

VITAMIN K DEFICIENCY AND BILIARY CIR-RHOSIS. The hemostatic abnormalities found in these two conditions are fairly similar. Vitamin K deficiency may be found: in biliary tract obstruction or biliary fistulae; prolonged antibiotic therapy particularly in children and the elderly; and anticoagulants of the coumarin or indanedione groups causing an effective vitamin K deficiency by metabolic blockage of vitamin K utilization.

Biliary tract obstruction itself can have varied hematological features. Chronic cholecystitis may have flare-ups, with neutrophilia; this is especially important since the clinical features of gallstones are notoriously vague (or absent). Ascending bacterial infection in the presence of obstruction can cause marked effects, e.g., Charcot's intermittent biliary fever characterized by intermittent jaundice, fever, prostration, and severe neutrophilia or leukemoid reaction. Complete obstruction is associated with vitamin K deficiency and a consequent bleeding tendency.

The Pancreas

There are only a few aspects of pancreatic disease of relevance in hematology, and those are some of the complications of acute pancreatitis, chronic pancreatitis, and pancreatic cancer.

1. **ACUTE PANCREATITIS**. The major hematological problem is the development of DIC and hyperfibrinolysis.
2. **CHRONIC PANCREATITIS**. The major hematological problem is the development of pancreatic insufficiency, with abnormalities in digestion and absorption of fats and of vitamins K and B_{12}.
3. **PANCREATIC CANCER**. This may be associated with hypercoagulability, particularly migrating thrombophlebitis (Trousseau's sign) and splenic vein thrombosis.

Malabsorption and the Malabsorption Syndromes

The impact of malabsorption should not be underestimated. Any of the four major nutrients relevant to blood diseases, i.e., iron, folate, and vitamins B_{12} and K may be deficient due to malabsorption, although the incidence varies with each. Of iron deficiencies 8% are due to malabsorption of iron; malabsorption of folate is a common cause of megaloblastic anemia; and vitamin B_{12} deficiency is primarily a disorder of absorption. Vitamin K deficiency due to malabsorption is common in certain circumstances only. Yet malabsorption is unfortunately very often an afterthought, especially in iron deficiency and bleeding tendencies. A major complication in the assessment of malabsorption is that many of the causes

and processes mentioned below can also lead to acute or chronic gastro-intestinal bleeding with iron deficiency, considerably complicating the diagnosis.

The causes of malabsorption may be grouped as follows:

1. **DISORDERS OF DIGESTION**
2. **DISORDERS OF THE ABSORPTIVE SURFACE**
3. **DISORDERS OF THE LYMPHATICS**
4. **DISORDERS OF MULTIPLE CAUSATION**
5. **DRUGS CAUSING MALABSORPTION**

All of the above may be associated with malabsorption of the four main hematological nutrients. Commonly malabsorption of these is due to more than one of the above. Note that, while the decrease in these nutrients may be part of a general malabsorption (i.e., many other nutrients also not being absorbed), **ISOLATED MALABSORPTION OF ONE OR MORE ONLY OF THESE HEMATOLOGICAL NUTRIENTS CAN OCCUR,** posing a special diagnostic problem, since one tends not to think of malabsorption in these circumstances.

Disorders of Digestion Causing Malabsorption

There are four general groups of conditions interfering with digestion: **GASTRIC PATHOLOGIES** producing either achlorhydria or hyperchlorhydria; **PANCREATIC DISEASE, DEFECTIVE INTRALUMINAL BILE SALT ACTIVITY**, and **INCREASED SPEED OF PASSAGE** of the gastro-intestinal contents ("intestinal hurry").

Gastric Disorders of Digestion

As mentioned, a complicating problem is that many of these diseases are also associated with bleeding, leading to iron deficiency through blood loss, as well as contributing to iron malabsorption. These disorders can be classed as

1. **CHRONIC GASTRITIS AND GASTRIC MUCOSAL ATROPHY**.
2. **INFILTRATIVE DISORDERS OF THE STOMACH**.
3. **THE COMPLICATIONS OF GASTRIC SURGERY**.
4. **HYPERACIDITY STATES**.

1. **CHRONIC GASTRITIS**. There are **THREE FAIRLY COMMON FORMS**, and these may in certain cases represent different stages of the same disease: **CHRONIC SUPERFICIAL GASTRITIS,**

CHRONIC ATROPHIC GASTRITIS, AND GASTRIC ATROPHY. In practice, chronic gastritis is divided into

a. **TYPE A CHRONIC GASTRITIS.** This involves the body and fundus and is associated with atrophy. It is regarded as an autoimmune condition. Pernicious anemia is primarily a type A gastritis.
b. **TYPE B CHRONIC GASTRITIS** is more common and typically is most severe in the antrum. It is usually associated with **H. PYLORI** infection.

In addition, there are six uncommon forms of chronic gastritis, only one of which is relevant to us here, viz.

c. **EOSINOPHILIC GASTROENTEROPATHY.** As the name suggests, it occurs anywhere in the GIT. It is idiopathic, causes pain, watery diarrhea, and protein loss, and is associated with prominent peripheral eosinophilia.

2. **INFILTRATIVE DISORDERS OF THE STOMACH.** These may cause symptoms in several ways:

a. Vague feelings of fullness may diminish appetite.
b. They may mechanically interfere with the mixing function of the stomach, with poor digestion.
c. They may be associated with achlorhydria, with an effect on the digestion of meat and the absorption of iron.
d. Systemic symptoms, due to the lesion itself.

3. **GASTRIC SURGERY MAY HAVE SEVERAL COMPLICATIONS AFFECTING DIGESTION AND ABSORPTION.** A lot depends on the type of surgery. These have been discussed above.

Pancreatic Disorders of Digestion

Proper digestion requires the following substances to emerge from the ampulla of Vater: lipase, proteases, HCO_3^{2-}, and bile salts. Pancreatic disorders may be primary or secondary.

PRIMARY PANCREATIC DISORDERS leading to defective digestion are chronic pancreatitis and pancreatic carcinoma. Among many other defects, deficiency of pancreatic lipase is an important cause of defective fat absorption and therefore of the fat-soluble vitamins, including vitamin K.

The most important cause of **SECONDARY PANCREATIC INSUFFICIENCY** is a gastrinoma, where constant high acid levels lead to inactivation of pancreatic lipase. Frequent associated peptic ulcers can lead to bleeding and iron deficiency.

Decreased Intraluminal Bile Salts

There are three broad groups of conditions:

1. **OBSTRUCTIVE LIVER DISEASE** especially biliary cirrhosis.
2. **DISEASE OR BYPASS OF THE DISTAL ILEUM**, interfering with the enterohepatic circulation of vitamin K and folate. Absorption of vitamin B_{12} is obviously also going to be compromised. Surgery for Crohn disease may do this, (thus adding the hematological complications of Crohn disease to the picture).
3. **BACTERIAL OVERGROWTH.** This has many effects, causing malabsorption by many different mechanisms (see later), but in this case it includes decreased deconjugation of bile salts.

Gastro-intestinal Hurry

Many conditions, particularly including certain forms of gastric surgery, can have as a complication very rapid movement of gastric contents down into the intestines (notably the "dumping syndrome"), with limited time for digestion. This significantly interferes with necessary processing of foods, preparatory to further absorption, and can affect all the relevant nutrients.

Disorders of the Absorptive Surface Causing Malabsorption

These may be divided into three groups: a decrease in the actual amount of surface; diffuse disease of the small intestine; and specific mucosal defects.

1. **DECREASE IN TOTAL ABSORPTIVE SURFACE.** This may be found in short-bowel syndrome (see Intestinal Surgery and Its Complications above) or fistulae.
2. **DIFFUSE DISEASE OF THE SMALL INTESTINE.** A large number of conditions are relevant:

a. Known or possible **IMMUNOLOGICAL INJURY**, such as gluten enteropathy and Crohn disease, and eosinophilic gastroenteropathy.
b. Known or possible **INFECTIONS**, such as tropical sprue, Whipple disease, bacterial overgrowth.
c. **INFILTRATIVE CONDITIONS** such as lymphoma and amyloidosis.
d. **FIBROTIC** conditions such as systemic sclerosis (scleroderma).

Only three conditions will very briefly be discussed: adult-onset gluten enteropathy, tropical sprue, and eosinophilic gastroenteropathy. Whipple disease and bacterial overgrowth cause malabsorption by multiple mechanisms and are briefly mentioned later.

Gluten Enteropathy (Celiac Sprue)

It is often thought that celiac disease is essentially a disease of children; however, while uncommon in adults, it is a distinct cause of nutritional anemias. The condition is due to hypersensitivity to gluten, with damage to and atrophy of the intestinal villi. In the adult it may not present typically and can demonstrate highly selective absorptive defects, such as of iron or folate alone.

Tropical Sprue

This is a disease of unknown etiology found in persons living in or even visiting certain areas, like Southeast Asia and the Caribbean. It can cause devastating epidemics. Features are typical but in addition there may be fever and anorexia. It typically affects vitamin B_{12} and folate. It responds dramatically to tetracycline therapy.

Certain Parasitoses

Notably **STRONGYLOIDES STERCORALIS**, may cause malabsorption, along with diarrhea and abdominal pain and are associated with a marked eosinophilia, although most cases are asymptomatic. This infection is common in Southeast Asia and is found also in expatriates living in the area and soldiers who had served there. It must be differentiated from eosinophilic gastroenteropathy, and this can be very difficult, since stool examination for ova is not very sensitive. Note that in the immune compromised, the eosinophilia tends to disappear, making the diagnosis even more difficult.

Eosinophilic Gastroenteropathy

There are different presentations, varying with the histological appearances, obstructive (mainly antral involvement), to classical malabsorption (mainly small bowel mucosa), to ascites (serosal involvement). The significant diagnostic factor is **PRONOUNCED PERIPHERAL EOSINOPHILIA**.

In the malabsorption form, there is evidence of iron deficiency, hypoproteinemia (with edema), hypocalcemia, increased fat in the stools, and an abnormal D-xylose test.

The condition responds dramatically to steroids, but it is strongly recommended that a course of albendazole be given before steroids.

Disorders of the Lymphatics Causing Malabsorption

Most disorders causing malabsorption because of lymphatic disease also have other pathological effects on the gut and are thus discussed under Multiple Mechanisms Causing Malabsorption.

Most lymphomas seem to affect the distal ileum, but stomach involvement is not rare. There is a variant called the "Mediterranean lymphoma" that predominantly affects the duodenum and jejunum.

Drugs Causing Malabsorption

1. **TETRACYCLINE**: **IRON** (by chelation)
2. **ANTACIDS**: **IRON** (by binding)
3. **PHENYTOIN**: **FOLATE** (by competitive binding)
4. **ALCOHOL**:

    a. **FOLATE** (toxic effect on mucosa)
    b. **VITAMIN B_{12}** (toxic effect on mucosa)

5. **METHOTREXATE**: **FOLATE** (competition for binding site)
6. **COLCHICINE**: **VITAMIN B_{12}** (mucosal damage)
7. **METFORMIN**: **VITAMIN B_{12}** (mucosal damage)

Multiple Mechanisms Causing Malabsorption

The following are the most important. Some have been discussed under other headings, indicating the predominant mechanism:

1. Post-gastrectomy steatorrhea
2. Bacterial overgrowth
3. Disease or bypass of the distal ileum
4. Scleroderma
5. Lymphoma
6. Whipple disease
7. Diabetes mellitus

Bacterial Overgrowth Syndromes

The lumen of the normal proximal small bowel contains $< 10^5$ bacteria per ml, mostly swallowed from the oropharynx. Excessive growth is normally prevented by active intestinal motility and gastric acid. It follows therefore that the two major causes of bacterial proliferation are **ACHLORHYDRIA** and **STASIS**.

STASIS can occur in many conditions, the most important being

1. After some forms of gastric surgery (especially Billroth II)

2. Blind intestinal loops developing as a result of post-operative adhesions
3. Diverticulae
4. Strictures, e.g., as a complication of Crohn disease and vascular disease
5. Scleroderma and amyloidosis

Note that vagotomy may result in bacterial overgrowth for reasons of both hypochlorhydria and motor insufficiency.

The major effect is malabsorption. This is a general malabsorption but particularly significant is the effect on vitamin B_{12}:

1. Bacterial hydrolysis of bile salts causes defective fat digestion and results in steatorrhea.
2. By-products of bacterial metabolism are toxic to the mucosa.
3. The bacteria consume free and bound vitamin B_{12}.

BACTERIAL OVERGROWTH SHOULD BE SUSPECTED IN ANY PATIENT WITH

1. Unexplained diarrhea,
2. Steatorrhea,
3. Weight loss,
4. Unexplained macrocytic anemia,

WHO ALSO HAS FEATURES SUSPICIOUS OF ANY OF THE FOLLOWING UNDERLYING CAUSES, i.e.,

a. Previous gastric or other abdominal surgery
b. Raynaud's phenomenon, dysphagia, and/or heartburn (scleroderma)
c. Known Crohn disease

Proving the diagnosis is difficult and requires referral. Treatment involves that of the underlying condition as well as tetracycline plus metronidazole.

Whipple Disease

This is a chronic condition characterized by arthritis and malabsorption with characteristic findings on small bowel biopsy. It is caused by a gram-negative organism, **TROPHERYMA WHIPELLI**; 50% of patients have fever and this may be the presenting symptom; ± 75% of patients have intermittent arthritis with acute attacks lasting for days to weeks. Over 90% of patients have small bowel disease resulting in malabsorption; the arthritis can antedate the malabsorption by years.

Other Features That May Be Clues to Malabsorption

Clinically one sometimes comes across one or more associated features that may suggest malabsorption and sometimes its cause.

1. **FEVER**: Possible inflammatory bowel disease and Whipple disease.
2. **LYMPHADENOPATHY**: Possible lymphoma or Whipple disease.
3. Skin manifestations:

   a. **DERMATITIS HERPETIFORMIS**: Possible celiac disease.
   b. **PYODERMA**: Possible inflammatory bowel disease.
   c. **HYPERPIGMENTATION** can occur.

A Summary of the Causes of Malabsorption of Hematological Nutrients

A very brief outline of the normal absorption of these elements has been given in Chapter 2. However, for malabsorption of these elements properly to be understood, a further brief review is in order, if only for reference.

The Absorption of Iron and Its Defects

1. **IRON IS ONLY ABSORBED IN THE FERROUS FORM**. Ingested iron can be in two forms – heme iron in red meat (already in the ferrous form) and inorganic (ferric) iron in dairy products and vegetables. While the iron in tablets and injections is in the ferrous form it is usually inorganic, although in recent years preparations of ferrous iron complexed with certain sugars are available; these are very effective but cannot be considered as organic iron from the physiological absorption point of view. Heme iron requires gastric acid for release of the heme. Thus in gastrectomy, gastric atrophy, and other causes of achlorhydria, iron derived from red meat is jeopardized. Similarly, acid is required for the reduction of ingested ferric iron.

2. **IRON IS MOSTLY ABSORBED IN THE DUODENUM AND UPPER JEJUNUM**. Thus extensive disease of these structures may be associated with iron malabsorption. These are relatively uncommon and include gluten enteropathy (with villous atrophy), extensive involvement by conditions such as Crohn disease, and infiltration by lymphoma (as mentioned, the so-called "Mediterranean lymphoma" primarily attacks the duodenum and jejunum).

   In addition, the antral, duodenal, and upper jejunal mucosa exert considerable control over how much iron can be absorbed.

3. **CERTAIN DRUGS CAN CAUSE MALABSORPTION**. These have been mentioned. To recap, tetracycline and antacids may bind ingested iron.

4. **CERTAIN FOOD COMPONENTS**. Some foods are known to interfere with iron absorption, such as tannin in tea, spinach, phosphates, some cereals.

The Absorption of Vitamin B_{12} and Its Defects

Dietary vitamin B_{12} is only found in red meat and liver. The raw vitamin is incapable of being absorbed, and the mechanisms that enable absorption are complex, relying on two other proteins: intrinsic factor (IF) and the so-called R-binders that are found in saliva, gastric juice, and bile. After its release from foods of animal origin by mastication, the vitamin binds to R-binders in the saliva. In this form it passes unchanged through the stomach (together with IF, which has been secreted by the parietal cells); vitamin B_{12} binds more avidly to R-binders than to intrinsic factor at **LOW** pH.

However, in the duodenum, pancreatic trypsin hydrolyzes the R-binders; the freed vitamin then binds to IF (the pH now having risen because of HCO_3^{2-} in the normal pancreatic juice) and this complex, being resistant to proteolysis, travels to the distal ileum.

In the ileum the complex binds to a specific receptor, the IF is shed and the vitamin once again binds to another R-binder, transcobalamin II, which carries it to the stores or wherever it is required (i.e., all cells undergoing mitosis, for DNA synthesis).

It is thus easy to see where potential defects in absorption can occur.

1. **IN THE MOUTH**, disorders causing defective chewing may have an effect. This effect is generally small except in the edentulous and those with ill-fitting dentures. Secretion of R-binders in the mouth may be poor in conditions causing xerostomia such as Sjogren's syndrome and in the aged because of frequent mouth breathing.

2. **THE STOMACH** is one of major sites for interference with the vitamin.

   a. **LACK OF PRODUCTION OF INTRINSIC FACTOR** (IF) is of course the proximate cause of pernicious anemia; the lack of IF in pernicious anemia is due to autoimmune destruction of the parietal cells, the producers of IF.

   b. However, **GASTRIC ATROPHY** from any other cause, if severe and extensive enough, will have a similar effect, as will total gastrectomy.

   c. **ACHLORHYDRIA** may be associated with normal absorption of aqueous vitamin B_{12} but defective absorption of protein-bound vitamin (the usual form), probably indicating the importance of peptic activity. This is one of the causes of a normal

Schilling test (see below) in the presence of total vitamin B_{12} deficiency; it is in fact a significant problem and has prompted attempts at developing a "food-Schilling" test. This test is evidently found to be very valuable in assessing vitamin status in gastric atrophy and unexplained low vitamin levels.

3. **THE DISTAL ILEUM** is the other major site of interference with the absorption of the vitamin. The major culprits here are Crohn disease and extensive resection of the ileum.

The Absorption of Folate and Its Defects

Most dietary folate is in the form of polyglutamates. However, absorption of monoglutamates is far more efficient, and thus deconjugation is an essential step. Folate conjugase is normally present only on the mucosal surface of the duodenum and jejunum, and consequently disease in this area will lead to malabsorption, the most important being tropical sprue, gluten enteropathy, and alcoholism. Rarely, malabsorption may be found in diabetes and chronic heart failure. However, if the ileum is healthy the conjugase can be induced on its surface. It cannot be induced in the colon, making rectal administration of folate (e.g., in the ICU) impracticable.

Note that the investigation and description of the tests for folate and vitamin B_{12} deficiency are to be found in Chapter 9. The investigation and the description of the tests for iron deficiency are to be found in Chapter 8. Vitamin K absorption has been adequately covered in Chapter 2.

The Investigation of Malabsorption

Some of the investigations are highly specialized and may only be available in large centers. For the generalist who suspects malabsorption, a start can be made by measuring stool fats in a 72 h collection. This is a very problematic test because of difficulty in stool collection, and frequently it is regarded as more precise to do a qualitative fat examination on a single sample plus serum carotene estimation:

1. If stool fats are > 6 g per 24 h or qualitative test for fats show increased excretion and the serum carotene levels are decreased, one proceeds to the D-xylose absorption test:

   a. If this is normal, diffuse mucosal disease is excluded, and the problem is most likely with pancreatic or bile salt excretion. Very sophisticated radio-active breath tests are now required for diagnosis.

b. If this is abnormal, this almost certainly indicates mucosal disease. The next step is to exclude bacterial overgrowth syndromes (see above).

c. If these are negative, intestinal biopsy is indicated.

2. If stool fats (and/or serum carotene levels) are normal, this does not exclude selective absorption defects, affecting especially iron, vitamin B_{12}, vitamin K, folate, and bile salts. Clearly one does not embark on these investigations without a reasonable suspicion (or perhaps as a last resort!). Often in practice, however, this situation presents itself in the opposite way: a patient diagnosed as having a deficiency of one of these elements by reference to other clinical features and for which none of the more obvious causes can be found and where there are none of the other classical stigmata of malabsorption is then considered a candidate for investigating for selective malabsorption:

a. If iron deficiency is present, a test for iron absorption is done.

b. If vitamin B_{12} deficiency is present, the Schilling test is performed.

c. If folate deficiency is present, tests for folate malabsorption are done.

d. Vitamin K deficiency is a special case, since vitamin K levels are not routinely measured. Diagnosis is made indirectly.

e. The investigation of suspected lactose intolerance and other abnormalities is outside the scope of this book.

A Summary of Blood Changes in Intestinal Disease Blood changes can play a valuable role in the evaluation of intestinal diseases:

1. **Anemia**. Anemia is found in many intestinal diseases:

   a. Microcytic anemia. This may be secondary to chronic blood loss, iron malabsorption, or chronic disease (or any combination of these).

   b. Macrocytic anemia. This is secondary to malabsorption of folate, or of vitamin B_{12}, such as in Crohn disease or blind loop syndromes.

   c. Dimorphic anemia. This is found where both a and b coexist.

   d. Normocytic anemia, as in a dimorphic picture, acute bleeding, etc.

2. **Raised hematocrit**. This can be due to dehydration from diarrhea.

3. **Leukocytosis**.

   a. Neutrophilia. There are numerous causes: any number of acute invasive bacterial infections; severe inflammatory bowel disease; appendicitis; pseudomembranous enterocolitis; amebic colitis; and paraintestinal abscesses, as in Crohn disease or diverticulitis.

   b. Neutropenia. This is most commonly due to drugs.

   c. Eosinophilia. Eosinophilic gastroentropathy and parasites.

   d. Lymphopenia. This may be found in conditions with excessive leakage of plasma proteins into the gut, such as lymphangiectasia.

4. **Thrombocytosis**. This may be found in a number of conditions, notably

   a. Celiac disease, associated with hyposplenism.

   b. Whipple disease.

   c. Ulcerative colitis.

5. **Prolonged prothrombin time**. Malabsorption of vitamin K (with fat).

Miscellaneous Conditions

1. **ESOPHAGUS**.

   a. **VARIOUS ESOPHAGEAL LESIONS** may seriously interfere with the ingestion of food, leading to numerous deficiencies.

   b. **CHRONIC IRON DEFICIENCY** itself is a cause of post-cricoid webs, leading to dysphagia.

   c. **ESOPHAGEAL CANDIDIASIS** is a fairly characteristic feature of AIDS.

2. **DUODENUM AND JEJUNUM**.

   a. **MUCOSAL ATROPHY**. There are numerous forms of atrophic enteropathy, the most important of which are celiac disease and tropical sprue.

   b. **POST-SHORT-CIRCUIT SYNDROME**. A very interesting and common syndrome has been observed in patients who have undergone a short-circuit operation for severe obesity. Within several months to years they may present with a chronic arthropathy affecting joints of all sizes, with anemia. The only solution is reversal of the bypass (which is strongly resisted by the patient!).

c. **INFESTATION WITH THE FISH TAPEWORM**. Dibothryocephalus latus is indigenous to areas around the Baltic Sea and New England. It seldom actually produces vitamin B_{12} deficiency; it does this by consuming ingested vitamin.

3. **CECUM AND COLON**. Clinical presentations are very different between the ascending and descending colons.

   a. **THE ASCENDING COLON AND CECUM**. Lesions here tend to present with iron deficiency, due to chronic bleeding from an otherwise silent lesion. Common lesions here are ulcerative colitis, polyps, Crohn disease, and carcinoma. Clearly the most ominous here is carcinoma – by the time the patient presents with iron deficiency, the disease is already quite advanced, and no time can be lost in properly investigating and treating the patient. See Case #14.

   b. **THE DESCENDING AND SIGMOID COLON**. These patients present with melena, hematochezia, or obstruction. They thus tend to be diagnosed earlier. Sigmoid diverticulosis and diverticulitis are common problems, and they may bleed profusely.

4. **RECTUM AND ANUS**. The major problem here from the hematological point if view is bleeding, and the major causes are **HEMORRHOIDS, VARICES,** and **CARCINOMA**.

   a. **HEMORRHOIDS**. Many people (including many surgeons) have the preconceived idea that the typical daily amount of bleeding from hemorrhoids is too small to cause significant iron depletion. As was pointed out in Chapter 2, absorption of iron is strictly controlled, normally by the amount of body iron. But even in severe iron deficiency, absorption can increase only to a maximum of about 4–5 mg/day. The effect is that, given a normal marrow and a good diet, increased absorption can cope with a daily loss of blood of about 5 ml, without iron deficiency ever developing or the stores being depleted. **ANY LOSS GREATER THAN THIS WILL START DRAINING THE STORES, AND DEPENDING ON THE SIZE OF THE STORES, WILL EVENTUALLY RESULT IN IRON DEFICIENCY.** Depending on how much blood is lost per day, it can take years for iron-deficiency anemia to develop. Hemorrhoids will classically take about 4 years to result in significant anemia.

   b. **VARICES**. Anal varices are a rare complication of portal hypertension.

c. **CARCINOMA**. This is an unusual cause of iron deficiency, since the other symptoms will usually lead to intervention before there is time for significant loss of blood to occur.

The Skin and Blood Diseases

Only the more common skin changes relevant to blood diseases will be discussed. Primary skin diseases are very seldom the cause of blood disease; a great many blood diseases or changes, however, manifest as or are associated with skin changes, permitting clinical suspicion or indeed diagnosis of blood disease. This includes skin changes as a result of therapy for blood diseases as well as hematological complications of treatment for other disorders. The basic clinico-pathological presentations are

1. **RASHES**. Rashes of hematological significance can be classified simply into

   a. **PURPURIC AND PSEUDO-PURPURIC**. These are discussed separately under Bleeding Manifestations and Vascular Disorders.

   b. **VESICULAR (BLISTERING)**. The four most important conditions here are herpes zoster, dermatitis herpetiformis, porphyria cutanea tarda, and porphyria variegata.

   HERPES ZOSTER: This is always suggestive of systemic disease, notably associated with immune deficiency. Many hematological diseases or changes can be associated:

   i. Chronic lymphocytic leukemia is one of the classic associations. The presentations are usually characteristic.
   ii. Both Hodgkin and non-Hodgkin lymphomas are also common associations. Clinical features are variable, and blood changes may not be present. The marrow may or may not be involved.
   iii. General immune deficiency diseases of various causes, such as AIDS (almost always indicating a very low CD4 count).
   iv. Myeloma.
   v. Collagen vascular diseases especially SLE.
   vi. Any underlying other malignancy.

   DERMATITIS HERPETIFORMIS. This is very frequently associated with gluten enteropathy with malabsorption and eosinophilia.

PORPHYRIA CUTANEA TARDA (PCT). This condition (along with porphyria variegata (PV)) is the only porphyria to affect the skin with any frequency. In PCT there is an enzyme defect leading to the accumulation of uroporphyrins I and III; these are water-soluble and therefore accumulate primarily in the skin. There are three types: type I, the pure acquired form (80% of cases); type II, with autosomal dominant inheritance (but often requiring an additional external cause to become clinically apparent); and type III, which is very rare. There are a number of external causes (relevant to both types), the most common being chronic alcoholic liver disease, although AIDS is rapidly catching up as a cause. AIDS may cause PCT directly, but more commonly via co-infection with other viruses, notably hepatitis B. Occasional causes are CMV infections, β-thalassemia, renal failure, and hemochromatosis. With respect to the latter, iron overload from any cause will aggravate the enzyme deficiency. Light (but **NOT** UV light) activates the porphyrins in the skin with release of free radicals, cellular damage, blistering, and eventually fibrosis of the dermis.

PORPHYRIA VARIEGATA. This is an inherited (autosomal dominant) condition, again due to an enzyme deficiency, with the accumulation of proto-, copro-, and uroporphyrins. These are both water- and lipid-soluble and consequently have skin involvement identical to that of PCT, as well as systemic involvement (mainly nervous). The only relevant hematological association is a tendency to iron overload.

c. **EXFOLIATIVE.** T-cell lymphomas of the skin characteristically show a widespread scaly rash, often with localized nodules and/or erythroderma. The blood and bone marrow may show no evidence of lymphoma, but sometimes characteristic lymphoma cells are seen; these cells may have a specific appearance, called Sezary cells, and the condition is then a variant of mycosis fungoides.

d. **ERYTHRODERMA.** The cutaneous T-cell lymphomas often begin with or present only with erythroderma.

e. **DRUG ERUPTIONS.** These occur frequently in blood diseases, either as a result of therapy for blood disease or where the reaction actually involves the blood components. They are discussed separately below.

f. **OTHER ERUPTIONS.**

Acanthosis nigricans is always suggestive of an underlying malignancy, primarily gastro-intestinal adenocarcinoma, particularly gastric. The hematological connection is that it must not be mistaken for purpura.

Acute febrile neutrophilic dermatosis (Sweet's syndrome) is not specific for any malignancy, but is said sometimes to be found in acute myeloblastic leukemia.

2. **PIGMENTARY DISTURBANCES.** Skin color is a composite effect of melanin pigmentation and the color of the blood flowing beneath and through it. The color of the blood clearly is primarily dependent upon the concentration of hemoglobin within it. Secondary causes, however, are found in certain hemoglobin abnormalities and other conditions:

a. **METHEMOGLOBIN** may be hereditary or acquired (discussed in Chapter 2). This causes the blood to take on a brownish hue, but when passing through the skin and mucosae appears blue – i.e., a false appearance of cyanosis. It may be accompanied by

b. **SULFHEMOGLOBINEMIA.**

c. **CARBOXYHEMOGLOBIN** is the effect on hemoglobin of carbon monoxide. Carboxyhemoglobinemia causes the skin to take on a cherry-red appearance.

d. **PLETHORA** and **PALLOR** will be extensively discussed in Chapter 5.

e. **JAUNDICE.** Any of the three types of jaundice – hemolytic, hepatocellular, and obstructive – may have implications for blood disease. See Chapter 5.

f. **PATCHY HYPOPIGMENTATION.** The most important condition from the hematological point of view is vitiligo. This is an autoimmune phenomenon and is frequently associated with pernicious anemia.

g. **DIFFUSE HYPERPIGMENTATION.** Important conditions from the hematological perspective are Addison disease, chronic renal failure, hemochromatosis, primary biliary cirrhosis, porphyria cutanea tarda, and porphyria variegata. Myeleran (busulphan)-induced hyperpigmentation was previously quite a common finding; myeleran is very seldom used these days. Also, myeleran is one of the drugs that may induce the development of porphyria cutanea tarda (other drugs that may do this are barbiturates and oral contraceptives).

h. **HEMOCHROMATOSIS.** The classical appearance of hemochromatosis is seen infrequently these days, because of earlier diagnosis. These comprise a dusky greyish (very seldom "bronze" as originally described) discoloration of the skin, with diabetes, heart failure, and endocrinopathies. These days the presentation is more commonly a **MILD** hyperpigmentation, difficult to distinguish from a suntan, with chronic arthritis of the first two MP joints. Over 20 different mutations have been described, but PCR methods are available only for the diagnosis of the two commonest ones.

3. **BLEEDING MANIFESTATIONS**. These may take the form of bruises, petechiae, typical purpura, and ecchymoses. There can also occasionally be hemorrhage into other skin lesions that are not normally hemorrhagic, considerably complicating diagnosis. Finally, specific patterns of bleeding may be very suggestive, such as the perifollicular bleeds in scurvy.

Many people are confused as to the nature of purpura, since its basically localized spotty appearance and absence of palpability seem strange. It will be remembered that the blood supply of the skin is into the dermis. The dermo-epidermal junction is characteristically papilliform, with a leash of vessels supplying each papilla. Figure 4.3 shows this in semi-diagrammatic form. The capillaries in each papilla are fairly fragile, and if they bleed there will be a localized little pool of blood, within the skin, producing the spotty appearance of typical purpura.

Purpura can take three forms: petechiae, classical purpura, and ecchymoses. Their differentiation is discussed in Chapter 5.

4. **VASCULAR DISORDERS**. Three vascular abnormalities are valuable in hematological diagnosis: telangiectases, angiomata, and various forms of vasculitis. The differentiation is discussed in Chapter 5:

a. **VASCULITIS** can take many forms.

   i. Leukocytoclastic. This produces the classic **P**alpable **P**urpura, which is often **P**ainful. Thus the most important hematological aspect is its differentiation from ordinary purpura. Henoch–Schönlein disease is a classic cause.
   ii. Non-inflammatory obliterative endarteritis, typically producing nailfold infarcts (as in SLE).
   iii. Necrotizing vasculitis, as in purpura with skin ulceration.

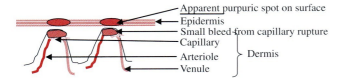

Fig. 4.3

iv. There are a few conditions that may indicate vasculitis, such as livedo reticularis (a highly significant sign in the antiphospholipid syndrome), and hemorrhagic vesicles and bullae.

b. **TELANGIECTASES**. These may be hereditary or acquired. Acquired forms include chronic liver disease and scleroderma. Hereditary hemorrhagic telangiectasia (Rendu–Osler–Weber syndrome) is an autosomal dominant disorder characterized by telangiectases in the skin, the mouth, the GIT, and vagina. In the tongue they are often mistaken for angiomata. Surgeons have also reported seeing them in connective tissue and muscle, considerably complicating their operative field. They may also develop pulmonary and cerebral arteriovenous malformations. They increase with age and, in females, with the menarche and pregnancy (due to the effect of estrogen) – occasionally they may present for the first time in young adulthood, especially in females. They bleed easily and typically present with iron deficiency.

The condition should be distinguished from ataxia telangiectasia. See under The Nervous System and Blood Diseases.

c. **THROMBOPHLEBITIS MIGRANS.** This is classically associated with carcinoma of the pancreas.

5. **CUTANEOUS MANIFESTATIONS OF DRUG REACTIONS OF DIRECT OR INDIRECT HEMATOLOGICAL SIGNIFICANCE.** There are two broad groups of cutaneous drug reactions: the non-immunological and those where an immunological pathogenesis is proven or likely. As far as the immune mechanisms are concerned, three of the four types of immune response may cause skin disease and be relevant to hematology. For further information regarding types of immune response, see under Immune Disorders and Infectious Disease and the Blood.

a) **TYPE I REACTIONS**. In the skin, these are characterized by urticaria (among other features). A common cause is hypersensitivity to the penicillins, which may also be associated, by a hapten-binding mechanism, with a hemolytic anemia.

b) **TYPE III REACTIONS** (vasculitis, e.g., drug-induced lupus erythematosis): such as associated with hydralazine. Penicillin-induced hemolysis can also be of this type.

c) **TYPE IV HYPERSENSITIVITY REACTIONS**. It is probable that one type of eruption associated with ampicillin and sometimes other penicillins is of this type. These eruptions clinically resemble contact dermatitis; indeed they tend to occur in sites of previous contact dermatitis.

Cutaneous drug reactions are of several types. Only those of hematological significance are mentioned:

a) **ACNEIFORM:** The only relevant drugs here are cortisone (and ACTH) used in the treatment of many blood diseases. Of importance is that the lesions are all in the same stage of development, unlike ordinary acne. Other drugs that may be relevant are oral contraceptives (which may cause a hypercoagulable predisposition) and dactinomycin, a commonly used chemotherapeutic agent.

b) **ALOPECIA.** The relevant issues here are two: diffuse alopecia may accompany oral anticoagulant therapy and drug-induced alopecia should be differentiated from primary alopecia. Many chemotherapeutic agents used in hematological (and other) malignancies cause a (reversible) alopecia.

c) **ECZEMATOUS ERUPTIONS:** Of relevance here are the eruptions associated with ampicillin and sometimes other penicillins, as discussed above.

d) **EXANTHEMATOUS ERUPTIONS.** These are the most common cutaneous drug reactions. Of hematological significance are allopurinol (used extensively in the supportive therapy of many chronic hematological malignancies), gold, and penicillins especially ampicillin. A specific type of rash occurs in the majority of patients with infectious mononucleosis (IM) who are given ampicillin (and to a lesser extent other penicillins), and different from the type discussed above: this is a rapidly developing generalized maculopapular rash. A similar phenomenon occurs in HIV-positive individuals taking trimethoprim-sulphamethoxazole. It can also be found in CMV infection and CLL.

e) **ERYTHRODERMA AND EXFOLIATIVE DERMATITIS.** Some drugs may cause exfoliation identical to that found in primary skin diseases (such as mycosis fungoides), and thus their differentiation can be very important. Important drugs are allopurinol and gold.

f) **FIXED DRUG ERUPTIONS.** These are rare in hematological practice – the only drug of relevance here is allopurinol.

g) **VASCULITIS.** Drug-induced vasculitis is classically of the leukocytoclastic type, presenting as a palpable purpura, which without proper examination can easily be confused with purpura itself. Important drug causes again are the penicillins and allopurinol.

h) **SKIN NECROSIS.** This can occur as a complication of coumadin therapy in patients with an underlying thrombophilia. See Chapter 21.

5. **BACTERIAL AND FUNGAL INFECTIONS.** A very large variety of surface infections can occur in the presence of immune depletion, such as in AIDS, induction of chemotherapy for hematological malignancies, lymphomas, myeloma, and neutropenia from many causes. In addition, primary infections such as erysipelas and cellulitis are usually associated with marked neutrophilia.

   PYODERMA GANGRENOSUM is a particularly serious complication of some deficiency states, such as myelodysplasia.

6. **NODULES AND PLAQUES.** Two groups of nodules and plaques may be of hematological relevance:

a. **MALIGNANT DEPOSITS.** Leukemic infiltrates in the skin occur in 3% of leukemic cases at presentation. Other types of nodules/skin infiltrations occur with Kaposi sarcoma and Langerhans cell histiocytosis (the current name for a group of conditions formerly known as eosinophilic granuloma, Letterer–Siwe disease, Hand–Schuller–Christian disease and histiocytosis X). The most common, however, are lesions secondary to lung cancer and breast cancer. From the hematological point of view, depending on the clinical background, search can be made for

   i. Acute or chronic leukemia (in the case of leukemids).
   ii. Concurrent bone marrow metastases (in the case of suspected cancer). Typically these are scattered, and straight X-ray and/or nano-colloid scanning of the skeleton may show areas suggestive of deposits, and which can then be biopsied for the greatest yield.
   iii. Immune deficiency (in the case of Kaposi sarcoma): notably AIDS, with a low CD4 count.
   iv. Langerhans cell histiocytosis. Skin involvement can occur, but the most prominent features are bony masses, sometimes causing great deformities.

b. **NODULES ASSOCIATED WITH JOINT DISEASES**, such as rheumatoid arthritis and gout, and hypercholesterolemia. Hematological implications for rheumatoid disease and gout are discussed under The Musculo-skeletal System and the Blood. Deposits of cholesterol (xanthomata and xanthelasma) may be associated with hypercoagulability.

7. **SCARS**. From the hematological point of view, the tissue-paper scars of factor XIII deficiency are noteworthy. Otherwise surgical scars may indicate previous procedures, such as gastrectomy, which may be relevant to the current hematological problem. Scarring is prominent in porphyria variegata.

8. **PRURITUS AND RELATED PHENOMENA**. There are a number of relevant conditions that are associated with pruritus. Many have already been mentioned. To summarize:

   a. **PRIMARY BLOOD DISEASES**: Polycythemia vera, Hodgkin disease, chronic lymphocytic leukemia.

   b. **SECONDARY BLOOD DISEASE**: Obstructive jaundice (bleeding tendency), chronic renal failure (bleeding tendency, chronic anemia, right shift of neutrophils), carcinoma of the lung (pancytopenia or leukoerythroblastic reaction), myxedema (macrocytic and/or microcytic anemia), pregnancy and oral contraceptives (thrombotic tendency), and some parasitic infestations.

9. **PHOTOSENSITIVE DISORDERS.** The most important conditions to consider here are SLE, dermatomyositis, and porphyria. These may be associated with sun-induced red wheals.

The Genito-urinary System and Blood Diseases

This is one of the systems where there are not very many potential hematological correlates, but those few are very important. They are chronic renal failure, renal adenocarcinoma, hydronephrosis, prostatic carcinoma, cystic disease, and uterine fibromata.

1. **CHRONIC RENAL DISEASE**. There are a number of distinct hematological correlates:

   a. **BLEEDING TENDENCY** (prolonged bleeding time)
   b. **CHRONIC ANEMIA**.
   c. **RIGHT SHIFT OF THE NEUTROPHILS**.

2. **RENAL ADENOCARCINOMA**. About 25% of these patients are anemic on presentation, whereas about 5% have erythrocytosis (due to inappropriate secretion of EPO). This tumor has a distinct tendency to metastasize to bone causing pancytopenia or a leukoerythroblastic reaction.

3. **POLYCYSTIC KIDNEYS.** Usually there is iron deficiency anemia due to hematuria; very occasionally they may produce EPO.

4. **HYDRONEPHROSIS**. These kidneys may produce inappropriate EPO, causing erythrocytosis.

5. **PROSTATE CANCER**. Bony secondaries tend to be sclerotic, making the bone very hard (when biopsied).

6. **UTERINE MYOMATA**. These can very occasionally produce EPO and erythrocytosis.

7. **CONTROL OF EXTRACELLULAR FLUID VOLUME**. Certain kidney diseases may be associated either with water (± electrolyte) losses, with dehydration possibly causing hemo-concentration and erythrocytosis. Similarly, water retention of renal origin may be associated with hemodilution and the development of **APPARENT** anemia.

Pregnancy and Changes in the Blood

Pregnancy has significant associations with hematology and the blood, and since pregnancy is very common something must be known about these.

In Chapter 3 the physiological changes occurring in pregnancy were outlined. To summarize:

1. **VALUES DECREASING IN PREGNANCY**:

   a. **HEMOGLOBIN, HEMATOCRIT, AND RED CELL COUNT**. This is spurious; in fact there is a mild true **INCREASE**, but this is masked by expansion of plasma volume, greater than the increase in the red cells. The plasma volume increases by ± 50% in the first and second trimesters while the red cell mass increases only by 20–30%. The net effect is that the Hb level falls to ± 10.5 g/dl (at sea level) from 16 to 40 weeks. The RCC, Hb, and Hct return to normal about 1 week after delivery.

   b. **FERRITIN** falls in early pregnancy and remains low throughout, even if supplementary iron is given.

2. **VALUES INCREASING IN PREGNANCY**:

   a. **A MODERATE NEUTROPHILIA** is common in pregnancy and reaches its maximum about 8 weeks before the birth. A left shift also is very common, with a significant increase in band forms.

   b. **THE ESR** increases steadily during pregnancy and can reach 25 mm/h without this necessarily indicating disease activity.

The following are common and clinically relevant findings in pregnancy:

1. **ANEMIA**. This can have numerous causes:

   a. **PHYSIOLOGICAL** – see above.
   b. **IRON DEFICIENCY**. The developing fetus requires ± 800 mg Fe^{2+}. This represents a massive

drain on the mother's stores. In addition the mother may lose blood from hemorrhoids.

c. **FOLATE DEFICIENCY**. The developing fetus requires an enormous amount of DNA synthesis. Since the normal mother's stores of Vitamin B_{12} are more than adequate, the provision of folate is the critical limiting factor in this regard. In addition, there is good evidence that autoantibodies to folate receptors in the jejunum can develop, especially in complicated pregnancies, thus aggravating folate deficiency (see under Autoantibodies in Pregnancy below).

Without supplementation the development of folate deficiency, with all its complications, is very common. The most important of these complications is the risk of neural tube defects in the fetus – note that this can happen even in the absence of clinical folate deficiency.

2. **THROMBOCYTOPENIA**. Thrombocytopenia is quite common in pregnancy. The problem is to decide what the cause is, since some of the causes can have ominous implications for the mother and the fetus. The causes are as follows:

a. **GESTATIONAL THROMBOCYTOPENIA**. This is generally regarded as almost physiological. It complicates 10% of pregnancies. It is mild, with the platelet count seldom below 80×10^9/l, and generally above 100×10^9/l. Occasionally it is associated with a (reversible) neonatal thrombocytopenia.

b. **IMMUNE THROMBOCYTOPENIA** (ITP). This is responsible for 3% of cases of thrombocytopenia in pregnancy and is commonly associated with raised anti-platelet IgG (but see Chapter 11 for a discussion on this). It may cause severe neonatal thrombocytopenia.

c. **DRUGS**. See Appendix A.

d. **PRE-ECLAMPTIC TOXEMIA** (PET) and **ECLAMPSIA**. Thrombocytopenia occurs regularly in PET. The cause is uncertain: in many cases excessive platelet aggregation can be seen on the smears, suggesting that the thrombocytopenia may be spurious in some cases. The question arises, however, as to why aggregation is so prominent in these cases, and it is likely that autoimmune mechanisms play a part – see below. There is a condition known as the HELLP syndrome that occurs in 10% of patients with eclampsia; HELLP stands for "**H**emolysis, **E**levated **L**iver enzymes, and **L**ow **P**latelets". This is a life-threatening condition with a very poor outcome for both mother and fetus.

e. **HEMOLYTIC-UREMIC SYNDROME** (HUS) and **THROMBOTIC THROMBOCYTOPENIC PURPURA** (TTP). These two conditions are currently regarded as pathologically related conditions, although their clinical features, especially when occurring in pregnancy, are different.

i. HUS typically occurs within 48 h after delivery of a normal pregnancy.
ii. TTP usually occurs before the 24th week of pregnancy.

These two conditions are briefly discussed in Chapter 23.

f. **DIC.** See later.

3. **COAGULATION DISTURBANCES**. In pregnancy, the finely controlled balance between pro- and anticoagulant processes is shifted somewhat toward the hypercoagulable state; this tendency is aided by venous stasis. Various changes occur:

a. There is an increase in the vitamin K-dependent factors ("1927"), in factor VIII, and in fibrinogen.
b. Fibrinolytic activity is decreased.
c. In addition there may be an increase in protein C, and a decrease in protein S and in antithrombin.

4. **DIC**. In Chapter 2 the pathogenesis of DIC was briefly outlined. Very important among the numerous elements that can trigger the activation of the coagulation mechanism within the circulation are abruptio placentae, intrauterine death, amniotic fluid embolism, sepsis, and eclampsia. The DIC due to amniotic fluid embolism has some unusual features: it typically occurs **IN THE COURSE OF A DIFFICULT DELIVERY** in a multipara and causes a chronic low-grade DIC.

5. **MORPHOLOGICAL CHANGES**. Most commonly, morphological changes will reflect the disorders and changes already mentioned. In summary, the following may be reported:

a. Neutrophilia with a left shift.
b. Thrombocytopenia.
c. The features of iron deficiency: see Chapter 8.
d. The features of folate deficiency: see Chapter 9.
e. The features of combined iron and folate deficiency: see Chapter 8.
f. Fragmented red cells, microspherocytes, decreased platelets: this picture can be found in DIC, HUS, and TTP.
g. The features of acute fatty liver of pregnancy: crenated red cells, basophilic stippling of red cells, and large platelets. Note that this condition is frequently associated with PET.

A few conditions require a further brief mention:

1. **THE ANTIPHOSPHOLIPID SYNDROME** (APS). This is an autoimmune condition most commonly

found in women ($9\female:1\male$) characterized by arterial and venous thrombosis and recurrent fetal loss (due to infarction of the placenta). Occasionally it presents as an ITP. From the point of view of pregnancy, it may present, or suspected to be present, in several ways:

a. Unexplained death of a morphologically normal fetus at 10 weeks or later.
b. Three or more consecutive miscarriages before 10 weeks.
c. One or more premature births of morphologically normal fetuses before 34 weeks due to PET, eclampsia, or severe placental insufficiency.

Apart from fetal loss, APS is also associated with infertility and other complications of pregnancy such as prematurity and stillbirths, and pregnancy-induced hypertension.

It has been recommended that women who have had proven APS should not take estrogen–progesterone oral contraceptives.

APS is further discussed in Chapter 21.

2. **HYPERCOAGULABLE STATES**. It was mentioned that pregnancy is normally a mildly hypercoagulable state. This may, however, be much more marked. It appears that the most common cause of this is **ACQUIRED ANTITHROMBIN (AT3) DEFICIENCY**. There are several known causes for this:

a. Associated liver disease.
b. DIC (consumption of AT3).
c. Renal loss in nephrosis.
d. Heparin therapy.

Note that 40% of pregnancies in AT3-deficient women will be complicated by venous thromboembolism.

3. **AUTOIMMUNE ASPECTS OF PREGNANCY** (and infertility). The relationship between pregnancy and autoantibodies is threefold:

a. There are a number of autoimmune disorders that unquestionably impact on the outcome of pregnancy:

   i. Antiphospholipid antibodies and APS. This is strongly linked to systemic lupus erythematosis (SLE) and thus to the anti-nuclear antibody (ANA). Note, however, that raised ANA without proven SLE is apparently not in itself associated with an adverse pregnancy outcome.
   ii. Raised levels of anti-angiotensin II type 1 receptor antibodies (AT1-AA) are found in nearly all women with PET.
   iii. There appears to be a high incidence of anti-folate receptor autoantibodies in women whose fetuses have neural tube defects.

b. As indicated earlier in the chapter, pregnancy probably plays a significant role in the development of autoantibodies and possibly in autoimmune disease. There is a much higher incidence of autoantibodies in the pregnant state. These can be of many types, such as anti-microsomal, anti-mitochondrial, and anti-nuclear. The practical effect of these is uncertain: some workers have claimed that some of these antibodies are associated with an adverse pregnancy outcome.

c. Pregnancy has a distinct effect on many, if not all pre-existing autoimmune disorders. As mentioned above, there is a modal shift in immune response in pregnancy, with the maternal immune responses shifted toward antibody-mediated responses and away from cell-mediated responses. Thus various autoimmune diseases are affected differently during pregnancy, exemplified by the following:

   i. Rheumatoid arthritis (primarily cell-mediated) tends to remit.
   ii. SLE (primarily associated with excess antibody production), tends to flare up, although generally speaking, this is not marked.

It is clear that diagnosis in pregnancy requires special care in the following circumstances:

1. The diagnosis of mild anemia.
2. The diagnosis of bacterial infection and the interpretation of neutrophilia.
3. The diagnosis of thrombocytopenia.
4. The investigation of apparent hemolysis.
5. The interpretation of many autoantibodies.

The Musculo-skeletal System and Blood Diseases

This system comprises a large number of distinct and in many cases unconnected conditions. As far as **THE MUSCULAR SYSTEM** is concerned, only one condition will be mentioned – dystrophia myotonica. This is a hereditary condition. The muscles of the face and chest are affected, the latter responsible for hypoventilation and compensatory **ERYTHROCYTOSIS**. ECG and EMG changes are very suggestive.

With respect to **BONE DISEASE**, again there are a limited number of relevant conditions.

1. **BONE METASTASES**. Certain primary carcinomas have a marked tendency to metastasize to bone, nl. breast, thyroid, kidney, prostate, and bronchus. In addition, myeloma in the later stages is classically a

disease affecting many bones (in the case of myeloma, the bones containing marrow: the vertex of the skull, the thoracic cage, the spine, and the pelvis). Pathological fractures may occur – indeed, myeloma may present for the first time with pathological fractures.

2. **ADVANCED HYPERPARATHYROIDISM** with the formation of osteitis fibrosa cystica. This may be so extensive as (rarely) to interfere with hematopoiesis.

3. **OSTEOPETROSIS** (marble bone disease) is known to cause a leukoerythroblastic reaction.

JOINT DISEASE. Use of this term is to some extent wrong, since so many of these rheumatological conditions affect other systems as well. There are a great many of these, and only general trends will be mentioned.

1. **RHEUMATOID ARTHRITIS** is overwhelmingly the commonest of these conditions. Hematological involvement is extensive:

   a. **ANEMIA** can be of many types:

      i. The commonest type of anemia is anemia of chronic disorders.
      ii. Iron deficiency anemia is relatively common, generally as a consequence of salicylate or NSAIDS gastric irritation
      iii. Macrocytic anemia is usually due to folate deficiency. This is most commonly found in patients with severe involvement of the hands and without social support, and who need to fend for themselves; they become folate deficient because their disability interferes with their ability to cook and prepare meals properly.
      iv. Combinations of the above are common, and the analysis of these FBCs requires accurate morphological comment plus other investigations.

   b. **THE GRANULOCYTES.** Neutrophilia may occur in the acute phases. Neutropenia is a hallmark of Felty syndrome. See Chapter 12.

   c. **THE PLATELETS.** Thrombocytosis commonly occurs as a result of active inflammation.

   d. **LYMPHOMAS.** The incidence of non-Hodgkin lymphomas is far higher than in the general population.

   e. Patients with clonal expansion of large granular lymphocytes with chronic neutropenia frequently have RA.

   Numerous **UNFAVORABLE PROGNOSTIC FEATURES OF RHEUMATOID DISEASE** are found in laboratory tests, such as the development of a **MARKED NORMOCYTIC ANEMIA** without there being evidence of a combined iron and folate

deficiency, **THROMBOCYTOSIS, EOSINOPHILIA, MARKEDLY RAISED ESR,** and **HYPOALBUMINEMIA.**

2. **SYSTEMIC LUPUS ERYTHEMATOSIS (SLE).** Hematological involvement is again extensive:

   a. Hemolytic anemia occurs in ± 15% of cases.
   b. Anemia from all causes develops in ± 75% of cases.
   c. Neutropenia occurs in ± 50% of cases.
   d. Lymphopenia occurs in ± 20% of cases.
   e. Thrombocytopenia occurs in ± 25% of cases.
   f. 15% of cases develop splenomegaly.

The above findings as well as a marked rise in ESR tend to indicate **ACTIVITY**. Also, **ADVERSE PROGNOSTIC INDICATORS** are the development of **AUTOIMMUNE NEUTROPENIA, NEUTROPHIL DYSFUNCTION,** and the features of **HYPOSPLENISM,** as well as late-onset **THROMBOCYTOPENIA.** The FBC thus has a valuable role in management.

The Endocrine System and Blood Diseases

Again there are few hematological correlates, but those can be very helpful. The important hormonal disorders of relevance to hematology or its tests are

1. **MYXEDEMA.** A great many hematological changes can be found in myxedema, almost all being different forms of anemia.

   a. **MACROCYTIC ANEMIA.** A mild macrocytic anemia with round macrocytes is the characteristic finding (this is related to the hypercholesterolemia that so commonly occurs). However, a true megaloblastic anemia (with oval macrocytes) may develop, either as a result of co-existent pernicious anemia or folate malabsorption.

   b. **MICROCYTIC ANEMIA** may develop as a result of chronic iron loss in the stools because of constipation, and menorrhagia in females. In subacute thyroiditis, anemia of chronic disorders may develop.

   c. **NORMOCYTIC ANEMIA** may develop from a number of causes:

      i. A combination of micro- and macrocytic anemia (of any of the causes as mentioned).
      ii. The development of an autoimmune hemolysis.
      iii. Early anemia of chronic disorders.

2. **ADDISON DISEASE.** The classic FBC pattern of Addison disease is a mild normocytic anemia and mild eosinophilia.

3. **CUSHING SYNDROME**. The classic FBC pattern of Cushing syndrome is a mild polycythemia or erythrocytosis, or mild neutrophilia, and eosinopenia.
4. **SIMMOND DISEASE** (hypopituitarism). A classic feature is a mild normocytic anemia.
5. **INCREASED ANDROGENS**. Whether endogenous or exogenous, a mild polycythemia or erythrocytosis is common.
6. **PHEOCHROMOCYTOMA**. The hematological implication is simply that it is a cause of marked pallor, which may be mistaken for anemia.

The Nervous System and Blood Diseases

There is a fairly restricted number of associations with the hematological system:

1. **CORTICAL DYSFUNCTION**. Apart from vague cognitive symptoms in any anemia, polycythemia, or erythrocytosis, two fairly typical presentations can occur in blood disease:

   a. **DEMENTIA**, sometimes agitated, can occur as a presenting feature of megaloblastic anemia (classically pernicious anemia – note that neurological complications almost never occur in folate deficiency).
   b. **DELIRIUM** can occur in the VAD regime for myeloma, due to the extremely high dose of methylprednisone.
   c. **PROGRESSIVE CORTICAL DEFICITS** occur in progressive multifocal leukoencephalopathy, the commonest causes of which are CLL and the lymphomas.

2. **CEREBELLAR DYSFUNCTION**. Two conditions in particular are relevant to hematology:

   a. **CEREBELLAR HEMANGIOBLASTOMA**. This is characteristically associated with erythrocytosis due to inappropriate secretion of EPO by the tumor.
   b. **ATAXIA TELANGIECTASIA** (AT). The hematological importance is that it should not be confused with hereditary hemorrhagic telangiectasia. Both conditions start in childhood but may present to adult physicians later. AT is very much more serious than HHT, with extensive features of spinal, cerebellar, and basal ganglia disturbance, later showing mental retardation. It has been said that a significant difference from HHT is that in HHT telangiectasis does not affect the conjunctivae: this is not true.

3. **THE MOTOR TRACTS**. These are almost always involved in transverse myelitis, one of the causes of which is pernicious anemia. The lateral motor columns are involved in subacute combined degeneration of the cord (SCDC) – see below.
4. **THE SENSORY TRACTS ESPECIALLY THE POSTERIOR COLUMNS.** The most characteristic disorder is SCDC. Typical motor signs are accompanied by loss of vibration sense and proprioception.
5. **PERIPHERAL NERVES**. One of the many causes of peripheral neuropathy is vitamin B_{12} deficiency. It is of interest that this can occur without overt evidence of pernicious anemia.

The Respiratory System and Blood Diseases

In this discussion our major concern is with the delivery of oxygen to the tissues. Diseases of the lungs can lead to hypoxia, followed by numerous adaptive mechanisms some of which are reflected in the FBC. On the other hand, and more interestingly, many disorders of the red cells are the cause of, or contribute to, defective oxygenation of the tissues.

The pathway of oxygen from atmosphere to mitochondrion is long and difficult, with numerous potential blocks as well as physiological adaptations: only one of the latter is provided by the red cell, although it is one of the most important. The red cell, its membrane, its contained hemoglobin and enzyme systems, and internal physico-chemical structure play a fundamental role in this regard. While the effects of defective oxidative metabolism are most dramatically seen in sepsis, SIRS, MODS, etc., it undoubtedly plays a role in chronic inflammatory disease, malignancies, and so on, as well as possibly a range of vague symptoms associated with anemia, etc.

ENERGY PRODUCTION IN THE MITOCHONDRIA depends on

1. The state of health of the mitochondria and its enzymes.
2. **ADEQUATE SUPPLIES OF OXYGEN** and other necessary nutrients.
3. Satisfactory disposal of CO_2 and H^{1+}. Note that the RBC, the Hb, and the flow characteristics of blood play a significant role here as well.

ADEQUATE OXYGEN SUPPLY REACHING THE MITOCHONDRIA depends on

1. **OXYGEN DELIVERY TO THE TISSUES**.
2. Healthy interstitial tissues that permit normal diffusion of O_2.

OXYGEN DELIVERY. There are two separate aspects to this:

1. Oxygen transport (TO$_2$) from heart to micro-circulation. This depends on

   a. **THE OXYGEN CONTENT OF THE BLOOD**.
   b. The pressure gradient between the heart and the micro-circulation.
   c. The state of the blood vessels.
   d. The rheological and flow characteristics of the blood.

2. Oxygen transport within the micro-circulation through the endothelium of the capillaries to the tissue cells. This depends on

   a. **THE OXYGEN CONTENT OF THE BLOOD**.
   b. The pressure gradient:

      i. Between the capillaries and the interstitial tissue.
      ii. Between the endothelium and the mitochondria.

   c. The state of the systemic capillary bed and the volume, hematocrit, and shear characteristics of the blood flowing through it.
   d. A clear diffusion path from RBC through endothelial cytoplasm through the interstitium to the mitochondria, and therefore the state of the interstitial tissues.
   e. Specific kinetic effects associated with the **FÅH-RAEUS EFFECT.**

3. The deformability of RBCs allowing a close fit of the RBC membrane to the endothelium.

4. Normal release (dissociation) of oxygen from hemoglobin.

   THE OXYGEN CONTENT OF BLOOD (Cao$_2$) depends on

1. **ATMOSPHERIC O$_2$ CONCENTRATION**.
2. **ALVEOLAR Po$_2$**.
3. **OXYGENATION OF VENOUS BLOOD IN THE PULMONARY CAPILLARIES.**
4. **Po$_2$ AND O$_2$ SATURATION (Sao$_2$) OF ARTERIAL BLOOD.**
5. **A MECHANISM BY WHICH LARGE VOLUMES OF OXYGEN CAN BE CARRIED WITHOUT CAUSING OXIDATIVE DAMAGE.**
6. **NORMAL ASSOCIATION OF OXYGEN WITH HEMOGLOBIN.**

   To create our context, the path is illustrated in Fig. 4.4. Our focus is on red cells and their contained hemoglobin – see Note 8.

The Respiratory Gas Path at Rest and at Sea Level

O$_2$ path in **RED**. CO$_2$ (and H^{1+} to a limited extent) path in **BLACK**.

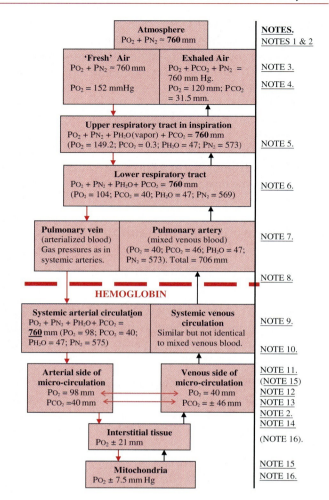

Fig. 4.4   The Respiratory Gas Path

Notes with respect to Fig. 4.4:

1. Oxygen moves in a direction and at a certain speed entirely dependent on a **PRESSURE GRADIENT**; this may be due to either (or both of)

   a) A direct pumping action as found in ventilatory movements.
   b) A difference in Po$_2$ between here and there, so to speak.

2. Where the O$_2$ has to diffuse through an area, additional **LIMITING FACTORS** are obtained, such as the thickness and structure of the diffusing medium.

3. Each gas in a mixture exerts a pressure as if it were alone (i.e., a **PARTIAL PRESSURE**), but the actual pressure is a proportional part of the total pressure, which can vary independently, e.g., with altitude. With increasing altitude, the partial pressure of each gas will

reduce proportionately. Therefore the partial pressure available for diffusion is reduced; hence the gradient and the volume of gas flow will be reduced. This decrease in Po_2 is not accompanied by an **EQUIVALENT** decrease in oxygen content – this phenomenon is discussed later. However, it can affect diffusion rate, since this is entirely dependent on Po_2.

4. **EXPIRED AIR** rapidly becomes partly dehumidified, the degree depending on the relative humidity and to some extent the temperature of the atmosphere.

5. **WATER VAPOR.** Molecules at a liquid/gas interface tend to escape into the gas phase, and this increases as the temperature rises; and the pressure of the vapor above the liquid depends directly on the temperature and is independent of the barometric pressure. The air in the upper respiratory tract becomes saturated with water, with a partial vapor pressure of 47 mmHg. Thus only $760 - 47 = 713$ mm Hg is available for the partial pressures of O_2, CO_2, and N_2. At 5000 ft above sea level the amount available drops to $620 - 47 = 573$ mm. Table 4.5 shows the difference in P_{H_2O} in severe hypothermia, severe pyrexia, and in health.

The effect of pyrexia on the available "space" for oxygen is clear. Note that temperature also has a significant effect on the hemoglobin oxygen-dissociation curve, and will be discussed later.

6. The gas in the lower respiratory tract is that which mainly occupies the terminal bronchioles and alveoli, and is generally referred to as **ALVEOLAR GAS**, equivalent to the residual capacity. Functionally it is a reservoir maintaining a reasonably stable composition in the face of marked changes in the constituent gases at the diffusion face.

7. The total **GAS PRESSURE IN THE MIXED VENOUS BLOOD** is only 706 mmHg. The total gas tension in venous blood is **ALWAYS** (in health) $\pm$ 55 mmHg lower than in arterial blood, because the reduction in the arterial/venous Po_2 is far more than the corresponding rise in the venous/arterial PC_{O_2}.

Normally, blood passing through a pulmonary capillary is fully saturated with oxygen by the time that it has traversed half the length of the capillary.

Table 4.5

Temperature, °C	P_{H_2O}, mmHg
37	47.0
30	31.8
	55.3
42	61.3

Thus there is a large diffusive reserve, and saturation of the blood is easily achieved. The impact of atmospheric Po_2 on oxygen supply to the systemic circulation is minimal until there is a significant ventilatory or diffusive defect, or interference with pulmonary blood supply, or people living at high altitudes, which would have dire consequences were it not for very sophisticated adaptive mechanisms.

8. A major element in the pathway has been omitted – the role of **HEMOGLOBIN IN DETERMINING OXYGEN CONTENT.** See how the Po_2 in the arterial blood remains high as a result of the functioning of the hemoglobin in red cells; since O_2 is so poorly soluble in water (or plasma), without Hb the Po_2 would drop precipitously (see below). **THE HB CAN WRONGLY ESTIMATE TISSUE OXYGENATION** to a lesser or greater degree in a number of pathological situations.

9. The total **GAS TENSION OF ARTERIAL BLOOD** is slightly lower than atmospheric pressure because of a small amount of the cardiac output normally passing from the right to the left side of the circulation without entering the alveolar capillaries. This causes the Po_2 to be reduced from $\pm$ 101 to $\pm$ 97 mmHg. In health this makes no practical difference to the interpretation of the Hb; however, in certain conditions the shunt can be very much larger, directly impinging on the oxygenation of Hb, and thus the Hb would tend to overestimate tissue oxygenation.

10. **OXYGEN TRANSPORT TO THE BEGINNING OF THE MICRO-CIRCULATION**. The amount of oxygen reaching the arteriole is more or less equal to oxygen content multiplied by blood flow, each with numerous factors affecting them.

11. **OXYGEN TRANSPORT IN AND THROUGH THE CAPILLARIES.** The amount of oxygen reaching the beginning of the micro-circulation is not the same as the amount of oxygen reaching the interstitial tissue because of the crucial part played by the red cells in their release of oxygen, the different circumstances within the capillary, the flow of blood, and the patency of the capillaries.

Up to the level of the arterial end of the capillary, flow is proportional to cardiac output (CO). Beyond that level, the major determinant is local regulation (by the tissues).

12. **THE Po_2 OF THE CAPILLARY BLOOD**. This, in relationship to the tissue Po_2, determines the diffusion gradient from the red cell to the interstitium. The Po_2, a plasma measurement, is in the first instance dependent on the alveolar Po_2 ($P_{A}O_2$); as oxygen diffuses outward, it is replenished from the red cell Hb-bound oxygen, and thus is secondarily dependent upon the O_2

content of the red cell, which in turn is dependent on the content of normal Hb. Note that oxygen diffusing though the endothelium does not directly come from the red cell but from the surrounding plasma, which is in a dynamic equilibrium with the Hb-bound oxygen. The release of oxygen from the Hb is due mainly to the nature of the Hb molecule (see later).

14. **THE DIFFUSION OF O_2 FROM THE RED CELL TO THE INTERSTITIUM.** For this discussion, we divide the gradient into two parts:

   a) **FROM HB MOLECULE THROUGH THE ENDOTHELIUM.**
   b) **FROM THE ENDOTHELIUM THROUGH THE INTERSTITIUM TO THE CELL.**

   A little later, items 14a and 14b are discussed separately, at length.

15. The marked **DROP IN P_{O_2}** from ±100 mmHg in the pulmonary veins to ±7.5 mmHg in the mitochondria illustrates one of the difficulties with O_2.

The Nature of the Flow of Blood and Its Relevance to Tissue Oxygenation

In Fig. 4.4, the role of hemoglobin has yet to be spelled out. As a preamble, consider what the state of tissue oxygenation would be if blood did not contain hemoglobin.

PLASMA HAS A LIMITED ROLE AS A CONVEYOR OF OXYGEN. Oxygen dissolves in plasma proportionately to the alveolar P_{O_2}. At a P_{O_2} of 97 mmHg, 0.3 ml oxygen will dissolve in the plasma of 100 ml of blood. Assuming the usual 5 l/min cardiac output, this means that 15 ml of dissolved oxygen per minute will reach the tissues, which is inadequate to sustain life in all but the lowliest (aerobic) multicellular organisms. And with strenuous exercise, normally the cardiac output may need to rise to 35 l/min because of increased oxygen requirements. By way of illustration, breathing pure oxygen at 3 atmospheres will produce a dissolved oxygen content of 7 ml/min – which is barely enough to sustain life at rest. Any form of unusual activity or other requirements would be impossible. In fact, **250 L** of blood **AT SEA LEVEL** would be required for adequate oxygen supply to the tissues to cope with normal stressful existence and the blood volume would have to be correspondingly huge.

Enter hemoglobin – one of the most astonishing molecules known. It is a transporter of oxygen *non-pareil*.

Hemoglobin permits a given volume of whole blood to **TAKE UP 65 TIMES AS MUCH OXYGEN AS AN EQUAL VOLUME OF PLASMA.** The special property of Hb is that it combines extremely **RAPIDLY** and **REVERSIBLY** with oxygen, loading it in the lungs and unloading it in the tissues without itself becoming oxidized (much) in the process. The presence of Hb completely alters the gas-containing characteristics of blood.

The P_{O_2} of 100 mm in the alveoli is not only to be found at sea level, where there is an atmospheric P_{O_2} of 140 mm: owing to numerous adaptive mechanisms, an alveolar P_{O_2} of ± 100 mmHg **CAN**, in normal circumstances, be found at altitudes up to 18,000 ft. But in the absence of adequate compensation (for example with rapid ascent) and at altitudes significantly above this, the P_{O_2} of blood falls; this fall is slight until the atmospheric P_{O_2} drops to about 70, for two reasons:

1. The nature of the binding of oxygen to hemoglobin.
2. The micro-anatomy and function of the lungs.

These will be discussed shortly. First, we must consider the effect of the hemoglobin on the blood. Naked hemoglobin would increase the osmolality of the blood to enormous levels, effectively making diffusion outward of fluid, etc., impossible. This is obviated by having the hemoglobin in red cells. But the number of red cells necessary to carry sufficient hemoglobin is enormous, and this has significant effects on the viscosity and hence flow – i.e., the rheological characteristics of the blood.

Rheology and the rheology of blood are very complex topics with great relevance to many diseases, especially vascular disturbances and in the critically ill. Blood is a very viscous fluid at rest. If an equivalent solution were made up of 45% ball bearings of 7 μm in diameter in a fluid of the viscosity of plasma, the resultant mixture would have a consistency almost of freshly mixed concrete (even if the ball bearings were of a very light material). Yet blood flows freely. This is accomplished by a number of factors, all of which have relevance to tissue oxygenation and many abnormalities which are known to cause many clinical and physiological disturbances. **THE MOST IMPORTANT OF THESE FACTORS ARE PHYSICAL CHARACTERISTICS OF THE RED CELL**, primarily its **AGGREGABILITY** and its **DEFORMABILITY**.

Shear Forces in a Cylindrical Tube

Any fluid flowing in any tube must be seen as a series of concentric cylinders flowing along. The wall – in our case the endothelium – exerts a drag (called a shear force) on the outer layer, with the result that this layer virtually adheres to the wall. This layer in turn exerts a drag on the next inmost layer, causing it to be retarded, and so on. The result is that the advancing column of fluid (blood) is parabolic, with the greatest shear forces on the outside and the lowest in the axis.

If the fluid contains deformable particles (red cells), any of these flowing near the periphery will come under the influence of the high shear forces and will be spun toward areas of lower shear – i.e., toward the axis. Thus in effect, the red cells form an axial column, leaving the periphery relatively clear, and hence the viscosity at the periphery drops markedly, permitting easier flow. However, this would not be enough to facilitate the ease of flow we see in blood – this requires special adaptation provided by the red cell, nl. the shape of the cell.

Because of their discoid shape, the red cells can aggregate by "stacking" on one another, like a roll of coins; these aggregates accumulate in the axis of the stream, making the density of the peripheral blood very much lower and permitting easy flow.

However, in the capillaries the red cells must disaggregate such that they can traverse the capillaries. Disaggregation normally occurs easily, since the bonds between cells in the axial aggregates are weak and can easily be broken when the shear forces rise in the arterioles as they become narrower. Of course, once reaching the venules, the shear forces change again, permitting reaggregation. Note in passing that there are many serious conditions causing abnormalities of the shear forces and flow characteristics, such as sepsis and diabetes, to name but a few.

It should be clear that if the red cells for some reason cannot disaggregate, for example due to **IMMUNE-MEDIATED AGGREGATION** (where the bonds are much stronger), they will not be able to negotiate the capillaries as successfully. This will result in defective tissue oxygenation unless compensatory mechanisms are adequate.

From a practical point of view, we can discuss oxygenation as occurring in two phases:

1. **INTRAVASCULAR**. Here the oxygen is carried by hemoglobin; the Po_2 remains very high; its transport is purely physical; and it is dependent only on **THE CHARACTERISTICS OF ARTERIAL AND CAPILLARY BLOOD FLOWS**.
2. **EXTRAVASCULAR**. Here the oxygen has dissociated from the hemoglobin and must move to the tissue cells by **DIFFUSION**. The amount of oxygen actually reaching the cells depends on

   a) The difference in pressures of oxygen between the blood (plasma) and the tissues.
   b) The solubility of oxygen in an aqueous solution – and this is poor.

The effect is that the Po_2 drops considerably en route to the tissue cells.

Arterial and Capillary Blood Flow

THE RATE AND VOLUME OF BLOOD FLOW per unit length of vessel in the arterial side of the circulation are thus very important: blood carrying a satisfactory amount of O_2 bound to normal Hb will not be of much use if it does not reach the capillaries in adequate volumes per unit time. There are numerous aspects to this:

1. **ARTERIAL AND ARTERIOLAR DISEASE**, reducing blood flow to the region, or causing turbulent flow, which decreases perfusion.
2. **ABNORMALITIES OF THE RED CELL**, notably where certain shapes prevent the proper axial aggregation of red cells; this increases the viscosity and decreases perfusion. Sickle cells are a prime example of this.
3. **BLOOD FLOW THROUGH THE CAPILLARIES**. This depends on

   a. **THE VISCOSITY**, determined mainly by the Hct. **THE HCT** in the capillaries is always lower than in the venous blood (where it is usually measured).
   b. **THE RATE OF FLOW**. This can play a large role. For example, in the hyper-dynamic flow that sometimes can occur in sepsis, the markedly increased flow can lead to decreased time for release of O_2.
   c. **THE VOLUME FLOW OF BLOOD**. Note that it is the total volume here that is relevant, not just that of the red cells – for example, in a dehydrated patient there may be adequate numbers of red cells (and Hb) but the decrease in plasma water can cause an increase in capillary hematocrit, with consequent sludging and considerable interference with oxygen release.
   d. **THE EFFICACY OF VENOUS AND LYMPHATIC DRAINAGE** of the micro-circulation. Diffusion into the tissues depends largely on the pressure gradient between the intravascular and extravascular spaces. The pressure in the extravascular space is affected by venous and lymphatic congestion. Thus the rate and volume of blood flow on the venous side is also relevant, albeit in a more indirect sense.
   e. **THE PATENCY, DIAMETER, AND TONE** of the capillaries.
   f. If a **SMALLER NUMBER OF CAPILLARIES IS OPEN** than are needed for the particular tissue's requirements, or if a larger proportion of blood is shunted past the capillary bed via the metarterioles

than is required, tissue hypoxia can supervene in the presence of adequate amounts of arterial oxygen.

g. **THE DEFORMABILITY OF THE RED CELL**. The red cell diameter is larger than the average capillary, and therefore must deform to pass through; in the process the red cell is closely applied to the endothelium, producing a very short diffusion path.

It can readily be seen that abnormalities of the red cell can significantly interfere with gas transfer, leading to tissue hypoxia. This further emphasizes the importance of morphology.

The Diffusion of Oxygen from the Hemoglobin Molecule Through the Endothelium

Despite what has been said about the importance of hemoglobin, the oxygen dissolved in plasma **IS** critically important; oxygen diffusing through the endothelium comes in the first instance from that dissolved in the plasma, where it exerts a pressure (the P_{O_2}), and not from that in the Hb. Although the **AMOUNT** of oxygen in the plasma at any one time is low, it exerts a considerable **PRESSURE** ($\pm$ 97 mmHg), and it is this pressure that is the driver of diffusion – oxygen bound to Hb exerts no pressure.

The plasma P_{O_2} of the blood entering the capillary is $\pm$ 97 mmHg. It encounters a tissue P_{O_2} of $\pm$ 40 mm. As a result of this pressure, and other things being equal, the O_2 will immediately start to flow into the tissues. As the P_{O_2} in the plasma drops, O_2 is released from the Hb, diffuses into the plasma, and restores the plasma P_{O_2}. This continues until either the P_{O_2} equals that of the tissues or the blood reaches the end of the capillary (±5 mm long), or as some think, the first part of the venule (and taking < 0.5 seconds).

(It follows that the nature of oxygen binding to Hb is of primary importance, and this will be discussed shortly).

However, other things are NOT always equal, and there are numerous factors that may interfere with the normal diffusion from Hb through the endothelium, one of the major ones being how firmly the Hb has bound the oxygen; thus even with an initially normal P_{O_2} (as the blood enters the capillary), effective capillary hypoxemia may develop with excessively tight binding (see below).

Figure 4.5 illustrates the diffusion path from the hemoglobin inside the red cell through the endothelium and into the interstitial space. Note that it is from the endothelium onward, after it has left the Hb, that the dramatic drop in P_{O_2} occurs in the gas path.

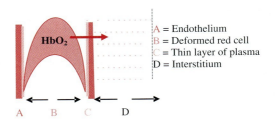

Fig. 4.5 The Normal Diffusion Path of O_2 from Hb through Endothelium.

Note in Fig. 4.5:

1. As the red cell ("B") enters the capillary, it deforms and in the process the red cell membrane, **IF NORMAL**, becomes closely apposed to the endothelium ("A"). The red cell goes into the capillary with the central pale area leading, in the process forming a parachute-shaped entity, and in this conformation provides a very large diffusing surface; the red cell must recover its normal discoid form once it reaches the venule, to enable it to aggregate again and thus reduce the viscosity.

2. Should the endothelium be swollen – a typical reaction to many stimuli such as sepsis – or the red cells be abnormal (see below), the red cells may not be able to traverse the endothelium at all. A healthy red cell in normal flow conditions will traverse the capillary in the above parachute shape, and it has been shown that in this shape it can successfully negotiate a diameter of 4 µm, which would otherwise constitute a significant narrowing of the capillary. It is clear therefore that in addition other factors are necessary for interference with passage; this is still under intense investigation, but almost certainly would encompass abnormal red cells and/or endothelial activation leading to adhesion of platelets and leukocytes, forming obstructions to flow.

3. There is a very thin layer of plasma ("C") (estimated at 1–2 µm thick) that "contains" the head of O_2 pressure (the P_{O_2}) for diffusion through the endothelium. (In fact, since the endothelium is not uniformly cylindrical as is often imagined, there are small "pockets" of plasma as well, usually due to the nuclei protruding into the lumen). This O_2 is constantly fed from the adjacent red cell, since the plasma P_{O_2} in the capillary is constantly falling as O_2 diffuses into the interstitium. The important role that shear forces play in vascular tone with respect to this layer was discussed before.

Thus, in summary, interferences with tissue oxygenation up to this point may result from

1. **ABNORMAL DISAGGREGATION**. Normal red cell aggregation is by WEAK bonds in the center of the

stream. These bonds, however, may be STRONG usually due to surface antibodies, especially cold agglutinins, causing difficulty in disaggregating.

2. **DEFECTS IN THE RED CELL.** The most important defect here is abnormal deformability, and this in turn has numerous causes. Deformability is a function of the red cell membrane and internal viscosity, and energy is required to restore the original discoid form after leaving the capillary. Causes of abnormal deformability can be due to membrane disorders or hemoglobin disorders. Note that most of these are morphologically identifiable.

a) **MEMBRANE DISORDERS** may be primary, as in **HEREDITARY SPHEROCYTOSIS**, or secondary as in **ACANTHOCYTOSIS** or due to incomplete antibodies on the red cell membrane (**HEMOLYSIS**). In Rh disease of the newborn, the oxygen delivery can be reduced by up to 15%. To what extent this occurs in adults with red cell surface antibodies is uncertain.

b) **HEMOGLOBIN DISORDERS** may be due to defective hemoglobinization, as in **IRON DEFICIENCY, ANEMIA OF CHRONIC DISORDERS, OR THALASSEMIA, OR DUE TO ABNORMALITIES OF THE GLOBIN CHAINS, WHICH CAN HAVE DIFFERENT PATHOPHYSIOLOGICAL EFFECTS:**

   i. **GLOBIN DISORDERS ASSOCIATED WITH DECREASED DEFORMABILITY (AMONG OTHER THINGS), SUCH AS SICKLE DISEASE IN WHICH THE RED CELLS ARE MORE RIGID THAN NORMAL (SINCE THE GLOBIN IS LESS SOLUBLE).**

   ii. **GLOBIN DISORDERS AS WELL AS CERTAIN ENZYME DEFICIENCIES LEADING TO INCREASED OXYGEN AFFINITY OF THE HEMOGLOBIN, AND THUS OXYGEN IS RELEASED TO THE HYPOXIC TISSUES WITH GREATER RELUCTANCE.**

c) **ENZYME DEFICIENCIES OR DEFECTS** leading to defective ATP production or abnormalities in oxygen affinity.

2. **INTERFERENCES FROM OTHER CELLS.** A very **HIGH WCC**, e.g., in chronic leukemia; so many WBC are present that they can actually block the capillary or can interfere with apposition of the red cells. A similar effect could occur with a very high platelet count.

3. **ENDOTHELIAL DISORDERS.** These can have a deleterious effect on tissue oxygenation, interfering with both flow and diffusion. Endothelial dysfunction is being implicated in more and more diseases, such as hypertension, diabetes mellitus, and so on. Also, apart from lipid peroxidative and cytokine damage, it is now clear that partial activation of the coagulation mechanism (as occurs in sepsis, etc.) results in soluble fibrin deposited on the endothelium, but without there being sufficient for factor XIII to cause cross-linkage and therefore insoluble fibrin formation. This fibrin has been shown to interfere significantly with oxygen diffusion.

4. **INTERSTITIAL DISORDERS** (see below).

Diffusion from the Endothelium Through the Interstitium to the Tissue Cell

A number of factors are relevant:

1. **THE TISSUE P_{O_2}.** Many factors can interfere with oxidative phosphorylation in the mitochondria and it is probable that this plays a significant role in anemia of chronic disorders, MODS, SIRS, and so on. The unutilized oxygen could accumulate in the interstitial space, causing increase in tissue P_{O_2} with a decreased diffusion gradient. Some or all of this oxygen could diffuse back into the venous side of the micro-circulation. Or of course it could be the source of reactive oxygen species, causing further tissue damage.

2. **THE TISSUE TENSION.**

3. **THE LENGTH OF THE DIFFUSION PATH TO TISSUE CELLS.** In this regard, one important issue is the presence of edema. Oxygen reaching the tissue cells does so entirely by diffusion. Diffusion of oxygen depends (because of poor solubility) on an adequate pressure gradient and a short distance. Normally the gradient from the capillary ($P_{O_2} \pm 100$ mmHg) to the cells ($P_{O_2} \pm 40$ mmHg) is about 60 mmHg. This is satisfactory since under normal circumstances no tissue cell is further than 50 µm from a capillary and the head of pressure is enough for rapid diffusion to occur. If the path length increases beyond 100 µm, it appears that diffusion drops off rapidly. This distance can easily be achieved in severe edema (think of the chronic skin changes in anasarca). Should there in addition be compromise in the gradient, there can be very serious consequences for tissue metabolism (**AND ALSO A POTENT SOURCE OF MISINTERPRETATION OF TISSUE OXYGENATION BY REFERENCE TO THE HB LEVEL**).

4. **THE STATE OF THE DIFFUSION PATH** to the tissue cells. Apart from edema, increase in fluid in the interstitial space may be inflammatory, containing large amounts of (plasma) proteins and inflammatory

cells. Here much oxygen clearly would be utilized by the neutrophils that have accumulated, with the production of vast amount of reactive oxygen species (ROS), aggravating the whole state of affairs. In severe infections, the neutrophil concentration in the exudates can easily be 1 million/mm^3. One million activated neutrophils can consume 2.2 mm^3 of O_2 – and one million cells is not much of an inflammatory exudate: it is the sort of response found in a boil. This will clearly impact on tissue oxygenation; on top of this, the ROS do considerable damage in the vicinity, interfering with oxygen utilization by the neighboring tissue cells. All this is particularly marked in cases of sepsis. The neutrophils can carry on easily metabolically, since they can exist anaerobically.

5. **DECREASED OXYGEN REACHING THE MITO-CHONDRIA TENDS TO RESULT IN THE PRODUCTION OF TOXIC METABOLITES.** These may diffuse back into the circulation, increase inflammation, and perhaps aggravate interstitial edema.

Oxygen Carriage and Transport

It is useful to compare the composition of arterial blood with that obtained in the venous side of the capillaries, since the values can be seriously abnormal in many disease conditions and are thus of diagnostic significance. See Table 4.6.

It can be seen that, in health and at rest, about one fourth of the O_2 delivered to the tissues is used. The 75% unused amount represents a considerable reserve that can be called upon (up to a maximum of $\pm 70\%$ extraction) in exercise and hypermetabolic states.

The loading and unloading of oxygen onto Hb requires the oxygen to combine with hemoglobin in a very specific way. Two very important aspects for the understanding of how this is achieved are

1. It is described by the oxyhemoglobin dissociation curve.

2. It is made possible by the physical and chemical nature of hemoglobin.

Oxygen binds to hemoglobin in a stepwise, self-reinforcing fashion. This is described by the oxygen-association/dissociation curve (ODC).

The association and dissociation of oxygen with and from hemoglobin are not linear. Study of the shape of this curve indicates the four-stage loading (and unloading) of oxygen (Fig. 4.6). It consists of four stages because each molecule of heme (consisting of four subunits) can bind four molecules of O_2 (i.e., one each). It does this in a very specific way, depending on the surrounding P_{O_2}.

The Oxygen-Dissociation Curve (ODC)

Figure 4.6 is a graphical representation of the ODC. Observe the following:

1. The **X**-axis represents the Pa_{O_2}, which essentially means the amount of oxygen theoretically available. But it is a pressure, and thus there is a driving force for O_2 to go either onto the Hb molecule or outward through the capillary endothelium. Note that the Pa_{O_2} affects the Ca_{O_2} by determining, together with pH and temperature, the Sa_{O_2} (the saturation).

2. The **Y**-axis represents to what degree the Hb is saturated with O_2 – essentially, how many molecules of O_2

Table 4.6

Amounts in the blood containing 15 g Hb/dl				
	ARTERIAL BLOOD: P_{O_2} = 98 MM HG P_{CO_2} = 40 MM HG HB 97% SATURATED		VENOUS BLOOD: P_{O_2} = 40 MM HG P_{CO_2} = 46 MM HG HB 75% SATURATED	
Gas	Dissolved	Combined	Dissolved	Combined
O_2	0.3	19.5	0.13	15.1
CO_2	2.5	46.5	2.96	49.6
N_2	0.97	0	0.97	0

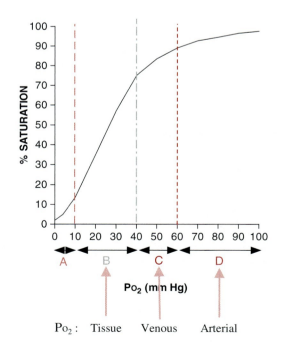

Fig. 4.6

are bound (reversibly) with Hb. This can be seen as the O_2 on multiple Hb molecules; however, for our purposes, it makes much more sense, as a start, to consider the chart as representing one single molecule of Hb only. Thus the amount of oxygen carried by Hb is a curvilinear function of P_{O_2}.

These measurements are all done on the following basis:

1. The P_H is 7.4, the temperature is 37 $^\circ$C, and the P_{CO_2} is 40. This is important because it will later be seen that these factors strongly influence the position and shape of the curve.
2. The Hb is functionally normal.
3. The curve is sigmoid (i.e., roughly S-shaped). There are four clinically significant parts of the curve:

   A: from a Pa_{O_2} of 0 to roughly 10 mmHg. In this area, with an increase in P_{O_2} the saturation (Sa_{O_2}) increases moderately, to about 10%. Thus a **MODERATE** increase in P_{O_2} is associated with a **MODERATE** increase in Sa_{O_2}. This part of the graph is relevant at a very LOW P_{O_2}; it is hardly ever found in life, regardless of the pathology. The normal tissue P_{O_2} is 40 mm. Dropping to < 20 mm would be life threatening.

   D: from a Pa_{O_2} of 60 to 100, the Sa_{O_2} increases only slightly, disproportionately little with respect to the increase in Pa_{O_2}. If the Pa_{O_2} were to increase significantly above 80 mmHg, the amount of oxygen **DISSOLVED IN THE PLASMA** would increase. This is of relevance in hyperbaric oxygen therapy – such therapy does not increase the oxygen saturation (unless it was abnormal before, and then only up to its maximum) – the extra oxygen goes into solution. This also has the effect of increasing intracellular P_{O_2}, resulting in increased superoxide formation.

   C: from a Pa_{O_2} of 60 to 40, the curve has started falling more rapidly, but not yet precipitously with decreasing Pa_{O_2}. This area is where, in a monitoring situation, one begins to be very proactive – improving oxygen supply at this stage can improve saturation still relatively easily.

   B: from Pa_{O_2} of 40 to 10, the saturation falls dramatically. It is clear that this is the clinically significant part of the graph. A small decrease in Pa_{O_2} leads to a marked drop in saturation and thus a marked increase in oxygen release from Hb. Note that the steepest part of the curve occurs at oxygen tensions that are found in the tissues (i.e., in that part labeled B). The steepest part is the most labile part, and here O_2 movement on and off Hb molecules is extremely active, depending on demand.

The region marked "D" is a useful rough way of dividing the curve clinically – to the left of the line, the curve can be considered the "tissue" part, and to the right is the "lung" portion. This part of the graph is relevant at a HIGH P_{O_2}, as found in the lungs. The curve is almost flat: the hemoglobin will be fully saturated or close to fully saturated with oxygen even if the alveolar Pa_{O_2} drops to about 65; also even most abnormal hemoglobins will be saturated.

In the region marked "B", found in the tissues, small alterations in the conditions can have a **MAJOR** effect on unloading of oxygen.

The shape of the curve can change in certain pathological states, affecting O_2 transport.

> Effectively, in the pulmonary capillaries the P_{O_2} dictates the oxygen content; in the systemic capillaries, the oxygen content dictates the P_{O_2}.

The actual position of the curve on the **X** and **Y** axes is a measure of the oxygen affinity of the Hb – i.e., oxygen's attraction to the O_2-binding sites.

> There are two critically important attributes of the ODC:
>
> 1. Its shape. This is due to the peculiar way that oxygen binds to hemoglobin, and is primarily because of the binding property hemoglobin displays called cooperativity.
> 2. Its position vis-à-vis the Y-axis; i.e., shifted to the left or right.

The key to understanding the sigmoidal shape is as follows: a fully saturated Hb molecule (four molecules of O_2 – one for each of the monomers) would give up one of these molecules when the P_{O_2} drops below a certain level (this is what is happening in region D of Fig. 4.6); the next one tends to be given off more easily, the third one even easier (region B of Fig. 4.6), and the last one virtually immediately thereafter (region A). (The opposite happens in the lung, i.e., in region "D".) This type of **ACCELERATING** process would clearly result in a sigmoidal pattern if plotted. The question, however, is how is this accomplished?

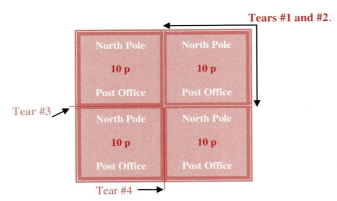

Fig. 4.7

There are several factors that contribute to the shape of the curve. The two most important are: **COOPERATIVITY** (the **MOST** important) and the action of **2,3-BPG**.

The Concept of Cooperativity

Cooperativity means the interactions between the globin sub-units. Students find the concept of cooperativity difficult. To explicate it, we shall use a four postage stamp analogy. (See Fig. 4.7.) Santa Claus has decided to respond to four of his young petitioners and requires four stamps. These he will remove from a block of four.

Note in Fig. 4.7: The first stamp requires **TWO TEARS (OR CUTS)**; a corresponding amount of time; and a modicum of energy – let us say 6 moles of ATP. **ONE STAMP** released.

The second stamp requires **ONE TEAR**; a shorter amount of time; and less energy – say 3 moles ATP. **ONE STAMP** released.

The third and fourth stamps also require **ONLY ONE TEAR**, but **TWO STAMPS** are released for the same energy. Thus, (see Table 4.7):

If you were to plot these figures, it can be seen that the relationship of how many stamps are released versus the number of tears would be (crudely) sigmoidal. The process described above represents the steps of oxygen release from Hb. **COOPERATIVITY IS THE EXACT OPPOSITE OF THIS PROCESS** (which is much more difficult to depict diagrammatically.

Table 4.7

Tear Number	Energy required	Stamps released
1	6	1
2	3	1
3	3	2

An important point needs to be made about this phenomenon: effectively every individual molecule of Hb is either fully saturated (oxyhemoglobin) or fully unsaturated (reduced hemoglobin) with O_2. But each normally hemoglobinized red cell contains 280,000,000 molecules of Hb and there are millions of red cells traversing a hypoxic area of tissue in the space of a second. Thus, **ON AVERAGE**, the Hb in an area (at the venous end of the capillary) is desaturated to the extent that requirements are met (normally the saturation at the venous end is about 75%).

COOPERATIVITY DEPENDS IN THE FIRST INSTANCE ON THE MOLECULAR STRUCTURE OF HEMOGLOBIN. THE HEMOGLOBIN MOLECULE IS BASICALLY A HIGHLY ORGANIZED AND COMPLEX TETRAMER. There are two α- and two β-globin (polypeptide) chains, coded for on separate chromosomes. Each chain (or monomer) in the Hb molecule contains on one end a heme molecule (a protoporphyrin ring plus an iron (Fe^{2+}) atom). Each heme/globin monomeric complex is so constructed that it forms a pocket within which one molecule of O_2 can be accommodated in a completely anhydrous form – being anhydrous will minimize any redox reaction, thus preventing the Fe^{2+} or the components of the pocket from becoming oxidized. The tetrameric form of Hb is critical, in that the four chains cooperate and indeed physically move on each other in the varying phases of oxygen carriage.

The binding of oxygen (potentially eight atoms per molecule) depends on the interaction of the four heme groups, i.e., cooperativity. This interaction is manifested by physical movements of the β-chains as oxygen moves in or out, one after the other. Closely coupled to this is the action of 2,3-BPG. See Fig. 4.8.

In Fig. 4.8(a) and (b) the effect of O_2 on the tetramer can be seen: when a molecule of O_2 is unloaded the β-chains are pulled apart permitting entry of 2,3-BPG. 2,3-BPG is generated in a side reaction of the glycolytic pathway (of the

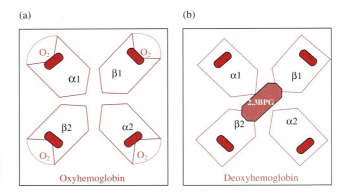

Fig. 4.8 (a) Hb in R conformation (b) Hb in T conformation

red cell, the neutrophil, and the eosinophil only) and binds avidly to elements of the β-chain of deoxyhemoglobin, resulting in a lower affinity for O_2 making release of the next molecule easier, and thereby enhancing tissue oxygenation. The 2,3-BPG stabilizes the molecule, and the deoxyhemoglobin form is called the T (for **TENSE**) structure. There are a number of factors that can alter the 2,3-BPG concentration, the best known being pH, temperature, and PCO_2. Let us look at some clinical conditions in which an increase of 2,3-BPG is found:

1. Hyperthyroidism.
2. Conditions associated with raised growth hormone levels.
3. Conditions associated with raised androgen levels.
4. Exercise, particularly in untrained subjects.
5. Ascent to high altitudes (see later).
6. Anemia.
7. Chronic hypoxic states.

In ascent to high altitudes, there is a **RISE** in P_H.

In uncomplicated anemias, there is no significant change in P_H, temperature, or PCO_2; the significant change is in DO_2.

In chronic hypoxic states, there can be complex changes in the above variables, depending on the cause and severity.

The only common denominator appears to be greater demand by the tissues for oxygen. Under conditions of hypoxia the 2,3-BPG levels can almost double, thus markedly decreasing O_2 affinity and improving tissue O_2 levels. It is essentially this process that is responsible for the sigmoid shape of the ODC.

In the lungs, as the blood becomes oxygenated, 2,3-BPG is released, resulting in increased oxygen affinity; this structure is called the R (for **RELAXED**) form.

THE OXYGEN-DISSOCIATION CURVE (ODC), in many respects, is independent of the amount of Hb present.

> The ODC can shift to the left or the right, as a physiological adaptation to varying demand or supply of oxygen to the tissues; or as pathological condition resulting from abnormal hemoglobins or occasionally from enzyme deficiencies or defects. The effects of the shifts vary greatly.

The Effect of a Shift to the Right

A SHIFT TO THE RIGHT means that affinity is decreased; thus more O_2 is released to the tissues at a given PaO_2. This can be understood in different ways:

1. There is a decrease in saturation at any given PaO_2. It is of minimal significance at the top of the curve (except at very high altitudes and/or very strenuous exercise), since the pulmonary micro-circulation (very different from the systemic one) is such that, in most cases, venous blood is more or less fully oxygenated. In the lower parts of the curve, **THE OXYGEN CONTENT IS DECREASED, BUT ITS RELEASE FROM HB IS MUCH EASIER.** Thus the effect is more obvious at a low PaO_2 – as in tissue hypoxia, and less obvious at high PaO_2, as in the lung. This can be found in physiological or pathological conditions. Clinically a right shift will tend to show mild anemia but without appropriate symptoms of anemia. Erythropoietin (EPO) secretion would be decreased.
2. A particular saturation requires a greater PO_2 than otherwise.
3. The tissues are better oxygenated at the same PaO_2.
4. Erythropoietin secretion is less stimulated than otherwise, therefore the Hb is lower than would otherwise obtain.

The overall effect is that more oxygen is given off to the tissues than otherwise.

> **The clinically significant effects of a shift to the right of the ODC are:** Good tissue oxygenation with a normal or even a low PaO_2, a low-normal or even decreased Hb, and low-normal or decreased erythropoietin levels.

The Effect of a Shift to the Left

A SHIFT TO THE LEFT means that affinity is increased; thus less O_2 is released to the tissues at a low PaO_2. This too can be understood differently:

1. At the same PO_2, more Hb is saturated than otherwise, since there are effectively more binding sites.
2. A particular saturation requires less PO_2 than otherwise.
3. More oxygen is carried back to the lungs.
4. In view of the tissue hypoxia, erythropoietin secretion is stimulated, tending in most cases to the development of erythrocytosis.

The O_2 pressure gradient is thus reduced and O_2 delivery becomes impaired. The overall effect is that less oxygen is given off to the tissues than otherwise.

This change is found mainly in pathological conditions, primarily abnormal hemoglobins, **AND PRESENTING, USUALLY, WITH COMPENSATORY ERYTHROCYTOSIS.**

> **The clinically significant effects of a shift to the left of the ODC are:** Tissue hypoxia with normal Pao$_2$, increased erythropoietin production and a tendency to erythrocytosis.

The shift in the ODC is a prominent part of the adaptation to anemia and hypoxia.

The Causes of a Right Shift in Clinical Terms

1. Hyperthermia.
2. Acidosis.
3. Hypercapnia.
4. Certain low affinity hemoglobins.
5. **CAUSES OF A RAISED 2,3-BPG:**

   a) Hypoxia.
   b) Anemia.
   c) Chronic lung disease.
   d) Cardiac failure.
   e) Blood loss.
   f) Thyrotoxicosis, hyperpituitarism in active phase, hyperandrogenemic conditions.
   g) Exercise increases the levels within an hour, but may not occur in the trained athlete.
   h) Ascent to high altitude, which is secondary to the rise in blood P$_H$.
   i) Acidosis inhibits glycolysis, thereby causing a reduced formation of 2,3-BPG.

It is, however, interesting that 2,3-BPG is not essential to life; in one case of hereditary absence, the "patient" was perfectly well apart from mild erythrocytosis.

The Causes of a Left Shift in Clinical Terms

1. Hypothermia.
2. Alkalosis.
3. Septic shock.
4. High-affinity hemoglobins. These include high levels of HbF, thus in certain thalassemias and hemoglobinopathies. As stated before, γ-chains (in HbF) bind 2,3-BPG very poorly. In these cases the leftward shift may be nullified by the effects of concomitant anemia.
5. Methemoglobinemia (presenting as cyanosis).
6. Carbon monoxide poisoning. Observe that carbon monoxide poisoning has multiple ways of causing hypoxia. This is dealt with below.
7. **CAUSES OF A DECREASED 2,3-BPG**. The effect of this is largely theoretical and possibly insignificant.

Hereditary deficiency of 2,3-BPG is exceedingly rare and evidently has little untoward effects. Bypassing of the Rapoport–Luebering shunt due to increased demand for ATP is a theoretical possibility but has not been, as far as I know, extensively researched.

Further Points with Respect to Hypoxemic Hypoxia

From the point of view of hematology, our major concern with respect to the respiratory system is hypoxemic hypoxia. There are several ways of classifying disorders of gas exchange, but to simplify, we can identify two broad groups:

1. **THOSE WITH DECREASED LUNG CAPACITIES** (volumes). Typical causes are obstructive disease (e.g., emphysema) and restrictive disease (e.g., pulmonary fibrosis). These all have V/Q (ventilation/perfusion) inequalities. Effectively this means areas of the lung are being perfused with blood from the pulmonary artery but not ventilated, and/or other areas are being ventilated but getting less blood than required to carry the respiratory gases.

2. **THOSE WITH NORMAL LUNG CAPACITIES**. There are two subgroups:

   a. (±) **PURE HYPOVENTILATION**. The most important causes are

      i. Depression of the respiratory center from drugs.
      ii. Structural abnormalities in the chest wall – deformities such as severe kyphoscoliosis and paralysis of chest muscles.
      iii. High altitude. The blood Po$_2$ steadily decreases with increasing altitude above sea level. In health, this only becomes significant when the altitude rises above 7000–8000 ft above sea level. At an altitude of 6000 ft the arterial Po$_2$ is about 620 mmHg (as opposed to 760 at sea level. Normal compensatory mechanisms are a rise in Hb by about 1.5 g/dl; levels of 2,3-BPG have increased; and the ODC has shifted to the right). Note that in commercial airliners, the ambient Po$_2$ is maintained at the equivalent altitude of 8000 ft.

   b. **DIFFUSION DEFECTS**. On their own, these seldom cause significant hypoxia.

THE ABOVE DOES NOT COVER ALL CAUSES OF TISSUE HYPOXIA. TISSUE HYPOXIA CAN INDEPENDENTLY BE CLASSIFIED AS

1. **ASSOCIATED WITH DECREASED LUNG CAPACITIES** – i.e., due to the causes of V/Q mismatch.

2. **ASSOCIATED WITH NORMAL LUNG CAPACI-TIES**. These are further subdivided into:

   a. **HYPOVENTILATION** (see above). Compensatory mechanisms are as described above.

   b. **INCREASED AFFINITY OF CIRCULATING HB FOR OXYGEN**. These may be hereditary but in practice are more often acquired, due to

      i. Massive transfusion of stored blood. Two significant relevant changes occur in stored blood:

         – The citrate used as an anticoagulant causes a decrease in 2,3-BPG.
         – The red cells become considerably less deformable, with poor capillary perfusion.

      ii. **EXOGENOUS BICARBONATE** administered in cases of shock of keto-acidosis.
      iii. **SEVERE HYPOTHERMIA**, acidosis, or hypophosphatemia.
      iv. **MYXEDEMA**.
      v. **CARBON MONOXIDE POISONING**.

In the above cases compensatory mechanisms either do not operate or take too long to become effective.

3. **HYPERVISCOSITY SYNDROMES**, such as P. vera, paraproteinemias, etc.
4. **ANEMIA**.

In a basically healthy patient, **THE RESPONSES TO HYPOXEMIC HYPOXIA** have been extensively discussed in this chapter. Only a few further points will be made:

1. The degree of compensation depends on tissue hypoxia and not on the oxygen tension in the blood.
2. The normal excess oxygen supply over requirement provides a considerable "store" of oxygen.
3. Extraction by the tissues increases if they are healthy.
4. Blood is redistributed unless micro-circulatory controls are lost (as in septic shock, etc).
5. The ODC shifts readily to the right – indeed, normal red cells and Hb molecules are a prominent part of the compensation.
6. Adaptation in skeletal muscle is a special case.

Other Lung Conditions of Relevance to Blood Disease

Three conditions require a brief mention:

1. **PULMONARY THROMBOEMBOLISM**. There are many hypercoagulable states. Some of these tend to affect the venous system predominantly, and thus pulmonary embolism (and perhaps eventual pulmonary hypertension) is a common complication. These are discussed in Chapter 21.
2. **PULMONARY EOSINOPHILIA**. There are a number of syndromes characterized by diffuse pulmonary infiltrates and peripheral eosinophilia. These are discussed in Chapter 15.
3. **PULMONARY HEMORRHAGIC SYNDROMES**. Intra-pulmonary bleeding (e.g., pulmonary hemosiderosis) is a very uncommon cause of iron deficiency.

The Hematology of Malignant Disease

We are here referring to non-hematological malignancies. These can and very frequently do cause marked changes both in the blood cells (i.e., seen in the FBC) and in the hemostatic mechanism (i.e., seen in the Hemostatic Screen). Numerous pathological processes can be responsible, and the main ones are

1. Blood loss.
2. Iron malutilization (anemia of chronic disorders).
3. Bone marrow infiltration by metastases.
4. Bone marrow depression due to therapy.
5. Autoimmune hemolysis.
6. Microangiopathic hemolysis.
7. Disseminated intravascular coagulation.
8. Other hypercoagulable states.

Blood Loss in Malignant Disease

By far the most common sites for bleeding from malignant disease are the gastro-intestinal tract and the uterus. Uterine bleeding is hardly a diagnostic problem. GIT bleeding, however, can be occult, and indeed iron deficiency may be the first sign of a slow chronic occult bleed, especially from certain sites, such as the cecum and ascending colon.

Metastatic Spread to Bones

This classically presents as a leuko-erythroblastic reaction, but sometimes as a pancytopenia.

Microangiopathic Hemolysis

The vessels in a malignant growth, especially in a rapidly growing tumor, are typically very abnormal. This tends to affect the blood cells passing through, causing crenation and even fragmentation and microspherocytes – it may be difficult to differentiate this from DIC. Sometimes an underlying occult malignancy has been suspected purely on the basis of a raised RDW.

Disseminated Intravascular Coagulation (DIC)

Many malignant cells, notably adenocarcinomas, tend to secrete procoagulants, such as tissue factor and what is known as "cancer procoagulant". Mucin from adenocarcinomas can also activate factor X. This may result in a frank DIC. Very rapidly growing tumors tend to undergo necrosis, and this too is a known trigger for DIC.

Hypercoagulable States

The link between cancer and thrombosis was first described by Trousseau over 100 years ago. The hypercoagulable tendency can take several forms:

1. Migratory thrombophlebitis (Trousseau's sign).
2. "Idiopathic" venous thromboembolism. The risk of a future malignancy in a patient with venous thromboembolism is nearly 10%. This risk increases to nearly 20% with recurrent VTE.
3. DIC.

A SUMMARY OF FBC MANIFESTATIONS OF MALIGNANCY

1. Anemia. This is found in over 50% of all advanced malignancies.
2. Erythrocytosis. Malignant causes to consider include renal cell carcinoma, cerebellar hemangioblastoma, and hepatoma.
3. Neutrophilia or leukemoid reaction. Any rapidly growing malignancy especially with much necrosis; carcinomas of lung, stomach, and pancreas.
4. Eosinophilia. Hodgkin disease, melanoma, and brain tumors.
5. Thrombocytosis. This can be found in many malignancies.
6. Thrombocytopenia. This is particularly prominent in lymphomas and CLL.

BLEEDING TENDENCY IN MALIGNANCY
This may be due to thrombocytopenia or acquired factor deficiencies, the most common

of these being factor X deficiency due to adsorption by paraproteins (e.g., myeloma and macroglobulinemia).

The Erythrocyte Sedimentation Rate (ESR)

This is an old, non-specific and very valuable test. The basic principle underlying this test is that red cells, being biconcave discs, have a tendency at relative rest to stack on each other, like a roll of coins, forming rouleaux. However, for this stacking to occur requires that the mutually repulsive negative surface charges be overcome; this is achieved by HMW proteins, especially those that are elongated and can thus bridge the gap. The most important of these proteins is fibrinogen.

Thus it can be expected that where fibrinogen levels are increased, there will be a greater tendency to rouleaux formation and thus a raised ESR.

It can also be expected that where significant numbers of red cells do not show the biconcave structure, the aggregation and packing into rouleaux and their subsequent settling will be impaired.

The rouleaux being relatively dense will sink to the bottom of the container more rapidly. A number of states will tend to promote rouleaux formation:

1. Normocytic anemia per se, since rouleaux can form more easily (anemia will cause a mild increase in ESR, never more than about 30 mm/h, with the very important exception of iron deficiency and other causes of rigid and/or very deformed red cells). Note that macrocytic anemias frequently have ESRs in the vicinity of 40–50 mm/h, but this is largely due to the nature of the underlying causes.
2. Inflammatory and infiltrative disorders, due to the production of so-called acute phase proteins. The ESR is thus classed as an "activity" test. The height of the ESR in these conditions varies roughly with the degree of tissue damage; however, very high ESRs (over 100 mm/h) are typically associated with: myeloma, tuberculosis, Hodgkin lymphoma, and collagen vascular disease.

It is worthwhile mentioning that **THE ESR CAN BE UNUSUALLY LOW** or perhaps lower than one would otherwise suspect, in certain conditions:

1. Polycythemia vera
2. Homozygous sickle disease

3. Massive leukocytosis, e.g., in chronic leukemias
4. Hypofibrinogenemia (of relevance in DIC, where one might expect a high ESR especially if caused by sepsis)
5. High-dose steroids
6. High-dose salicylates

Other Activity Tests

This is a convenient place to briefly mention other tests of activity – the acute phase reactants. These, in contrast to the ESR, are all chemical tests (although some are performed by immunological methods). They are in general no more specific than the ESR (and a great deal more expensive), but have the advantage that they are not affected by anemia as well as being more rapid in their response to disease onset and offset. The most widely used are the C-reactive protein (CRP) and serum amyloid A (SAA). In hematological practice they are particularly useful in evaluating the significance of various leukocytoses and of ferritin levels in cases where the distinction between iron deficiency and anemia of chronic disease is important. There are three important caveats:

1. Steroids and non-steroidal anti-inflammatory drugs can significantly lower the levels.
2. Decreasing levels are not always indicative of successful therapy but can be due to hepatic failure (this is a particular practical problem in the ICU with severe sepsis).
3. There is major inter-laboratory variation. As with so many other tests, use the same lab for follow-up testing.

The CRP is probably the commonest of these tests. Some comments are appropriate:

1. Moderate increases (10–100 mg/l) occur in viral, spirochetal, mild, or early bacterial infections, and some parasitoses. Surgical procedures similarly will cause a moderate rise, but this falls rapidly in the absence of bacterial infection.
2. Marked increases are virtually pathognomonic of significant bacterial infections.
3. Group B streptococcal infections are frequently associated with a poor CRP response.
4. As mentioned, a fall in the level in bacterial infection is not necessarily a sign of good response to therapy, but may be due to liver failure as part of the sepsis syndrome.

There have been very many suggestions (and even directives in this regard), that the ESR should be retired and replaced by plasma viscosity and/or other activity tests, notably the CRP and the SAA. Yet like a bad penny, the ESR keeps turning up in the request list of the laboratory, and for very good reasons:

1. It is cheap and technically robust. The viscometers keep breaking down. One manufacturer has already stopped servicing them.
2. It can be done as an office procedure, and with due care will give reproducible results.
3. It has specific utility in a number of conditions where the CRP is normal, such as temporal arteritis.
4. The body of clinical knowledge relating to its interpretation is enormous.

Note, however, that

1. There is only a reasonable correlation between the plasma viscosity (PV) and the ESR. There are advantages to both methods, but in no sense can any one of them be seen to replace the other. For example, steroid treatment can normalize the PV but not the ESR.
2. While the ESR is indeed slower to rise and slower to fall than the CRP and PV, this is really only of relevance in specialized circumstances, such as rheumatological disorders, especially in the follow-up of acute exacerbations.

To summarize the causes of an increase in any of the activity tests, it is useful to remember the rule of "I's": Injury, Incision, Infection, Inflammation, Infarction, Infiltration.

Summary

This chapter discusses two broad fields in hematology:

1. A number of general pathophysiological processes or states that cannot conveniently be discussed elsewhere and which are of central importance in the understanding of certain changes in hematological reports.
2. Clinical interactions of the hematological system with other systems. Understanding these interactions are very important not only for the diagnosis of many blood diseases but to understand the clinical pictures that may present in practice.

General Pathophysiological Processes

1. The physiological response to hemorrhage. This shows itself as a sequence of changes, usually thrombocytosis, neutrophilia, and then anemia with reticulocytosis. The individual changes can be severe enough to cause diagnostic confusion.

2. The response of the blood cell system to hypoxia. This depends on whether the hypoxia is normobaric, i.e., with a normal arterial P_{O_2} (e.g., due to anemia), or hypobaric – i.e., with a decreased P_{O_2}. The difference is manifest in the rate and constancy of secretion of EPO and hence the development of reticulocytosis.

3. The raised hematocrit. This is a common FBC presentation and numerous disparate causes, from dehydration to myeloproliferative disorders. It is important to be able to distinguish these causes.

Clinical Interactions of the Blood with Other Systems

Diagnosis in blood diseases is very unusual in that almost all the evidence looked for and interpreted is secondary – i.e., in other systems. Also, it is important to know just how pathology in other systems may reflect or cause blood disease. Consequently, each of the other systems is looked at from this point of view. It is astonishing just how profound these interactions can be.

A Final Word!

Clinical laboratories provide vital and essential services for doctors in all fields. Properly, the relationship between clinicians and the laboratory should be one of partnership, of mutual respect. The laboratory is manned by very highly educated specialists who have a great deal to offer. There are a steadily increasing number and complexity of tests available; there is also great pressure on all concerned to contain costs. Cooperation will maximize the appropriateness, both medical and financial, of tests requested, as well as the timing, sequence, and interpretation of the tests.

Exercise 4.1

A quick self-test (Answers below)

True	False	Questions
		1. Anemia is logically the immediate response to acute hemorrhage
		2. Neutrophilia can be a purely physiological response, such as in reaction to hemorrhage
		3. Patients with a normal Hb and blood P_{O_2} can still have hypoxic tissues
		4. In hypobaric hypoxia erythropoietin secretion is constantly raised
		5. Erythrocytosis refers only to a raised red cell count
		6. Dehydration per se is a common cause of anemia
		7. Type III immune reactions are the only ones not associated with blood disease
		8. Drug-induced hemolytic reactions can be of the autoimmune type
		9. For an antibody to activate complement C1 it must bridge at least three antigenic sites
		10. The Coomb test detects only antibodies of autoimmune origin
		11. Thrombocytopenia in chronic liver disease may be due to endothelial activation
		12. The investigation of suspected malabsorption can only be done in specialized units
		13. Adverse prognostic features in systemic lupus erythematosus are autoimmune neutropenia, neutrophil dysfunction, and hypersplenism
		14. The characteristic blood picture of Addison disease (hypocorticalism) is mild normocytic anemia and eosinophilia
		15. The proper diagnosis of purpura is by laboratory testing
		16. The body's mitochondria consume 600 l of O_2 per day
		17. The oxygen-dissociation curve can be divided into three functional zones: tissue, venous, and arterial

Exercise 4.2

Match the items in columns 1 and 2 (Answers below)

Column 1	Column 2
A. Isolated thrombocytosis	1. May be found in dehydration, hypoxia, or chronic myeloproliferative disease
B. An appropriate reticulocyte response to a hemorrhage	2. The commonest form in Africa and typically the most severe
C. Hypoxia from the hematological point of view	3. Frequently involve the hematological system
D. A raised hematocrit	4. Can complicate chronic myeloproliferative diseases
E. Bronchopulmonary aspergillosis	5. May be the result of an active hemorrhage
F. Cold-type autoantibodies to red cells	6. Leukopenia, lymphopenia, hemolytic anemia, thrombocytopenia, raised ESR
G. Complicated pregnancies	7. Usually IgM complete antibodies
H. P. Falciparum malaria	8. By diffusion, with a maximum length physiologically of 100 μm
I. Pulmonary arterial hypertension	9. May be due to thrombocytopenia or acquired factor deficiency
J. Malabsorption syndromes	10. Either hypobaric or normobaric
K. Pregnancy	11. One that will restore the previous Hb within 2–3 weeks
L. Important indicators of activity in systemic lupus erythematosus	12. Have been implicated in the pathogenesis of autoimmune diseases
M. The oxygen supply path from the endothelium to the mitochondria of tissue cells	13. Associated with multiple changes in the blood, both physiological and pathological
N. A bleeding tendency in malignant disease	14. A typical example of an Arthus-type (type III) immune reaction

Answers

Exercise 4.1

1F; 2T; 3T; 4F; 5F; 6F; 7F; 8T; 9F; 10F; 11T; 12F; 13T; 14T; 15F; 16F; 17T.

Exercise 4.2

A5; B11; C10; D1; E14; F7; G12; H2; I4; J3; K13; L6; M8; N9.

Further Reading

Andreoli TE, Bennett JC, Carpenter CCJ, Plum F (eds) (1997). Cecil Essentials of Medicine. 4th edn. Philadelphia: WB Saunders.

Epstein RJ (1996). Medicine for Examinations. 3rd edn. London: Churchill Livingstone.

Hoffbrand AV, Catovsky D, Tuddenham EGD (eds) (2005). Postgraduate Haematology. 5th edn. Oxford: Blackwell Publishing.

Hoffbrand AV, Pettit JE (2001). Essential Haematology. 4th edn. Oxford: Blackwell Science.

Mammen EF (1994). Coagulation defects in liver disease. Med. Clin. N. Am. 78: 545–551.

Roitts I (1997). Essential Immunology. Berlin: Blackwell Wissenschaft-Verlag GmbH.

References

1. Gomez-Cambronero J (2001). The oxygen-dissociation curve of hemoglobin: bridging the gap between biochemistry and physiology. JCE 78: 757.
2. Hsia CW (1998). Respiratory function of hemoglobin. N. Engl. J. Med. 338: 239–247.

Her pure and eloquent blood,
Spoke in her cheeks, and so distinctly wrought
That one might say her body thought.

(John Donne)

Preview *Most students and many of their tutors do not know how (or indeed, why) to perform a systematic clinical examination in cases of suspected blood disease, on the assumption that the clinical features are not important and that the laboratory tests will give the diagnosis. Clinical methodology in blood diseases has unique aspects that need to be understood for an effective clinical approach to the patient. Thus it will be necessary to review briefly the general process of clinical diagnosis, a topic we generally take for granted, otherwise the hematological diagnostic approach will not be properly understood. Basically, the pathological diagnosis is achieved in three stages – the anatomical (or first-stage) diagnosis, the general pathology diagnosis, and then the special pathology diagnosis. Included is a discussion of how tests can reflect disease and how to use the results to make clinical decisions and ultimately a diagnosis. The concept of a constantly narrowing clinical search space is presented, and its relation to Bayes' theorem. These principles are then applied with considerable adaptation to the diagnosis of blood diseases. The result is a sensible and sound patient-orientated approach to blood diseases.*

More specifically, with respect to blood diseases, the clinical approach is discussed in three sections:

1. *How to suspect clinically that a patient has a blood disease.*
2. *Relevant issues in the clinical history.*
3. *The clinical examination. Each of the features is discussed with reference to the findings in the first-line tests.*

It should be understood that effective diagnosis in hematology requires broad clinical expertise.

It will be recalled that the theme of this book is the integrated clinical and laboratory approach to hematological problems and their tests. **THE APPLICATION OF CLINICAL METHODOLOGY TO BLOOD DISEASES HAS SOME UNIQUE ASPECTS**. Students in learning clinical methods naturally take a great deal for granted, without giving much thought to the actual process. But integrating blood diseases into the clinical realm is not quite straightforward, and a conscious understanding of what we do in a clinical encounter will be necessary to achieve this integration.

It is therefore necessary to describe the traditional clinical methodology in broad outline, as well as investigate currently popular statistics-based methods, particularly Bayes' theorem. Enormous amounts of research into these topics have been performed. The subsequent discussion of clinical and diagnostic methods in blood diseases will thus be placed in a proper context, enabling some unusual and complex concepts to be understood; this is essential if a properly integrated assessment is to be achieved.

The Nature of Traditional Clinical Diagnosis

Traditionally the student has always been taught that first he takes a history (with several subsections); then he does the clinical examination (usually a complete examination of all systems); and finally he does such special investigations

O.N. Beck, *Diagnostic Hematology*, DOI 10.1007/978-1-84800-295-1_5,
© Springer-Verlag London Limited 2009

that seem relevant. This is all very well as a discipline, but the real world does not work this way; generally the clinician is faced with the patient, greets him, and makes him comfortable. In the process, even before a word has been spoken, numerous observations have been made that frequently cause him to think in certain directions, and these initial assessments become more and more accurate with experience. This direction has many aspects:

1. Are there any features that indicate or suggest that the patient has a disease? If so, do the features suggest what type of process is operating?
2. How seriously ill is the patient – the actual question being: is the patient ill enough that urgent intervention is required and therefore postpone the systematic parts of the history and examination?
3. What sort of disease and which system are involved?

The range of considerations also depends on the circumstances: seeing a patient in an office in a chair across a desk from the clinician gives a more restricted list of possibilities than if he were lying in bed, for example, in the first case he is exposed only to the head and neck, and perhaps the hands. This also to some extent determines the order of doing things. In essence, however, the history and examination are undertaken more or less concurrently.

In practice we must first and foremost suspect that a patient has a disease – in our case a blood disease. We must then systematically follow up the suspicious finding. With experience this pattern is often observed virtually as a single entity (the so-called "spot" diagnosis); this should always be confirmed by further systematic study of the patient.

All experienced clinicians are aware that any one fact elicited in the history or examination tends to suggest at least a **RANGE** of possibilities. They will then seek further data that may confirm or refute the suspicious possibilities. Conversely, a specific disease possibility may be suggested by several findings in different parts of the body.

The effect is that the subsequent search is more directed so as to find more features that could be relevant to his original suspicion. This "direction" is such that, having a suspicion or a provisional diagnosis, any further examination, procedure, or test (these will be all referred to as "tests" as a generic term) must be evaluated in terms of whether it increases or decreases the likelihood of the suggested diagnosis being correct. These two states, before and after the particular test, and known as pre-test and post-test degree of certainty, are further discussed later in the section on Statistical Aspects of Diagnosis: Bayes' Theorem.

The rational approach to diagnosis in **ALL** diseases and systems generally goes through several stages:

1. **THE IDENTIFICATION OF FEATURES THAT MAKE ONE SUSPECT THAT A DISEASE IS PRESENT**. This provides a general direction in which one thinks based upon these features. In this case the provisional diagnosis/es would be an inference, **WORKING FROM THE PARTICULAR (THE OBSERVATION OF A SPECIFIC FEATURE) TO THE GENERAL (ONE OR MORE PROVISIONAL DIAGNOSES)**. Numerous methods exist:

   a. **OBSERVATION**. The appearance of the patient or a part of him may be enough to raise suspicion. This suspicion may be more or less specific.
   b. **A SPECIFIC COMPLAINT** by the patient. This may be very difficult to elicit, for various reasons.
   c. **AN INCIDENTAL FINDING** during questioning or examination. This may be as simple as a throwaway line such as "I don't feel the left side of my body normally," or a simple finding like koilonychia.
   d. **A FINDING IN A BLOOD TEST** requested for another reason. For example, in a life insurance examination, the incidental finding of a raised MCV in an otherwise normal FBC may be found.

2. **SYSTEMATIC INVESTIGATION – MAKING THE PATHOLOGICAL DIAGNOSIS**. Any of the above should lead to a systematic search, via questioning and examination, for confirmatory or contradictory features (a primarily clinical, stepwise, logical process). It involves making the pathological diagnosis by the gathering of relevant data. A finding may point not only to a disease being present but to its general nature, for example, urea frost points not only to the fact that the patient is ill, but also directly to renal failure. The process involves answers to three distinct questions:

   a. **WHERE IS THE PATHOLOGY?** That is, which organ, tissue, or compartment is the seat of disease? This is the first-stage or **ANATOMIC DIAGNOSIS**. Its importance cannot be overstated: for example, if a mass in the left loin were identified as an enlarged kidney rather than an enlarged spleen, a completely different direction of further investigation would be followed from that were it an enlarged spleen. Note that in most cases, **EXCEPT IN HEMATOLOGY,** the first-stage diagnosis is entirely clinical (even in hematology it is occasionally possible to make a firm first-stage diagnosis entirely clinically; for examples see later in this chapter under The Pathologic Diagnosis in Blood Diseases). Note also that the first-stage diagnosis generally comprises a list of possibilities, and subsequent clinical investigation is directed toward finding features that tend to confirm or refute each possibility.
   b. **WHAT POSSIBLE GENERAL PATHOLOGY PROCESSES OF A LESION IN THAT**

ANATOMICAL SITE COULD BE RESPONSIBLE? Examples are infective, inflammatory, degenerative, structural/metabolic (hereditary), neoplastic, and the like. This requires knowledge of general, organ, and tissue pathology. But actually **GETTING TO THE GENERAL PATHOLOGY DIAGNOSIS DEPENDS HEAVILY ON CLINICAL INPUT**: selecting the right questions to ask and the sites to examine and for what, and hence deciding what investigations are warranted, if any. **WITHOUT THE FIRST-STAGE DIAGNOSIS IT WOULD BE VERY DIFFICULT INDEED TO KNOW HOW TO PROCEED IN THIS WAY.** Note that the general pathology diagnosis generally also subsumes a list of possible **SPECIFIC** pathologies. Each of the possibilities is then weighed up, for and against.

c. **WHAT IS THE SPECIFIC CAUSE OF THE PATHOLOGY AT THAT SITE?** This very often requires special investigations, the choice of which is again determined by the general possibilities.

> The pathological diagnosis fits into a broader diagnostic context:
>
> 1. The pathological diagnosis.
> 2. The etiology.
> 3. The complications.
>
> In general clinical work these are often made clinically but reinforced and *sometimes* replaced by technology.
>
> 4. Purely clinical issues of prognosis, decisions of management, etc.

Finding the pathology is central to standard, scientific medicine; it is what sets us apart from all the "alternative" disciplines. Correlation of pathology with clinical features is in its turn the basis of our clinical practice; clinical features that are known to reflect pathological changes enable us to infer the pathology from the clinical examination. An example will make things clearer.[1] A male patient 50 years of age presents with a right-sided hemiplegia and motor aphasia:

1. That **HE HAS A DISEASE** is without doubt. It is of the nervous system and numerous general possibilities cross one's mind, including causes in the cardiovascular system and so on.
2. **THE ANATOMICAL DIAGNOSIS** also is straightforward: it is a lesion in the left motor cortex or subcortex. This then also functions as the pre-test diagnosis. But, given only this information, this is **ALL** that one can say. To advance we need more information, and the information we seek is **DEPENDENT UPON,**

DIRECTED BY, THE ANATOMICAL DIAGNOSIS. Every piece of information of whatever type that we select to find an answer for – i.e., a "test" – is chosen strictly on the basis that it will increase or decrease the post-test level of certainty.

3. How we choose these tests is dependent upon the pathological possibilities. **THE POSSIBLE GENERAL PATHOLOGY CAUSES** in the above-mentioned case are vascular, neoplastic, infective, inflammatory, and so on. We weigh up the possible general causes, in terms of probability and on the basis of evidence for and against each possibility. Finding this evidence requires considerable pathological and clinical knowledge – it is a highly intellectual process that we undertake almost automatically and take largely for granted. Directed enquiry and examination again follow. Thus, should we now elicit the additional information about this patient that the hemiplegia came on **SUDDENLY**, we could put a **VASCULAR CAUSE** high up on the list of probable general pathology causes (even an acute bleed into a neoplasm is still, in this context, a vascular lesion). What we cannot yet do is say what specific type of vascular lesion it is – hemorrhage, thrombosis, or embolism – not without further information. Once again this is gained by eliciting further relevant information, **DIRECTED BY THE PREVIOUS STAGES**. The possibilities are now considerably fewer than with only the anatomical diagnosis – indeed, without the correct anatomical diagnosis, arriving at the general (and then specific) diagnosis would be immeasurably more difficult. In addition the level of certainty is considerably greater.

4. **THE SPECIFIC (OR SPECIAL PATHOLOGY) DIAGNOSIS** in this patient is easily reached after the following data are obtained – the patient is severely hypertensive, there is projectile vomiting, and the level of consciousness is very low and deteriorating. Thus one could confidently conclude that the lesion is a hemorrhage.

Note in the above case that one is working from the general ("stroke") to the particular ("cerebral hemorrhage"), i.e., a deductive process, with the diagnostic considerations becoming ever less. We can thus speak of a constantly narrowing search space. A practical example with hematological connotations illustrates the process: a middle-aged female patient presents. She on first sight is very obese. We could speak of "obesity" as the anatomical diagnosis. There is a very wide range of causes of obesity, only a minority of which are not due to caloric imbalance, and the number of pre-test possibilities is large.

What is NOT acceptable is saying that, since caloric imbalance is the commonest cause of obesity, the obesity should in the first instance be treated as such, and that

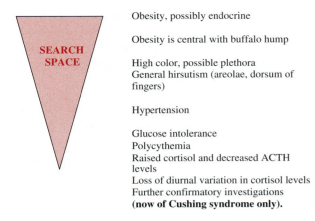

Obesity, possibly endocrine

Obesity is central with buffalo hump

High color, possible plethora
General hirsutism (areolae, dorsum of fingers)

Hypertension

Glucose intolerance
Polycythemia
Raised cortisol and decreased ACTH levels
Loss of diurnal variation in cortisol levels
Further confirmatory investigations
(**now of Cushing syndrome only**).

Fig. 5.1

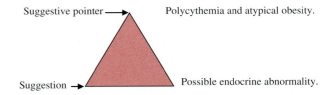

Fig. 5.2

only if this is unsuccessful is the rest of the diagnostic process engaged upon (a standard HMO type of approach, depending entirely on prevalence and cost–benefit ratios). A patient with myxedema, for example, could be placed in considerable jeopardy if this process were adhered to. Thus we are constrained to exclude these other causes of obesity, and a thorough clinical examination would go far to achieve this.

In this process, we wish to find features that could identify the general cause; therefore we look for them actively, based on our knowledge of obesity. We note that the patient has a moon face and a flourishing moustache. While these could be incidental, a flag is raised in our mind of the possibility of an endocrine disturbance (such as Cushing syndrome, Stein–Leventhal syndrome, etc.). See Fig. 5.1 – this illustrates some of the steps and findings in the further stepwise examination and thinking.

Note in Fig. 5.1 that the search becomes ever more concentrated, with increasingly greater specificity with respect to the ultimate diagnosis, and less and less chance of being wrong. The figure lists a **FEW** of the findings that have enabled us to reach the specific diagnosis (of Cushing syndrome). Note that as the search space constantly narrows, each finding suggests a more specific feature of the disease (more or less).

Observe that the above paradigm is, in logic, essentially deductive – i.e., from the general (provisional list of possible diagnoses) to the particular.

However, not all patients with Cushing syndrome have the classical appearance. It may be (as has happened to the author) that a male patient presents with generalized obesity and none of the other stigmata of Cushing. The patient had been referred for stabilization and an assessment of antibiotic prescription since he had pneumonia. Two specific observations were crucial: in the FBC the (expected) neutrophilia was accompanied by a raised Hct and platelet count (see Chapter 15); and when interviewing his relatives

it was observed that only the patient was obese – indeed, the rest of the family were decidedly skinny. Thus the primary observations or entry points into the paradigm were primarily the polycythemia (which could have had a simple explanation) and then the atypical obesity. A (very) tentative diagnosis of Cushing syndrome was entertained (and later proven biochemically).

Here the general provisional diagnostic possibility was provided by observation of one or more particular features. In this part of the process in this case it can be seen that the logical process is essentially inductive – i.e., from the particular to the general. Induction is portrayed in Fig. 5.2. And in the deductive part of the process that follows, the entry point is lower in the paradigm of obesity/Cushing syndrome; properly one not only continues "down" the space, but also backtracks to check on the possible existence and interpretation of previous findings.

In effective clinical work, both forms of logic – deductive and inductive – are used seamlessly. For example, at any point in the process we may come across a feature that does not belong to the pattern or one that in fact tends to contradict our previous findings. This would then operate as a new pointer to another possibility (induction), which then is investigated formally (deductive).

At any and every point in the clinical encounter, the doctor has to decide

1. Whether disease exists or not
2. Whether to order a test or not
3. Whether to institute treatment or not

It is here that operating characteristics of the various clinical and laboratory findings can be of great assistance. They cannot, however, supplant clinical judgment. In our description of clinical methodology in blood diseases, we shall see how the above template is extremely useful.

The Pathological Diagnosis in Blood Diseases

On the one hand there are considerable similarities in the diagnostic approaches to blood disease compared with other systems. For example, a patient has what appears to be a rash consisting of dark spots most noticeable around the axillae; if this were misdiagnosed as purpura instead of **ACANTHOSIS NIGRICANS** (which we have seen done, and by a postgraduate!), there is no way that the true nature of the pathology would be elucidated.

However (and this is where diagnosis in hematology is markedly different from other specialties), purpura happens to be one of the very few anatomical diagnoses in hematology that can be made entirely clinically. Generally in hematology the anatomical diagnosis poses a problem. Hematological conditions are largely functional in terms of their clinical presentation, and there is not an obvious anatomical equivalent of say anemia. However, if, e.g., anemia were defined as a reduction in the total red cell mass, then that can function as an **ABSTRACT** anatomical structure (and indeed one formal definition of anemia is a reduction in total red cell mass).

So, utilizing this concept in conjunction with the results of **THE FIRST-LINE TESTS**, one can talk of a number of "anatomical," **FIRST-STAGE DIAGNOSES**, for example,

1. Microcytic anemia
2. Severe eosinophilia
3. Thrombocytosis
4. and so on

This makes the approach in hematology almost unique, and constitutes the major difference from other clinical diagnostic activities.

Using the process described, we are putting the results of our first-line tests into a strictly clinical methodology. It is said by many that, for example, "anemia" is not a diagnosis, but a symptom. The author disagrees: it **IS** a diagnosis, albeit only a first-stage diagnosis, just as "massive splenomegaly" is a first-stage diagnosis, which needs further to be clinically defined.

In the vast majority of cases, the first-stage diagnosis in hematology (e.g., "microcytic anemia") is achieved *via the blood tests*: without reaching this diagnosis accurately, one could not expect to rationally proceed further to the diagnosis of say iron deficiency and thence perhaps to carcinoma of the cecum.

There are occasions, however, when a firm or reasonably firm first-stage diagnosis can be made clinically. A few examples:

1. *Henoch–Schönlein "purpura."* The typical clinical picture is classical.
2. *Severe hemophilia.* At least the differential diagnosis of hemophilia A and B can be made reasonably confidently.
3. *Iron-deficiency anemia.*
4. *Pernicious anemia.*

5. *The toast-and-tea syndrome.*
6. *Hypoxic plethora.*

In the above conditions the clinical features can be so convincing that the diagnosis is obvious.

However, any attempt to make a purely clinical first-stage diagnosis in hematology is to be discouraged except for the very experienced. Even then and if only for medico-legal reasons, the relevant first-line blood test/s must be requested.

For various reasons, the concept of the first-stage diagnosis in the bleeding disorders is different, and poses some special problems. It will be discussed later. Therefore, for the rest of this section we concentrate solely on the disorders involving the blood cells (but since this includes the platelets, there will inevitably be some involvement of bleeding).

Thus, the first question is: where is the pathology? In the case of hematology this is an abstraction, and relies very heavily on the results of the first-line tests.

Once the anatomical diagnosis has been made, the main problem in practice is **WHAT TO DO WITH THE FIRST-STAGE DIAGNOSIS**. Properly, this is followed by a consideration of the general pathology.

The General Pathology Diagnosis

The possibilities here depend on the system involved and on the first-stage diagnosis. And it is at this stage that clinical acumen is most crucial.

In the case of say anemia, the **GENERAL CAUSES** would be post-hemorrhagic, nutritional deficiency, extravascular hemolysis, decreased production, and so on (see Chapter 6). Let us say that we find in a patient that the anemia is normocytic (the "anatomical" diagnosis – the possible general causes of a normocytic anemia are listed in Chapter 10). In an attempt to identify the general pathology triggered by this anatomical diagnosis (**AND THIS IS AN ENTIRELY CLINICAL PROCEDURE**), we now elicit the story that the patient has had chronic recurrent anemia and jaundice for years, has an enlarged spleen, reticulocytosis, and a history of a relative who had had the same problem and was "cured" by splenectomy: the provisional **GENERAL DIAGNOSIS** of a **CHRONIC HEREDITARY EXTRAVASCULAR HEMOLYSIS** would be very high on the list. What we cannot say, without further information, is what the specific diagnosis will be.

THUS THE CLINICAL INPUT AT THE STAGE OF THE GENERAL PATHOLOGY DIAGNOSIS is extremely significant; and this is one of the areas where clinical acumen is central; sometimes, however, the firm diagnosis requires **ADDITIONAL** ancillary laboratory and radiological efforts.

> Thus the second question is: what are the general types of pathology (the nature of the process) that a lesion of this kind could be?

The Special Pathology Diagnosis

It generally requires special investigations, but sometimes in certain systems, a specific diagnosis can be made clinically with reasonable certainty, as for example in our patient with stroke. In blood diseases, by contrast, the specific diagnosis is almost always an exclusively laboratory activity, requiring more or less extensive further tests to identify the exact cause of the general process – but the major point to be made is that ONLY THOSE TESTS NOW NEED TO BE DONE (as opposed to a shotgun approach). The diagnostic clincher is always made at this stage, and can take various forms.

In our patient with chronic anemia, jaundice, and splenomegaly, numerous spherocytes in the smear of our patient would strongly suggest hereditary spherocytosis, which would be confirmed by other specific tests. Thus it is the task of the next stage of diagnosis to identify what is going on, by requesting the appropriate tests (and **ONLY** these tests).

> Thus, the third question is: what is the cause of this general process?

In ending this section, it is always useful to ask yourself two traditional clinical questions:

1. "What kind of disease is this patient likely to get?"
2. "What kind of patient is this disease likely to attack?"

Unfortunately most teaching in hematology (including books) stops at or becomes skimpy after the first-stage diagnosis. It may seem difficult to reach the anatomical diagnosis on the basis of the first-line tests (although this book will show that this should not usually be a problem), but arriving at the general pathology diagnosis (a primarily clinical process) can indeed be difficult. The key to the whole process is **WORK SYSTEMATICALLY AND LOGICALLY THROUGH THE STAGES**.

Traditional clinical diagnosis as discussed above is regarded in some quarters as superfluous (in truth probably as requiring too much effort and mental discipline), and many shortcuts are described, most of them statistical. A common one, to be avoided at all costs, is to say that, since a majority of blood diseases are secondary to nutritional deficiencies, one can conclude that the other causes are not of practical significance. This error has led to the focusing on those features of the tests (notably the FBC) that are typical of nutritional disorders, without recognizing that **THE SAME OR SIMILAR FINDINGS CAN REFLECT OTHER TYPES OF DISEASE**. This can (and commonly does) lead to absurd and potentially dangerous practices such as treating say a thalassemia (a microcytic anemia) with an iron preparation or an aplastic anemia (characterized by a mild macrocytosis) with vitamin B_{12} injections! What has happened here?

1. The examiner stopped thinking as soon as he saw that the anemia was microcytic or macrocytic, as the case may be.
2. There was no system to the investigation.
3. There was a very restricted view of blood disease. Imagine a gynecologist deciding that, since the commonest cause of menorrhagia in a 30-year-old woman is endocrine imbalance, it is not necessary to exclude myomata! He would not dream of doing this, yet colleagues of his persuasion have been known to apply this type of thinking to hematology.
4. There was no recognition of the importance of the clinical input.

Another shortcut is to attempt to find methods of making a diagnosis of a blood abnormality exclusively on the basis of blood tests and bypassing the clinical evaluation; this is a major source of error and unnecessary further testing. These methods also depend on the **STATISTICAL MIND-SET**.

However, it must be emphasized that statistical and probability studies have considerably enriched the traditional methods, in terms of validation and quantification of the different stages. These methods are discussed next.

Clinical Assessment in Hematology: a Perspective

Considerable research has quantified the value added by each stage of the clinical evaluation in many specialties. For instance in neurology, the physical examination constitutes a very significant part of reaching the final diagnosis, in the order of 60 or 70%. The situation in hematology is very different.

In hematology, the history on average contributes about 25% to the diagnosis, and thus its importance cannot be exaggerated – indeed, it has happened time and time again that a careful history has provided a clear (and ultimately accurate) estimate of the final diagnosis before a finger (or syringe) was laid on the patient.

The physical examination adds only about 5%, but this 5% can be extremely valuable in certain circumstances.

The laboratory tests contribute around 65% (frequently a lot more). However, it should be remembered that the FBC plays a dual role – it is both a diagnostic and confirmatory test, and has a very significant role in actually deciding whether or not a blood disease (in the broadest sense) exists.

Since changes in the blood such as anemia may be (and indeed very commonly are) the result of disease in another system, it will be *that* system that deserves the focus, and therefore the clinical methodology of that system must be known. The type of hematological change found in these cases may throw light on the nature of the primary disease, e.g., the anemia of chronic disorders suggests that a chronic disease in that system be looked for.

On the other hand, changes in one of the other systems may be directly attributable to disease in the blood, e.g., factor V_{Leiden} deficiency, which can be responsible for recurrent pulmonary emboli. The clinical features in other systems are often of relevance in assessing the severity of the blood disease: for example, the severity of anemia is a clinical decision, arrived at by evaluating changes in other systems.

Statistical Methods of Diagnosis: Bayes' Theorem[2]

As mentioned before, considerable research has been done to elucidate the diagnostic process. One of the most fruitful lines has been the application of Bayes' theorem. This has become an important contemporary topic, and something should be known about it. The theorem itself is highly theoretical, and only a general description will be given here. Note that its use derives from the statistical mind-set. The essential fact to mention is that in its pure form, as an algorithm, it very commonly is successful, but the time taken is totally unpractical. Therefore only aspects are used, and used very successfully.

Let us consider a highly relevant part of the diagnostic process, which is seeking a state that maximizes $p(D|S)$, that is, the probability (p) of the disease (D), given the sign or symptom or test result (S). It is very difficult to calculate $p(D|S)$ from instances of S. Bayes' theorem provides a way of calculating it from three other quantities, $p(D)$, $p(S|G)$, and $p(S)$. Thus

$$p(D|S) = \frac{p(D) \times p(S|D)}{p(S)}$$

where

1. $p(D)$ is the **A PRIORI PROBABILITY THAT D IS CORRECT**
2. $p(S)$ is the **A PRIORI PROBABILITY OF S BEING PRESENT**
3. $p(S|D)$ is the **PROBABILITY OF OBSERVING S GIVEN THE DISEASE D**

Consider the diagnosis of cerebral hemorrhage and its relation to hypertension:

$p(S|D)$ requires a knowledge of the chance of finding hypertension in cases of cerebral hemorrhage.

$p(S)$ requires a knowledge of what is the probability of hypertension is, being present in otherwise normal people and regardless of any diagnosis. Obviously if a large number of people are hypertensive without any symptoms or sequelae, finding hypertension in a case of sudden hemiplegia loses a lot of validity as a diagnostic finding. (This point and way of thinking puts hypertension – and other signs – into a considerably different perspective. It is one of the major benefits and intellectual contributions to clinical thinking provided by Bayes' theorem. It also applies to the interpretation of blood tests. Note, however, that in this example the **SEVERITY** of the hypertension has not been taken into account).

The major problem in this exercise is calculating or determining $p(D)$, i.e., whether cerebral hemorrhage is present. Current thinking in many quarters is that this is provided by knowledge of the prevalence of the

Fig. 5.3 Bayes' Theorem in clinical diagnosis

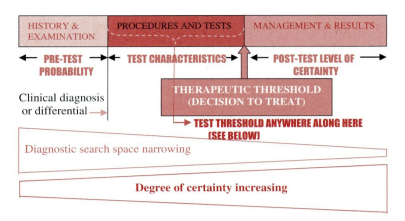

disease in the community, and this is where the author respectfully disagrees; while prevalence of a disease is a necessary consideration, it cannot be used as the sole criterion for a pre-test diagnosis. A proper clinical examination plus logic will in most cases provide this pre-test diagnosis. But the rest of the Bayesian paradigm is extremely useful. A modified schema is shown in figure 5.3.

The Bayesian Stages of Diagnosis To summarize briefly and broadly, there are four stages in this diagnostic paradigm, each with its own set of criteria, processes, and dangers:

1. The pre-test probability of a diagnosis
2. Testing
3. Therapeutic threshold
4. Post-test probability

THE PRE-TEST PROBABILITY of a diagnosis is provided **BY THE CLINICAL HISTORY AND EXAMINATION**, influenced by knowledge of incidence and prevalence of disease. It is essentially based on the clinician's **CLINICAL** estimate of the diagnosis **BEFORE ANY CONFIRMATORY TESTS ARE DONE**, and is a process of generating hypotheses about the nature of the illness presented to us. How the pre-test diagnostic probabilities are reached has already been discussed.

TESTING strictly speaking involves any clinical or other test or procedure to change the pre-test diagnosis. From our point of view, the most important tests involve laboratory or radiological investigations. Once again, one attempts to quantify their contribution.

THE THERAPEUTIC THRESHOLD is reached when we have sufficient certainty to initiate therapy.

THE POST-TEST LEVEL of certainty.

This paradigm, in a very simplified form, is depicted in Fig. 5.3. In general, the figure depicts the sequence of events usually followed, and each stage reached usually narrows the "search space" within which to look for the final answer.

The different stages shown are all decision thresholds, and they are reached depending on

1. The operating characteristics of the test or clinical procedure (see Chapter 4)
2. The risk of the test or procedure
3. The efficacy and risk of the proposed therapy

One thus attempts to weigh up the benefit versus risk of any procedure, test, or treatment. The greater the risk, the more certain the diagnosis must be. When benefits equal costs/risks, the treatment threshold probability is 0.5. If disease probability is lower than this, the doctor can either **ORDER A TEST** or **DO NOTHING**. When these choices have an equal probability, one has reached the **TEST THRESHOLD.**

Actually determining these thresholds mathematically is a very complicated procedure, and in at the general level, only the principles should be known:

1. Decide on a treatment threshold (the probability above which you would treat and below which you would wait). How you do this depends very much on you – your training, your experience, and so on – and on the circumstances – the patient in context, economic considerations, etc.
2. Decide on the likelihood ratio of a positive test (LR + or sensitivity/false-positive rate) and of a negative test (LR– or false-negative rate/specificity).

What the above boils down to is that our decisions are (or should be) determined by **PROBABILITY AND UTILITY**. So, in practice, determine the most common diagnosis first, then check for "a diagnosis you cannot afford to miss."

Thus, depending on the skill and experience of the practitioner, the history and examination will generate one or more hypotheses about the probability of disease being present and its characterization:

1. If the probability is say <5%, no further tests are indicated and the patient is reassured and sent home.
2. If a disease can be identified with a probability of say >80%, treatment is instituted without further ado.
3. However, the usual scenario is that the probability of an identifiable disease is around 50%. In this case the hypotheses generated influence the choice of tests to be done (a tiny subset of all possible tests). However, to be able to do this, the nature of the relevant tests, their characteristics, and **HOW TO INTERPRET THEM** must be known. Again, to reiterate, the laboratory, with the best will in the world, can seldom make the final decision: the pathologist has not seen the patient and the results must be correlated **BY THE CLINICIAN** with the clinical features to make them truly relevant.

A Note About "Testing" in Hematology

Apart from each specific question and examination method in the clinical examination being a "test," laboratory and radiological tests play a very large role in the diagnosis of blood diseases, particularly the first-line tests. The FBC or hemostatic screen may be done or requested at any stage of the proceedings, depending on the presentation.

The patient may even present with a FBC. There are many cases, usually presenting to the family practitioner, of very vague symptoms – simply a feeling of debility, malaise, chronic tiredness, perhaps lack of concentration. There are many possible causes, but if on history and examination nothing contributory is found, it is extremely common for a few blood tests to be requested, the most important undoubtedly being the FBC, since it has potentially so much to offer.

One point must be stressed: there must be some justification for requesting any test. When done in this way, the tests should be interpreted as part of the full clinical examination.

How to Suspect that a Patient Has a Blood Disease

It will be remembered that we are using the term "blood disease" in its broadest sense, i.e., either a reactive, a secondary, or a primary blood disease.

Note that this is an entirely clinical enterprise, except in the case where a first-line test, almost always the FBC, has been performed as a "routine." In this sort of case the FBC may provide a (provisional and partial) diagnosis of a blood disease, which may be either reactive, secondary, or primary. This would then be the starting point of the clinical process and would be followed by the same sort of thinking as that described below, but a little more directed in nature. For example, the features may suggest iron deficiency (see Chapter 8); directed search would now be made for sources of bleeding (perhaps occult or ignored by the patient), for dietary inadequacies, and for evidence of malabsorption. In the rest of this discussion, however, we concentrate on the more standard clinical presentation – i.e., a specific symptom, a set of symptoms, or signs, that suggest blood disease.

> Bear in mind that the operating characteristics of many of the clinical features described in the next few pages have not been extensively researched, and traditional clinical judgment is necessary.

Symptoms Volunteered by or Elicited from the Patient that Suggest a Blood Disease

1. Proneness to easy bleeding, bruising, bleeding into the skin, gums [?bleeding disorder]
2. Pruritus [?polycythemia vera, especially when associated with cold water, ?obstructive biliary disease, ?Hodgkin lymphoma]
3. Painful mouth and tongue [?iron, B_{12}, or folate deficiency]
4. Post-prandial bloating especially with wheat, barley, and oats products [?adult-onset gluten enteropathy with iron and/or folate deficiency]
5. Recurrent Painful swelling of the joints [?hemophilia, ?collagen disease]
6. Bone Pain [?myeloma, ?leukemia, ?bone secondaries (breast, kidney, lung, thyroid, prostate), ?hyperparathyroidism]
7. Pain or weakness in legs, gait [?vitamin B_{12} deficiency, ?amyloidosis]
8. Passage of dark urine [?red cells, usually renal pathology; ?myoglobin, as in rhabdomyolysis; ?hemoglobin, most commonly due to intravascular hemolysis]
9. Dysphagia [?iron deficiency, especially if localizable to the upper chest]
10. Dyspnea on effort relieved by lying flat [?anemia]

11. **R**ecurrent thrombosis [?hypercoagulability, usually venous]
12. **R**ecurrent infections [?immune deficiency, either in the white cells or in specific plasma proteins]
13. **R**ecurrent jaundice [?hemolysis]
14. **R**aynaud's phenomenon [?immune hemolysis, ?scleroderma, ?cryoglobulinemia]

Signs Found on Inspection that Suggest a Blood Disease

1. **P**allor [?anemia]
2. **P**lethora [?**P**olycythemia]
3. **P**urpura [?bleeding disorder or vasculitis]
4. Other **P**igmentary disturbances, such as lemon-yellow jaundice [?hemolysis, ?megaloblastosis], cyanosis [?chronic chest disease with erythrocytosis, ?methemoglobinemia]
5. **P**ruritus, especially associated with cold water [?**P**olycythemia vera].
6. **P**erifollicular hemorrhages [?scurvy]
7. Severe **P**yrexia and other features of se**P**sis [?immune deficiencies – AIDS, lymphoma, myeloma, etc.]
8. **P**eutz–Jegher syndrome [?iron deficiency]
9. **P**eriorbital bleeding [?hemophilia, ?acute leukemia]
10. **P**ainful red tongue [?iron, B_{12}, or folate deficiency]
11. **P**eriodontal infiltration and bleeding [?scurvy, ?monoblastic leukemias, ?epanutin intoxication (megaloblastic anemia)]
12. S**P**oon-shaped nails (koilonychia) [?iron deficiency]
13. Raynaud's **P**henomenon [?immune hemolysis, ?scleroderma, ?cryoglobulinemia]
14. **P**regnancy [?iron and folate deficiency, ?pre-eclampsia with thrombocytopenia, ?hemolytic anemia, ?bleeding disorder (acquired factor VIII deficiency), ?antiphospholipid syndrome]
15. **P**ickwickian syndrome and obesity in general [?hypoventilation with erythrocytosis, ?Cushing syndrome with polycythemia]
16. Multiple sternal **P**unctures [?bone marrow diseases characterized by difficult aspiration, such as myelofibrosis, hairy cell leukemia]
17. Enlarged s**P**leen [?hereditary red cell disorders with chronic hemolysis, ?amyloidosis, ?hypersplenism with cytopenias]
18. **P**ortal hypertension [?chronic liver disease with anemia, bleeding tendency, cytopenias]
19. **P**rostatic enlargement [?carcinoma with bone metastases (cytopenias)]
20. **P**arasitoses [various presentations, plus eosinophilia]
21. **P**ainful swollen joint [?hemophilia, ?septic arthritis (?immune depleted)]
22. **P**eripheral neuropathy [?vitamin B_{12} deficiency, ?amyloidosis – ?palpable nerves]
23. **P**sychosis [?vitamin B_{12} deficiency, ?VAD therapy for myeloma]
24. **S**ternal or other bone tenderness [?myeloma, ?leukemia (especially sternal tenderness), ?bone secondaries (breast, kidney, lung, thyroid, prostate), ?hyperparathyroidism]
25. **C**yanosis. This may be true cyanosis and may be associated with erythrocytosis, or false cyanosis, suggesting methemoglobinemia; this characteristically is not accompanied by dyspnea.

There are a few others that are rare – you can add to the list as you see fit. These characteristics are discussed in full later. Suspicion may arise as soon as the encounter begins or it may arise in the course of the full examination. Obviously, suspicion is immeasurably strengthened when two or more of the features pointing to the same possibility are found.

"Listen to the patient – he is giving you the diagnosis". (Sir William Osler)

The Clinical History

If a FBC or hemostatic screen has been done, they may provide considerable assistance in the taking of the history and may provide a first-stage diagnosis at this early stage. Care must be exercised, however, that the focus is not too narrow as a result of having these results.

The following points should ideally be included in the history from all your patients, bearing in mind that many can be symptoms of disease in many different systems. The examples given for each symptom are obviously hematological, to illustrate their importance, even though causes in other systems are often more common. Clearly, if suspicion was raised about a blood disease, as described above, those parts of the history will be concentrated upon, in the first instance.

Note that, in terms of our search-space paradigm, we would not necessarily follow these descriptions in the order given – we would instead use the ones suggested by the pointer and by the previous facts elicited.

Constitutional and General

1. **"TIREDNESS," "WEAKNESS."** These are very common complaints and can be very difficult to assess, particularly in the less articulate. These terms can sometimes be a misinterpretation by the patient of dyspnea, actual muscular weakness, or lassitude/malaise.

   HEMATOLOGICAL CONDITIONS TO CONSIDER: **ANEMIA**, particularly with lassitude and dyspnea; **AN UNDERLYING CHRONIC DISEASE**, such as a malignancy or a parasitic infestation (classical examples here being hookworm infestation in children and schistosomiasis).

   REMEMBER TO ASK FURTHER: Diet, bleeding diathesis, travel, family history, residence, pica, chronic disease, sore mouth, diarrhea.

2. **FEVER, RIGORS**.

   HEMATOLOGICAL CONDITIONS TO CONSIDER: There is really an enormous list of possibilities. Important ones are an **UNDERLYING IMMUNE DEPLETION**, such as hypogammaglobulinemia or neutropenia, especially in a patient with malignancy; **A SIDE EFFECT OF SOME DRUGS**, e.g., l-asparaginase; **A TRANSFUSION REACTION**; **MALARIA, SEPTIC SHOCK WITH DIC, SOME MALIGNANCIES**.

3. **NIGHT SWEATS**.

   HEMATOLOGICAL CONDITIONS TO CONSIDER: HODGKIN LYMPHOMA, often accompanied by other features – and which are in contradistinction to non-Hodgkin lymphoma unless in the late stages: weight loss, malaise, pruritus (see later); other causes of night sweats should not be forgotten (TB, brucellosis, alcoholic withdrawal, nocturnal hypoglycemia, nightmares (Epstein 1996)), some of which could have hematological implications).

4. **WEIGHT LOSS**.

   HEMATOLOGICAL CONDITIONS TO CONSIDER: **HODGKIN LYMPHOMA** is a classic hematological cause; **MANY NON-HEMATOLOGICAL CAUSES** (TB, AIDS, malignant disease) are associated with secondary hematological effects; **POSSIBLE MALABSORPTION** – a valuable symptom here in a patient with weight loss is that the patient has a voracious appetite and indeed ingests huge numbers of calories.

Neurological, Mental, and Psychological Symptoms

1. **VAGUE SYMPTOMS, ESPECIALLY COGNITIVE**, can be found in any number of conditions, such as chronic anemia, polycythemia, chronic parasitic infestation, hyperviscosity syndromes, recurrent minor ischemic episodes, and so on.

2. **MORE SPECIFIC SYMPTOMS INCLUDE**

   a. **PAIN LOCALIZED TO A DERMATOME**, with lower limb paresthesiae and ascending weakness, sphincter dysfunction; later flaccid paralysis and total sensory loss. These suggest **TRANSVERSE MYELITIS.**

      HEMATOLOGICAL CONDITION TO CONSIDER: **VITAMIN B_{12} DEFICIENCY**, among very many others.

   b. **PAIN AND PARESTHESIAE OF A GLOVE-AND-STOCKING DISTRIBUTION** suggest peripheral neuropathy.

      HEMATOLOGICAL CONDITIONS TO CONSIDER: **VITAMIN B_{12} OR FOLATE DEFICIENCY**; **AMYLOIDOSIS** (one would remember to see if there are palpable nerves and to check for autonomic neuropathy); **AIDS** (frequently a painful neuropathy). A motor neuropathy may be caused by **LEAD POISONING** (classically associated with a normo- or microcytic anemia).

   c. **AGITATED DEMENTIA** may be caused by **VITAMIN B_{12} DEFICIENCY**.

   d. **A COMBINATION OF MOTOR WEAKNESS WITH CLUMSINESS OF FINE MOVEMENTS**, and a "cotton-wool" sensation over the skin, may indicate subacute combined degeneration of the cord.

      HEMATOLOGICAL CONDITION TO CONSIDER: **VITAMIN B_{12} DEFICIENCY**.

   e. **TRANSIENT ISCHEMIC ATTACKS (TIA's)**. These are focal episodes of neurological insufficiency, lasting for a few minutes to an hour or so, and are followed by complete functional recovery. Although blood diseases are not the commonest cause of TIAs, they are common enough for certain disorders to be considered in every case. These patients are unlikely to present to the clinician during an attack, and thus the history is very important. There are two broad groups:

      TIA's AFFECTING THE INTERNAL CAROTID ARTERY DISTRIBUTION. About $1/3$ of these are associated with carotid artery stenosis on the ipsilateral side, most of the rest being due to emboli from the aortic arch or the heart.

      CLINICAL FEATURES are very variable, depending on where in the distribution the micro-occlusion occurs. Fairly common patterns are

      i. Hand-arm or face-hand-arm **PARESIS** without sensory loss.

ii. **APHASIA** and/or hemiparesis.

iii. **AMAUROSIS FUGAX**. This is a rapidly developing unilateral graying-out of vision in one eye, lasting for seconds to minutes, followed by full recovery. It may take the form of a central scotoma. Fundoscopic examination during an attack will show narrowing of both arteries and veins, sometimes accompanied by yellowish refractile spots, which are cholesterol crystals.

iv. It is extremely important to note that disturbances of consciousness are **NOT** features of carotid TIA's.

v. Note also that recurrent attacks in the same person tend to be the same every time, unlike with vertebro-basilar disease.

vi. A **BRUIT** is frequently heard over the carotid, usually at the site of the bifurcation.

   Carotid artery stenosis has in recent years been closely associated with hyperhomocysteinemia. This condition is a known predisposition to arterial thrombosis. However, its impact appears not to be nearly as significant as previously thought, except (probably) in the case of carotid stenosis.

   TIA's AFFECTING THE VERTEBRO-BASILAR DISTRIBUTION. The possible presentations are extremely variable, and tend to vary in the same patient during different attacks.

   CLINICAL FEATURES: Common presentations are

   i. **AMNESIA**
   ii. **"ABSENCES,"** resembling but not to be confused with petit mal attacks
   iii. **DIPLOPIA**
   iv. **EPISODIC DROWSINESS**
   v. **ATAXIA**
   vi. **DYSARTHRIA**
   vii. **ATYPICAL MIGRAINE** attacks
   viii. **CERVICAL SPONDYLOSIS** or osteoarthritis is often present, especially in the elderly
   HEMATOLOGICAL CONDITIONS TO CONSIDER: As mentioned, hematological causes are the minority. They should always be considered and excluded, since most are treatable. The hematological causes of relevance are

   i. **THROMBOCYTHEMIA**, particularly with platelet counts over 1,000,000 /mm^3
   ii. **POLYCYTHEMIA VERA**
   iii. **MARKED LEUKOCYTOSIS**, generally > 500,000/mm^3

   iv. **PLATELET HYPERAGGREGABILITY**
   v. **SICKLE DISEASE**
   vi. **WALDENSTRŌM MACROGLOBULINEMIA** and myeloma especially IgM
   vii. **ANTIPHOSPHOLIPID SYNDROME**
   viii. **HYPERHOMOCYSTEINEMIA**.

Cardiovascular, Respiratory, and Performance Status

1. **PERFORMANCE STATUS**. It is always advisable to document the patient's performance status. Often some clear patterns can emerge with time. Modified ECOG (Epstein 1996) criteria are satisfactory for general purposes:

   a. **GRADE 0**: asymptomatic
   a. **GRADE 1**: symptomatic, fully ambulant
   b. **GRADE 2**: symptomatic, ambulant in over 50% of the waking hours
   c. **GRADE 3**: symptomatic, in bed for more than 50% of the waking hours
   d. **GRADE 4**: symptomatic, confined to bed

   In addition to the above, two other features can be helpful in the assessment of physiological reserves, especially in anemic patients – dyspnea and angina.

2. **DYSPNEA ON EFFORT THAT IS RELIEVED BY LYING DOWN FLAT**. This is very suggestive of anemia, as opposed to the dyspnea of say left ventricular failure. The amount of effort required to bring on dyspnea of this nature is a rough guide to how severe the anemia is and how rapidly it is progressing. For example, if one gets the history that a month previously the patient could climb one flight of stairs before experiencing dyspnea and now gets short of breath after walking 10 m, one can say with confidence that if the dyspnea is due to anemia it is progressing quite rapidly, which would in turn inform the urgency of your intervention. Note that the patient with anemia almost never has dyspnea when lying down at rest, no matter how severe (unless there are co-existent other causes).

3. **ANGINA**. One of the causes is severe anemia. Numerous cases are referred to cardiologists erroneously. Remember that the majority of patients over 50 years with severe anemia present with angina.

4. **RECURRENT THROMBOEMBOLIC EPISODES**, especially in odd sites, or heart attacks and stroke at a relatively young age.

5. **RECURRENT EPISTAXIS.** While this is commonly due to dilated veins in Little's area, important

hematological causes are hereditary hemorrhagic telangiectasia (in which epistaxis is the most prominent symptom), and bleeding disorders, especially thrombocytopenia.

Skin, Bone, Muscles, and Joints

1. **JAUNDICE.** A history of jaundice can be significant.

   a. A recent episode, possibly associated with abdominal pain, may indicate acute hepatitis or cholecystitis (?pigment stones in chronic hemolysis).

      HEMATOLOGICAL CONDITIONS TO CONSIDER: Chronic extravascular hemolysis, such as hereditary spherocytosis or vivax malaria. Subsequent development of pancytopenia might be linked to the hepatitis, suggesting aplastic anemia.

   b. Recurrent attacks of jaundice. Many possibilities exist:

      i. Hemolytic jaundice. Recurrence suggests a chronic extravascular (usually hereditary) hemolytic disease.
      ii. Alcoholism, suggesting binges (classically associated with macrocytic anemia).
      iii. Chronic liver disease with intermittent insufficiency.

2. **PRURITUS.**

   HEMATOLOGICAL CONDITIONS TO CONSIDER: POLYCYTHEMIA VERA (pruritus particularly in relation to contact with cold water) and **HODGKIN LYMPHOMA**. In addition, dermatitis herpetiformis is an extremely itchy eruption classically associated with **GLUTEN ENTEROPATHY (WITH IRON AND/OR FOLATE MALABSORPTION** among others) and with **INTESTINAL LYMPHOMA. OBSTRUCTIVE JAUNDICE** is classically pruritic and often has hematological implications.

3. **MARKED PHOTOSENSITIVITY.**

   HEMATOLOGICAL CONDITIONS TO CONSIDER: Systemic lupus erythematosis (SLE), porphyria cutanea tarda, and porphyria variegata.

4. **EASY BRUISING OR PROLONGED BLEEDING** after injury (including during and after surgery).

   HEMATOLOGICAL CONDITIONS TO CONSIDER: Moderate (or even mild) hemophilia, von Willebrand disease, thrombocytopenia, platelet function disorders.

5. **BLOODY SPOTS OR AREAS** on the skin.

HEMATOLOGICAL CONDITIONS TO CONSIDER: As under 4.

6. **ARTHRITIS IN A PATIENT WITH SYMPTOMS OF MALABSORPTION.** This could suggest Whipple disease, among others.

   HEMATOLOGICAL CONDITIONS TO CONSIDER: Iron and/or folate deficiency; lymphoma.

7. **ACUTE VERY PAINFUL SWELLING OF A JOINT** especially without a history of trauma and particularly in a male.

   HEMATOLOGICAL CONDITIONS TO CONSIDER: Hemarthrosis due to hemophilia. Hemarthrosis may also be found in acute leukemia, the severe (rare) variety of von Willebrand disease, anticoagulant therapy, and thrombocytopenia.

8. **LARGE, INAPPROPRIATE (TO THE DEGREE OF TRAUMA) MUSCLE HEMATOMATA.**

   HEMATOLOGICAL CONDITIONS TO CONSIDER: Hemophilia, the severe variety of von Willebrand disease.

9. **BONE PAIN.**

   HEMATOLOGICAL CONDITIONS TO CONSIDER: Acute leukemia, myeloma, and hyperparathyroidism (osteitis fibrosa cystica can rarely produce pancytopenia or a leukoerythroblastic reaction).

Gastrointestinal and Nutritional History

Some specific conditions mentioned are discussed later in Chapter 4 under The Gastrointestinal Tract and Blood Disease. Many symptoms and features are particularly relevant to blood disease:

1. **A DETAILED DIETARY HISTORY** should be taken. Features relevant to blood diseases (in brief) are

   a. **NUMBER OF PORTIONS OF RED MEAT** per week (the minimum is 3, else iron and vitamin B_{12} deficiency may arise).

   b. **PORTIONS OF FRESH SALAD AND VEGETABLES** per day (should be at least once per day, else folate deficiency may arise, particularly in the presence of other factors – see Chapter 4).

   c. **HOW VEGETABLES ARE PREPARED.** See Chapter 4. Steaming is the best.

2. **PICA (A CRAVING MOST COMMONLY FOR ICE OR SOIL).** This is characteristic of iron deficiency.

3. **A SORE MOUTH AND TONGUE.** This is particularly associated with nutritional anemias.

4. **DIFFICULTY IN SWALLOWING**. If the dysphagia is experienced high up in the chest, post-cricoid webs should be considered, although a very sore mouth due to other deficiencies may be so severe as to make swallowing difficult. Irradiation and iron deficiency are important causes. The triad of dysphagia due to a post-cricoid web, glossitis, and iron deficiency is known as the Plummer–Vinson or Kelly–Paterson syndrome; this condition is typically found in pre-menopausal women of northern European extraction. Other causes of dysphagia (e.g., carcinoma) may cause anemia due to decreased nutrient intake, as well as due to the disease itself.

5. **NAUSEA, HEARTBURN**. These may be part of dyspepsia or suggest hiatal hernia that can bleed slowly, chronically and sub-clinically.

6. **EPIGASTRIC DISCOMFORT, PAIN**. Apart from dyspepsia, of possible hematological import these features could indicate

    a. **CHOLECYSTITIS** secondary to pigment gall stones, presenting sometimes as colic but sometimes very vaguely.
    b. Some forms of **HEPATITIS** such as due to alcohol may be directly related to changes in the blood (in this case a macrocytic anemia and thrombocytopenia, and rarely hemolytic anemia).
    c. A large **ABDOMINAL ANEURYSM** may leak slowly, causing pain and iron deficiency.

7. **OTHER ABDOMINAL PAIN**. Vague abdominal pain associated with blood disease or changes may be

    a. **SICKLE DISEASE** abdominal crises
    b. **LEAD POISONING**
    c. **ACUTE INTERMITTENT PORPHYRIA**
    d. **DIVERTICULITIS**
    e. **ALCOHOL-INDUCED PAIN** in Hodgkin lymphoma affecting abdominal nodes

8. **EARLY SATIETY**. This interesting symptom can be a subtle pointer to either a infiltrative lesion of the stomach, such as a MALT lymphoma, or indicate a mass pressing on the stomach from the outside, the most common being an enlarged spleen or a pancreatic pseudocyst.

9. **BLEEDING.** The gastro-intestinal tract and the uterus in females are the source of the bulk of cases of chronic bleeding leading to iron deficiency, and since iron deficiency is the commonest disease in the world, it is important that the pathology be understood. There are two broad groups of presentation of gastro-intestinal bleeding:

First, the obvious and well-known presentations, such as hematemesis, melena, and hematochezia, and second, a group of conditions where the bleeding is occult, from a variety of causes, some of which more commonly present in a more typical fashion.

a. **HEMATEMESIS**. The common causes are **GASTRIC EROSIONS, GASTRIC AND DUODENAL ULCER, CARCINOMA, LYMPHOMA, VARICES, GASTRO-ESOPHAGEAL TEARS** (the Mallory–Weiss syndrome – this is usually **BUT NOT ALWAYS** preceded by extensive vomiting and is most common in alcoholics). An associated history of dyspepsia, heartburn, or exposure to gastric irritants serve as strong pointers. Also, the massive bleeding from varices may be suspected by recognizing the features of portal hypertension and its causes. Very rarely, hematemesis may be due to a bleeding disorder.

b. **MELENA, HEMATOCHEZIA**. Traditionally these indicate a local lesion in the colon, rectum, or anal canal. Characteristically, these would be associated with a change in bowel habits, constipation, pain and urgency at defecation, or noticeable hemorrhoids with blood coating the stools. Important causes are carcinoma, diverticulosis, inflammatory bowel disease, hemorrhoids, anal fissures, and proctitis (usually in homosexual men). Difficulties are found, however, with a number of occult lesions that are clinically silent and **PRESENT** with iron deficiency, such as **ISCHEMIC COLITIS** (usually in the elderly), **ANGIODYSPLASIA**, and **CARCINOMA AND OTHER LESIONS OF THE CECUM AND ASCENDING COLON**. Again, uncommonly, bleeding disorders may present in this way.

10. **BLOATING, DISTENTION**. A wide variety of pathologies can be responsible, such as gallstones. However, of particular relevance to blood disease is malabsorption.

11. **FEATURES WHICH MAY SUGGEST MALABSORPTION**. Malabsorption is an important and complex topic (for example, ± 8% of all iron deficiencies are due to malabsorption). Even in the late stages the condition is difficult to suspect, let alone diagnose, since so many other conditions can produce similar symptoms. A high index of suspicion is required. We provide some guidelines, but correlation with the clinical findings and blood tests is crucial.

a. **THE PATHOPHYSIOLOGICAL CONSEQUENCES** of malabsorption may be the clearest indicators of possible malabsorption:

- A very important "red light" feature is **THE PATIENT WHO LOSES WEIGHT WHILE ENJOYING A GOOD (OR INCREASED) APPETITE** and food intake. In severe cases there may be **WASTING**, often with edema. These are, at least in part, related to hypoalbuminemia.
- **PARESTHESIAE AND TETANY**. These are associated with hypocalcemia that may be followed later by secondary hyperparathyroidism, osteopenia, and pathological fractures.
- **MUSCLE CRAMPS** are due to magnesium deficiency (a prominent feature in most cases of malabsorption).
- **PERIPHERAL NEUROPATHY**, night blindness (vitamin A deficiency).
- **BLEEDING TENDENCIES**, usually due to vitamin K deficiency.
- **ANEMIA** may be of any type, reflecting different possible nutrient deficiencies.

b. **CHRONIC DIARRHEA** is frequently associated with malabsorption. It may vary from 10 watery stools per day to 1 stool per day that is putty-like, and floats on the water (**STEATORRHEA**). The stool **MASS** is invariably increased.

c. **FLATULENCE, BLOATING AND BORBORYGMI** are common. Flatulence is mainly due to fermentation of dietary carbohydrate. Distention may be due to impaired absorption of intestinal contents, excessive gas formation, or actual secretion of fluid into the bowel, as in celiac disease and tropical sprue.

d. **WORSENING OF SYMPTOMS** with the ingestion of wheat, barley, and oats products.

e. **ABDOMINAL PAIN** is common in Crohn disease, diffuse intestinal lymphoma, and chronic pancreatitis, all of which may be associated with malabsorption.

f. **PERSISTENT NON-SPECIFIC GASTROINTESTINAL "UPSET"** may indicate celiac disease.

12. **ALTERED BOWEL HABITS**. This may be associated with many disorders of the bowels, such as diverticulosis. Of major importance, however, is the possibility of carcinoma of the colon, particularly of the transverse and descending colon.

13. **PAINFUL, MUCOUS STOOLS**. Inflammatory bowel disease has numerous and diverse secondary effects on the blood.

Previous Medical and Surgical

1. **A PREVIOUS DIAGNOSIS** of anemia or bleeding disorder (or indeed any abnormality in a first-line test) should always prompt further investigation.

2. **A HISTORY OF HAVING REQUIRED REPEATED BLOOD TRANSFUSIONS**, except for traumatic hemorrhage. Important details are how many, how often, over how many years, were chelating agents (most commonly desferrioxamine) administered at the same time? This would strongly suggest a chronic anemia, of many possible causes. The issue of chelating agents is important, since regular blood transfusion can lead to iron overload (each unit of red cells provides ± 250 mg of iron, which the body cannot get rid of except by bleeding or chelation therapy).

3. **IS THE PATIENT, OR HAS HE BEEN, A BLOOD DONOR**? How often, for how long? At what intervals? When was the last donation? It should be remembered that donation of more than three units per annum results in depletion of iron stores. This is not a significant problem except

   a. Overt iron deficiency can occur in females of child-bearing age.
   b. Should an underlying occult bleeding lesion develop, iron deficiency can develop more quickly.

4. **VERY FREQUENT AND MULTIPLE PREGNANCIES** (depletion of iron stores, folate).

5. **COMPLICATIONS OF PREGNANCY.** Venous thrombosis, multiple miscarriages (? antiphospholipid syndrome), acute cerebral episode post-partum.

6. **RECURRENT PAINFUL SWELLING** of a single large joint, typically the knee and typically after playing a contact sport, in a boy with no other bleeding disorder (moderate hemophilia being one of the causes – i.e., this would then be a "target joint"; see Chapter 18).

7. **PREVIOUS SURGERY (OR IRRADIATION OF THE RELEVANT ORGAN**).

   a) **SPLENECTOMY**. If this was done for a hematological reason, one must suspect a chronic extravascular hemolytic anemia, a lymphoma/chronic leukemia, or occasionally myelofibrosis (in which case the liver will be very large). In addition, splenectomy for any reason tends to cause changes in the FBC (see Chapter 4).

   b) **CHOLECYSTECTOMY**. One of the reasons for cholecystectomy is the presence of pigment stones, as found in the chronic extravascular hemolytic states. One would suspect this when other suggestive features are present, and especially when the cholecystectomy was done in a young patient (even the teens). Note that when splenectomy is done for chronic extravascular hemolysis, it is quite common practice to do a cholecystectomy at the same time, regardless of whether pigment stones are causing complications.

c) **GASTRECTOMY**. To an extent, the hematological consequences of gastrectomy depend on the type of gastrectomy and the reason for it. Thus an attempt should be made to ascertain the details of the operation.

d) **MASTECTOMY, THYROIDECTOMY, AND NEPHRECTOMY** (for malignant disease): Metastases in the bones (and marrow) may occur years after the operation, producing a number of blood pictures, classically the leuko-erythroblastic reaction (see Chapter 15).

e) Similarly, **PROSTATECTOMY** may be associated later with the development of bone secondaries. These are characteristically sclerotic, producing very hard bones, and this may be suspected when one does a marrow biopsy (with osteopetrosis as a differential).

f) **SMALL BOWEL RESECTION**. This may have been done for mesenteric thrombosis (and which in turn suggests investigation for a hypercoagulable state). The possible results are manifold, including hypoproteinemia and vitamin B_{12} and folate deficiency.

g) **OOZING IN THE OPERATION SITE** is a very important symptom. It may be found in diverse bleeding disorders, including telangiectasia, mild to moderate hemophilia, von Willebrand disease.

Ethnic, Geographical, and Travel History

Note that only general trends are presented – one will always find sporadic cases in any population, and there are often variations within a region:

1. **MEDITERRANEAN LITTORAL**: β-Thalassemia (typically β^0 or severe β^+ – see Chapter 7); G6PD type A⁻ deficiency.
2. **AFRICA: GENERAL**: α-Thalassemia, G6PD deficiency. **SCHISTOSOMA MANSONI** infection is endemic – see below.
3. **AFRICA: NORTH AND WEST AFRICA:** HbC trait and disease; HbC/β-thalassemia; HbS/β-thalassemia (the thalassemia is β^+, resulting in mild disease – see Chapter 7 for an explanation).
4. **CARIBBEAN:** As under 2 and 3.

5. **SOUTH AMERICA: SCHISTOSOMA MANSONI** infections are endemic – see below.
6. **AFRICA: WEST AFRICA**: HbS (sickle trait and disease); HbC, HbSC, hereditary elliptocytosis (one form).
7. **MIDDLE EAST**, including Yugoslavia and Romania: β-thalassemia, Southeast Asian ovalocytosis.
8. **SOUTHEAST ASIA** (including southern China, Thailand, Malaysia, Papua New Guinea, Philippines, Pacific islands): β-Thalassemia, Southeast Asian ovalocytosis, HbH disease (Hb constant spring), HbE trait and disease, HbE/β-thalassemia, G6PD Canton deficiency in southern China. **STRONGYLOIDES STERCORALIS** infection is common, and is a common cause of eosinophilia. **SCHISTOSOMA JAPONICUM** and **MEKONGI** infections are endemic.
9. **INDIA**: β-Thalassemia, Southeast Asian ovalocytosis.
10. **FAR EAST IN GENERAL**: Hypercholesterolemia and diabetes mellitus – relevant from the point of view of thromboembolic disease.
11. **NORTHERN EUROPE:** Hemochromatosis type I (HFE gene), especially Ireland, Scotland, Wales, Brittany (thus possibly suggesting Celtic origin) and Scandinavia.
12. **FINLAND** (but sporadically general); Imerslund–Gräsbeck disease (megaloblastic anemia in infants).
13. **CAUCASIANS IN GENERAL:** Caucasian-type G6PD deficiency.
14. **ASHKENAZY JEWS:** Gaucher's and Niemann–Pick diseases, factor XI deficiency, Bassen–Kornzweig disease.
15. **RESIDENCE AT AN ALTITUDE SIGNIFICANTLY DIFFERENT TO ONE'S OWN.** The reference ranges for the red cell indices vary with altitude, and healthy patients with indices near the limits of the reference ranges for their altitude may be erroneously diagnosed as anemia or erythrocytosis when at another altitude.

TRAVEL HISTORY. Travel either to or from areas that are known to have endemic infections, or to or from a very different altitude, can be a significant pointer to blood disease. Any patient that develops a fever after traveling to an endemic area should prompt search for a number of important conditions, many of which are hematological in many respects. They are, more or less in order of frequency: malaria, salmonellosis (typhoid, etc.), hepatitis A and B, and amebiasis. There is a long list of uncommon infections: rickettsial infections such as Q fever, viral infections such as dengue (the hemorrhagic form is very severe and is characterized by thrombocytopenic bleeding, etc.), hemorrhagic fevers, yellow fever, HIV; and other protozoa such as trypanosomiasis and kala-azar, both of which have significant hematological features.

1. **MALARIA**. Clinical presentation can aid, to some extent, in identifying which plasmodium is responsible. Urgent laboratory identification is always necessary since the prognosis and urgency of intervention depends to a great extent on this:

   a. **PLASMODIUM FALCIPARUM**. There is generally no cyclical pattern to the fever. It presents within 3 months of infection, sometimes within a few weeks. It commonly presents with high fever, anemia, jaundice, mental confusion, and renal failure. Overt DIC may develop. Hemoglobinuria ("blackwater fever") may occur.

   b. **PLASMODIUM OVALE** tends to exhibit a "tertian" cycle, i.e., fever every 48 h. It is typically not very severe clinically.

   c. **PLASMODIUM VIVAX** also tends to exhibit a "tertian" cycle. It commonly presents with persistent splenomegaly and anemia; 10% of cases present over a year after exposure; symptoms may recur every few months for 10 years. Splenic rupture is common.

   d. **PLASMODIUM MALARIAE** exhibits a fever of "quartan" pattern – i.e., every 72 h. A complication found only in this form is an immune complex chronic glomerulonephritis, presenting as the nephrotic syndrome.

      Note that thrombocytopenia is common in all forms of malaria. A moderate leukopenia may also occur, sometimes with a monocytosis.

2. **FILARIASIS**. This is often associated with marked eosinophilia. Two species of filaria are particularly relevant to hematology. See Chapter 4.

   Both of them cause marked lymphatic obstruction. They are also responsible for one form of pulmonary eosinophilia.

3. **TRYPANOSOMIASIS** (sleeping sickness). Transmitted by the tsetse fly, this condition is found only between 15°N and 20°S of the equator. Clinical features are somewhat different in infection with the two species responsible.

4. **SCHISTOSOMIASIS**. This is the most common cause of hepatosplenomegaly in the world, and can lead to portal ("pipe-stem") fibrosis, portal hypertension with bleeding varices, and hypersplenism (with anemia and/or leukopenia and/or thrombocytopenia).

5. **TROPICAL SPRUE**. This is endemic in most countries lying between the Tropics of Cancer and Capricorn. Expatriates from these areas can develop symptoms months to years after leaving. Travelers from temperate climates can be affected. It presents as a malabsorption syndrome (e.g., of iron, folate).

6. **TRAVELER'S EOSINOPHILIA**. The returning traveler may, after having experienced vague symptoms **WEEKS TO MONTHS AFTER RETURNING** may be found to have a significant eosinophilia in the blood. The usual causes of this are filariasis and oncocerciasis.

7. **STRONGYLOIDES STERCORALIS INFECTION**. Clinical features are very variable, but eosinophilia is a constant characteristic, except in the immune compromised. While often asymptomatic, it may present with diarrhea and the features of malabsorption.

Family History

1. **A "BLOOD DISEASE" OR BLEEDING TENDENCY**. There are a very large number of hereditary blood diseases, some of which can be seen in adults. The most common from the point of view of adult medicine are

   a. **HEREDITARY SPHEROCYTOSIS** (hemolytic anemia)
   b. **G6PD DEFICIENCY** (hemolytic anemia)
   c. **THALASSEMIAS** (complex presentations)
   d. **SICKLE DISEASE** (complex presentations)
   e. **VON WILLEBRAND DISEASE** (quite a common bleeding disorder)

2. **A FAMILY HISTORY OF A THROMBOTIC TENDENCY**. Many conditions, in and out of the blood system, can predispose to abnormal thrombosis, i.e., an increased thrombotic tendency. There are many pointers suggesting this:

   a. **THROMBOSIS AT A YOUNGER AGE** (< 40 years)
   b. **THROMBOSIS IN PECULIAR SITES,** e.g., the axilla or the hepatic vein (Budd–Chiari syndrome)
   c. **RECURRENT THROMBOSIS** at different sites
   d. **THROMBOSIS WHILE ON ANTICOAGULANT THERAPY**

3. **A FAMILY HISTORY OF A "HIGH COLOR"** (or a high color from childhood). This may indicate a **HIGH-AFFINITY (FOR OXYGEN) HEMOGLOBIN**.

Drugs, Previous Therapies, Habits

1. **DRUGS CAN CAUSE FEATURES SUGGESTIVE OF ORIGIN IN THE HEMATOLOGICAL SYSTEM**. By far the most important of these are drugs causing cytopenias, presenting clinically as pallor, recurrent infections (including infections due to

unusual organisms such as fungi), or purpura, or various combinations of these. There is a very large list of drugs doing this (see Appendix A). There are numerous mechanisms, notably direct damage to the marrow, direct damage to the circulating cells, and immune mechanisms either via the drugs acting as haptens, forming immune complexes, or by initiating autoimmune activity. Direct damage may be via physico-chemical trauma to the cells themselves or via interference with metabolism such as DNA synthesis.

2. **DRUGS THAT CAN CAUSE MALABSORPTION OF**

   a. **IRON:** Tetracycline (by chelation); antacids (binding)
   b. **FOLATE:** Phenytoin (competitive binding); alcohol (toxic effect on mucosa, competition); methotrexate (competition for binding site)
   c. **VITAMIN B$_{12}$:** Ethanol; colchicine; metformin (mucosal damage)

3. **DRUGS AND OTHER THERAPIES USED PREVIOUSLY FOR BLOOD DISEASES** may play an important part in the assessment of the current presentation. This applies especially to cortisone preparations, immune suppressants, heparin, coumadin, and cyclokapron (why, for how long, what dosage?), and chemotherapeutic agents and irradiation.

4. **DRUGS MAY CAUSE DEFECTS IN THE HEMOSTATIC MECHANISM.** Platelet dysfunction may be caused by aspirin and NSAIDS. Coumadin and heparin are well known as causes of changes in the coagulation tests.

5. **EXCESSIVE TEA DRINKING:** Tannin binds ingested iron. Tea should not be taken within 1 h before and after a meal.

6. **EXCESSIVE ALCOHOL USAGE.** This can have many effects on the hematological system, and will be discussed later in the chapter.

7. **SMOKING.** This has many deleterious effects on the body, including the blood. This is further discussed in Chapter 16.

a) **OXIDANTS.** There are many products potentially responsible. Aniline is probably the best known. It can cause acute or chronic methemoglobinemia, and sometimes hemolytic anemia, characterized by the presence of Heinz bodies in the red cells. The latter is particularly prone to occur in G6PD deficiency.

b) **CHLORATE SALTS**, used in pesticides and herbicides. It has also been described in dialysis patients where the water has been contaminated by chloramines. They cause a severe methemoglobinemia and hemolysis.

2. **HEMOLYSIS ASSOCIATED WITH EXPOSURE TO HEAVY METAL COMPOUNDS.** The most important of these are arsine, lead, and copper:

   a) **ARSINE** causes a severe acute intravascular hemolysis with hemoglobinuria.
   b) **LEAD.** Apart from all the other effects of lead (see later), it too can cause an acute intravascular hemolysis.
   c) **COPPER.**

3. **PORPHYRIA.** A large number of chemicals has been associated with porphyria, and can take the form of several known patterns. Hexachlorobenzene and lead are probably the best known.

4. **DECREASED OXYGEN SATURATION.** Carbon monoxide is the primary villain here.

5. **TOXINS AFFECTING HEMOPOIESIS.** Conditions known or suspected to be relevant here are aplastic anemia, myelodysplasia, and thrombocytopenia.

   a) **APLASTIC ANEMIA.** Benzene is well known. Others are ionizing radiation, TNT, and lindane.
   b) **MYELODYSPLASIA.** Industrial toxins and pesticides are widely suspected of playing a role in MDS, but proof is still being awaited.
   c) **THROMBOCYTOPENIA.** A number of chemicals have been implicated, the best known probably being vinyl chloride.

Occupational History

There is a very large number of occupational hazards that can affect the blood. Only a very brief overview is given:

1. **METHEMOGLOBINEMIA AND HEMOLYSIS.** There are two groups of chemical that can be responsible: oxidants (by far the largest group) and chlorates.

Bleeding and Thrombosis

1. **SPONTANEOUS OR VERY READY BLEEDING** from an anatomical site, e.g., epistaxis, or after surgery or trauma (see Chapter 17).
2. **BLEEDING** may be secondary to systemic disease. A classical example is severe bleeding tendency in uremia.
3. **PERSISTENT OOZING** after extraction.

4. There may be a clear history of **PROLONGED BLEEDING** after a cut, abrasion, or laceration. These features are described later.
5. **TRANSIENT ISCHEMIC EPISODES**, amaurosis fugax.
6. **RECURRENT ABORTIONS** (miscarriages) (?anti-phospholipid syndrome).

Once the history is taken, a list of possibilities can be drawn up.

The Clinical Examination

Although the clinical examination only provides on average 5–10% of the information ultimately required for diagnosis, positive clinical features can facilitate the diagnosis enormously, in the process minimizing the need for expensive and time-consuming (and sometimes painful) investigations. On occasion the clinical examination can lead one very close to the final answer. The clinical examination is therefore discussed extensively.

Typically a number of preliminary assessments are made prior to the formal examination:

1. **PYREXIA. PYREXIA OF UNKNOWN ORIGIN** (PUO) is a rather uncommon but serious finding. The criteria are a fever of 38.5°C or more on several occasions for at least 3 weeks. The most important causes are infections, malignant disease, collagen diseases, and granulomatous diseases. It is important to find out about a past history of rheumatic fever, TB, and splenectomy; intravenous drug use; recent foreign travel; sexual practices; and exotic foods. These may provide a pointer, but otherwise one is dependent on blood tests. Obviously dozens of tests could be ordered, but this is one case where the first test **MUST** be the FBC. Numerous syndromes can be described. A few examples:

   a. **RETROPERITONEAL SARCOMA**, presenting characteristically with pyrexia, tachycardia, and moderate to severe **NEUTROPHILIA**.
   b. **MALIGNANT NEURAL CREST TUMORS**, with diverse clinical features but typically showing a moderate to severe **NEUTROPHILIA**.
   c. **LYMPHOMAS**, especially involving deep sites. **ANEMIA** is the most prominent finding.
   d. **ACUTE LEUKEMIAS**, especially the so-called "aleukemic" leukemias.

   e. In **THE CANCER PATIENT**, pyrexia may be due to **NEUTROPENIA**, hypogammaglobulinemia, the effects of certain drugs, or a **TRANSFUSION REACTION**. Various pyrexial patterns can be seen in Hodgkin lymphoma.
   f. Low-grade, especially intermittent pyrexia, may indicate a **CHRONIC INFECTION**, frequently due to intracellular organisms. These may be associated with widespread granulomatous disease including in the marrow, and presenting with low-grade **ANEMIA, INTERMITTENT LEUKOCYTOSIS, AND/OR THROMBOCYTOPENIA**. It may take the form of a hemophagocytic syndrome.
   g. **A DEEP UNDERLYING INFECTIVE FOCUS**, such as a sub-phrenic abscess, may only be suspected by intermittent fever and neutrophilia.

2. **HEIGHT, WEIGHT, AND CERTAIN OTHER MEASUREMENTS.** These include chest and abdominal girth measurements. These might provide information with respect to a number of conditions:

   a. A tendency to thromboembolic disease, in terms of obesity and the suspicion of diabetes mellitus and the metabolic syndrome.
   b. Chronic intra-abdominal bleeding (for example, in DIC) may be suspected because of a gradually increasing abdominal girth.
   c. Various structural disorders of the chest wall, either congenital or acquired, may be associated with hypoxia and erythrocytosis.

The clinical examination is depicted in Fig. 5.4. It follows the traditional sequence, but of course this may be changed depending on the severity and the triggers as outlined above. In this figure, features pointed to refer only to those associated in one way or another with a blood disease (whether reactive, second, or primary), including disorders due to abnormal bleeding and thrombosis: with the latter, however, there are additional considerations, and they are further expanded upon in Fig. 5.8. These schemata should be integrated into your general clinical examination.

The nervous system has a block of its own, despite the fact that some aspects are discussed in individual blocks. The examination of the nervous system cannot really be tied to a region. Nervous system signs are fairly common in some blood diseases, are potentially serious but many are potentially curable if diagnosed and treated timeously, and can be of assistance in diagnosis.

In the text following the figure, the causes of the various findings plus the essential differentiating features (in

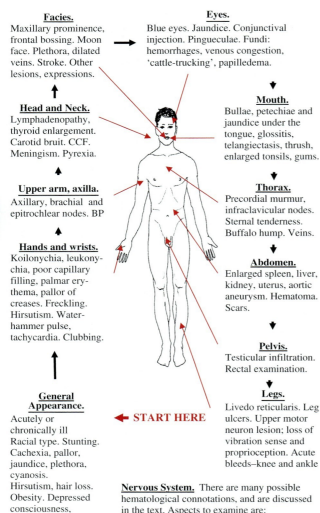

Facies.
Maxillary prominence, frontal bossing. Moon face. Plethora, dilated veins. Stroke. Other lesions, expressions.

Head and Neck.
Lymphadenopathy, thyroid enlargement. Carotid bruit. CCF. Meningism. Pyrexia.

Upper arm, axilla.
Axillary, brachial and epitrochlear nodes. BP

Hands and wrists.
Koilonychia, leukonychia, poor capillary filling, palmar erythema, pallor of creases. Freckling. Hirsutism. Water-hammer pulse, tachycardia. Clubbing.

General Appearance.
Acutely or chronically ill Racial type. Stunting. Cachexia, pallor, jaundice, plethora, cyanosis. Hirsutism, hair loss. Obesity. Depressed consciousness, delirium, confusion. Skin: scars, pigmentation, nodules, exfoliation, bruising, purpura.

Eyes.
Blue eyes. Jaundice. Conjunctival injection. Pingueculae. Fundi: hemorrhages, venous congestion, 'cattle-trucking', papilledema.

Mouth.
Bullae, petechiae and jaundice under the tongue, glossitis, telangiectasis, thrush, enlarged tonsils, gums.

Thorax.
Precordial murmur, infraclavicular nodes. Sternal tenderness. Buffalo hump. Veins.

Abdomen.
Enlarged spleen, liver, kidney, uterus, aortic aneurysm. Hematoma. Scars.

Pelvis.
Testicular infiltration. Rectal examination.

← START HERE

Legs.
Livedo reticularis. Leg ulcers. Upper motor neuron lesion; loss of vibration sense and proprioception. Acute bleeds–knee and ankle

Nervous System. There are many possible hematological connotations, and are discussed in the text. Aspects to examine are:
1. State of Consciousness and Mentation.
2. Cerebellar function.
3. The Motor Tracts.
4. The Sensory Tracts especially posterior columns.

Fig. 5.4 The general examination

brackets) are summarized. More details can be found in various chapters, in square brackets, e.g. [12].

The General Examination

1. **THE CHRONICALLY ILL APPEARANCE. HEMATOLOGICAL CONDITIONS TO CONSIDER**:

   a. **LOW-GRADE LYMPHOMA, CLL** [22, 15]. (Pruritus, weight loss, night sweats)

   b. **BLAST CRISIS IN CHRONIC MYELOCYTIC LEUKEMIA** [15]. (Previously diagnosed CML: pallor, purpura)

   c. **MYELOMA** [22]. (Bone pain (70%))

   d. **MYELOFIBROSIS** [16]. (Previous treatment for polycythemia vera or concurrent plethora)

   e. **MYELODYSPLASIA**. (Chronic transfusion-dependent anemia, a severe bleeding tendency for no apparent reason)

   f. **MALIGNANT DISEASE (NON-HEMATOLOGICAL PRIMARY)** [4]

   g. **THALASSEMIA MAJOR** [8]. (Stunting of growth, jaundice, duskiness from frequent transfusions, maxillary over-growth, frontal bossing)

   h. **MEGALOBLASTIC ANEMIA** [9]. (? Pernicious anemia: premature grayness, blue eyes, vitiligo, difficulty in walking; ? chronic alcoholism: typical facies, difficulty in walking; pregnancy)

   i. **PARASITOSES** [15]. (Residence in or recent visit to a tropical area)

2. **THE ACUTELY ILL APPEARANCE.**
   Conditions to consider:

   a. **SEPTICEMIA**. (Recent pneumonia, urinary tract infection, or abdominal/pelvic surgery; purpura)

   b. **ACUTE HEMOLYSIS** [4, 10]. (? Mainly extravascular hemolysis: loin pain, shock, previous episodes of jaundice, a history of recent ingestion of certain drugs, a family history of jaundice and pallor, ethnic origin in West and North Africa; ? Mainly intravascular or combined extra- and intravascular hemolysis: passage of red or pink urine, blanching and coldness of fingers and toes)

   c. **ACUTE LEUKEMIA/HIGH-GRADE LYMPHOMA** [15]. (A history of lassitude, recurrent infections, easy bruising, and bleeding).

   d. **HEMORRHAGIC SHOCK**. It is important that hemorrhagic shock be differentiated from acute severe dehydration

   e. **ACUTE DEHYDRATION** [4]

3. **STATE OF CONSCIOUSNESS.**
   Conditions to consider:

   a. **CLOUDING, CONFUSION**. Particular features of potentially hematological significance are malignant disease, myxedema, hypoxia (e.g., pulmonary emboli), and TIA's (of the vertebro-basilar distribution).

   Liver and kidney failure are frequently accompanied by severe disturbances of consciousness.

b. **DELIRIUM AND DEMENTIA**. There are several hematological connotations, with different clinical features:

   i. Vitamin B_{12} deficiency: this is typically an agitated dementia [9].
   ii. VAD regime for myeloma (due to the high dosage of dexamethasone) [22].
   iii. Primary and secondary cerebral HIV infection [4].
   iv. Secondary malignant brain disease.

c. **EPISODIC ABNORMALITIES**. The most important are transient ischemic attacks. These are unlikely to present during an attack and the history is most important. Note that hematological causes are the minority. They should always be considered and excluded, since most are treatable.

4. **CACHEXIA**. This is frequently equated with wasting and the chronically ill appearance; however, it is essentially **A CHANGE OF COMPLEXION TOWARD SALLOWNESS AND PALLOR,** usually (but not always) with progressive weight loss. Associated findings: achlorhydria (of relevance to iron absorption), diffuse hyperpigmentation (melanoderma) also of mucosae and neutrophilia (but often leukopenia in the late stages).
Conditions to consider:

a. **MYELOFIBROSIS** (advanced). See 1d
b. **MALIGNANT DISEASE**. See 1f
c. **LIVER FAILURE**.
d. **KIDNEY FAILURE**.
e. **CHYLOUS ASCITES**. Cachexia usually only occurs after repeated paracentesis
f. **KALA-AZAR**. (Far East, especially Indian subcontinent and vicinity)
g. **MALARIAL CACHEXIA** (usually in endemic areas)
h. **SEVERE HOOKWORM INFESTATION**

5. **STUNTING OF GROWTH, DEFORMITIES**.
Conditions to consider:

a. **THALASSEMIA MAJOR** [8].
b. **SICKLE DISEASE** [10]. (Ethnic origin in West Africa, family history, painful crises, episodes of severe pallor and weakness, transfusion dependency, deformities, and decreased movements of the hip and legs, due to avascular necrosis of the femoral head).
c. **FANCONI'S ANEMIA** [13]. (Slow and retarded growth (with a spurt at puberty in males); chronic anemia, transfusion dependency; short stature;

café-au-lait spots; deformities of the radii and/or thumbs).
d. **CELIAC DISEASE**. The features tend to differ quite markedly depending if the onset is in childhood or not. We concentrate on adult-onset disease [4].
e. **DEFORMITIES OF MUSCLES AND JOINTS** may be the result of recurrent bleeding, especially in hemophiliacs. Untreated or poorly managed severe hemophiliacs will eventually have severe, even crippling deformities of many joints. Recurrent bleeds into muscles will eventually result in severe contractures. Rheumatoid arthritis is very commonly followed by severe deformities especially of the hands.
f. **CHEST WALL DEFORMITIES.** Chest wall deformities may be sufficiently serious to interfere with aeration of the lungs and thus predispose to hypoxia and erythrocytosis.

6. **EVIDENT RACIAL BACKGROUND**. This matter has been discussed under the history. However, a racial/geographical history is advisable even when there are no suggestions of a relevant racial type.

7. **OBESITY**.
Conditions to consider:

a. **THE "PICKWICKIAN SYNDROME"** (as it used to be called) [17]. (Plethora, cyanosis and sleep disturbances)
b. **CUSHING SYNDROME** [16]. (Obesity with a characteristic distribution – central obesity, a moon face, and the buffalo hump; hirsutism; purple striae; plethora; hypertension; single crop acne)
c. **MYXEDEMA** [9]. (A history of cold intolerance, mental dullness, apathy, constipation, menorrhagia)

8. **PALLOR, JAUNDICE, PLETHORA, AND CYANOSIS.** For practical reasons these are discussed under "Head and Neck" below.

9. **HAIR**. Disturbances relevant to hematology may be hirsutism, generalized hair loss, and dry, coarse hair.
Conditions to consider:

a. **HIRSUTISM: CUSHING SYNDROME**.
Hirsutism can be a very difficult diagnosis to make, especially in the male. Obvious increased hairiness on the dorsum of the middle and distal phalanges is significant.
b. **GENERALIZED HAIR LOSS: HYPOPITUITARISM** [10]. (Pigmentary disturbances, pallor, a prematurely aged appearance, secondary amenorrhea. Mild normocytic anemia).
c. **DRY, COARSE HAIR: MYXEDEMA** [9].

10. **SKIN**. Many clues to blood diseases, primary, secondary, and reactive, may be found in the skin. The disorders or findings may be rashes, alterations in pigmentation, vascular abnormalities, scars and scarring, various dermatoses, and malignant disease. The lesions of the porphyrias affecting the skin are most prominent in the face and hands, because of sun exposure: these are thus discussed under "Face."

Conditions to consider:

a. **VITILIGO**. This is a common accompaniment of pernicious anemia.

b. **PATCHY DEPIGMENTATION: HYPOPITUI-TARISM** (Normocytic anemia).

c. **HYPERPIGMENTATION:**

   i. **ADDISON DISEASE**. (Melanotic hyperpigmentation under pressure areas (belt line, watchstrap, etc.)), areolae, inside the mouth. In the late stages this can be generalized. Hypotension. Mild normocytic anemia, mild eosinophilia, hyponatremia, and hyperkalemia).

   ii. **CHRONIC RENAL FAILURE**. (Normocytic anemia and bleeding tendency).

   iii. **HEMOCHROMATOSIS**. See below.

   iv. **PRIMARY BILIARY CIRRHOSIS**.

   v. **PORPHYRIA CUTANEA TARDA**.

d. **BRONZING/DUSKINESS: HEMOCHROMA-TOSIS** [20]. (Arthritis especially of first two MP joints of the hands, cardiac failure, diabetes, endocrine failure. Raised ferritin and iron saturation. The FBC is typically normal).

e. **FINDINGS SUGGESTIVE OF T-CELL LYM-PHOMAS OF THE SKIN** [4, 22]. (Erythroderma (redness of skin), features of folate deficiency, lymphadenopathy in the majority of cases).

f. **HERPES ZOSTER**. May point to underlying lymphoma and collagen diseases.

g. **DERMATITIS HERPETIFORMIS**. This is a condition characterized by intensely itchy herpes-like vesicles over the extensor aspects of the knees, elbows, and buttocks, and eosinophilia, and is characteristically associated with gluten enteropathy, with malabsorption of iron, folate, and vitamin K.

h. **LEUKEMIDS**. Leukemic infiltration of the skin occurs in 3% of cases at presentation. They can take various forms, from nodules to necrotic ulcerative lesions.

i. **METASTATIC DEPOSITS: NODULES**. Commonly from breast, lung, and colon carcinomas. (Leukoerythroblastic reaction may be seen, particularly in the former two).

j. **HELIOTROPE RASH AROUND THE EYES**. This suggests dermato- (poly-) myositis, associated in the adult with a high incidence of malignant disease. Other findings are Grotton's papules (violaceous nodules on the dorsal surface of the proximal interphalangeal joints, and muscle weakness).

k. **POINTERS IN THE SKIN SUGGESTING OR INDICATING A BLEEDING DISORDER:**

   i. **MULTIPLE BRUISES** without a history of significant trauma.

   ii. **TELANGIECTASES: RENDU–OSLER–WEBER SYNDROME** [8]. There may be a history of persistent oozing during and after surgery, or epistaxis. There may be features suggesting chronic iron deficiency.

   iii. **PURPURA AND PERIFOLLICULAR HEMORRHAGES**. Their characteristics are discussed later.

   iv. **TISSUE-PAPER SCARS**. These are characteristic of factor XIII deficiency [18].

l. **POINTERS IN THE SKIN SUGGESTING DRUG-INDUCED SKIN DISORDERS OF HEMATOLOGICAL SIGNIFICANCE. SEE THE BOX FOLLOWING.**

Summary of Presentations of Common Drug-Induced Cutaneous Disorders of Hematological Import

1. Penicillins

   a. Urticaria (Type I hypersensitivity reaction) – ?associated hemolytic anemia
   b. Vasculitis (Type III hypersensitivity reaction) – differentiate from purpura
   c. Contact dermatitis (Type IV hypersensitivity reaction)
   d. Eczematous eruption
   e. Exanthematous eruption – check for infectious mononucleosis, HIV positivity, CMV, and CLL

2. Gold (?associated neutropenia)

   a. Cytotoxic (Type II hypersensitivity reaction)
   b. Exanthematous eruptions

3. *Allopurinol* (used in many blood diseases)

   a. Exanthematous
   b. Exfoliative dermatitis
   c. Fixed drug eruptions
   d. Vasculitis

4. *Corticosteroids* (used in many blood diseases)

   a. Acneiform eruptions
   b. Hirsutism
   c. Plethora

5. *Methyldopa*. Autoimmune hemolytic anemia
6. *Hydralazine*. Drug-induced lupus
7. *Oral contraceptives*. These may precipitate bullous eruptions in porphyria cutanea tarda

Hands and Wrists

1. **PALMAR ERYTHEMA.** This is often found in

   a. **POLYCYTHEMIA** [16] **AND ERYTHROCYTOSIS** [17].
   b. **PREGNANCY.** There are various possible hematological associations, discussed in Chapter 4.
   c. **RHEUMATOID DISEASE AND SLE.** See below under "Arthritis."

2. **PALMAR CREASE PALLOR.** If the palms are pale and the creases are equally pale, one can be reasonably confident that the Hb is 9 g/dl or below.
3. **FRECKLING OF THE PALMS (AND SOLES).** This suggests the Peutz–Jeghers syndrome (see under "The Face," since the typical lesions are most likely to be observed there first).
4. **NAIL CHANGES.** There are many changes of possible hematological significance in the nails:

   a. **CLUBBING.** Hematological associations are celiac disease, Crohn disease (with vitamin B_{12} and iron deficiency); cyanotic heart and lung disease (with erythrocytosis); lung cancer (with possible bone metastases).
   b. **TELANGIECTASES AND NAILFOLD INFARCTS.** Hematological associations are collagen diseases (with manifold possible abnormalities in the blood); vasculitis (not to be confused with purpura).
   c. **"HALF-AND-HALF"** nails suggest renal failure.
   d. **LEUKONYCHIA** suggests liver disease.

   e. **BLUE LUNULES** are found in Wilson's disease. Possible hematological association: hepatosplenomegaly with hypersplenism.
   f. **KOILONYCHIA.** In a pale patient this is almost diagnostic of iron deficiency.
   g. **CAPILLARY REFILLING.** If a nail is compressed and then released, the time taken for it to become pink again reflects two things – the state of the local vessels and the amount of hemoglobin. Any significant delay will mean an abnormality; however, a delay of longer than 4 s will almost always be due to a vascular problem.

5. **HIRSUTES.** A difficult diagnosis. Suggestive features in a female: hair around areolae, abnormal pubic distribution, hair on knuckles, obvious facial hair. Suggestive features in a male: hair on dorsum of distal phalanges.
6. **ARTHRITIS.** The clinical characteristics of the arthritis must clearly be identified, i.e., the distribution, associated characteristic deformities, associated nodules, etc.

   SUBSEQUENT FEATURES TO LOOK FOR: Swollen joints, nodules (see below), subluxation of hand joints, arthritis mutilans, ulnar deviation, enlarged spleen, malar rash, pericarditis, pulmonary nodules. Chronic arthritis in the first two carpo-metacarpal joints is characteristic of hemochromatosis.

   POSSIBLE BLOOD FINDINGS: Micro-, macro-, or normocytic anemia, neutropenia (with enlarged spleen, consider Felty syndrome). Rheumatoid and anti-nuclear factors positive in certain patterns.

7. **NODULES.**
   Nodules over the joints and tendons are typically associated with rheumatoid disease and gout, but can be xanthomatous. Rarely, violaceous nodules over the interphalangeal joints suggest dermatomyositis.
8. Lesions of **THE PORPHYRIAS**.
9. **THE PULSE.** Two features of the pulse are relevant – the rate and the volume.
   BRADYCARDIA may reflect myxedema.
   TACHYCARDIA. Various types of tachycardia have relevance to blood disease:

   a. **MILD TO MODERATE TACHYCARDIA** is a typical response to exertion in anemia, the degree of tachycardia and the time taken for the pulse rate to return to its previous level after exertion being a measure of its severity.
   b. **A FULL VOLUME, BOUNDING PULSE** may occur with septic shock, but otherwise, in the anemic patient it may indicate severity, especially if it has a water-hammer character and there is associated an increased pulse pressure. This is a

hyper-dynamic circulation. However, note a significant qualification: as the anemia worsens the pulse pressure gets wider; **BUT**, once the heart begins to fail, the cardiac output begins to drop and the pre-load begins to increase, resulting in a decrease in pulse pressure, and with the blood pressure tending to **RETURN TO A MORE NORMAL LEVEL; THIS INDICATES AN EXTREMELY SEVERE AND LIFE-THREATENING ANEMIA**. It is clear that one must be on one's clinical toes with a pale patient. The blood pressure as a whole tends to drop in these circumstances.

Upper Arm, Axilla

1. **THE BLOOD PRESSURE.** This has been discussed above.
2. **AXILLARY AND EPITROCHLEAR NODES.** These must be evaluated as part of the assessment of lymphadenopathy – see page 158. Enlarged epitrochlear nodes are particularly important: if part of a widespread lymphadenopathy, they are in favor of a non-Hodgkin lymphoma. An interesting cause of axillary and epitrochlear adenopathy is cat-scratch disease, since most scratches are on the upper limb. It can sometimes present as an infectious mononucleosis-like syndrome.

Head and Neck

While color changes in a patient are really a general observation, in practice one mostly decides on these by reference to the head and face:

1. **PALLOR** is a very common and clinically vague sign. It can be found in a very large variety of disparate clinical (and physiological) conditions. Because of this it is often regarded as a relatively useless sign unless it is very obvious, and is not given much attention in clinical primers. Yet, when considered in relation to other features, it can be a very useful pointer in the correct clinical direction. It is one of the first features we notice about another person, even in a social context, and often at a subliminal level. It is also the prime clinical feature suggesting anemia. It is useful to distinguish mild from moderate and severe pallor:

   a. **MILD TO MODERATE PALLOR:** Apart from the obvious exceptions of stress, fear, and causes of vasomotor syncope, the important causes are

   i. **ANEMIA**
   ii. **CONGESTIVE CARDIAC FAILURE**
   iii. **SEVERE CORONARY ARTERY DISEASE**
   iv. **CONVALESCENCE**
   v. **SYNCOPE**
   vi. **MYXEDEMA, HYPOPITUITARISM,** and **HYPOGONADISM**

   b. **MODERATE TO SEVERE PALLOR:**

   i. **ANEMIA**
   ii. **SYSTEMIC ILLNESS**
   iii. Severe **SHOCK** states
   iv. **PHEOCHROMOCYTOMA.** Pallor is a characteristic feature, and can sometimes be very severe. Both the nor-adrenaline- and adrenaline-secreting types are pale; the adrenaline-secreting type may have intermittent flushing. See page 164 for the other features.

A frequent problem is when to consider ordering a FBC in cases of pallor. A thorough clinical examination, bearing the important causes in mind, will often prevent one from falling into the trap of reflexively ordering a FBC or consulting a blood specialist whenever a pale patient presents herself. It has happened more than once that the consultant is requested to see a patient in hospital who is very pale, and who turns out to be in cardiac failure, with a normal FBC. The main features to search for in any pale patient are those that tend to indicate that the pallor is due to anemia (and they also are markers of severity):

   a. Features of a hyper-dynamic circulation
   b. Delayed capillary refilling
   c. Pallor of palmar creases
   d. Dyspnea on effort relieved by lying flat

2. **JAUNDICE.** Jaundice of hematological significance is typically light lemon-yellow in color, characteristic of unconjugated bilirubin. The three major causes are **EXTRAVASCULAR HEMOLYSIS, INEFFECTIVE ERYTHROPOIESIS,** and **HEPATITIS**. The commonest cause of ineffective hematopoiesis presenting with jaundice is megaloblastic anemia. Note that very early or very late jaundice may only be noticed under the tongue. However, hepatocellular jaundice (**HEPATITIS, ALCOHOLISM**) may also have a pale jaundice. Obstructive jaundice (**GALLSTONES, PANCREATIC CARCINOMA, PRIMARY BILIARY CIRRHOSIS, SCLEROSING CHOLANGITIS**) can have hematological associations.

With **EXTRAVASCULAR HEMOLYSIS**, one **LOOKS FOR** pallor, enlarged spleen, family history, acrocyanosis, Raynaud's phenomenon.

With **MEGALOBLASTIC ANEMIA**, one **LOOKS FOR** pallor, glossitis, neurological abnormalities (see later), and vitiligo.

Superficially, extravascular hemolysis and megaloblastic anemia can look very similar, particularly in cases where the features are not all present.

CLINICAL FEATURES IN FAVOR OF HEMOLYSIS and **AGAINST MEGALOBLASTOSIS** are splenomegaly, leg ulcers, family history.

CLINICAL FEATURES IN FAVOR OF MEGALOBLASTOSIS and **AGAINST HEMOLYSIS** are neurological symptoms and signs, glossitis, alcoholic background, pregnancy, and absence of splenomegaly.

Blood tests are essential to clinch the diagnosis as well as further to identify the type of process. [9].

3. **PLETHORA AND CYANOSIS.** Plethora can be a very misleading finding. It generally implies a fullness of color (a "high" color), and is generally applied to the facies and conjunctive, and very often the palms. The usual cause that comes to mind is polycythemia or erythrocytosis (i.e., a raised hematocrit), but

a. It should be distinguished from **ERYTHRODERMA** from any number of causes (including cutaneous T-cell lymphoma), and chronic exposure to the sun and/or to alcohol in persons with certain complexions.

b. It should be distinguished from **CONGESTION**. This is particularly relevant when this affects the upper body, as may be found in the superior vena cava syndrome and sometimes in the subclavian steal syndrome.

THE FEATURES OF THE SUPERIOR VENA CAVA SYNDROME: Non-pulsatile neck veins, plethora and cyanosis of head, neck, and upper chest with dilated veins over the chest wall draining downward, absence of plethora over the lower body, facial edema, chemosis, tachypnea, perhaps Horner syndrome. A critical differentiating finding is the absence of hepatojugular reflux. Note that, despite the apparent plethora, the patient is usually anemic.

FEATURES OF SUBCLAVIAN STEAL: Different blood pressure in the two arms, fainting or other vague neurological deficit when exercising the arm on the side of the occlusion (there is usually no obvious difference in pulse volume). In these patients a mild erythrocytosis is common in blood taken from an arm.

c. True plethora almost certainly indicates **A RAISED HCT**. If this is found in the FBC, the task is to identify the nature of this rise. This is further discussed in Chapter 4 ("The Raised Hematocrit") and in Chapter 16.

CENTRAL CYANOSIS may be an accompaniment of primary types of polycythemia and erythrocytosis, or be the consequence of chronic chest disease leading to secondary erythrocytosis. This form is further discussed in Chapter 16. It may also occur as a result of methemoglobinemia; this is further discussed in Chapter 21.

4. **THE NECK VEINS.** Distended neck veins that pulsate are of course classically associated with right-sided failure; this may also be seen in severe anemia. However, distended neck veins without pulsation are a very significant finding, since they suggest obstruction to venous return from the head, and the most important of these is the superior vena cava syndrome – see above. This is generally due either to lymphoma or bronchogenic carcinoma in the mediastinum.

5. **ENLARGED LYMPH NODES.** The neck is the commonest place to find enlarged lymph nodes. The general approach to lymphadenopathy is discussed on page 158. In this section we shall mention only the involvement of the neck in the lymphomas and leukemias, and certain classical non-malignant causes:

a. **THE LYMPHOMAS.** The characteristic pattern of adenopathy in the lymphomas (and CLL) is discussed on page 157.

b. **THE LEUKEMIAS.** Apart from CLL, adenopathy in the leukemias is generally unimpressive.

c. **INFECTIOUS MONONUCLEOSIS.** Glandular fever is characterized by tender cervical (and other) lymphadenopathy and pharyngitis. However, it should not be inferred that the adenopathy is secondary to the pharyngitis.

d. **TOXOPLASMOSIS.** This is a classical cause of often prominent cervical lymphadenopathy, which is non-tender and due to an infective cause.

e. **THERE IS A GROUP OF RARE CAUSES** whose malignant status is not clear.

6. **THYROID ENLARGEMENT.** The only significant point here is thyromegaly due to malignancy, since thyroid carcinoma has a pronounced tendency to metastasize to bone and cause a leukoerythroblastic blood picture.

7. **EVIDENCE OF STROKE.** The various appearances of gross abnormality should be well known. The

significance is the possible existence of hypercoagulability or carotid stenosis, usually causing a bruit (and particularly associated, it is said, with homocystinemia). TIA's can produce very subtle changes – minor degrees of diplopia, mild dysphasia, and so on.

8. **MENINGISM.** In patients with acute leukemia, meningeal infiltration is far commoner in ALL than in non-ALL varieties. Other conditions can be considered in the very ill patient (e.g., AIDS), such as cryptococcal or tuberculous meningitis.

Face, Mouth, and Eyes

1. **GENERAL.** Facial appearances can be very revealing. Most of these have already been mentioned in passing:

   a. **CUSHINGOID FEATURES** when well developed are quite obvious: the moon face, often plethoric, and hirsute.

   b. **MYXEDEMA.** The established case is easy to spot.

   c. **THALASSEMIA MAJOR.** The facies of thalassemia major is quite typical, with maxillary overgrowth, frontal bossing, jaundice, hyperpigmentation (due to iron overload).

   d. **EVIDENCE OF STROKE** especially TIA's.

   e. **PLETHORA.**

   f. **CHRONIC ILLNESS.**

2. **SPECIFIC CHANGES.** Many of these can have relevance to hematology.

   a. **PIGMENTARY DISTURBANCES**, such as in hypogonadism, thalassemia, Addison disease, hemochromatosis, jaundice, cyanosis.

   b. **EDEMA.** This may occur in dermatomyositis, associated with a heliotrope rash around the eyes, muscle weakness and tenderness, and frequent underlying malignancy (in adults); the other classic cause is myxedema.

   c. **CENTRAL FACIAL RASHES.** SLE (anemia of chronic disorders, autoimmune hemolytic anemia, thrombocytopenia, leukopenia, hypercoagulability), dermatomyositis (underlying malignancy with spread to bone marrow), porphyria cutanea tarda.

   d. **FACIAL TELANGIECTASIS.** Relevant conditions to be considered here are scleroderma (anemia both from chronic disease and malabsorption, thrombocytopenia); hereditary hemorrhagic telangiectasia (easy bleeding including from operation sites – note that ataxia telangiectasia should be excluded); chronic liver disease; scleroderma, chronic liver disease (spiders).

   e. **ABNORMALITIES OF FACIAL EXPRESSION** can sometimes be a clue to blood disease or an abnormality in the FBC. Apart from the apathetic dull expression of myxedema, the akinetic, expressionless facies of dystrophia myotonica is striking: due to weakness of respiratory muscles, these patients eventually develop erythrocytosis.

3. **THE LIPS.** Three appearances warrant mention:

   a. **FRECKLING OF THE LIPS** (and palms) is strongly suspicious of the **PEUTZ–JEGHERS SYNDROME.**

   b. **CROHN DISEASE** may affect the mouth and lips, causing a severe cheilitis with edema. The presence of megaloblastic anemia due to vitamin B_{12} deficiency would tend to reinforce any clinical indication that the ileum is involved.

   c. **B VITAMIN DEFICIENCIES IN GENERAL** cause cracked painful lips, which may interfere with eating.

4. **THE EYES.** The eyes warrant careful attention. **BLUE EYES** are characteristically associated with pernicious anemia (along with **PREMATURE GRAYING OF THE HAIR**); **BLUE SCLERAE** on the other hand can be found in chronic iron deficiency (as well as fragilitas ossium). **JAUNDICE** is easily seen in the eyes (except under artificial lighting). **CONJUNCTIVAL INJECTION** is a feature of all the causes of plethora. (Note that the color of the conjunctivae is very unsatisfactory for the assessment of anemia, although considerable work has recently been done, tending to show that it is the anterior rim of the conjunctiva rather than the body that should be looked at – see Chapter 6). **DISORDERS OF CRANIAL NERVES III, IV, AND VI** can occur with TIA's, and are often very subtle. There may be evidence of Horner syndrome (possible superior vena cava syndrome, usually from a Pancoast tumor). The **FUNDI** may show congestion in plethoric patients; "cattle-trucking" and even papilledema can occur in some hyperviscosity states. **PINGUECULAE** are regularly found in Gaucher disease: these are triangular patches of yellowish lipid material adjacent to the **EXTERIOR** limbus and must not be confused with pterygia, found at the **INNER** limbus – see Fig. 5.5. Gaucher disease classically presents with a large spleen and pancytopenia in Ashkenazy Jews.

5. **THE MOUTH.** Changes in the mouth are very common in blood diseases:

   a. **PURPURA** may manifest itself as blebs, bullae, and classical purpura on the palate and under the tongue.

b. **GLOSSITIS** is a common accompaniment of nutritional anemias: in megaloblastic anemia the whole mouth interior is bright red, and the tongue is smooth and painful; in iron deficiency the tongue, while smooth and painful does not have the bright-red color – it may indeed be pale. This can be so severe as to interfere with eating and swallowing.

c. **TELANGIECTASES** and cherry angiomata may be obvious in the mouth. They may represent similar malformations throughout the gut as part of the **RENDU–OSLER–WEBER SYNDROME** [8].

d. **THRUSH.** This may indicate an immune deficiency – esophageal candidiasis should then be suspected, which is a prominent feature of AIDS.

e. **ENLARGED TONSILS** in an elderly person should prompt the suspicion of CLL.

f. **MACROGLOSSIA** may indicate amyloidosis.

g. **TUMORS, INFECTION, AND SEPSIS** in the mouth may result in bleeding or inadequate intake and/or defective digestion (poor release of iron).

h. **NEUTROPENIA AND OTHER FORMS OF IMMUNE DEFICIENCY** are typically associated with infections of the mouth, e.g., periodontitis. In the latter case, esophageal candidiasis (and therefore AIDS) should always be excluded.

i. One of the classic presentations in **HEMOPHILIA** is **CHRONIC BLEEDING FROM THE FRENUM OF THE TONGUE OR THE LOWER LIP** as a result of a fall. The problem is that it is impossible adequately to compress and immobilize such lesions.

6. **THE TEETH AND GUMS.**

a. **HYPERTROPHIC, OFTEN BLEEDING GUMS** can be found in a number of conditions, most commonly periodontal disease. However, two conditions of hematological import should be considered: acute monoblastic or myelomonocytic leukemia and chronic epanutin administration which can be associated with megaloblastic anemia.

b. **VITAMIN C DEFICIENCY** results in a bleeding tendency, with gum bleeding a prominent presentation.

7. **THE THROAT.**

a. **ACUTE TONSILLITIS** may seriously interfere with appetite and with swallowing. See Case #8.

b. **INFECTIOUS MONONUCLEOSIS SYNDROMES** typically are associated with acute pharyngitis and stomatitis.

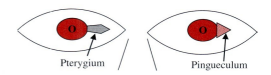

Fig. 5.5

The Thorax

1. **DILATED VEINS.** These may be found in two important conditions, and the direction of flow is extremely important:

a. **SUPERIOR VENA CAVA SYNDROME.** The veins drain downward.

b. **PORTAL HYPERTENSION** (caput medusae). The veins drain outward from the umbilicus.

2. **SKIN LESIONS.** Purpura, telangiectases, angiomata, and nodules commonly are seen on the chest skin.

3. **STERNAL TENDERNESS.** Characteristic of acute leukemia, but also seen in hyperparathyroidism.

4. **INFRACLAVICULAR NODES.** When involved are typical of Hodgkin lymphoma and CLL.

5. **CARDIAC EXAMINATION.** The hyper-dynamic circulation (as found in severe anemia, thyrotoxicosis, late pregnancy, large AV communications) is characterized by harsh murmurs over the precordium.

6. **BUFFALO HUMP.** This is characteristic of Cushing syndrome.

The Abdomen and Pelvis

In the abdomen, the enlargement of various organs, diagnosed either by palpation of sonography, can be very helpful.

1. **THE ENLARGED SPLEEN.** Typically it enlarges diagonally across the abdomen, even right into the right iliac fossa; in this case its diagnosis seldom presents a problem. Sometimes, however, it enlarges straight downwards and may then have to be differentiated from an enlarged kidney. In this case, differentiation is usually easy – if you can get a finger between the paravertebral muscles and the mass posteriorly, it is a spleen (since the spleen is not a retroperitoneal organ). The diagnostic problem is that there are numerous and disparate causes of enlargement, both hematological and non-hematological. Figure 5.6 depicts a good clinical approach to splenomegaly. Some points to note:

a. A spleen greater than 20 cm in size is regarded as a "massive" splenomegaly. This is a valuable distinction, since such a spleen is always significant and serious and frequently hematological in origin.

b. A truly enormous spleen, extending into or close to the iliac fossa, has a limited range of causes: chronic myelocytic leukemia, myelofibrosis, kala-azar; very occasionally other causes of a massive splenomegaly, such as CLL, can reach this size.

SPLENOMEGALY CAN PLAY A CRUCIAL ROLE IN AIDING THE DIFFERENTIATION OF BLOOD DISEASES, AND THESE WILL BE DEMONSTRATED IN THE DISCUSSION OF DIFFERENT PRESENTATIONS IN CHAPTERS 8–22.

In Fig. 5.6, it is taken for granted that the previous sequence, as depicted in Fig. 5.2, has been followed. Thus only issues specific to the spleen and splenomegaly are discussed.

2. **ABDOMINAL ANEURYSM.** Aneurysms greater than 5 cm in diameter are regarded as serious. They can present as iron deficiency due to slow oozing and chronic abdominal pain.

3. **ENLARGED KIDNEY.** This can be associated with a normocytic anemia or, paradoxically, erythrocytosis due to inappropriate secretion of erythropoietin (EPO). This enlargement does not have to be malignant.

4. **ENLARGED UTERUS.** The most significant point here is myomata causing chronic menorrhagia and iron deficiency. Occasionally they produce EPO with erythrocytosis.

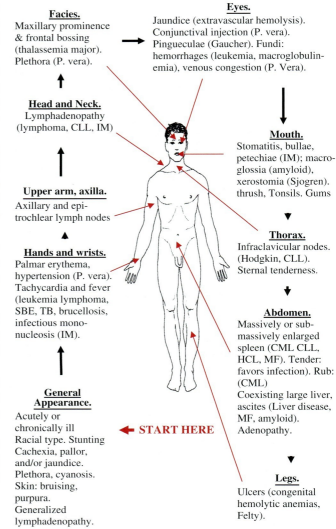

Facies.
Maxillary prominence & frontal bossing (thalassemia major). Plethora (P. vera).

Head and Neck.
Lymphadenopathy (lymphoma, CLL, IM)

Upper arm, axilla.
Axillary and epitrochlear lymph nodes

Hands and wrists.
Palmar erythema, hypertension (P. vera). Tachycardia and fever (leukemia lymphoma, SBE, TB, brucellosis, infectious mononucleosis (IM).

General Appearance.
Acutely or chronically ill Racial type. Stunting Cachexia, pallor, and/or jaundice. Plethora, cyanosis. Skin: bruising, purpura. Generalized lymphadenopathy.

Eyes.
Jaundice (extravascular hemolysis). Conjunctival injection (P. vera). Pingueculae (Gaucher). Fundi: hemorrhages (leukemia, macroglobulinemia), venous congestion (P. Vera).

Mouth.
Stomatitis, bullae, petechiae (IM); macroglossia (amyloid), xerostomia (Sjogren). thrush, Tonsils. Gums

Thorax.
Infraclavicular nodes. (Hodgkin, CLL). Sternal tenderness.

Abdomen.
Massively or submassively enlarged spleen (CML CLL, HCL, MF). Tender: favors infection). Rub: (CML) Coexisting large liver, ascites (Liver disease, MF, amyloid). Adenopathy.

← **START HERE**

Legs.
Ulcers (congenital hemolytic anemias, Felty).

Fig. 5.6 The enlarged spleen

The Lower Limbs

Chronic, often pigmented leg ulcers in the context of an anemic patient may suggest a chronic extravascular hemolysis, especially sickle disease. They are rarely found in Felty syndrome (neutropenia, rarely pancytopenia).

Livedo reticularis is most prominent in the legs. It is a reticulated (lacy) erythema, found in many collagen disorders and the antiphospholipid syndrome.

The Nervous System

There are many hematological associations:

1. **DEMENTIA.** In vitamin B_{12} deficiency, this is characterized by a chronic confusional state with poor memory, severe attention deficit but no aphasia or apraxia, distinguishing it from Alzheimer's disease.

2. **OPTIC NEUROPATHY.** This again can complicate vitamin B_{12} deficiency, often presenting as red desaturation.

3. **STROKE AND ISCHEMIC EPISODES.** The features can vary from various paretic syndromes to epilepsy to blindness, and even migraine.

4. **CEREBELLAR DISEASE:**

    a. **V**ertigo

    b. **A**taxia

    c. **N**ystagmus

    d. **I**ntention tremor

    e. **S**canning speech

f. **H**ypotonia.

Cerebellar signs in a plethoric patient suggest a cerebellar hemangioblastoma. Cerebellar dysfunction may occur in AIDS.

5. **TRANSVERSE MYELITIS**. Pain localized to the sensory level (dermatome), with lower limb paresthesiae and ascending weakness, sphincter dysfunction; later flaccid paralysis and total sensory loss. In a patient with a macrocytic anemia, vitamin B_{12} deficiency is a strong possibility. There are many other causes, however – cervical spondylosis, epidural abscess, spinal tumor, viruses, and radiation.

6. **SUBACUTE COMBINED DEGENERATION**. A prominent cause of this is vitamin B_{12} deficiency:

   a. **DORSAL COLUMNS**: "Cotton wool" sensation over skin, clumsy fine movements, loss of proprioception, and vibration sense.

   b. **LATERAL COLUMNS**: Typical upper motor neuron features.

   c. **THE GAIT** seems to be a combination of "stamping" and "scissors."

7. **PERIPHERAL NEUROPATHY**. Predominantly sensory (glove and stocking). Patients on high-dose pyridoxal (vitamin B_6 – up to 200 or even 300 mg per day) for the treatment of some forms of the myelodysplastic syndrome often develop a very severe peripheral neuropathy, which tends to be relatively permanent.

The Assessment of Lymphadenopathy

There are very many causes of lymphadenopathy. In our approach, the main task is to distinguish benign from malignant causes.

1. **NON-MALIGNANT ENLARGEMENT**. Factors in favor of a non-malignant cause: localized enlargement, tender, less than 2 cm in diameter, non-matted, non-adherent, in the drainage area of an obvious infection.
2. **MALIGNANT ENLARGEMENT**. These nodes tend to be larger, often matted and fixed, hard rubbery consistency, and non-tender.

With the exception perhaps of small mobile non-tender nodes in the inguinal region, **NO LYMPHADENOPATHY CAN BE IGNORED**. The diagnosis almost always involves pathological tests, including very often biopsy.

Lymphadenopathy localized to **ONE** of the 13 clinical areas (see later) could easily be benign, draining an infected area (which can sometimes be difficult to find). Occasionally, however, localized enlargement, particularly if very large, could have a malignant cause (e.g., a very large mediastinal node due to lymphoma or cervical adenopathy draining a malignant neoplasm in the retina, mouth or throat).

By contrast, generalized lymphadenopathy is commonly malignant, but exceptions do occur, such as IM. Also secondary syphilis and toxoplasmosis can have generalized lymphadenopathy without tenderness.

WE ARE HERE CONCERNED ONLY WITH LYMPHADENOPATHY THAT IS FOUND IN, OR IS LIKELY WITHOUT TREATMENT TO EXTEND INTO, MORE THAN ONE SITE.

Figure 5.7 shows the distribution of normal lymph nodes from a clinical point of view. There are 13 clinical groups of nodes, 8 bilateral and 5 midline.

In a (potentially) generalized lymphadenopathy, every group must be examined and assessed, many requiring sonography or CT scanning. This is critical for staging and other purposes. A number of patterns can be recognized (with a great deal of overlap):

1. **HODGKIN LYMPHOMA**. Two thirds of cases start in the neck. Constitutional symptoms are prominent with weight loss, fever, night sweats, pruritis, sometimes pain in one or more sites almost immediately after ingestion of alcohol. Any of the sites can be involved, but it is noteworthy that epitrochlear nodes are hardly ever involved in Hodgkin lymphoma, and the infraclavicular group is unusually frequently involved. Note that extranodal involvement is very rare.
2. **NON-HODGKIN LYMPHOMA**. Less than 50% of cases commence in the neck. The epitrochlear nodes are involved unusually often. Extranodal involvement, even presentation, is very common. Constitutional symptoms occur but late in the disease.
3. **CHRONIC LYMPHOCYTIC LEUKEMIA**. Any nodes can be involved. In addition, the spleen is almost always involved. Should an elderly patient present with a chronic sore throat and enlarged tonsils, CLL should be considered early.

We are not going to discuss staging – it is a specialist activity.

Clinical Evaluation of Enlarged Lymph Nodes

A great deal depends on the presentation, especially:

1. **THE DISTRIBUTION**.
2. **THE SIZE**. It has been found that a node that is, in any projection, greater than 2 cm is to be regarded as suspicious – not necessarily of malignancy but possibly

Fig. 5.7 The lymph nodes

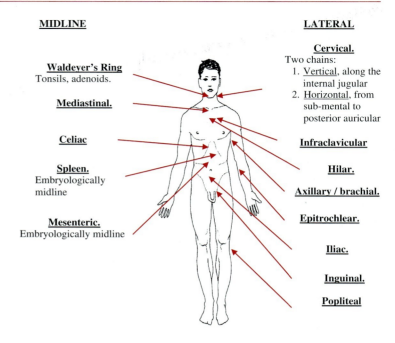

MIDLINE

Waldeyer's Ring
Tonsils, adenoids.

Mediastinal.

Celiac

Spleen.
Embryologically
midline

Mesenteric.
Embryologically midline

LATERAL

Cervical.
Two chains:
1. Vertical, along the
   internal jugular
2. Horizontal, from
   sub-mental to
   posterior auricular

Infraclavicular

Hilar.

Axillary / brachial.

Epitrochlear.

Iliac.

Inguinal.

Popliteal

also of one of the many strange and rare causes of lymphadenopathy that have been described. Sometimes enlarged nodes are discovered (usually serendipitously) only in the deep chains, such as abdominal or hilar. When these are discovered by sonography it should be realized that the technique is not very accurate for sizing purposes, and unless the nodes are indisputably larger than 2 cm, their size should always be confirmed by CT scanning, with contrast.

3. **THE CHARACTERISTICS BY PALPATION.** Matted glands are not of very great assistance in differential diagnosis. Tenderness (or pain), however, is. Tender glands are very seldom malignant. Fixity to underlying structures is a very strong indicator of malignancy.

4. Whether there is **A LOCAL INFLAMMATORY OR MALIGNANT LESION** that the enlarged nodes are possibly draining. This may be difficult to find – and indeed, in the case of a malignancy, the enlarged glands may occur after the primary has been removed, sometimes years before (e.g., a melanoma of the choroid).

5. **SUGGESTIVE FEATURES IN THE FBC.** Sometimes one can reach the answer in this way, at least provisionally, such as in CLL and infectious mononucleosis.

Except in cases of CLL, malignant lymphadenopathy must always be confirmed by biopsy – no oncologist or clinical hematologist would treat a patient without this.

The Clinical Examination in the Bleeding Disorders

There are several crucial clinical points of difference between general blood diseases and the bleeding disorders:

1. Most of the diseases the FBC tests for are not susceptible of another explanation outside the hematological system – for example, in anemia, the proximate cause and nature of the anemia will be found within the blood cell system: the production, damage to, or disposal of the red cells and/or hemoglobin. Thus, abnormal findings in the FBC will almost always directly point at some abnormality in the blood cells, blood-forming organs, and organs concerned with disposal of cells. By contrast, a bleeding presentation in a patient need not (in fact usually does not) indicate any disorder within the hemostatic system. There are many distinct clinical patterns of bleeding that are due to a local cause (e.g., hematemesis and melena due to peptic ulceration) but which can unusually be a manifestation of say a coagulation factor defect. Thus the approach to bleeding presentations clearly requires a strong clinical grounding **TO DETERMINE THE NATURE OF THE BLEEDING.** This can range from epistaxis to hematuria to menorrhagia to intracranial bleeding; all these **MAY, UNCOMMONLY,** be due to a bleeding disorder.

Head and Neck.
Lymphadenopathy,
Bald (?chemotherapy)

Upper arm, axilla.
Axillary, brachial and
epitrochlear nodes.
Joint swelling, defor-
mity. Ulnar nerve
palsy. Defective shoul-
der movements. Com-
partment syndrome

Hands and wrists.
Hypotension, shock,
tachycardia, fever.
Deformities, swelling.

**General
Appearance.**
In acute pain.
Chronically ill,
cachectic. Mal-
nourished (scurvy)
Cushingoid (bruis-
ing, purpura).
Obvious deformity.
Obvious purpura or
bruising. Palpable
purpura (vasculitis)
Persistent bleeding
or oozing from a
site. Adenopathy.

Eyes.
Conjunctival telangiec-
tases, hemorrhages.
Fundi: hemorrhages,
Jaundice (?Evans
syndrome). raccoon
eyes, nerve lesions.

Mouth.
Bullae, petechiae
under the tongue,
telangiectasis, enlarged
tonsils. Persistent
oozing from cut lip,
frenum of tongue,
macroglossia-amyloid

Abdomen
Massively or sub-
massively enlarged
spleen (CML, CLL,
HCL, MF). Large
liver: amyloid.
Bruises. Masses. ?
bleeds, with nerve
lesions. Compartment
syndrome.

Legs.
Acutely painful and
swollen knee or ankle.
Compartment syn-
drome. Evidence of
spinal cord lesion.

← **START HERE**

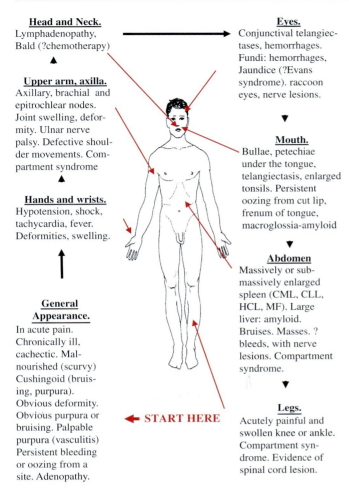

Fig. 5.8 Examination: bleeding tendency

So, before one can even think of a hemostatic mechanism underlying the bleeding, one must make a decision as to whether the bleeding is in fact pathological (i.e., not due to trauma or some form of tissue damage).

2. The symptomatology of the blood diseases is relatively straightforward and predictable: neutropenic patients can be expected to show one or more of a fairly restricted range of clinical features; this would apply also to patients with say polycythemia vera; but the symptoms referable to neutropenia would only very exceptionally apply to polycythemia, and vice versa.

In the bleeding disorders this does not hold, and the reason for this is to be found in the nature of pathological bleeds. There are two broad groups of presentation in the bleeding disorders that can be identified – the "purpuric," and the "coagulation defect" (which in the vast majority of cases is a coagulation factor defect). However, there are very many cases that do

not fit in with these typical appearances, or there are some features of both present.

3. It is very uncommon for the FBC to be normal with a significant blood disease, whereas some bleeding disorders have a completely normal HS.

In summary, therefore, it follows that the clinical assessment of a bleeding disorder is more complex (and even more necessary) than with other disorders.

It involves two separate decisions:

1. Whether the bleeding disorder that is presenting is in fact due to a disorder of hemostasis.
2. Once having decided that abnormal bleeding indeed exists, the clinical features **MAY** strongly suggest the nature of the abnormality. But one is some-times surprised, and it is often wise to screen both elements of hemostasis (the platelet-vascular aspect and the coagulation-fibrinolytic aspect) even if one thinks one is certain of the nature of the bleeding.

What Features Can Suggest that Bleeding Is Pathological?

1. The most obvious indicator of abnormal bleeding is bleeding at or from a particular site and which, after appropriate investigation, shows **NO EVIDENCE OF AN ANATOMICAL LESION**. Epistaxis is a prime example.
2. As a general rule, if any bleed, e.g., epistaxis, menor-rhagia, hemarthrosis, hematemesis, etc., which nor-mally can be explained by a local pathology, has **ANY UNUSUAL FEATURES** whatsoever, one should think of a bleeding disorder sooner rather than later. In all these cases the HS is essential (and indeed, this is where it is a **SCREEN** in the true sense of the word).
3. Similarly, a **PARTICULAR AND KNOWN PAT-TERN OF BLEEDING** occurring in a patient in whom this pattern is completely unexpected. An example is a recent case that comes to mind – a well, cared-for, and happy child (i.e., no evidence of abuse) of 13 months presenting with hematemesis and melena; she turned out to have a hereditary factor X deficiency.
4. Post-operative, post-extraction, or umbilical stump **BLEEDING OR OOZING THAT PERSISTS** for more than 24 h (unless it is severe, when intervention must take place immediately).
5. Obvious spontaneous **PURPURA.**

6. **ACUTE HEMARTHROSIS, MUSCLE, AND/OR SOFT TISSUE BLEEDS IN THE ABSENCE OF TRAUMA, OR AFTER INAPPROPRIATELY SMALL TRAUMA.** These are highly significant presentations, in that they tend strongly to suggest a coagulation-defect bleed, particularly in a male.

A NUMBER OF THESE PRESENTATIONS REQUIRE SPECIAL DESCRIPTION. THE PATHOLOGY AND PATHOGENESIS HAVE BEEN DISCUSSED IN CHAPTER 4. HERE WE CONCENTRATE ON THE MOST CHARACTERISTIC CLINICAL PRESENTATIONS, ALTHOUGH IT MUST BE EMPHASIZED THAT FREQUENTLY THE CLINICAL FEATURES ARE INCONCLUSIVE. THE TYPICAL FIRST-LINE LABORATORY FINDINGS ARE PRESENTED IN CHAPTER 5.

Hemarthrosis

Hemarthrosis is the classical appearance of hemophilia A and B (factors VIII and IX, respectively). However, it should be realized that hemarthrosis occurs in many other bleeding disorders, with the incidence varying from very rare to quite common. What is of major importance, however, is that the approach to and management of hemarthrosis is the same regardless of the type of bleeding disorder.

There are two broad presentations of hemophilic joint disease: the acute, generally single joint involvement, and chronic destructive arthropathy involving usually many joints, which may or may not involve actual bleeding into the joint. It is the acute presentation that requires specific discussion, and this can be a very difficult diagnosis.

> Hemarthrosis should always be regarded as a medical emergency. The major reason is that it may be due to a bleeding disorder, and unless appropriate treatment is instituted immediately, irreparable damage to the joint will follow. This is particularly relevant to the first time the patient presents: the patient usually presents to a family practitioner, who thinks that because hemophilia is rare, he need not know about it and therefore does not know how to institute treatment. He also probably does not know that diagnostic aspiration of a hemophilic hemarthrosis should be avoided if at all possible.

> It is thus necessary to discuss the issue of how this diagnosis is made clinically. Clearly one must, as far as possible, exclude the other causes of hemarthrosis and of a very painful swollen joint.

The Acute, Very Painful Swollen Joint (Essentially a Monoarthritis)

The most important causes of this are

1. Septic arthritis
2. Sero-negative and "reactive" arthritis (ankylosing spondylitis, psoriatic arthropathy, inflammatory bowel disease, Reiter syndrome, Behcet syndrome)
3. Hemarthrosis
4. Crystal arthropathy (gout and pseudogout)

Establishing the cause is in the first instance a very clinical business, and serological tests are of great value. But before diagnostic aspiration is done (if considered essential), hemophilia **MUST BE EXCLUDED**, especially if the patient is a young boy, and the joint involved is a hinge joint (knee, ankle, or elbow). All that is required is for blood to be sent urgently for a PTT – this can be done within 30–60 min, depending on the lab and its distance. Even in the bush, a Lee–White coagulation time is easy (see Appendix C) and will provide a general answer.

See the box on page 161 for the commonest causes of hemarthrosis. In practice, the most important differential is between septic arthritis and hemarthrosis, since both are extremely painful and both are associated with pyrexia. In the diagnosis, one tries to make do with the associated clinical features, and this requires considerable judgment. Typically, there should be no problem with a first-time tense very painful swollen joint, usually a knee, in a boy without a history of remembered trauma and without systemic evidence of a septic focus – this must in the first instance be considered hemophilic. However, the maximum pyrexia compatible with hemophilia is 38.5°C – anything more than this is presumptive evidence that this is not hemophilic (diagnostic aspiration is not contra-indicated in non-hemophilic hemarthrosis). Nevertheless sepsis is always a worry. It is always advisable to seek specialist advice here – urgently.

The emergency treatment of hemophilic hemarthrosis is detailed in Chapter 17.

> ### The Commonest Causes of Hemarthrosis
>
> 1. Trauma (?underlying fracture)
> 2. Villonodular synovitis
> 3. Charcot's joint, especially due to diabetes
> 4. Hemophilia
> 5. Anticoagulant therapy
> 6. Myeloproliferative disorders
> 7. Thrombocytopenia

Acute on Chronic Hemarthrosis

Unless the acute hemarthrosis is managed properly, the joint will slowly develop a chronic arthropathy, very prone to bleeding thereafter. Sometimes, particularly in moderate hemophilia, a single joint will be repeatedly affected. This is called a "target" joint – here there may be **NO OTHER** clinical stigmata of hemophilia (see Chapter 19).

Chronic Arthropathy in the Bleeding Disorders

Patients who have had recurrent hemarthroses and whose treatment and general management have been inadequate will tend to have recurrent episodes of joint swelling, with pain. These may of course be further bleeds, but in many cases the fluid in the joint contains little or no blood; presumably the latter reflect a non-specific reaction to the joint damage. It is often a very difficult matter to decide whether the patient needs factor or not.

Massive Bruising After Inappropriately Small Trauma

Since the blood does not clot easily, it tends to track extensively under gravity. Large amounts of blood can be lost into the tissues.

Acute Muscle and Soft Tissue Bleeds

These can be very difficult to diagnose if deep. They can mimic numerous other clinical presentations – for example, ilio-psoas hemorrhage may clinically mimic acute appendicitis; large intra-abdominal bleeds may track up through the diaphragm and present as a pleural effusion. Since the blood clots poorly, these hematomata tend to become very large and may cause nerve compression syndromes and compartment syndromes. Some examples of how they can present are given in Chapter 19.

Raccoon Eyes (Periorbital Bleeding)

This is a well-known presentation. The major differentials are a fracture of the base of the anterior fossa and acute leukemia (in this case, usually associated with proptosis).

Laceration of the Frenum of the Tongue or Lower Lip

These can occur after a fall, and can ooze for days. The problem is that these sites cannot be immobilized.

Multiple Hemangiomata

The most important of these is **HEREDITARY HEMORRHAGIC TELANGIECTASIS** (the Rendu–Osler–Weber syndrome). Multiple telangiectases are usually easy to spot, commonly in a child. However, there are two problems:

1. Sometimes the lesions are mainly internal, and they can present with a variety of signs – often post-operative oozing. Surgeons will sometimes report having seen plenty of the lesions in the operative field.
2. Although hereditary, the lesions will sometimes only present with bleeding – usually chronic – later in life, particularly in young females (because of the influence of estrogen causing the lesions to get larger and more wide spread).

Multiple hemangiomata are also a feature of cirrhosis. These do not, however, seem to be a significant cause of bleeding.

Liver Disease

The existence of underlying liver disease may be obvious, and the full HS would be indicated, including the D-dimer and FDP assays. However, sometimes it is not obvious, and one requires a considerable index of suspicion to investigate for this. Indeed, it is here that the clinical features of the underlying disease may be very helpful.

Thus in very general terms the effects of liver disease on hemostasis can be divided into

1. Hepatocellular damage, affecting production of all factors as well as often causing thrombocytopenia
2. Cholestatic disease and interferences with vitamin K metabolism

For example, a patient with features very strongly suggestive of obstructive jaundice with a bleeding tendency would probably bring to mind the possibility of a functional deficiency of factors II, VII, and X, since they are vitamin K dependent and vitamin K is a fat-soluble vitamin. If typical features of liver disease are present there is usually no difficulty, especially if portal hypertension is present. Chronic stable liver disease can, however, be a problem. The liver's involvement in hemostasis is extensive and has been discussed in Chapters 1 and 3.

Disseminated Intravascular Coagulation (DIC)

In DIC the underlying cause may be obvious, and the full HS is indicated, including the D-dimer and FDP assays (as well as the FBC). However, sometimes they are not obvious, and one requires a considerable index of suspicion to investigate for these. Indeed, it is here that the clinical features of an underlying disease may be very helpful. **DIC** can vary considerably from the clinical point of view. Should the coagulation mechanism be inappropriately activated within the circulation, widespread fibrin formation occurs particularly in the smaller vessels. It is caused most commonly by sepsis, obstetric accidents, and the presence of necrotic and traumatized tissue. These may be clinically obvious.

Other Hematological Diseases with Bleeding

These may affect both the platelet-vascular component and, more rarely, the coagulation component.

1. **DISORDERS INVOLVING THE PLATELET-VAS-CULAR COMPONENT.** The most important here are myelodysplasia, aplastic anemia, and leukemia. In myelodysplasia the platelet count may well be on the low side, but bleeding tends to be disproportionately severe, because of functional defects in the platelets. In aplastic anemia, the usual cause of bleeding is severe thrombocytopenia. In the leukemias, both thrombocytopenia and functional platelet disorders may be responsible for bleeding.

2. **DISORDERS INVOLVING THE COAGULATION COMPONENT.** Hyperfibrinolysis can occur secondary to certain malignancies. The abnormal plasma proteins in some of the paraproteinemias, e.g., myeloma, can adsorb on to their surface some of the coagulation factors – factor X seems to be particularly affected in this regard.

Miscellaneous Presentations

1. **PERIFOLLICULAR HEMORRHAGE** is characteristic of scurvy. Typical associated features are swollen bleeding gums and deep tenderness in the long bones, due to periosteal bleeds. True purpura may occur.

2. **PURPURA** can be a difficult diagnosis. Traditionally purpura is recognized as a skin lesion, but in fact it also occurs in the mucosae, albeit usually in different forms – blebs, blisters, and bullae. A characteristic early place to look for them is under the tongue (occasionally the only place they may be seen). **IN THE SKIN** purpuric lesions are intradermal bleeds that may be petechiae (pinhead bleeds), purpura proper (up to 2 mm diameter lesions), or ecchymoses (more extensive or coalescing lesions).

Since there is no laboratory test that can identify a lesion as purpuric, we outline the characteristic clinical features. A purpuric lesion:

   i. Occurs spontaneously.
   ii. Is not palpable (cf. vasculitis, bruises).
   iii. The blood in it cannot be pressed away (it is best to use a glass slide to press, so you can see the lesion) (cf. hemangiomata).
   iv. Is not painful (cf. vasculitis).
   v. Is not tender (cf. vasculitis, bruises).
   vi. Does not itch (cf. fleabites). It is extraordinary how some surface appearances can be misdiagnosed as purpura. We have seen the following, even by postgraduates:

   i. Bruising.
   ii. Multiple hemangiomata
   iii. Acanthosis nigricans ⎱ unlike purpura, these
   iv. Café-au-lait spots ⎰ lesions will not clear up within a few days.

   v. Fleabites.

vi. Vasculitis. Some forms of vasculitis may bleed into the skin and strongly resemble purpura.

vii. Scurvy. True purpura can, however, also occur in scurvy.

Other Characteristic Clinical Features

Two clinical features that are sometimes extremely helpful are how any wounds bleed and more importantly how they stop bleeding, and the family history:

1. **BLEEDING FROM WOUNDS AND ITS DIAGNOSTIC VALUE.** Particular attention must be paid to **THREE TYPES OF WOUND: ABRASIONS, LACERATIONS, AND INCISIONS**.

   a) **PLATELET-VASCULAR** ("purpuric-type") bleeding. All the wounds commence bleeding immediately and continue to bleed, but usually stop with adequate pressure for adequate time, and treatment with vasoconstrictors and other hemostatics. (Bruises may also occur, but are usually in relation to trauma, albeit minimal. Bruising, however, is not a classical feature, since it occurs in the coagulation-defect disorders as well.)

   b) **COAGULATION-DEFECT** bleeding:

      i. Abrasions will usually stop bleeding with local pressure, but sometimes requiring vasoconstrictors and other hemostatics.

      ii. Lacerations will stop bleeding normally after 5 min or so, but then, after a variable period – anything up to an hour – **THEY WILL START BLEEDING AGAIN, AND NO AMOUNT OF PRESSURE WILL STOP THIS. THIS IS A CARDINAL FEATURE OF HEMOPHILIA.**

      iii. The behavior of incisions depends largely on the depth: if less than about 2 mm, they will behave like abrasions; otherwise like lacerations.

2. **THE FAMILY HISTORY AND ITS DIAGNOSTIC VALUE:**

   a) **IN THE PLATELET-VASCULAR BLEEDS** there usually is no family history except in the case of functional platelet disorders, which usually have a normal platelet count. A history of a recent viral infection in such a patient may suggest a thrombocytopenia.

   b) **THE CLASSICAL HEMOPHILIAS** (deficiencies of factors VIII or IX) are X-linked, and thus will have a typical family history pattern. The personal history is also valuable – usually in that there is a relevant history going back to childhood (**BUT BEWARE, NOT ALWAYS**).

   c) All the other hereditary bleeding disorders including von Willebrand disease show autosomal inheritance, usually dominant.

Figure 5.8 illustrates specific aspects of the examination of a patient in whom a bleeding tendency is known or suspected; clearly it is part of the overall examination is as is depicted in Fig. 5.4.

> Even if a causal relationship between changes in the blood and disease in other systems cannot be proven, a regular correlation between these is very helpful – indeed, the establishment of clinical correlates is (and has always been) a fundamental aspect of the clinical method.

Common Clinical Patterns in Blood Diseases

With experience we try to integrate various clinical findings into **PATTERNS**. There are many patterns that cause one to suspect a blood disease.

A. In a distinct minority of cases, a pattern of signs and symptoms may strongly suggest or even indicate a known hematological disorder, such as many cases of pernicious anemia, iron deficiency, chronic (and occasionally acute) extravascular hemolysis, factor VIII or IX deficiency, and so on. Note that the relative prevalences of diseases play a big role here. For example, a boy presenting with an acute hemarthrosis in the absence of significant (or any) trauma is suggestive of a coagulation-defect bleeding disorder; whilst many factor deficiencies can do this, most of them are very rare indeed, particularly presenting in this way. One will almost certainly think of factors VIII or IX deficiencies, to the exclusion of the others. On the other hand, if the patient were female, the considerations would be very different.

B. There may be presentations of a patient with features suggesting one or other blood abnormality in the presence of a systemic (non-hematological) disease.

C. Finally, there are (possibly the majority of) cases where there is clear or suggestive evidence of a blood disorder without any other features indicating its nature.

One can classify the clinical features of groups A and B into six rough groups:

1. **PATTERNS STRONGLY SUGGESTIVE OF A KNOWN BLOOD DISEASE.** There are a few classic pictures like this. As clinicians you are already aware of the value and interpretation of signs and symptoms. So it would be useful here for the reader to pick out essential features of the clinical examination and make them directly relevant to hematology. Many other detailed examples will be given in the individual chapters. For example,

a) A pale patient with a sore tongue, pica, and koilonychia (or perhaps with dysphagia localizable to the upper third of the chest). This would be strongly indicative of iron deficiency. This would be strengthened in a patient who has say hemorrhoids or menorrhagia.

b) The middle-aged patient with prematurely gray hair, pale, with a severe glossitis and stomatitis and a smooth painful tongue, diarrhea, and significant neuropathy of various possible types, perhaps in cardiac failure or with delirium/dementia. This would be strongly suggestive of pernicious anemia (i.e., vitamin B_{12} deficiency – note that megaloblastosis due to folate deficiency very seldom causes significant neuropathy).

c) The pregnant patient (typically one who has not been attending at an antenatal service) or the alcoholic, presenting with many of the features described under (b). This would be strongly suggestive of folate deficiency, and in the case of the pregnant patient, associated iron deficiency, especially in a multipara.

d) The elderly person living on their own in a tiny room on a very limited income, surviving on toast and tea, can present with features as in (c) above, and with the same basic cause.

e) The basically fit patient presenting with pallor, light jaundice, loin pain, an enlarged spleen, and a story of an relative who had been "cured" of the same problem by splenectomy; the diagnosis of chronic extravascular hemolysis can be made (although the classical cause is hereditary spherocytosis, this is not always the case).

f) A similar patient could present with purpura and deteriorating pallor – the strong suspicion is raised of secondary aplastic anemia.

g) A patient can present with an acute onset of pallor and jaundice and loin pain, with shock and a palpable spleen. An acute hemolytic episode can be inferred.

h) Acute or chronic intravascular hemolysis can sometimes present in a very suggestive manner, with hemoglobinuria (on dipstix), pallor, and perhaps Raynaud's phenomenon.

i) A youngster may present with a painless rash resembling purpura over the buttocks and down the back of the legs. There may be associated abdominal pain or renal dysfunction. These features would be very suggestive of Henoch–Schönlein purpura.

j) A male child may present with a serious bleeding disorder, particularly with hemarthroses. These would be very suggestive of one of the hemophilias.

k) A malnourished person may present with easy bleeding from the gums and from trauma. There are purpuric spots in various places, but some of these spots, particularly on the thighs, can actually be seen to be perifollicular hemorrhages. These features would be very suggestive of scurvy.

l) Myeloma. A typical patient would be over 50, and present with severe bone pain, pallor, and renal failure.

2. **PATTERNS SUGGESTING BLOOD DISEASE ASSOCIATED WITH OR DUE TO A SYSTEMIC ILLNESS.** This list is considerably longer. These presentations are really just expressions of hematological complications or manifestations of disease in other systems. Note that since the clinical focus is on the systemic illness, the hematological features may be overlooked. It is worthwhile to bear these in mind, since the patient may derive benefit from having these treated independently, and also their presence may help in the diagnosis or management of the systemic illness. A few examples (in brief) are

a) Pallor in association with rheumatoid arthritis, lymphoma, other malignant disease, AIDS, etc.

b) Pallor, weight loss, chronic diarrhea, or steatorrhea: malabsorption

c) Purpura in association with drug toxicity, viral infections, etc.

d) **H**eadache, **H**ypertension, **H**ypotension (orthostatic, **H**eartbeat awareness (palpitations), **H**yperhidrosis (sweating): **P**heochromocytoma

e) Weight loss, night sweats, lassitude, pruritis, enlarged cervical nodes: possible Hodgkin Lymphoma

3. **PATTERNS INDICATING THE SEVERITY OF A PROCESS OR STATE.** For example, cardiac failure due to anemia indicates **SEVERE** anemia.

4. **PATTERNS INDICATING COMPLICATIONS OR EFFECTS** that can **SOMETIMES** occur in a disease or process. For example, amaurosis fugax in thrombocytosis.

5. **PATTERNS ESPECIALLY VALUABLE IN FOL-LOW-UP**, such as the band cell count.
6. **PATTERNS THAT ASSIST IN THE INTERPRE-TATION OF THE TESTS**.

There is considerable overlap in these; for example, amaurosis fugax is in favor of (malignant) thrombocythemia rather than (reactive) thrombocytosis, in a patient presenting with a high platelet count. **THE LARGER GROUP, I.E., GROUP C, COMPRISES THOSE WITH LITTLE IF ANYTHING TO INDICATE WHAT, IF ANY, BLOOD DISEASE IS PRESENT**. This is where sensible interpretation of the FBC becomes critical. From the point of view of this book, this is the most important group, and is discussed in Chapter 5.

Indications for Ordering a FBC

It is very difficult to prescribe the indications for doing a FBC in clinical practice. Because anemia, the commonest presenting disorder, is frequently so difficult to diagnose, one may be tempted to do more FBCs than are warranted. The following are suggested indications. On the other hand, one does not want to miss an anemia.

Absolute Indications

1. Any chronically ill patient should have an FBC done at least once.
2. An obviously pale patient.
3. A patient with a family history of "blood disease."
4. A patient presenting with purpura or unexplained bruising where there is no evidence of sepsis.
5. An ill or pale patient in or from an endemic area, such as the Mediterranean, the Indian subcontinent (thalassemia), or West Africa (Sickle and HbC disease), Africa as a whole (thalassemia, HIV, trypanosomiasis, malaria, etc.).
6. A patient with a hyper-dynamic circulation that is not obviously thyrotoxic or pregnant.
7. A patient with lymphadenopathy, splenomegaly, or possibly hepatomegaly.
8. A patient with bone pain, especially if pale and in obvious renal failure (myeloma).
9. A patient over 50 presenting for the first time with angina.
10. A patient with effort dyspnea without evidence of cardio-respiratory disease, especially of the dyspnea is relieved by lying flat.

11. A patient with recurrent hematemesis, melena, menorrhagia.
12. A patient with weight loss, especially of accompanied by night sweats and has lymphadenopathy.
13. A patient with obvious chronic liver disease.

Relative Indications

1. Any patient consulting you for the first time
2. A patient with an acute infection of any type
3. A patient with an acute monoarthritis
4. A patient with suspected renal disease

> We are now in a position to apply and complete the epidemiological approach discussed in Chapter 4 to the problem of a Hb of 13.1 g/dl that was presented in that chapter.

An Application of the Epidemiological Approach

WE RETURN TO OUR PATIENT WITH THE HB OF 13.1 G/DL, AS AN ISOLATED, SINGLE RESULT. We approach this (highly simplified) example according to the steps described in Chapter 4.

TASK #1: IS IT NORMAL? Clearly this will depend on a number of factors. We first consider the basic causes of the different values Hb can have, i.e., altitude, gender, and age:

1. If the patient is at sea level, then the Hb, for both males and females, falls within the reference range, and the Hb **COULD BE** (truly) normal. All that is required now is to correlate this with the clinical features: if there are features in any way suspicious of a cause of anemia, they should then be followed up appropriately
2. If the patient is at 2,500 or 5,000 ft above sea level, then gender and age become relevant:

   a) If the patient is an adult female, then the Hb falls within the reference range. If the patient is an adult male, the Hb is below the given reference range and the patient **COULD BE** anemic.
   b) If the patient is over ±70 years, then the Hb falls within the reference range.

Our patient is an adult male of 40 years and resident at 5,000 ft. He therefore could be anemic.

TASK #2: HOW VALID IS THE RESULT? Here we consider possible pre-analytic variables:

1. Pregnancy and old age are not relevant.
2. The blood was drawn in the morning, with the patient recumbent.
3. He is a smoker, which potentially is a serious confounder:

   a) Chronic smokers frequently show a raised Hct. Thus in this patient his true Hb could well be lower, and thus more significant.
   b) Chronic smokers are prone to numerous complications, including malignancies, which here could be a cause of the suspected anemia.

4. The blood was drawn at 10 am, the specimen was transported in a cool-box, and the test was performed at 12 midday. The laboratory reports that the tube was adequately filled. The time the specimen was drawn, the delay in delivery, the mode of delivery, and the adequacy of tube filling are, however, not relevant to the Hb estimation unless:

   a) The tube was received frozen
   b) The tube was received by the laboratory more than about 2 days later
   c) The blood was obviously infected or hemolysed

No adverse factor was found in our patient that might cause one to think that the possibly abnormal result could have a non-disease cause.

Third, we consider possible analytic variables. Here we are in the hands of the laboratory. On enquiry we are told that the QC for Hb for that day was well within the prescribed limits, and we can thus assume that the result is valid.

TASK #3: WHAT ARE THE LIMITATIONS OF A TEST IN TERMS OF ITS PURPOSE? To see just how the test (Hb) reflects actual pathology, two issues need to be addressed:

1. Does this result outside the given reference ranges necessarily mean an abnormality?
2. What are the operating characteristics of the test.

The answer to 1 is of course "NO." The only ways to get a reasonable answer based on figures alone would be

1. To repeat the test.
2. Is there a previous Hb with which to compare?
3. Are there any other tests available from the results of which we might infer an abnormality?

The answers to 2 and 3 are "NO." The only other test available is a total white cell count, which is normal. Thus the question of possible normality of this result is open, and must be answered at some stage.

The Operating Characteristics of the Hb Test

Our major concern is whether there is in fact an anemia. – i.e., what is the likelihood? To calculate this we require the sensitivity and specificity of the Hb result for anemia in an adult male at this altitude. We look up a table and see that the sensitivity at this level is about 0.28 – i.e., not very sensitive, and the specificity is 0.89.

The positive predictive value $[p(D^+|T^+)]$ is about 0.35, i.e., there is a reasonable chance that the patient is in fact anemic, and since anemia is a common condition in any community, this should be taken seriously.

What then of the likelihood ratio, i.e., effectively the likelihood that the Hb test has altered the pre-test probability of disease?

$$\text{Positive LR} = \frac{p(T^+ \text{ if diseased})}{p(T^+ \text{ if not diseased})}$$
$$= \frac{\text{Sensitivity}}{1 - \text{Specificity}}$$
$$= \frac{0.28}{1 - 0.89}$$
$$= 2.55$$
$$\text{Negative LR} = \frac{p(T^- \text{ if diseased})}{p(T^- \text{ if not diseased})}$$
$$= \frac{\text{Specificity}}{1 - \text{Sensitivity}}$$
$$= \frac{0.89}{0.72}$$
$$= 1.23$$

There is thus a fairly small chance that further testing will change the pre-test diagnosis. An FBC was requested (see below), with the object of looking at the MCV. This was 80 fl, which was really of no help. What was one now to do? According to the operating characteristics, it would be pointless to investigate further. However, the clinical side has hitherto been ignored. **CAN WE AFFORD TO IGNORE THIS HB OF 13.1? THE GREAT VALUE OF THE CLINICAL INPUT CAN NOW BE SEEN.**

TASK #4: HOW SIGNIFICANT IS THE RESULT FROM THE CLINICAL POINT OF VIEW?

The patient, a 40-year-old man, was booked for extensive periodontal surgery. He had told the anesthetist that he had been feeling off-color for a few months, with episodes of dull abdominal pain. The anesthesiologist felt it wise to request a Hb and total white cell count. The WCC was entirely normal, but the Hb was the source of the above uncertainty. While it is entirely possible that the mild anemia was due to low-grade chronic sepsis, it is not wise to assume so without further ado.

Accordingly and after consultation, an FBC was performed and evaluated. While the MCV was at the lower limit of normal, the MCH was slightly decreased, the RDW was somewhat increased, and the smear showed a population of mildly hypochromic cells. Once again there was the possibility that this was due to low-grade sepsis, particularly since iron studies suggested a malutilization pattern. But the (much-derided) clinical "feel" was that there was something else. An extensive clinical examination revealed only a vague fullness in the umbilical region; sonography revealed enlarged para-aortic lymph nodes, confirmed by CT (and which later turned out to be a lymphoma).

The critical point to be made in the above exercise is that clinical considerations can override any epidemiological or statistical considerations.

Summary

1. The application of standard clinical methodology to the diagnosis of blood disease has many unique features and offers many benefits so long as these unique aspects are understood and adapted to. The clinical approach has the greatest benefit in terms of the following:

    a. Identifying the features that make one suspect that a patient has a blood disease.
    b. The clinical history is often very convincing as to the nature of the process.
    c. The clinical examination sometimes reveals features pointing to the underlying disease.
    d. In the interpretation of the first-line tests, the clinical features are very often decisive.

2. The pathological diagnosis is made in three stages:

    a. The anatomical diagnosis, almost always made by reference to a first-line test, which is almost unique to hematology.
    b. The general pathology diagnosis. In principle this means identifying one of the classical general pathologies, such as vascular, infective, etc.; in blood diseases these categories are considerably modified to fit in with the dynamics of the hematological system. Clinical input is most important at this stage.
    c. The special pathology or specific diagnosis. In hematology this almost always is done by specific further laboratory tests. It is very important to realize that one should always try to work systematically through these stages, rather than reaching immediately for the final diagnosis.

3. In keeping with modern trends as well as because hematology is so dependent on laboratory results, statistical analysis and a clinical epidemiological approach are strongly encouraged so as to maximize the utility of the laboratory tests as well as of some clinical features.

4. The clinical history and examination in blood diseases are subsets of those in general medicine.

5. As experience grows, one learns to identify patterns of blood disease that may sensibly improve efficiency.

6. A practical example of using standard clinical epidemiological analysis applied to a simple FBC abnormality is shown.

A Final Word

"The technically trained physician, as distinguished from the educated physician, may try impulsively, by the unwise and neurotic multiplication of tests and superfluous instrumentations to achieve the illusion of certainty, and such behavior may only be a manifestation of another type of superstition, *blind faith in the laboratory report*. Such a physician, technically overloaded but inadequately educated in the humane sense, is often constrained to maintain a phony attitude of omniscience".[3] (My italics)

Exercise 5.1

A quick self-test (Answers below)

True	False	Questions
		1. Making the anatomical diagnosis is in most cases the most fundamental step in reaching a diagnosis
		2. Only the deductive form of logic is of relevance in the diagnosis of blood disease
		3. The anatomical diagnosis in blood diseases always refers to the bone marrow or spleen
		4. It is not important to make the first-stage diagnosis in bleeding disorders because they are all due to hereditary causes
		5. The physical examination typically contributes only 5% to the final diagnosis and is therefore not worth doing
		6. Amaurosis fugax is a transient disturbance of vision in one eye and is always followed by full recovery
		7. Pigment gallstones due to chronic hemolysis are unusual in that they may resolve spontaneously
		8. Depletion of iron stores due to blood donation only occurs after donation of more than 5 units per annum
		9. Tetracycline and antacids may cause malabsorption of iron
		10. Vitamin B_{12} deficiency may present with agitated dementia
		11. A common association of cachexia is achlorhydria and therefore of folate deficiency
		12. Pheochromocytoma is characterized by marked pallor due to bleeding from the tumor
		13. Statistical methods are a valuable aid in diagnosis
		14. A classical symptom of anemia is dyspnea relieved by sitting up
		15. 80% of iron deficiency cases are due to malabsorption
		16. Transient ischemic episodes are almost always diagnosed on the history
		17. Gold therapy is a well-known cause of neutropenia
		18. Vitiligo is a common accompaniment of pernicious anemia due to folate deficiency
		19. A common association of cachexia is achlorhydria, which may contribute to iron deficiency
		20. The suggested logical approach to diagnosis means that the history, physical examination, and special investigations be performed in strict sequence
		21. Vivax and ovale malaria typically follow a tertian fever pattern
		22. Dysphagia in the iron-deficient patient is most commonly due to bleeding from a carcinoma at the gastro-esophageal junction
		23. Differentiating between a very large spleen and a very large left kidney can reliably be made clinically

Exercise 5.2

Match the items in columns 1 and 2 (Answers below)

Column 1	Column 2
A. Making a clinical diagnosis	1. Recurring attacks are the same every time.
B. Nutritional deficiency	2. Is provided mainly by the history and physical examination, with reference to the prevalence of disease in the community.
C. The pre-test probability of a diagnosis	3. Commonly associated with malabsorption of iron and folate.
D. Subacute combined degeneration of the cord	4. An example of a general pathology diagnosis in hematology.
E. Transient ischemic attacks as a result of disease affecting the internal carotid distribution	5. Usually caused by filariasis or oncocerciasis.
F. Hematological causes of pruritus	6. A medical emergency
G. Dermatitis herpetiformis	7. Classically caused by vitamin B_{12} deficiency.
H. *Plasmodium vivax* malaria	8. Characteristically associated with iron deficiency
I. Traveler's eosinophilia	9. Is a stepwise process
J. Peutz–Jegher syndrome	10. Suggests hemochromatosis.
K. Falciparum malaria	11. Characteristically presents with persistent splenomegaly and anemia.
L. Arthritis of the first two MP joints	12. Hodgkin disease, polycythemia vera

Answers

Exercise 5.1

1T; 2F; 3F; 4F; 5F; 6T; 7F; 8F; 9T; 10T; 11F; 12F; 13T; 14F; 15F; 16T; 17T; 18F; 19T; 20F; 21T; 22F; 23T

Exercise 5.2

A9; B4; C2; D7; E1; F12; G3; H11; I5; J8; K6: L10

References

1. Pappworth MH (1984) A Primer of Medicine. 5th edn. Boston: Butterworths.

2. Cohen PR, Feigenbaum EA (eds) (1982). Handbook of Artificial Intelligence, Volume III. Pitman.
3. Whitehorn JC (1961). N. Engl. J. Med. 265: 301.

Further Reading

Andreoli TE, Bennett JC, Carpenter CCJ, Plum F (eds) (1994). Cecil Essentials of Medicine. 4th edn. Philadelphia: WB Saunders Company.

Duthie RB, Rizza CR, Giangrande PLF, Dodd CAF (eds) (1994). The Management of Musculoskeletal Problems in the Haemophilias. 2nd edn. Oxford University Press.

Epstein RJ (1996). Medicine for Examinations. 3rd edn. Churchill Livingstone.

Hoffbrand AV, Catovsky D, Tuddenham EGD (eds) (2005). Postgraduate Haematology. 5th edn. Oxford: Blackwell Publishing.

Pappworth MH (1984). A Primer of Medicine. 5th edn. Boston: Butterworths.

Rosenstock L, Cullen MR (eds) (1994). Textbook of Clinical Occupational and Environmental Medicine. Saunders.

A Practical Approach to the FBC and Hemostatic Screen

The Bone Marrow Report

Not learning but doing is the principal thing.
(Perkay Abat)

Preview *The groundwork has been laid in terms of both the diagnostic process and the significance of the first-line tests. In this chapter, we present a practical approach to these tests. Building on the diagnostic approach as outlined in Chapter 5, the first decision to make is "what is the 'anatomical' diagnosis?" How to arrive at this is explained. The approach to this anatomical diagnosis is then handled in the relevant chapter, but the principles are outlined here. Thereafter, the essentials of the bone marrow examination are presented, purely from the point of view of the clinician.*

In Chapter 5, we emphasized the important role clinical assessment plays in the interpretation of the blood tests. Reaching the first-line diagnosis however is most commonly via interpreting the first-line tests. Also, there are very many cases where the clinical features are of no help at all, or in fact the patient **PRESENTS** with an abnormal test. Therefore, knowledge of an interpretive assessment of these tests **ON THEIR OWN (I.E., PRESENTING WITHOUT CLINICAL INPUT)** is of great importance.

The primary goal is making the **"ANATOMICAL" DIAGNOSIS** (as defined previously). This diagnosis then will refer you to Chapters 8–18, the chapter headings of which are in fact either anatomical diagnoses per se, for example "Microcytosis: the Microcytic Anemias," or groups of anatomical diagnoses, such as "The Leukocytoses" which then will include in the discussion individual anatomical diagnoses, such as "Neutrophilia." In this chapter, we place the whole process in context, outlining it and its advantages, and illustrating the essentially **LOGICAL** nature of the process. We also discuss general causes of blood diseases as a whole.

2. On the basis of the anatomical diagnosis, consider the possible **GENERAL** causes, using the approach outlined in Chapter 5. State the possibilities.
3. Look for such other features that strengthen each possibility.
4. Look for such other features that are against each possibility.
5. Weigh up the different possibilities and list them in the order of likelihood.
6. Investigate further each one according to probabilities.
7. Do such clinical and laboratory investigations that will clinch, or point you to, your final pathological diagnosis – the **SPECIFIC** cause.

The complete diagnosis is more than just the special pathological diagnosis – questions of etiology, complications, prognosis, assessment of management options, etc. are required, but these are aspects of clinical hematology that are largely outside the scope of this book, since they are so dependent on the individual circumstances of each patient. They are discussed, however, in many of the teaching cases where tests aid in deciding them.

! The Full Blood Count: Summary of the Approach

1. Make the **"ANATOMICAL"** diagnosis – the main subject matter of this chapter.

A Critically Important Concept! It should clearly be understood that the FBC should properly be looked at as a whole. It consists of a battery of results, and any one of these by themselves **!**

frequently provides far less information than does looking at patterns of results. Unfortunately, most work on operating characteristics are to do with only one or perhaps two of these measurements, in the process not only losing a lot of information but instilling a very utilitarian, reductionist, and anti-intellectual view of medical diagnosis.

How to Make the Anatomical Diagnosis

EXAMINE ALL THREE CELL LINE COUNTS, with the proviso that with the red cell series, we look first at the Hct rather than the Hb or RCC because of the complication created by varying red cell sizes. Thus:

1. **WHAT IS THE HEMATOCRIT (HCT)?**
2. **WHAT IS THE WHITE CELL COUNT (WCC)?**
3. **WHAT IS THE PLATELET COUNT (PC)?**

With an increase in Hct, there are two possible first-stage diagnoses: "erythrocytosis" (where the other cell concentrations are normal) and "polycythemia" (all three cell lines are increased). "Raised Hct" as a first-stage diagnosis is to be discouraged.

IF ALL THE COUNTS ARE WITHIN THE NORMAL RANGE, YOU CANNOT STOP THERE, since certain abnormalities can be detected by reference to other features, or suspicions raised about possible abnormalities, despite normal counts. There are certain measurements in each cell line that need to be looked at, regardless of normal counts – the important ones are

1. **THE RDW.** A raised RDW in an otherwise normal count deserves attention, and morphological comment should be asked for.
2. **REVERSAL OF THE NEUTROPHIL:LYMPHOCYTE RATIO.** Even though the individual counts are in the reference range, this reversal has significant implications. It is discussed in Chapter 15, even though it is not strictly speaking a leukocytosis – or if you like, it can be considered a **RELATIVE LYMPHOCYTOSIS**.
3. **CERTAIN CLINICAL DISORDERS WHERE THE EXPECTED CHANGES ARE NOT IN EVIDENCE.** This could suggest a functional disorder of the marrow or spleen, and morphological features may support this – for example, infective/inflammatory disorders with a persistently normal WCC.
4. **PURPURIC BLEEDING WITH A NORMAL PLATELET COUNT** – the morphology of the platelets may suggest a functional disorder.

In these cases, however, the anatomical diagnosis now becomes a very problematic issue, and will need specialist opinion. These cases however will be in a distinct minority.

IF MORE THAN ONE OF THE COUNTS ARE ABNORMAL then look for a particular pattern. Recognizable patterns include pancytopenia, polycythemia, bicytopenia (specified). Within this pattern, you then characterize the changes in each of the cell lines separately as discussed below. With greater experience, you would end up with a more elaborate anatomical diagnosis, such as say a "pancytopenia with macrocytic red cells." For the time being, we will stick with the basic observation as your anatomical diagnosis.

> **A Word of Warning!** In the initial assessment of an abnormal FBC, there is a tendency for one's attention to be drawn to one abnormal feature and concentrate on that alone, without realizing that associated abnormalities are often very informative. Thus, one may, for example, notice a raised Hct and concentrate on that, and if the associated increase in WCC and PC were not seen, an unnecessary amount of investigation would be done, at least in the first instance.
>
> After all, in clinical work, the observation of say a very slow regular pulse could prompt extensive investigation. This could be considerably lessened if an obvious myxedematous facies were noticed. Why should the same mental processing not be as effective in assessing a FBC?

Once a pattern involving more than one cell line is defined, you then proceed to examining the specific type of change in each of the cell lines.

NEXT, EXAMINE EACH CELL LINE SEPARATELY – and this applies even if the counts as such are normal – for certain essential measurements. Each abnormality is characterized.

1. **IF IT IS AN ANEMIA**, is it **MICROCYTIC, MACROCYTIC,** or **NORMOCYTIC**?
2. In many cases, the **SEVERITY** has diagnostic importance, e.g., **SEVERE** eosinophilia has a different range of causes than a **MILD** case. In general, the severity of a laboratory result should bear some relationship to clinical severity and not merely be derived from the statistical spread of data. Many of these ranges are fairly arbitrary and approximate, such as for neutrophilia, and the different causes given are based on clinical experience; but others have been thoroughly

researched in terms of their clinical, etiological, and epidemiological implications, such as with eosinophilia. An additional problem arises with respect to anemia, since severity of anemia is a clinical definition. The severity of each type of change is indicated in the specific chapter dealing with that change.

THE ANATOMICAL DIAGNOSIS SHOULD THEN, IF POSSIBLE, BE CLEARLY STATED, IN FORMAL TERMS. Anatomical diagnoses can be classified into three groups:

1. **STRAIGHTFORWARD, SINGLE ABNORMALITIES**:

   a. **ERYTHROCYTOSIS**
   b. Any one of **NEUTROPHILIA, MONOCYTOSIS, EOSINOPHILIA, LYMPHOCYTOSIS**, and whether it is **MARKED, MODERATE, OR MILD**
   c. **THROMBOCYTOSIS, MARKED, MODERATE, OR MILD**
   d. Any one of **NEUTROPENIA, LYMPHOPENIA**, and whether it is **MARKED, MODERATE, OR MILD**
   e. **THROMBOCYTOPENIA, MARKED, MODERATE OR MILD**
   f. **MICROCYTIC, MACROCYTIC**, or **NORMOCYTIC ANEMIA**
   g. **MICROCYTIC** or **MACROCYTIC RED CELL PICTURES** (i.e., no obvious anemia)

2. **STRAIGHTFORWARD, MULTIPLE ABNORMALITIES**:

   a. **POLYCYTHEMIA**
   b. A **LEUKOCYTOSIS** (i.e., increase in many or all of the different white cell series, or their precursors)
   c. A **LEUKOPENIA** (i.e., decrease in many or all white cells)
   d. **PANCYTOPENIA** or **BICYTOPENIA.**

3. **COMPLEX AND MIXED PICTURES**. There are many possibilities. The anatomical diagnosis here is frequently a succinct description. Only the commoner ones will be mentioned here. Very confusing patterns should be referred, either to a clinical specialist or for consultation with your laboratory.

   a. **MICROCYTHEMIA**: this means an increase in the red cell count but the red cells are microcytic. This is an important diagnosis, and is discussed under Microcytosis: the Microcytic Anemias (Chapter 8).
   b. **LEUKEMOID REACTION**: this means a markedly raised neutrophil count with a marked left shift.
   c. **LEUKO-ERYTHROBLASTIC BLOOD PICTURE**: this means both a marked left shift in the neutrophils and the presence of normoblasts (red cell precursors).

THE TERMS LEFT AND RIGHT SHIFT *Left Shift* broadly means the appearance of leukocytic precursors in the blood. However the term is not used for acute leukemia; while it is true that blasts as so on are precursors, the clinical emphasis is very different.

In all other cases, the presence of any precursors is regarded as a left shift. Most commonly it takes the form of band cells. If the left shift consists only of band cells, then the criteria are the following: 5% of the neutrophils show 2 lobes or fewer; the more there are of these, the more marked the left shift would be. However, sometimes few band cells are present, but there are metamyelocytes, myelocytes or even promyelocytes: this is regarded as a very marked left shift.

Right shift means that the neutrophils (and this can also be applied to eosinophils) show more lobes than normal. The criteria are 5% of neutrophils show five or more lobes.

While a left shift almost always implies younger than normal neutrophils, a right shift does *not* imply older cells.

Making the General Pathology Diagnosis

With the anatomical diagnosis in hand, the next step will be the general pathology diagnosis – i.e., the possible causes of the change observed in terms of **GENERAL PROCESSES, AND INFORMED BY CLINICAL FINDINGS**. Each anatomical diagnosis will have a set of possible general causes (which are summarized a little later, and more fully discussed in the relevant chapters. And in the relevant chapter, further investigation is suggested as to how to most effectively reach the **SPECIAL PATHOLOGY DIAGNOSIS** – i.e., the specific, proximate cause of the original presentation).

Thus the anatomical diagnosis provides a clear direction in which to think and to discover how to proceed further: for example, an anatomical diagnosis of a microcytic anemia would not in the first instance suggest that you should start looking for bone marrow infiltration. If, after going down the diagnostic path for a microcytic anemia (as will be described), you find inherent contradictions, you can then retrace your steps to that previous step where you

WERE certain and look for a new path. But all this is basic clinical thinking, and need not be expanded upon, except to stress that the process should be logical and systematic.

The set of possible causes is specific for each anatomical diagnosis. These causes are subsets derived from a master list, which follows.

The Master-set of General Pathology Causes of Anatomical Diagnoses Made from the FBC Findings

1. Acute myeloproliferative disease
2. Chronic myeloproliferative disease
3. Acute lympho-plasma-immuno-proliferative disease
4. Chronic lympho-plasma-immuno-proliferative disease
5. Defective production of cells
6. Abnormal production and/or development of cells
7. Defective physiological stimulus of cell numbers or function
8. Nutritional deficiency
9. Functional disorders of cells
10. Intravascular destruction of cells
11. Intravascular sequestration of cells
12. Abnormal extravascular destruction of cells
13. Technical aberrations (NOT a pathology, but since hematology is so dependent on laboratory testing, this has to be included).

As mentioned before, the presenting picture can be very complex, involving changes in more than one cell line, with no particular pattern. The anatomical diagnosis for this type of problem would frequently be descriptive, such as "A leukoerythroblastic pattern with tear-drop poikilocytes and fragmentation." The unraveling of the general diagnosis then becomes a systematic following through of the different findings to enable, if possible, a coherent and integrated view. Of course, as in all complex clinical problems, this is sometimes not possible, and the disease picture will have to be handled piece-meal. We have attempted to deal with some of these in Chapter 23, which deals with complex cases.

Making the General Pathology Diagnosis: an Example

To exemplify the process, we use an easy example: THROMBOCYTOPENIA. The patient (a young male student) is completely asymptomatic (an entry condition). The blood was drawn as part of a project studying oxygen utilization in pre-examination stress. See Table 6.1

Table 6.1

Case #4			Reference range	
	Value	Units	Low	High
Red cell count	5.1	$\times 10^{12}/l$	4.5	5.5
Hemoglobin (Hb)	15.3	g/dl	13	17
Hematocrit (Hct)	0.45	l/l	0.4	0.5
Mean cell volume	88	fl	80	99
Mean cell Hb	30.0	pg	27	31.5
Mean cell Hb conc.	34.1	g/dl	31.5	34.5
Red cell dist. width	12.1	%	11.6	14
White cell count	7.3	$\times 10^9/l$	4	10
Neutrophils abs.	4.23	$\times 10^9/l$	2	7
Lymphocytes abs.	2.18	$\times 10^9/l$	1	3
Monocytes abs.	0.45	$\times 10^9/l$	0.2	1
Eosinophils abs.	0.38	$\times 10^9/l$	0.02	0.5
Basophils abs.	0.06	$\times 10^9/l$	0.02	0.1
Platelet count	**4.2**	$\times 10^9/l$	150	400

Discussion

1. We look at all three cell lines: only the platelets are abnormal – i.e., this case is of an ISOLATED THROMBOCYTOPENIA, and therefore most likely not part of a complex problem.
2. We turn to Chapter 11 and see firstly that this represents a SEVERE THROMBOCYTOPENIA. This then is the ANATOMICAL DIAGNOSIS.
3. We now consider the possible GENERAL causes of a severe isolated thrombocytopenia, as per our list above

   a. Acute myeloproliferative disease
   b. Chronic myeloproliferative disease
   c. Acute lympho-plasma-immuno-proliferative disease
   d. Chronic lympho-plasma-immuno-proliferative disease
   e. Defective production of platelets
   f. Abnormal production and development of platelets
   g. Defective physiological stimulus of platelet numbers or function
   h. Nutritional deficiency
   i. Functional disorders of platelets
   j. Intravascular destruction of platelets
   k. Intravascular sequestration of platelets
   l. Abnormal extravascular destruction of platelets
   m. Technical causes of APPARENTLY decreased platelets.

Discussing Briefly Each Possibility:

It is important to estimate the likelihood of each general cause as being responsible; therefore features for and against the cause are weighed up. Thus, we look for supporting or detracting evidence in:

1. **THE REST OF THE FBC** including the morphology IF this is supplied (if not and morphology is adjudged important, you either demand one or try to make do with whatever flags are reported).
2. **OTHER (NON-HEMATOLOGICAL) TESTS.** Some tests in particular can be of great assistance, e.g., liver functions, thyroid functions, autoimmune profile, etc.
3. **THE CLINICAL FEATURES.** Apart from the clinical features per se, facts such as age, race, sex, family history (particularly patterns of inheritance), recent transfusion, place of domicile, regions recently visited, can be enormously helpful.

Acute Myeloproliferative Disease, Such as an Acute Leukemia.

FEATURES IN FAVOR: this is a well-known albeit uncommon cause of thrombocytopenia, otherwise none.

FEATURES AGAINST: the rest of the FBC is completely normal. Nevertheless, in the absence of a morphological comment and a clinical examination, the **OUTSIDE** possibility must be retained.

Chronic Myeloproliferative Disease.

FEATURES IN FAVOR: this can cause thrombocytopenia, otherwise none.

FEATURES AGAINST: these diseases can cause thrombocytopenia but only **LATE** in the disease. Here, the rest of the FBC is completely normal.

The above remarks apply also to:

Acute Lympho-Plasma-Immuno-Proliferative Disease and Chronic Lympho-Plasma-Immuno-Proliferative Disease.

These are all extremely unlikely.

Defective Production of Platelets.

(e.g., aplastic anemia, megakaryocytic hypoplasia, myelodysplasia).

FEATURES IN FAVOR: none. But a fairly common cause is direct damage to megakaryocytes (and/or platelets) by drugs, chemicals, or radiation. This is unlikely in this patient, but it cannot be excluded. Therefore **LOW** on the list.

FEATURES AGAINST: it is unusual in the extreme for marrow failure (drugs and toxins excluded) to present with such a FBC, especially with such a very low platelet count and completely normal other indices.

Abnormal Production and Development of Platelets.

(e.g., myelodysplasia).

FEATURES IN FAVOR: none.

FEATURES AGAINST: it is unusual for say myelodysplasia to present with such a FBC. Thus it is very unlikely, but it cannot be excluded. Therefore **LOW** on the list.

Defective Physiological Stimulus of Platelet Numbers or Function.

Not much is known about the role of physiological stimulus of platelet production. The role of thrombopoietin in platelet production is far more complex than that of EPO in red cell production. Thus we must keep this cause in (very much at the back of) one's mind.

Nutritional deficiency.

FEATURES IN FAVOR: none.

FEATURES AGAINST: it would be very unusual indeed for nutritional deficiencies (such as vitamin B_{12} or folate) to present only with thrombocytopenia and no positive clinical features. Film morphology would be extremely helpful.

Functional Disorders

These very seldom present with thrombocytopenia. Morphology would be very helpful in identifying macrothrombocytopenia (a feature of group of rare diseases).

Intravascular Destruction of Platelets

(such as DIC, some antibodies).

FEATURES IN FAVOR: none. Without a detailed history, however, one cannot be sure. Important here would be a history of recent transfusion or drug therapy.

FEATURES AGAINST: DIC is generally a severe disease. Occasionally it may occur in a more-or-less sub-clinical fashion, as with certain viral infections (especially arboviruses), but usually one would expect anemia as well as morphological evidence of fragmentation and spherocytes – however, no morphology was supplied. Patients **MAY** be asymptomatic with cirrhosis, but one would expect a round macrocytosis in the blood, perhaps with target cell formation – again, without morphology we are handicapped. These are thus fairly **LOW** on the list (mainly because of the lack of morphological comment).

Intravascular Sequestration of Platelets

(such as giant hematomata (Kasabach–Merritt syndrome – generally found in small children)).
FEATURES IN FAVOR: None.
FEATURES AGAINST: Giant hematomata are almost always visible on the surface. Sequestration may also occur in some malignant circulations. Thus this cause would be **LOW** on the list.

Abnormal Extravascular Destruction or Sequestration of Platelets

Platelets may be attacked by antibodies (as in ITP), and the complexes then removed by the spleen, etc. Certain drugs may aggravate this process, usually acting as haptens. Finally, an enlarged spleen may destroy or sequester platelets (hypersplenism). Thus:

1. **DESTRUCTION OF PLATELETS BY ANTIBODIES** – ITP.
   EVIDENCE IN FAVOR: none, but then there frequently is not.
   EVIDENCE AGAINST: none.
   HIGH on the list (because it is a common cause – that is to say, a high pre-test probability).
2. **DRUG REACTION**
   EVIDENCE SUPPORTING: none.
   EVIDENCE AGAINST: no history of drug ingestion (entry condition).
   LOW on the list.
3. **HYPERSPLENISM.** The sine qua non of this condition is an enlarged spleen, but we are not given any details. Usually the causes of an enlarged spleen are clinically significant, so in this patient it is unlikely.

Technical Causes of APPARENTLY Decreased Platelets

   FEATURES IN FAVOR: none really, except that there is no suggestion whatsoever of any disease. Because of the frequency of this problem, it is **HIGH** on the list.
   FEATURES AGAINST: NONE.

The next task was to collect further relevant information as to the probable causes in terms of likelihood. As soon as the FBC was seen, the patient was examined. Important points in the history were

1. The patient felt in excellent health. There was no story of a recent viral infection. A positive history of a viral infection would add somewhat to the possibility of an ITP.
2. The diet was very good, and he used minimal alcohol. There was no pica, sore tongue, or dysphagia. These would be somewhat against nutritional deficiency or liver disease.
3. There had been no exposure to drugs, chemicals, or radiation, and he had never been transfused. These would be against marrow failure and transfusion-related thrombocytopenia.

On examination:

1. He appeared in excellent health, with excellent physical reserves. There was no evidence of infection. The skin was normal.
2. There was no lymphadenopathy or hepatosplenomegaly, and no bony tenderness.
3. There was no glossitis or koilonychia.

All these features were strongly against most of the possibilities. The order of likelihood therefore, **IN THE ABSENCE OF MORPHOLOGY**, was something of the order of: ITP > Spurious > Drug reaction > Cirrhosis > Atypical DIC > Bone Marrow disease.

The patient was referred back to the lab for a platelet count to be done from a citrate tube (the tube normally used for coagulation studies), and a morphological assessment of the smear. The repeat platelet count was 198×10^9/l and the morphological comment was "The red cells are normochromic and normocytic, without abnormal forms. The white cells were normal in number and distribution. There was marked platelet satellitism". Thus **THE GENERAL DIAGNOSIS** was "Technical: spurious thrombocytopenia", and the **"SPECIFIC"** cause, if one can use the term here, was **PLATELET SATELLITISM** (a benign film manifestation of technical origin).

The value of morphology is again demonstrated. If examination of the smear had not revealed spurious thrombocytopenia, it would still have been of enormous help in the assessment of DIC, cirrhosis, Kasabach–Merritt syndrome, and bone marrow disease.

OBSERVE THE VALUE OF THIS METHODICAL AND LOGICAL PROGRESSION FROM ANATOMICAL TO FINAL DIAGNOSIS:

1. The clinical search space steadily narrows. The process directs one's attention along specific pathways without much danger of taking a wrong route – and, should it become clear that the route **IS** wrong, it is easy to **BACKTRACK TO A POSITION OF CERTAINTY**, and progress again from there. **THERE IS A GREAT**

TEMPTATION TO PROCEED DIRECTLY FROM THE "ANATOMICAL" DIAGNOSIS TO THE SPECIFIC CAUSE, AND THE DANGERS INHERENT IN THIS CANNOT BE OVERSTRESSED: usually there is more than one cause of an "anatomical" change. These are often not all remembered, and in practice it means that only the causes most readily to hand will be considered. These may be at hand not because they are necessarily the most likely, but are the ones most recently seen or read about, or are a hobby-horse of the practitioner. An important less common cause may then be overlooked, and only returned to after extensive (and perhaps painful) investigations have failed to confirm the original cause. In the process, time and money have been wasted.

2. It may save the patient from unnecessary and sometimes painful investigations, since the temptation to leap at the most easily remembered cause is reduced; for example, in the above case, the systematic procedure obviated someone jumping to the conclusion that the diagnosis is most likely ITP, and therefore subjecting the patient to an unnecessary bone marrow aspiration.

3. It may save the patient from unnecessary therapy – the probabilistic approach as discussed in case #3 in Chapter 3 may well have led to the patient being put on steroids for 6 months, with all the complications possible.

The above example demonstrates the value of the clinical assessment in the evaluation of an FBC.

> **!** Any patient presenting with a low platelet count and is otherwise healthy with a normal FBC, or has a condition wherein thrombocytopenia is unexpected, should, in the first instance be referred back to the lab for a citrate tube-based platelet count and morphological assessment.

Clinical Input in Diagnosis (of the FBC) Summarized

There is a set of clinical features that are of particular value in the interpretation of the FBC: they point one in certain directions, and can often short circuit the process, at least provisionally. Table 6.2 shows a number of the commoner clinical features that, if present, will aid greatly in differentiating various FBC appearances (they are somewhat over-simplified, and exceptions exist in all cases). It is assumed that no other cause of the clinical feature exists.

Table 6.2 Helpful Clinical Features in the Interpretation of the FBC

FBC feature	Clinically	These favor	As opposed to
Microcytosis	Pica, bleeding, dysphagia, koilonychia.	Iron deficiency	Anemia of Chronic Disorders, Thalassemias.
Microcytosis	Chronic inflammatory/infiltrative disease	Anemia of chronic disorders	Iron deficiency, thalassemias.
Microcytosis	Malar prominence, poor growth, "hair-on-end" appearance on X-ray	Thalassemia major	Iron deficiency, anemia of chronic disorders.
Macrocytosis	Liver or thyroid disease	Liver or thyroid causes	Megaloblastic anemia.
Macrocytosis	Premature greying, diarrhea, jaundice without splenomegaly, other autoimmune (vitiligo)	Pernicious anemia	Folate deficiency, extravascular hemolysis, liver disease.
Macrocytosis	Delirium, transverse myelitis, neuropathy, subacute combined degeneration	Vitamin B_{12} deficiency	Folate deficiency
Macrocytosis	Pregnancy, alcoholism, poor diet (various)	Folate deficiency or liver disease (or both).	Vitamin B_{12} deficiency
Normocytic anemia, other cytopenias	Large spleen, ± evidence of portal hypertension	Hypersplenism	Hemolysis, renal failure, nutritional anemias, some endocrine.
Normocytic anemia	Renal failure	Renal anemia	As above or hypersplenism.
Normocytic + microcytes and macrocytes	Combined deficiency of iron and folate/B_{12}	Nutritional disorder	As above.
Erythrocytosis	Chronic chest disease	Chronic hypoxia	Inappropriate EPO, myeloproliferative
Erythrocytosis	Renal mass or obstructive uropathy	EPO-producing tumor/lesion	Chronic chest disease
Erythrocytosis	Clinical dehydration	Apparent erythrocytosis	True erythrocytosis
Erythrocytosis	Cerebellar signs	Inappropriate EPO hemangioblastom	Reactive or stress
Granulocytosis ± increased platelets	Very large spleen plus many failed marrow punctures	Myelofibrosis	Chronic myelocytic leukemia
Leuko-erythroblastic reaction	Large spleen	Myelofibrosis	Acute marrow stress
Lymphocytosis with atypical lymphocytes	Recent viral infection (e.g., infectious mono nucleosis)	Benign lymphocytosis	Lymphoma or chronic lymphocytic leukemia
Eosinophilia	Features of iron deficiency	Hookworm infestation	Hypereosinophilic syndrome, allergy
Eosinophilia	Endocardial fibrosis, CCF	Hypereosinophilic syndrome	Reactive eosinophilia
Eosinophilia	Multiple neurological lesions	Hypereosinophilic syndrome	Reactive eosinophilia
Neutropenia	Associated autoimmune disease	Autoimmune neutropenia	Marrow disease
Neutropenia	Rheumatoid disease	Drug exposure or Felty syndrome	Marrow disease
Thrombocytosis	Petit mal attacks, amaurosis, migraine, etc	Thrombocythemia	Reactive thrombocytosis
Thrombocytopenia	Prosthetic valve	Mechanical destruction	ITP, etc
Thrombocytopenia	Renal failure, neuro signs	TTP or HUS	ITP, etc.
Pancytopenia	Large spleen	Hypersplenism, BM infiltration.	Aplasia
Polycythemia	Pruritus, large spleen	Polycythemia vera	Dehydration, Cushing's
Polycythemia	Cushingoid features	Hypercortisolism	Polycythemia vera, dehydration
Acute leukemia	Meningism	ALL	AML
Acute leukemia	Gum and tissue infiltration	Acute monoblastic or myelomonocytic Leukemia	Other types of non-lymphoblastic leukemia

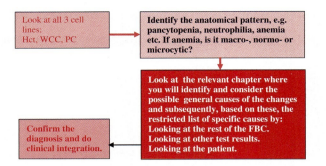

Fig. 6.1. Flowchart Summary of the approach as discussed.

Making the Specific Diagnosis

The identification of the specific nature of the general causes is usually very much a laboratory affair. It is very occasionally possible, with experience, to reach a final diagnosis in blood diseases entirely clinically.

The Final Diagnosis

THE COMPLETE DIAGNOSIS IS ESSENTIALLY A CLINICAL AFFAIR – IT CANNOT BE LEFT TO THE LABORATORY. If not already available from the investigations already considered, it is often necessary to do further tests to confirm etiology, complications, and issues relevant to management and prognosis. These will also be handled in the relevant chapters, where appropriate (Fig. 6.1).

The Integrated Assessment

Hematological diagnosis has two connotations, one clinical, the other in the tests. Two examples will be used to illustrate these, and the critical importance of using **BOTH** modalities. The first example is a single patient with separate approaches from the clinical, the FBC, and the integrated point of view. The second consists of two different patients presenting almost identically but with very different pathologies.

   EXAMPLE #1 (CASE #5). The patient is a pale 25 weeks pregnant woman (P5G6). It is decided that she is anemic. What is the cause? The approach to the diagnosis could be

1. **VIA CLINICAL ASSESSMENT ONLY** i.e., derived from the signs and symptoms of the patient, which often enables at least a provisional anatomical diagnosis independent of the tests, and from which a consideration of possibilities and further evaluation of possible general pathology causes, and thence to special pathology causes, can be made. Our patient is found to have had

her five children in the space of 4½ years and is from a poor socio-economic and psychological background; in addition, she has a poor dietary history. She presents with severe pallor and exhaustion. The first impression is that of **ANEMIA.** Further investigation reveals koilonychia and severe glossitis and diarrhea. A provisional **GENERAL DIAGNOSIS OF FOLATE DEFICIENCY COMBINED WITH IRON DEFICIENCY** is entertained (since this is a typical presentation in pregnancy, i.e., the pre-test probability is high). This is then confirmed by folate and iron studies in the blood. It is also **CONFIRMED** by an FBC – i.e., the diagnosis is not **MADE** by the FBC.

2. **ON THE BASIS OF AN FBC ALONE.** The considerations of general and specific pathologies are often different from those in the purely clinical approach, which can lead to confusion. The FBC in the above patient is unlikely to be straightforward; the anatomical diagnosis could vary considerably. But to use a typical single FBC appearance as an example, let us say that the picture is that of a pancytopenia with a very wide RDW, large and small ovalocytes, and a prominent right shift of the neutrophils. This picture is complex, and while a **GENERAL DIAGNOSIS OF MEGALOBLASTOSIS PLUS IRON DEFICIENCY IS POSSIBLE**, there are other more ominous possibilities such as myelodysplasia. Proceeding toward the special diagnosis is now more complex, possibly requiring bone marrow aspiration and biopsy, blood folate and vitamin B_{12} levels and iron studies, before certainty is reached.

3. **THE INTEGRATED APPROACH** would be to take into account the pre-test probability on the basis of the clinical features (i.e., of a combined deficiency), note that the FBC features are markedly compatible, and then, depending on resources, either confirm the deficiencies or institute therapy and follow-up. **IT CAN BE SEEN THAT THE COMBINED APPROACH AS AN INTEGRATED PROCESS WILL SAVE A LOT OF TIME AND A LOT OF MONEY.**

> **Assessment of Example #1** In this case, the value of the FBC is less than that of the clinical approach and far less than the combined approach. To emphasize: *the role and value of the FBC varies a lot in different circumstances.* This applies particularly in cases that present very similarly clinically and where the anatomical diagnoses appear to be very similar but have fundamentally different pathologies. The mutual interdependence of the clinical and laboratory is stressed, and in examples #2 and #3, the two approaches exemplify this.

EXAMPLES #2 AND 3. The patients (A and B) are men of 50 who are brought to you with a story of having suddenly passed a great deal of blood per rectum. In each of the two approaches, there is **A DIFFERENT PATHOLOGY**; they present similarly, but the FBC findings are very different and indeed the value of the FBC is very different. Each is presented first from the clinical point of view, and then from the FBC point of view. Note the interdependence and varying value of the two approaches in the two presentations.

EXAMPLE #2 (CASE #6) (PATIENT A).

1. **CLINICAL ASSESSMENT ONLY**. Without further information, all one can say is there is a lesion or process in the gastro-intestinal tract (GIT), most likely the lower GIT. This then is the **ANATOMICAL DIAGNOSIS** from the clinical point of view, and, with the data given, this is ALL one can say. The possibilities (general pathology) are many: traumatic, inflammatory, vascular, malignant, bleeding tendency, and so on. These serve to focus the mind in a certain direction – there would for example be hardly any point in now turning one's attention to the central nervous or cardiovascular systems in an attempt to identify the pathology. The patient is somewhat hypotensive with a thready pulse and is sweating.

   Further questioning reveals that he has had alternating constipation and diarrhea for over a year that has been getting worse, as well as a fair amount of weight loss. Examination reveals an enlarged nodular liver, with some of the nodules being possibly umbilicated. These findings would make one think very strongly of a carcinoma of the descending or transverse colon, but other possibilities also exist, such as double pathologies (of the liver and gut, for example), or cirrhosis with portal hypertension and secondary varices. These various possibilities are weighed up, for and against, with further clinical data being sought.

   Colonoscopy reveals a large fungating, ulcerated, bleeding mass in the descending colon, close to the splenic flexure. Biopsy confirms a carcinoma. Laparoscopy and biopsy confirm the metastatic nature of the hepatic nodules.

2. **THE FBC ONLY** is looked at, without reference to the patient – assume you know nothing about the patient except his age and sex and that he presents with rectal bleeding (note that this is the situation that the laboratory hematologist is usually faced with, and this example will illustrate why it is often so difficult, if not impossible, for the laboratory hematologist to give you the final diagnosis. The fault here lies **NOT** with him, but with the clinician for providing him with insufficient information. But even with sufficient information, the unique circumstances of the patient would require his comments to be re-evaluated).

The initial FBC is taken 30 min after admission of the above patient (about 2 h after the bleeding appears to have started), and reveals the following (Examine Table 6.3):

NOTES ON Table 6.3

a. The anemia is normocytic. There are a large number of possible causes (see Chapter 10), but there is very little in the FBC to indicate which one it is.

b. The thrombocytosis could be compatible with the recent bleed, but could also be a non-specific reaction (or both).

c. The FBC is really only of assistance in the diagnosis of this case in a negative sense – i.e., there is no evidence of a primary blood disease being the cause of the bleeding – specifically, it is not due to thrombocytopenia. The absence of dysplastic changes is against this being a myelodysplasia, which can produce very dysfunctional platelets without any morphological alteration in the platelets.

Table 6.3

Case #6			Reference range		Permitted range	
	Value	Units	Low	High	Low	High
Red cell count	**4.11**	× 10¹²/l	4.64	5.67	3.99	4.23
Hemoglobin (Hb)	**11.3**	g/dl	13.4	17.5	10.9	11.7
Hematocrit (Hct)	**0.33**	l/l	0.41	0.52	0.32	0.34
Mean cell volume	80	fl	80	99	78.4	81.6
Mean cell Hb	27.5	pg	27	31.5	26.9	28.0
Mean cell Hb conc.	34.4	g/dl	31.5	34.5	33.7	35.1
Red cell dist. width	**16.3**	%	11.6	14	15.8	16.8
Retic. count	0.61	%	0.26	0.77	0.6	0.6
Retic. absolute	25.1	× 10⁹/l	26	100	23.2	27.0
White cell count	12.1	× 10⁹/l	4	10	11.19	13.01
Neutrophils %	81.3	%				
Band cells %.	0	%				
Lymphocytes %	9.6	%				
Monocytes %	4.2	%				
Eosinophils %	3.8	%				
Basophils %	1.1	%				
Neutrophils abs.	**9.84**	× 10⁹/l	2	7	9.10	10.58
Lymphocytes abs.	1.16	× 10⁹/l	1	3	1.07	1.25
Monocytes abs.	0.51	× 10⁹/l	0.2	1	0.47	0.55
Eosinophils abs.	0.46	× 10⁹/l	0.02	0.5	0.43	0.49
Basophils abs.	0.13	× 10⁹/l	0.02	0.1	0.12	0.14
Normoblasts	0	/100 Wbc	0	0		
Platelet count	**671.0**	× 10⁹/l	150	400	435.7	506.3
Sedimentation	**37**	mm/hr	0	10	29	33
Morphology:	There is a mild anemia. The red cells show anisocytosis and anisochromia with numerous irregular and crenated cells. The granulocytes appear normal. Several giant platelets are seen.					

d. The morphological comment is actually confusing – until one knows the clinical background; in which case, the thrombocytosis and neutrophilia are compatible with a very recent bleed. The anemia however, is not, unless there was a previous sub-clinical bleed; an underlying chronic condition could be responsible.

Thus **THE ANATOMICAL DIAGNOSIS VIA THE FBC** would be

a. Mild normocytic anemia with anisochromia
b. Mild neutrophilia and thrombocytosis.

The **GENERAL PATHOLOGY DIAGNOSIS** would consist of a few possibilities:

a. Iron deficiency, anemia of chronic disorders, or both
b. Sideroblastic anemia as an outside possibility
c. Superimposed acute hemorrhage.

The **SPECIAL PATHOLOGY DIAGNOSIS** would require a fairly large number of investigations to clinch the diagnosis.

The FBC report is in fact a complex picture, when seen in isolation, no matter how good the morphological comment is.

3. We now examine the **COMBINED CLINICAL AND LABORATORY APPROACH**.

   a. The **ANATOMICAL DIAGNOSIS** of **THE COMBINED APPROACH** would remain a lesion or process in the gastro-intestinal tract (GIT), most likely the lower GIT.
   b. The **GENERAL PATHOLOGY DIAGNOSIS, BY REFERRING TO BOTH THE CLINICAL AND FBC DATA,** could quite reasonably be narrowed down to:

       i. Malignant disease of the colon with acute on chronic hemorrhage.
       ii. Chronic liver disease with portal hypertension and acute on chronic bleeding.
       iii. Other possibilities such as inflammatory bowel disease and angiodysplasia would be kept in the back of one's mind.

   c. The **SPECIAL PATHOLOGY**, to identify the specific pathology, now requires only a few highly selected investigations.

Example #3 (Case #7) (Patient B)

Another man of the same age presents with a history of having suddenly passed a lot of fresh blood per rectum,

and once again the anatomical diagnosis is that there is a lesion or process in the gastro-intestinal tract (GIT), most likely the lower GIT.

1. **CLINICAL ASSESSMENT ONLY.** As before, the general pathology possibilities are traumatic, inflammatory, malignant, vascular, bleeding tendency, and so on. The patient is similarly somewhat shocked. However, the subsequent investigation takes a very different direction. Further questioning reveals that he has been growing steadily weaker over the last few months, with severe lassitude and effort intolerance. This he has ascribed to the effects of chronic chest disease, and which has apparently been responding poorly to home treatment. Also, he has been troubled by numerous episodes of epistaxis and bleeding gums. He stops bleeding normally after a cut.

Table 6.4

Case #7	Value	Units	Reference Range Low	Reference Range High	Permitted Range Low	Permitted Range High
Red cell count	3.01	× 10¹²/l	4.64	5.67	2.92	3.10
Hemoglobin (Hb)	8.1	g/dl	13.4	17.5	7.8	8.4
Hematocrit (Hct)	0.25	l/l	0.41	0.52	0.24	0.26
Mean cell volume	83	Fl	80	99	81.3	84.7
Mean cell Hb	26.9	Pg	27	31.5	26.4	27.4
Mean cell Hb conc.	32.4	g/dl	31.5	34.5	31.8	33.1
Red cell dist. width	15.7	%	11.6	14	15.1	16.2
Retic. count	1.71	%	0.26	0.77	1.7	1.8
Retic. absolute	51.5	× 10⁹/l	30	100	47.6	55.3
White cell count	3.11	× 10⁹/l	4	10	2.88	3.34
Neutrophils %	33.0	%				
Band cells %.		%				
Lymphocytes %	57.5	%				
Monocytes %	6.1	%				
Eosinophils %	1.2	%				
Basophils %	2.2	%				
Neutrophils abs.	1.03	× 10⁹/l	2	7	0.95	1.10
Lymphocytes abs.	1.79	× 10⁹/l	1	3	1.65	1.92
Monocytes abs.	0.19	× 10⁹/l	0.2	1	0.18	0.20
Eosinophils abs.	0.04	× 10⁹/l	0.02	0.5	0.03	0.04
Basophils abs.	0.07	× 10⁹/l	0.02	0.1	0.06	0.07
Blasts %		%	0	0		
Promyelocytes %		%	0	0		
Myelocytes %		%	0	0		
Metamyelocytes %		%	0	0		
Normoblasts	2	/100 Wbc	0	0		
Platelet count	53.3	× 10⁹/l	150	400	78.1	88.3
Sedimentation	41	mm/hr	0	10	39	43
Morphology	There is a pancytopenia with normocytic red cells. The red cells are normochromic and show mild anisocytosis. The neutrophils show prominent dysplastic changes.					

Examination shows considerable pallor and scattered petechiae over the chest and thighs. There is no organomegaly. The general pathology possibilities now change, but the picture is vague. The available evidence is somewhat suggestive of a bleeding disorder but this must remain very tentative. **MUCH GREATER RELIANCE IS PLACED ON THE FIRST-LINE TESTS IN THIS PARTICULAR CASE.**

2. **THE FBC ONLY**. The FBC taken 30 minutes after admission and about 2 h after the bleeding appeared to have started is shown (Examine Table 6.4).

   NOTES ON TABLE 6.4

   a. **THERE IS A PANCYTOPENIA**. The further approach to a pancytopenia is discussed in Chapter 13; very briefly, however, the general causes are

   i. Bone marrow failure or replacement
   ii. Peripheral destruction, e.g., hypersplenism
   iii. Intramedullary destruction, e.g., megaloblastosis or myelodysplasia.

   However, a platelet count of 53 is typically most unlikely to lead to gastro-intestinal bleeding, unless in addition they are functionally abnormal. The morphological comment about the dysplastic white cells is thus very significant. A bone marrow examination revealed a myelodysplastic picture; it is known that platelets can be markedly dysfunctional. It also explains the pancytopenia – it is due to intramedullary hemolysis. Normal platelet morphology is the usual finding.

   b. The FBC is rather complex:

   i. Because the underlying disease is complex.
   ii. Because the picture has been complicated by the reaction to the bleeding.
   iii. The chronic chest disease itself can confuse the FBC picture.

   WITHOUT MORPHOLOGICAL COMMENT, YOU WOULD HAVE BEEN SEVERELY AT A LOSS.

   Assessment of Examples #2 and 3. It is clear that the relative value of the FBC is very different in the two cases. In example #2, there is no way by which the final diagnosis could be reached by means of the FBC – indeed, it had not even a confirmatory role – it merely indicated that "there was something going on." In example #3, however, the diagnosis could not have been reached *at all* without the FBC (etc). As with all the cases presented in this book, try to see the relevance of the clinical features in arriving at the final diagnosis.

   The above cases have adequately illustrated a very important point with respect to the FBC – its clinical utility in the diagnosis of hematological problems varies considerably from case to case. This could perhaps be demonstrated as a spectrum of utility. At the one end, the FBC gives the total answer (an unusual occurrence); at the other end, the clinical assessment gives the full answer, also very unusual. Most cases require an admixture of both approaches. To illustrate, see Fig. 6.2.

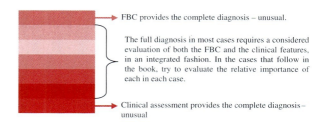

FBC provides the complete diagnosis – unusual.

The full diagnosis in most cases requires a considered evaluation of both the FBC and the clinical features, in an integrated fashion. In the cases that follow in the book, try to evaluate the relative importance of each in each case.

Clinical assessment provides the complete diagnosis – unusual

Fig. 6.2

TO RETURN TO THE FBC MORPHOLOGICAL DESCRIPTION AND COMMENTS. THESE ARE GENERALLY VERY USEFUL, EVEN IN A NEGATIVE SENSE. IN MANY CASES, THEY ARE DECISIVE.

As has been mentioned, it is increasingly uncommon to be given a proper description and interpretation of the morphological features. Basically, there are four types of report with respect to morphology:

1. **A COMPLETE REPORT**, containing, apart from the numerical results, a description of the changes found, a provisional interpretation based on these findings, and a list of suggestions for further investigations. The interpretation is necessarily provisional, since a full interpretation requires a proper clinical assessment – which is your job. The quality of this type of report is very much dependent upon the clinical data you supply to the laboratory at the time of requesting the investigation.

2. **NO DESCRIPTION OR INTERPRETATION** whatsoever. You have a problem and are dependent on your own resources. Of course, the FBC may be entirely normal, in which case a comment

can be foregone (but with reservations). It is up to you to make sure that there are no clues that suggest the count may be abnormal after all. Important features here are the RDW, the MCHC, the plateletcrit, and so on. These will be or have been discussed elsewhere.

3. **A LIMITED SORT OF REPORT CONSISTING OF A LIST OF FLAGS** reported by the counter. There is a restricted number of common flags produced by the instruments and their meaning must be explained. You will notice that they are often somewhat confusing, but they can be very helpful if clearcut. However, these instruments are by no means infallible in this regard. The same observations can occur within a proper morphological report, where their significance is likely to be more meaningful. These flag reports will only be found in level 3 and 4 laboratories; their meanings follow in the next sections (note that they tend to be reported semi-quantitatively with plusses, e.g., "++").

4. **A SEMI-QUANTITATIVE LIST OF CERTAIN OBSERVATIONS**, often made by a technologist. This type of report is clearly better than the instrument-generated one, and is often technically outstanding – the problem is that it is seldom clinically orientated. Examples will be included in the relevant chapters.

The latter two categories are very common, and an attempt therefore is now to be made to assist with this problem.

Unfortunately, there is no easy way to remember the meanings of the morphological changes or indeed to simplify the descriptions; and some knowledge of this is essential. Some of the above-mentioned types of report have to be discussed further.

A Note on Morphology Comments

THE "COMMENT" MAY BE QUASI-MORPHOLOGICAL, CONSISTING ONLY OF FLAGS. This type of comment is reported by the instrument alone. It is worthwhile to see the flags in perspective: most of the flags are triggered if the deviation from "normal" is very small. Thus if there is a sub-population of red cells that are smaller than normal and it accounts for a mere 2% of cells, there will be a flag reporting "Microcytosis +." I suspect that, especially with multiple flags triggered in this

way, most users will find the resulting "report" too confusing. For example, to make something of the following report one would need fairly considerable knowledge, which the average practitioner might not have.

Microcytosis +
Macrocytosis ++
Anisocytosis ++

One point – unfortunately – must be made: it is known that some laboratories use the flags produced by the instrument and generate a written report from it, making it appear that the smear was studied when in fact it was not (and it is astonishing how many students and clinicians assume that these flags mean that the slide has been examined!)

Please note that not all the flags discussed below are produced by all the instruments available. **THE FLAGS MAY BE DIVIDED INTO RED CELL FLAGS, WHITE CELL FLAGS, AND PLATELET FLAGS.**

Red Cell Flags

ANISOCYTOSIS. THIS IS PROBABLY THE COMMONEST FLAG REPORTED BY MODERN INSTRUMENTS. It is also the easiest to understand. It is triggered whenever the RDW is $\geq 14\%$ (this is the coefficient of variation).

MICROCYTOSIS AND MACROCYTOSIS ARE PROBABLY THE TWO MOST IMPORTANT RED CELL FLAGS. At first sight, it would seem that these flags merely restate the MCV, but this is not so. In fact a complex algorithm is used based on the MCV and MCHC. What these flags are actually reporting is the presence of a **POPULATION** of microcytic or macrocytic cells, or indeed both. Therefore, it can be found even if the **MCV IS NORMAL**, indicating a population or tail of small and/or large cells, respectively. How to interpret this is of course another matter.

"MICROCYTOSIS" NOT ACCOMPANIED BY "MACROCYTOSIS.' There are two possibilities:

1. **THE MCV IS DECREASED.** Here you should have no problem – the anatomical diagnosis is "Microcytic anemia" if the Hb is decreased or "Microcytic red cell picture" if normal. The RDW could be normal but is usually increased.

2. **THE MCV IS NORMAL.** This means a **TAIL** of microcytic cells, which would suggest an associated mild iron deficiency, chronic disease, or fragmented cells, among others, as part of a more complicated pathogenesis. The RDW would be increased.

"MACROCYTOSIS" WITHOUT "MICROCYTOSIS" AS A COMMENT. Again, there are two possibilities:

1. **THE MCV IS INCREASED**. Here you should have no problem – the anatomical diagnosis is "Macrocytic anemia" if the Hb is decreased or "Macrocytic red cell picture" if normal. The RDW may be normal or increased.
2. **THE MCV IS NORMAL**. This means a **TAIL** of macrocytic cells, which would suggest an associated reticulocytosis, liver disease, hypothyroidism, or early or partially treated megaloblastosis as part of a more complicated pathogenesis. The RDW is often nearly normal.

BOTH "MACROCYTOSIS" AND "MICROCYTOSIS" REPORTED. Since there are obviously both large and small cells, the MCV is going to give an indication as to which group of cells predominates, if any. Consider a few examples:

1. **MCV = 109 FL**: here the macrocytic cells predominate. The basic approach is the same as for "macrocytosis," but with the proviso that the small group of small cells must be explained, possibly as a co-existing iron deficiency, anemia of chronic disorders, or fragmentation, and so on. The RDW could well be nearly normal.
2. **MCV = 78 FL.** The opposite holds. The RDW is likely to be raised.
3. **MCV = 89 FL.** Other things being equal, the groups of large and small cells are roughly equal – i.e., it is a normocytic blood picture, and should be approached as such. The RDW is likely to be moderately increased.

HYPOCHROMIA. As with microcytosis, a report of "hypochromia" by an instrument reflects a fairly complex algorithm involving the MCV, the MCH and the MCHC. It does not necessarily mean that the red cells are microcytic, as is commonly thought. It is triggered when the number of hypochromic cells is $\geq 4\%$, and will be further discussed under Target Cells a little later.

HYPERCHROMIA. Similarly, this flag is triggered when the number of hyperchromic cells is $\geq 4\%$. It can be found in two situations:

1. Some forms of macrocytes where the red cell is thicker than normal and the MCHC, e.g., megaloblastic anemia.
2. In spherocytosis, where the red cell is thicker than normal and the MCHC is increased.

RED CELL FRAGMENTS. Red cell fragmentation **CAN** be reported as a flag by some instruments, but this is such a significant finding that a morphological reassessment is probably mandatory. They are identified by their size, and the instruments cannot differentiate between red cell fragments and platelets. Thus falsely high platelet counts can occur.

Considerable degrees of fragmentation always indicate intravascular red cell damage. Varying lesser degrees can occur with a number of other conditions, such as megaloblastosis, myelofibrosis, iron deficiency, certain forms of hereditary elliptocytosis, thalassemia. Certain types of intravascular damage may show only moderate to mild fragmentation, particularly in the cardiac hemolytic anemias such as with artificial heart valves or valvular leakage associated with turbulent left ventricular flow.

You will note in all the above examples that without a proper morphological comment, it is very difficult indeed to reach a proper diagnosis. In the absence of such a comment, very many more investigations are likely to be necessary to reach an answer.

White Cell Flags

On some instruments, alterations in the numbers of the different white cells below or above the reference range are merely repeated in word form, such as **LEUKOCYTOSIS, NEUTROPHILIA, MONOCYTOSIS, LYMPHOCYTOSIS, EOSINOPHILIA, BASOPHILIA, LEUKOPENIA, NEUTROPENIA, MONOPENIA, LYMPHOPENIA, AND SO ON.** These are more or less simply "commercials."

LEFT SHIFT. This refers to the presence of granulocyte (usually neutrophil) precursors. The instruments from different manufacturers and of different vintages vary in their accuracy in this regard.

IMMATURE GRANULOCYTES/BAND CELLS. This flag is identical to the previous one, but on a different instrument.

BLASTS. On the very latest instruments, this has been found to be a reliable flag, with one or two caveats.

ATYPICAL LYMPHOCYTES. There are actually different types of atypical lymphocytes and they can be anything from "viral" lymphocytes to lymphoma cells. Here too, the instruments vary considerably in their accuracy.

NUCLEATED RED CELLS. These can be identified with a fair degree of accuracy.

Platelet Flags

LARGE PLATELETS AND PLATELET CLUMPS. These are generally accurately reported because of their light-scattering properties. Platelet clumping usually results from an interaction in certain individuals between the platelets and the EDTA anticoagulant.

The Report May Be a Semi-quantitative List of Certain Observations Made Microscopically

The report may well include descriptive words that CAN be reported by the instrument as well, such as "Microcytosis," and the approach will be the same as in the section above. **THE PROBLEM IS TO IDENTIFY THE REPORT AS NOT BEING AN INSTRUMENT-GENERATED ONE**; the most practical way is to realize which one-word comments or brief descriptions CAN be reported by the instrument. The list is as follows:

Microcytosis
Macrocytosis
Hypochromia
Hyperchromia
Anisocytosis
Leukocytosis
Neutrophilia
Monocytosis
Lymphocytosis
Thrombocytopenia
Thrombocytosis
Large platelets.

Some instruments can report the following; however, with the current technology they cannot be relied upon. Your own judgement is essential.

Red cell fragments
Blasts
Immature leukocytes.

ANY OTHER FINDING INDICATES THAT THE SLIDE WAS EXAMINED BY SOMEONE (I.E., NONE OF THE INSTRUMENTS AVAILABLE TODAY CAN RECOGNIZE THESE CHANGES, OR THEY RECOGNIZE THEM VERY UNRELIABLY). HAVING RECEIVED SUCH A REPORT, IT IS POSSIBLE TO MAKE A GOOD ESTIMATE OF WHAT IS GOING ON IN THE MORE STRAIGHTFORWARD CASES.

The trick is to put all the various little comments together into a meaningful assessment as to the pathological possibilities. Complex cases can be very difficult and may require specialist experience. Consequently, the more complex the case, the more urgent is the need for a proper professional assessment.

However, to give you a taste of what can be achieved at a simple level, consider the following reports (without any counts as such, although clearly having the counts would enormously assist this process). This is the type of report that would be produced by a technologist who is capable of recognizing the changes but not putting them together as a coherent report.

1. Anisocytosis ++
   Microcytosis++
   Anisochromia++
   Micro-ovalocytes ++
   Pencil cells +
   Target cells: occasional
   Neutrophils: right shift.
   ANSWER: A typical iron-deficiency picture; anemia of chronic disorders and thalassemia to be excluded.
2. Anisocytosis +++
   Oval macrocytes ++
   Tear-drop poikilocytes +
   Fragmentation +
   Neutrophils: right shift +++
   ANSWER: A typical megaloblastic picture.
3. Anisocytosis +
   Diffuse basophilia (or "polychromasia")++
   ANSWER: Strongly suggestive of **H**emorrhage, **H**emolysis, **H**ypoxia, response to **H**ematinics.
4. Anisocytosis ++
   Diffuse basophilia ++
   Autoagglutination ++
   Spherocytes +
   Neutrophils: left shift and toxic granulation.
   ANSWER: Acute immune hemolysis.
5. Anisocytosis ++
   Irregular cells and crenated cells ++
   Spherocytes +
   Target cells ++
   Howell–Jolly bodies +
   ANSWER: Suggestive of a post-splenectomy picture.
6. Anisocytosis ++
   Two populations of cells.
   Hypochromic population with oval microcytes ++
   Normochromic population showing some autoagglutination +
   ANSWER: Suggestive of a recent transfusion for iron deficiency.

A Note on the Use of Elements of the FBC in Isolation

Subsets of the FBC are often requested, such as the Hb or Hct only, the WCC or WCC plus differential, or the platelet count. This practice needs some comment:

1. When used in monitoring progress or therapy, for example the Hct in cases of previously diagnosed and characterized erythrocytosis and the platelet count in

cases of known ITP, it is quite satisfactory, with the proviso's that one must maintain constant awareness that other elements of the FBC may change at any time, and that this practice is not followed where the disease causes, or can cause, changes in other cells lines, such as polycythemia vera.

2. Where the clinical picture very clearly indicates that the pathology will lie only in one cell line, such as the WCC and differential in cases of acute infection in an otherwise well patient and where the clinical possibilities are restricted. Nevertheless, one is frequently surprised when an FBC in these cases reveals other changes.

3. Uninformed hospital or medical insurance administrators, trying to save money, have been known to insist that doctors use only those parts of the FBC that are "relevant" (placing an impossible burden on the clinician and the lab). Apart from the clinical dangers of the practice, as mentioned above, they fail to understand the practical economics: the FBC is not a "battery" of tests, like say liver functions which consists of a group of numerous **INDEPENDENTLY PERFORMED TESTS**; earlier-generation blood counters cannot be "programmed" to perform only an Hb, say – the instrument must do **ALL** the components of the FBC. So, if only say a platelet count is requested, all the tests are done, willy-nilly, and only the platelet count is then reported (and charged for); and this is very unfair to the laboratory. Consequently, the fee charged for any one component of the FBC is very much higher than pro rata as a proportion of the whole fee. All counters from level 2 upwards **MUST** do, with every count, the following: Hb, RCC, MCV, WCC and PC; level 3 counters typically also (must) do the so-called three-part diff, and later models an optional full diff. If the fee for a FBC is, for argument's sake, $10.00, the fee for the Hb alone is necessarily far higher than 1/6 of $10.00. It can be very difficult to make administrators see this point.

Note that the fee for an FBC does not specifically include that for a morphological comment, nor is there a separate fee structure for this. Thus, since they are not going to get paid for it anyway, there is a great temptation to forgo the morphological assessment.

The Hemostatic Screen in Practice

There are some fundamental conceptual differences between the FBC and the hemostatic-screen (HS).

1. The FBC is a full-fledged first-line test for the majority of blood diseases, whereas the HS is used for a very restricted presentation – bleeding. (The thrombotic disorders have a different approach entirely – see Chapter 21).

2. The FBC is a standard test and the components are, to all intents and purposes, the same in all circumstances. The HS however can differ:

   a. From the laboratory point of view, it consists of the bleeding time (BT, which has accompanied the blood for testing), the platelet count (PC), the PT and PTT, the thrombin time (TT), and the fibrinogen. Depending on the results of these tests, further confirmatory tests are done automatically by the laboratory, and the report issued.

   b. From the clinician's point of view, the basic screen consists of the BT, the PC, the PT, and the PTT (further tests will or should be done automatically by the lab). There is a temptation to be too selective in the HS, but this is unwise. For example:

      i. In a case of purpura with a proven very low platelet count, one tends to think that there is no point in doing the BT. In fact, most people get away with not doing the PT or PTT either. However, the clinical features may warrant these, e.g., in apparent sepsis or von Willebrand disease.

      ii. A boy presenting with an acute hemarthrosis, a story of a typical pattern of bleeding and a typical X-linked family history, is most likely to be a hemophilia, and the BT and PC are usually superfluous. Again, however, it is always wise to do these, even if only to have a baseline.

3. The distinction between general and specific pathology diagnoses is not as clear-cut as in the disorders approached via the FBC. For example, the PTT and PT are often necessary for both aspects of the pathological diagnosis.

ANYTHING ATYPICAL SHOULD BE REFERRED.

How to Make the First-Stage Diagnosis

From the foregoing, it follows that the concept of the first-stage diagnosis in the bleeding disorders is less clear-cut than it is with the FBC. Once having decided that abnormal bleeding indeed exists, the clinical features may strongly suggest the nature of the abnormality. But one is sometimes surprised, and a great deal of care is necessary.

Nevertheless, the logic is comparable. In most cases, the first-stage diagnosis is very general and often tentative – it commonly boils down to "Probable bleeding disorder". This, however, is extremely valuable, since it performs the task of the first-stage diagnosis – pointing you in the right direction.

There are certain situations where the diagnosis must be made as soon as possible. Unfortunately, because of the perceived rarity of these disorders, great opportunities to prevent lasting damage may be missed. The prevalent erroneous impression that bleeding disorders are rare apart from thrombocytopenia, and that therefore they deserve little attention, may derive largely from the fact that most students seem to equate the bleeding disorders with the **INHERITED** disorders of coagulation, which are indeed rare (although the clinical impact of one or two, such as von Willebrand disease, are underestimated). The acquired disorders of hemostasis are far from rare. But even if the inherited forms are rare, their impact, and the critical role that primary carers like family doctors can and should play in preventing lifelong deformities is so important that awareness of these conditions should be heightened.

The initial clinical assessment thus must include an assessment of severity, complications, and management – particularly how urgently therapy must be instituted. However, it is unfortunate that there is a great tendency to rely exclusively on the blood tests for the diagnosis; this tendency derives from the confusion about hemostasis that existed for centuries. If we consider some of the bleeding diseases, one can be overwhelmed with the various patterns that are found. Consider the following pattern:

BT prolonged; PT prolonged; PTT prolonged; PC decreased; D-dimers increased. This pattern can be found in a number of widely different conditions, namely DIC, liver disease, and as a complication of massive transfusion. Yet, why bother to remember this pattern when there is in the vast majority of cases an obvious clinical difference in these conditions? Similarly, it is most unlikely that the diagnosis of a boy with an X-linked family history presenting with an acute hemarthrosis in a knee is likely to be confused with thrombocytopenia.

We thus will continue with a strictly clinical approach in the first instance. The difficult cases can be dealt with as exceptions. It is in only in these cases that it would be necessary to screen both elements of hemostasis (the platelet-vascular aspect and the coagulation-fibrinolytic aspect) as a routine.

The General Pathology Diagnosis

As with the FBC, the first-stage diagnosis in bleeding disorders will be found in a set of possible general causes.

The Master-set of General Pathology Causes of First-Stage Diagnoses in the Bleeding Disorders

1. Deficient production or production of defective procoagulant factors (which here includes platelets). To facilitate clinical thinking in this category, it may be convenient to subdivide these as follows:

   a. Deficient/defective procoagulant production (platelet numbers)
   b. Deficient/defective procoagulant production (platelet defect)
   c. Deficient/defective procoagulant production (vitamin K-dependent coagulation factors)
   d. Deficient/defective procoagulant production (other coagulation factors)
   e. Deficient/defective procoagulant production: combinations

2. Increased production or activity of anticoagulant factors
3. Increased production or activity of fibrinolytic factors
4. Abnormal consumption of procoagulant factors
5. Defects in vascular structure or function.

   We now use this list and illustrate each point with the commonest disorders, their typical presentations, and their typical test results. The abbreviations used are as follows:

BT = Bleeding Time
PT = Prothrombin Time (generally rendered as the INR)
PTT = Partial Thromboplastin Time
PC = Platelet Count
DD = D-dimers
N   = Normal
P   = Prolonged
I   = Increased
D   = Decreased
(U) = Usually

Deficient/Defective Procoagulant Production (Platelet Numbers)

COMMONEST DISORDERS: Aplastic anemia, leukemia, myelodysplasia.
TYPICAL PRESENTATIONS: Purpura, spontaneous bleeding, oozing after trauma.
TYPICAL TEST RESULTS: BT = P; PT = N; PTT = N; PC = D.

Deficient/Defective Procoagulant Production (Platelet Defect)

COMMONEST DISORDERS: Effect of aspirin/NSAIDS ingestion, renal failure, storage pool disease, myelodysplasia.

TYPICAL PRESENTATIONS: Purpura, spontaneous bleeding, bruising, oozing after trauma.

TYPICAL TEST RESULTS: BT = P; PT = N; PTT = N; PC = N.

Deficient/Defective Procoagulant Production (Vitamin K-Dependent Coagulation Factors)

COMMONEST DISORDERS: Cholestatic liver disease, coumadin anticoagulation, malabsorption of vitamin K.

TYPICAL PRESENTATIONS: Spontaneous bleeding, bruising, oozing after trauma.

TYPICAL TEST RESULTS: BT = N; PT = P; PTT = P; PC = N (note that with coumadin anticoagulation, the PT prolongs first, and only later, in a few weeks, does the PTT also prolong).

Deficient/Defective Procoagulant Production (Other Coagulation Factors)

COMMONEST DISORDERS: Hepatocellular liver disease, heparin anticoagulation, and hemophilia.

TYPICAL PRESENTATIONS: Spontaneous bleeding, bruising, secondary oozing after trauma, hemarthrosis in some.

TYPICAL TEST RESULTS: BT = N; PT = N; PTT = P; PC = N.

Deficient/Defective Procoagulant Production (Combinations)

COMMONEST DISORDERS: Cirrhosis, von Willebrand disease.

TYPICAL PRESENTATIONS: Purpura, spontaneous bleeding, bruising, oozing after trauma.

TYPICAL TEST RESULTS: BT = P; PT = P; PTT = P; PC = D (PT is normal in von Willebrand disease).

Abnormal Consumption of Procoagulant Factors

COMMONEST DISORDERS: DIC, TTP, HUS, and large vascular malformations.

TYPICAL PRESENTATIONS: Purpura, spontaneous bleeding, bruising, oozing after trauma.

TYPICAL TEST RESULTS: BT = P; PT = P; PTT = P; PC = D; DD = I.

Defects in Vascular Structure or Function

COMMONEST DISORDERS: HHT, scurvy, large vascular malformations.

TYPICAL PRESENTATIONS: Purpura, spontaneous bleeding, bruising, oozing after trauma, perifollicular bleeding in scurvy.

TYPICAL TEST RESULTS: BT = P; PT = N; PTT = N; PC = N; DD = N.

The Special Pathology (Specific) Diagnosis

It can readily be seen that proceeding from the test results directly can be very confusing. We have seen by looking at the sets of results that very similar results may be found in disorders of widely different pathogenesis. It would be very unproductive to try to reach the diagnosis via the tests, when in most cases the clinical features are so different and easily recognizable.

Thus, the clinical features of most of these conditions are reasonably obvious. The tests are then used for confirmation. Uncommonly, these will be confusing – it is only then that the tests must be used in the first instance, and interpretation is then sometimes difficult. In any case, they require specialist expertise.

Once again it is instructive to look at an actual case. See case # 8. This case demonstrates the overriding importance of the clinical assessment and a good history; there are nevertheless some uncertain aspects.

Table 6.5

Patient	Age	Sex	Race	Altitude
Miss P v B	10 yrs	Female	White	2,500 ft

This girl, from a small country town, had presented to her GP with a severe sore throat, high fever, and prostration. He diagnosed an acute bacterial tonsillitis, and commenced treatment with a broad-spectrum antibiotic. Because of dysphagia and loss of appetite, she ate virtually nothing for several days, subsisting largely on ice water and carbonated drinks. On the 7th day she began to feel better, and went for a ride on her bicycle. She fell off and hurt her right hip and hand. The apparent injury was minor and no notice was taken of it. The next day she was astonished to see an enormous bruise over her right side, extending down into the thigh and knee. The GP felt that the size of the bruise was inconsistent with the degree of injury and suspected an associated bleeding disorder, and ordered some investigations. He then urgently telephoned for advice and faxed the results from the local laboratory. He confirmed that there was no purpura. She had had no cuts or lacerations. A vitamin K1 injection was recommended, and she was referred the next day in person. The following tests were the ones performed in her hometown.

	Value	Units	Reference range Low	Reference range High	Permitted range Low	Permitted range High
Red cell count	4.55	$\times 10^{12}/l$	3.91	4.94	4.41	4.69
Hemoglobin (Hb)	13.1	g/dl	12.4	15.5	12.6	13.6
Hematocrit (Hct)	0.40	l/l	0.37	0.47	0.38	0.41
Mean cell volume	87	fl	80	99	85.3	88.7
Mean cell Hb	28.8	pg	27	31.5	28.2	29.4
Mean cell Hb conc.	33.1	g/dl	31.5	34.5	32.4	33.8
Red cell dist. width		%	11.6	14	0.0	0.0
White cell count	9.1	$\times 10^9/l$	4	10	8.42	9.78
Neutrophils abs.	7.19	$\times 10^9/l$	2	7	6.65	7.73
Lymphocytes abs.	1.00	$\times 10^9/l$	1	3	0.93	1.08
Monocytes abs.	0.55	$\times 10^9/l$	0.2	1	0.51	0.59
Eosinophils abs.	0.27	$\times 10^9/l$	0.02	0.5	0.25	0.29
Basophils abs.	0.09	$\times 10^9/l$	0.02	0.1	0.08	0.10
Platelet count	405.0	$\times 10^9/l$	150	400	364.5	445.5

Case #8 (Tables 6.5 and 6.6)

Table 6.6

Test	Value	Units	Reference Range	
Bleeding time	4.5	minutes	3	7
Platelet count	405	$X10^9/l$	140	400
PT	27	Seconds	12	13
PTT	29	Seconds	23	36

Discussion

The possible clinical diagnoses are

1. Purpuric bleeding (despite the absence of clinical purpura).
2. Coagulation-defect bleeding.

Note that extensive bruising can be a feature of both platelet deficiency or disorder, and of a coagulation disorder. Also we had no knowledge of

1. Whether she had been exposed to any anticoagulant drugs.
2. A personal history or family history of this disorder.

Clinical experience suggested that coagulation-defect bleeding was far more likely in this patient. It was clear however that this was a case in which both the purpuric and coagulation-defect aspects of the screen were necessary, mainly because of the bruising.

THE FBC: Looking at all three cell lines: all the indices are within normal limits. This does not exclude a functional platelet disorder.

THE (REST OF THE) HEMOSTATIC SCREEN: We see that the bleeding time is normal and there is an isolated prolongation of the PT. We can now be reasonably certain that this is a coagulation defect, because

1. Functional platelet disorders seldom present with massive bruising.
2. The bleeding time is normal.
3. There is a marked abnormality in the coagulation screen.

So, for the time being, we state our anatomical diagnosis as a **COAGULATION-DEFECT BLEED**. We can always return to this point (of relative certainty) if we encounter a contradiction. We thus for the time being ignore the general causes relevant to the FBC and concentrate on the general causes of bleeding disorders.

We now turn to Chapter 18 and see the possible **GENERAL** causes of a coagulation-defect bleed. The only likely ones are

1. Deficient production or production of defective procoagulant factors
2. Deficient production or production of defective fibrinolytic control factors
3. Increased production or activity of anticoagulant factors
4. Increased production or activity of fibrinolytic factors
5. Abnormal consumption of procoagulant factors.

Discussing Briefly Each Possibility:

Again, we look for supporting or negating evidence in the rest of the hemostatic screen and in the FBC; in any other (non-hematological) tests that are available; and in the clinical features.

DEFICIENT PRODUCTION OR PRODUCTION OF DEFECTIVE PROCOAGULANT FACTORS (INCLUDING PLATELET FUNCTION). In this case, we distinguish between the likelihoods of a platelet disorder and a coagulation factor disorder. Having for the time being ignored platelet dysfunction, we concentrate on coagulation defects. We would return to platelet function if no adequate answer emerges.

FEATURES IN FAVOR:
The prolonged PT and the clinical bruising with minimal trauma
The exposure to broad-spectrum antibiotics
FEATURES AGAINST: None.

DEFICIENT PRODUCTION OR PRODUCTION OF DEFECTIVE FIBRINOLYTIC CONTROL FACTORS.

FEATURES IN FAVOR: None.
FEATURES AGAINST: These are extremely rare conditions, particularly in an apparently otherwise healthy person.
INCREASED PRODUCTION OR ACTIVITY OF ANTICOAGULANT FACTORS. There are no well-defined conditions where the natural anticoagulants are increased. We thus concentrate on administered anticoagulants.
FEATURES IN FAVOR: None. If it came to the worst, we would later have to come back to this point and look at ingestion of one of the coumadins.
FEATURES AGAINST: None.
INCREASED PRODUCTION OR ACTIVITY OF FIBRINOLYTIC FACTORS.
FEATURES IN FAVOR: None.
FEATURES AGAINST: This is a very rare condition, particularly in such a patient.
ABNORMAL CONSUMPTION OF PROCOAGULANT FACTORS.
FEATURES IN FAVOR: None. There is no evidence of giant hematomata but this is something to consider; a DIC type of process is most unlikely, if only because the platelet count is normal.
FEATURES AGAINST: The patient is reasonably well, and the platelet count is normal.
THE POSSIBILITIES IN ORDER OF LIKELIHOOD would be something like: abnormal production of the vitamin K-dependent factors due to the ingestion of broad-spectrum antibiotics > Surreptitious ingestion of coumadin-type anticoagulants > platelet function defect > Hereditary factor VII defect.

By the time she was seen by the clinical hematologist (18 h later), the bruise (according to the patient) had not enlarged. There was no other bleeding or bruising history, and her periods had been normal. There was no relevant family history. She felt ill, and felt that this was different from the malaise she had experienced with the tonsillitis. The FBC and hemostatic screen were repeated (Examine Tables 6.7 and 6.8).

Comments

1. The FBC clearly shows features strongly in keeping with a recent substantial bleed (see Chapter 3). It is frequently not recognized just how much blood can be lost in extensive bruising.
2. The PT has improved.
   The provisional diagnosis of depleted vitamin K-dependent coagulation factors was made. The patient

Table 6.7

Case #8 cont.	Value	Units	Reference range Low	High	Permitted range Low	High
Red cell count	3.47	× 10¹²/l	3.91	4.94	3.37	3.57
Hemoglobin (Hb)	10.1	g/dl	12.4	15.5	9.7	10.5
Hematocrit (Hct)	0.29	l/l	0.37	0.47	0.29	0.30
Mean cell volume	85	fl	80	99	83.3	86.7
Mean cell Hb	29.1	pg	27	31.5	28.5	29.7
Mean cell Hb conc.	34.2	g/dl	31.5	34.5	33.6	34.9
Red cell dist. width	13.6	%	11.6	14	13.6	13.6
Retic count	0.71	%	0.25	0.75	0.7	0.7
Retic absolute	24.6	× 10⁹/l	26	100	23.9	25.4
White cell count	11.1	× 10⁹/l	4	10	10.27	11.93
Neutrophils abs.	8.10	× 10⁹/l	2	7	7.50	8.71
Band cells abs.	0.48		0	0	0.43	0.53
Lymphocytes abs.	1.64	× 10⁹/l	1	3	1.52	1.77
Monocytes abs.	0.65	× 10⁹/l	0.2	1	0.61	0.70
Eosinophils abs.	0.10	× 10⁹/l	0.02	0.5	0.09	0.11
Basophils abs.	0.12	× 10⁹/l	0.02	0.1	0.11	0.13
Normoblasts	0	/100 WBC	0	0		
Platelet count	721.0	× 10⁹/l	150	400	648.9	793.1
Sedimentation	27	mm/h	0	20	26	28

Table 6.8

Test	Value	Units	Reference range	
Bleeding time	3.7	min	3	7
Platelet count	721	× 10⁹/l	140	400
PT	18	s	12	13
PTT	32	s	23	36

was given further vitamin K1 and followed up. The tests normalized completely. No further episodes of abnormal bleeding were reported. The anemia responded very well to oral iron therapy.

Miscellaneous Notes

LACK OF LABORATORY FACILITIES. Occasionally you may find yourself in primitive circumstances and faced with a bleeding problem, with the nearest laboratory out of practical reach. You can get quite a long way with the following:

1. **THE WHOLE BLOOD CLOTTING TIME**. This will pick up the presence of any significant factor deficiency. Emergency treatment can if necessary be instituted (i.e., fresh frozen plasma). For the technique, see Appendix C.
2. **THE BLEEDING TIME**. This will pick up clinically significant platelet or vascular causes of prolonged bleeding. See Appendix C.
3. You may have a simple **BLOOD STAIN** with you – make a film, stain it, and look for platelets, fragmentation, leukemia, and so on.

CIRCULATING ANTICOAGULANTS are not to be confused with the heparins, oral anticoagulants, or other therapeutic anticoagulants. They refer to inhibitors to specific coagulation factor/s, and are antibodies.

EVEN WITH ESTABLISHED ORAL ANTICOA-GULANT THERAPY, the PT is more prolonged than the PTT.

MASSIVE TRANSFUSION is discussed in Chapter 19.

Sex Differences in the Bleeding Disorders

ITP is **SLIGHTLY** more common in the female (of no real diagnostic assistance). When it comes to coagulation-defect bleeding, there is a tendency to concentrate only on the hemophilias as such and assume that they are very rare in females. To some extent, this is true. However, coagulation-defect bleeding can occur in females, from several causes:

1. **CLASSICAL HEMOPHILIC BLEEDS**. This is very rare, and can only occur when the father is a hemophiliac and the mother is a carrier.
2. **A MILD HEMOPHILIC-TYPE PRESENTATION**. This is usually only picked up by finding a slightly prolonged PTT, and is due to variations in the lyonization phenomenon: it will be remembered that one of the

X-chromosomes in all the cells in a female is inactivated in a totally random fashion. In a hemophilic carrier, this usually results the production of sufficient factor VIII or IX, as the case may be, for the patient to be asymptomatic. Sometimes the inactivation will, purely by chance, favor a majority of the normal X-chromosomes, and the production of factor will be correspondingly less. Very occasionally this is extensive enough to result in a moderate hemophilic presentation.

3. **DEFICIENCIES OF FACTORS OTHER THAN VIII, IX, AND VON WILLEBRAND FACTOR**, while rare, are inherited autosomally, and thus have an equal chance of occurring in a female. (The common varieties of von Willebrand disease are also autosomally inherited.)
4. **ACQUIRED HEMOPHILIAS**, especially VIII deficiency, are also rare, but can occur, and indeed seem to be more common, in females.

The Bone Marrow Aspiration and Report

At the general level, only very few points need be made. The bone marrow report from a laboratory is akin to a histopathological report in that a full pathological description plus interpretive comment and where possible, a pathological diagnosis is provided by the laboratory. Your only task, as with all laboratory reports, is to make the report relevant to that particular patient – you cannot expect the lab to do this, not having seen the patient clinically.

It goes without saying that **RELEVANT CLINICAL INFORMATION** as well as a summary of diagnostic problems and clinical differential diagnosis are critically necessary for the laboratory hematologist. It is also necessary to indicate

1. **WHETHER SUCTION PAIN WAS PRESENT.** If it was absent (and you are sure the needle was in the marrow cavity), this is highly suggestive of marrow fibrosis (and in which case you probably should proceed directly to a biopsy).
2. **WHETHER UNUSUAL DIFFICULTY WAS EXPERIENCED IN GETTING MARROW**, e.g., whether numerous attempts had to be made. This finding, particularly when coupled with the FBC findings, can be very suggestive of certain diagnoses, such as **MYELOFIBROSIS, HAIRY CELL LEUKEMIA**, and occasionally **ACUTE LEUKEMIA**, where the cells are so densely packed that aspiration is difficult. Except in the case of leukemia (and here the FBC should help you out), you have good motivation to proceed to a biopsy.

3. **THE SITE OF ASPIRATION.** This is sometimes useful. If for example a hypoplastic marrow is found in a sternal aspirate, the fact that the patient has had previous radiotherapy to the chest would prompt the suggestion that the aspirate be repeated from say the pelvis, with the implication that the specimen submitted is not representative because of radiation-induced local aplasia.

4. If you want a good report, you must provide a good specimen. The quality of the specimen is extremely important. Marrow is a semi-solid gelatinous material consisting of a stroma and a multitude of cells. The process of aspiration breaks this up into small fragments suspended in some blood. To minimize the admixture of blood, **ONLY TWO OR THREE DROPS** should be aspirated. These drops are expressed on to slides. On the slide, you should be able to see the fragments; these comprise the material to be examined. To make a good specimen, the fragments on each slide are smeared along, leaving a trail of marrow cells. These are what will be examined. Note that you need to move quickly in making the smears, since marrow clots quickly. **IN THE ABSENCE OF FRAGMENTS (PARTICLES), MANY CRITICAL ASPECTS OF A FUNCTIONAL INTERPRETATION CANNOT BE GIVEN.**

Note that for the hematologist to make a more meaningful interpretation, he needs a FBC done at roughly the same time, plus an indication of findings in previous FBCs (and marrows).

The report once received will fall broadly into one of two categories:

1. **A FINAL PATHOLOGICAL DIAGNOSIS** is given, such as acute leukemia or myelodysplasia. From your point of view, this is the easiest, since very little further clinical integration is required, and the patient can be referred after stabilization.

2. **A COMMENTARY, PERHAPS WITH A DIFFERENTIAL DIAGNOSIS THAT REQUIRES AN INSIGHT INTO THE DYNAMICS OF THE PATIENT'S HEMATOLOGICAL PROBLEM,** is provided. The more relevant data the hematologist is given, the better will she be able to understand this. Nevertheless, the final integration must be yours or whomever you refer the patient to. It is this type of report that needs clinical integration on the part of the clinician.

Basically you want to correlate marrow function with peripheral blood findings together with an assessment of the pace of disposal of the various cell types. Thus, you want to

1. Explain the peripheral blood concentration of the cells.
2. Explain the morphology of the peripheral cells.

The Peripheral Blood Concentration of Cells

It is necessary to relate the concentrations of **EACH CELL LINE** with marrow production. The essential questions are

1. Does the peripheral count appropriately reflect marrow activity?
2. Or is the marrow activity greater than the peripheral count would suggest? This latter case would suggest peripheral destruction of cells with attempt at compensation by the marrow. If there were an increased peripheral count, one would expect to see an increase in the relevant precursors in the marrow.

Thus, depending on the cell line/s involved, one wants to know if the degree of activity of the precursors in the marrow (i.e., the cellularity of those precursors) is proportional to the peripheral count of that particular line.

1. **IF THERE IS AN ANEMIA**, are the red cell precursors (i.e., is erythropoiesis) decreased, which would indicate that the anemia is due to diminished production; or are they increased, which would indicate that there is peripheral destruction or loss and the marrow is trying to compensate?

2. **IF THERE IS A LEUKOPENIA**, are the white cell precursors decreased, which would indicate that the leukopenia is due to diminished production; or are they increased, which would indicate that there is peripheral destruction or loss and the marrow is trying to compensate?

3. **IF THERE IS A THROMBOCYTOPENIA**, are the platelet precursors (i.e., megakaryocytes) decreased, which would indicate that the thrombocytopenia is due to diminished production; or are they increased or normal, which would indicate that there is peripheral destruction or loss and the marrow is trying to compensate?

However, there are a few little complications that need first to be addressed:

1. When we assess the cellularity of the marrow, because of the density of the cells in the marrow particles, we only look at the mass of cells and cannot in fact make

out the individual cells. These masses of cells need not in fact be normal hemopoietic cells, but instead could be metastases or proliferated primitive cells such as blasts (i.e., leukemia). To identify the nature of the cellularity, we look at the cell trails left by the smearing process. You will note that if there are no particles, we cannot reliably comment on cellularity, and if you have submitted poor smears, we cannot reliably comment on the morphology.

2. In Chapter 2, it was said that the marrow has an important function with relation to release of cells from the marrow, and that certain types of very abnormal cells tend to be removed by the marrow before they can get into the circulation; and that this occurs especially in megaloblastosis and myelodysplasia. This function is conveniently thought of as being a separate compartment. But in these cases, even though the proximate cause of the decreased counts lies in the marrow, the marrow still attempts to compensate, and thus is hypercellular.

To illustrate all this as well as what has been said previously, let us look at pancytopenia, in this case due to megaloblastosis. (Examine Fig. 6.3).

So it can be seen that the interpretation of marrow cellularity is critically important as a functional assessment, which is why it is usually the first comment in a marrow aspiration report.

To complete this functional assessment, one will look at the following elements of the report:

1. The **MEGAKARYOCYTES**, whether they are present in sufficient numbers, and to be correlated with platelet numbers.
2. The **MYELOID:ERYTHROID RATIO** (M:E). This will give you an idea whether these two cell production lines are normal in relationship to each other (M:E = 2.5:1 to about 4:1), and if not, which one is affected. Where the ratio is abnormal, one wants to see if the affected lines are absolutely increased (or indeed decreased). And this is where the cellularity comes in again.

3. **CELLULARITY.** Evaluating absolute changes in production of a particular cell line will require you to correlate the M:E ratio with the cellularity. A few examples to illustrate will be given a little later. An increase in cellularity, as already indicated, means one of three things:

   a. **INCREASED COMPENSATORY PRODUCTION.** Using the M:E ratio, one can soon see which of the cell lines is hyperactive. It also means that you should have or look for increased peripheral breakdown or loss.

   b. **INCREASED PRIMARY PRODUCTION.** Again, by reference to the M:E, you can see which line is being over-produced. This is found in myeloproliferative conditions, and the morphology and comment should clarify the situation for you. There is no evidence of peripheral breakdown or loss, but **THERE IS ONE IMPORTANT CAVEAT**: peripheral breakdown or loss can be so well compensated that the cell counts are normal. You must always therefore consider whether there is **CLINICAL** evidence of such loss.

   c. **REPLACEMENT BY ABNORMAL CELLS**, particularly malignant cells.

IT MAY BE OF ASSISTANCE TO SUMMARIZE THE POSSIBLE RELATIONSHIPS BETWEEN MARROW CELLULARITY AND THE PERIPHERAL COUNTS. SEE TABLE 6.9.

In Summary

1. **A NORMAL PERIPHERAL COUNT MAY BE FOUND IN ASSOCIATION WITH**

   a. **A NORMOCELLULAR MARROW**: either normal or (very occasionally) when infiltrated

   b. **A HYPERCELLULAR MARROW** as with compensation for peripheral loss, or occasionally when the marrow is infiltrated.

2. **A DECREASED PERIPHERAL COUNT MAY BE FOUND IN ASSOCIATION WITH**

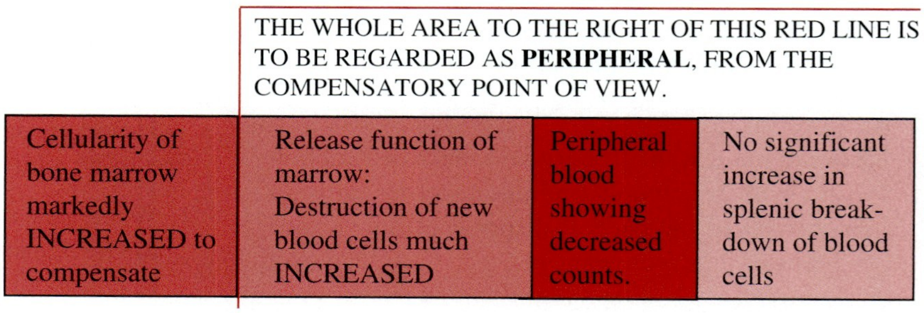

Fig. 6.3 Illustration of the bone marrow dynamics in megaloblastosis.

THE WHOLE AREA TO THE RIGHT OF THIS RED LINE IS TO BE REGARDED AS **PERIPHERAL**, FROM THE COMPENSATORY POINT OF VIEW.

| Cellularity of bone marrow markedly INCREASED to compensate | Release function of marrow: Destruction of new blood cells much INCREASED | Peripheral blood showing decreased counts. | No significant increase in splenic breakdown of blood cells |

Table 6.9

Marrow cellularity	Marrow characteristics	Peripheral blood counts
Normocellular	Normal	Normal
	Infiltrated by non-hemopoietic cells	Decreased (typical); normal; increased (rare)
	Infiltrated by abnormal hemopoietic cells	Increased (typical); normal; decreased
Hypercellular	Otherwise normal	Normal: marrow compensating fully. Decreased: marrow not compensating adequately
	Abnormal	Decreased: either poor release of cells, or replacement of hemopoietic tissues Increased: myeloproliferative disorders
Hypocellular	Otherwise normal	Decreased (aplastic anemia)
	Abnormal	Decreased: hypoplastic myelodysplasia, hypoplastic leukemia
		Increased: e.g., myelofibrosis

Table 6.10a

Case #9			Reference range		Permitted range	
	Value	Units	Low	High	Low	High
Red cell count	2.5	$\times 10^{12}$/l	3.8	4.8	2.19	2.81
Hemoglobin (Hb)	7.3	g/dl	12	15	7.0	7.6
Hematocrit (Hct)	0.21	l/l	0.36	0.46	0.20	0.22
Mean cell volume	88	fl	80	99	78.8	97.2
Mean cell Hb	29.2	pg	27	31.5	26.1	32.3
Mean cell Hb conc.	34.8	g/dl	31.5	34.5	34.1	35.5
Red cell dist. width	17	%	11.6	14	17.0	17.0
Retic count	29	%	0.25	0.75	26.8	31.2
Retic absolute	725.0	$\times 10^9$/l	26	100	652.5	797.5
White cell count	9.4	$\times 10^9$/l	3.5	10	8.46	10.34
Neutrophils abs.	6.49	$\times 10^9$/l	1.5	7	5.84	7.13
Lymphocytes abs.	2.63	$\times 10^9$/l	1	3	2.37	2.90
Monocytes abs.	0.28	$\times 10^9$/l	0.2	1	0.25	0.31
Eosinophils abs.	0.00	$\times 10^9$/l	0.02	0.5	0.00	0.00
Basophils abs.	0.00	$\times 10^9$/l	0.02	0.1	0.00	0.00
Normoblasts	3	/100 WBC	0	0		
Platelet count	489.0	$\times 10^9$/l	150	400	440.1	537.9

Table 6.10b
Peripheral Blood MARROW

Diagnosis	Cellularity	ME ratio	Morphology
Hemolytic anemia	Increased	0.6:1	Normal

a. **A HYPOCELLULAR MARROW**, such as aplasia, etc.
b. **A NORMOCELLULAR MARROW** due to infiltration
c. **A HYPERCELLULAR MARROW**, due to abnormal release of cells, such as megaloblastosis, or inadequate compensation for peripheral loss.

3. **AN INCREASED PERIPHERAL COUNT MAY BE FOUND IN ASSOCIATION WITH**

   a. **A HYPERCELLULAR MARROW**, due to a myeloproliferative disorder
   b. **A NORMO- OR HYPOCELLULAR MARROW**, as in myelofibrosis.

   ### ILLUSTRATIVE EXAMPLES

We consider a black woman of 40 years, at sea level, in a level 4 laboratory.

She has developed an acute severe hemolytic anemia (Examine Table 6.10).

Here one sees the hyperplasia of the erythropoietic elements, due to compensation for the hemolysis – reflected in part by the reticulocytosis. (Note that one does **NOT** (in the first instance) do marrow aspirates on uncomplicated hemolytic anemias!! This case is presented for teaching purposes only.)

Case #10.

Here instead the patient has developed pure red cell aplasia. (Table 6.11).

Table 6.11a

Case #10			Reference range		Permitted range	
	Value	Units	Low	High	Low	High
Red cell count	2.1	$\times 10^{12}$/l	3.8	4.8	1.84	2.36
Hemoglobin (Hb)	6.1	g/dl	12	15	5.9	6.3
Hematocrit (Hct)	0.19	l/l	0.36	0.46	0.18	0.20
Mean cell volume	85	fl	80	99	76.1	93.9
Mean cell Hb	29.0	pg	27	31.5	26.0	32.1
Mean cell Hb conc.	32.1	g/dl	31.5	34.5	31.5	32.7
Red cell dist. width	12	%	11.6	14	12.0	12.0
Retic count	0.1	%	0.25	0.75	0.1	0.1
Retic absolute	2.1	$\times 10^9$/l	26	100	1.9	2.3
White cell count	7.7	$\times 10^9$/l	3.5	10	6.93	8.47
Neutrophils abs.	4.70	$\times 10^9$/l	1.5	7	4.23	5.17
Lymphocytes abs.	2.39	$\times 10^9$/l	1	3	2.15	2.63
Monocytes abs.	0.31	$\times 10^9$/l	0.2	1	0.28	0.34
Eosinophils abs.	0.23	$\times 10^9$/l	0.02	0.5	0.21	0.25
Basophils abs.	0.08	$\times 10^9$/l	0.02	0.1	0.07	0.08
Normoblasts	0	/100 WBC	0	0		
Platelet count	312	$\times 10^9$/l	150	400	290.0	329.0
Sedimentation	29	mm/h	0	20	28	30

Table 6.11b
Peripheral Blood MARROW

Diagnosis	Cellularity	ME ratio	Morphology
Normocytic anemia	Decreased	15:1	Normal

Here there is **HYPO**plasia of the erythropoietic elements, due to aplasia – observe the marked reticulocyto-**PENIA**, which reflects this hypoactivity. The peripheral blood diagnosis is necessarily at the anatomical stage, since this diagnosis can only be made on the bone marrow. Note also the raised ESR, due solely to the anemia.

CASE #11.

Here instead the patient has developed erythrocytosis due to an EPO-secreting renal adenocarcinoma (Table 6.12).

Table 6.12a

Case #11			Reference range		Permitted range	
	Value	Units	Low	High	Low	High
Red cell count	**5.7**	× 10¹²/l	3.8	4.8	4.99	6.41
Hemoglobin (Hb)	**17.1**	g/dl	12	15	16.5	17.7
Hematocrit (Hct)	**0.53**	l/l	0.36	0.46	0.51	0.55
Mean cell volume	91	Fl	80	99	81.4	100.6
Mean cell Hb	30.0	Pg	27	31.5	26.9	33.2
Mean cell Hb conc.	32.3	g/dl	31.5	34.5	31.6	32.9
Red cell dist. width	12	%	11.6	14	12.0	12.0
Retic count	1.2	%	0.25	0.75	1.1	1.3
Retic absolute	68.4	× 10⁹/l	26	100	61.6	75.2
White cell count	3.6	× 10⁹/l	3.5	10	3.24	3.96
Neutrophils abs.	1.69	× 10⁹/l	1.5	7	1.52	1.86
Lymphocytes abs.	1.62	× 10⁹/l	1	3	1.46	1.78
Monocytes abs.	0.25	× 10⁹/l	0.2	1	0.23	0.28
Eosinophils abs.	0.00	× 10⁹/l	0.02	0.5	0.00	0.00
Basophils abs.	0.04	× 10⁹/l	0.02	0.1	0.03	0.04
Normoblasts	0	/100	0	0		
		WBC				
Platelet count	331.0	× 10⁹/l	150	400	297.9	364.1
Sedimentation	0	mm/h	0	20	0	0

Table 6.12b
Peripheral Blood MARROW

Diagnosis	Cellularity	ME ratio	Morphology
Erythrocytosis due to EPO-secreting renal adenocarcinoma	Increased	0.5:1	Normal

Note that the RDW is normal, since there is nothing wrong with the red cell-producing mechanism. Erythropoiesis is being chronically over-stimulated by the EPO. Also, there is little or no reticulocytosis, since this is a very chronic process. The ESR is low, due to the erythrocytosis, despite there being an underlying chronic disease.

Note also that the diagnosis is complete. The finding of erythrocytosis would have led, among other things, to the estimation of EPO. Once found to be raised, the underlying cause would be sought. In other words, marrow examination is NOT necessary for the diagnosis. The case was used for illustrative purposes only. Erythroid hyperplasia is the cause of the hypercellularity.

Case #12.

Here instead our unfortunate patient presented with a marked leukocytosis with mild anemia and thrombocytosis (Table 6.13).

Table 6.13a

Case #12			Reference range		Permitted range	
	Value	Units	Low	High	Low	High
Red cell count	**3.5**	× 10¹²/l	3.8	4.8	3.06	3.94
Hemoglobin (Hb)	**10.8**	g/dl	12	15	10.4	11.2
Hematocrit (Hct)	**0.31**	l/l	0.36	0.46	0.30	0.32
Mean cell volume	**106**	fl	80	99	94.9	117.1
Mean cell Hb	30.9	pg	27	31.5	27.6	34.1
Mean cell Hb conc.	34.8	g/dl	31.5	34.5	34.1	35.5
Red cell dist. width	15.8	%	11.6	14	15.8	15.8
Retic count	0.81	%	0.25	0.75	0.7	0.9
Retic absolute (abs.)	28.4	× 10⁹/l	26	100	25.5	31.2
White cell count	**101.3**	× 10⁹/l	3.5	10	91.17	111.43
Neutrophils abs.	**40.52**	× 10⁹/l	1.5	7	36.47	44.57
Lymphocytes abs.	**9.12**	× 10⁹/l	1	3	8.21	10.03
Monocytes abs.	**1.01**	× 10⁹/l	0.2	1	0.91	1.11
Eosinophils abs.	**4.05**	× 10⁹/l	0.02	0.5	3.65	4.46
Basophils abs.	**5.07**	× 10⁹/l	0.02	0.1	4.56	5.57
Blasts	**1**	%	0	0		
Promyelocytes	**3**	%	0	0		
Myelocytes	**15**	%	0	0		
Metamyelocytes	**13**	%	0	0		
Band cells	**9**	%	0	0		
Normoblasts	**5**	/100	0	0		
		WBC				
Platelet count	**501.0**	× 10⁹/l	150	400	450.9	551.1
Sedimentation	**47**	mm/h	0	20	45	49

Table 6.13b
Peripheral Blood MARROW

Diagnosis	Cellularity	M:E ratio	Morphology
Probable chronic myelocytic leukemia	Increased	19:1	Basophil leukocytosis and blasts in keeping with CML

Note: the diagnosis on the peripheral blood is only probable since the result of the chromosome studies is being awaited. Bone marrow aspiration is not needed for the diagnosis from the morphological point of view; it is necessary however if chromosome studies on the marrow are needed, and to see the blast count (see Chapter 15). The MCV is raised for technical reasons that will be discussed in Chapter 9. The high ME ratio indicates that the hypercellularity is due to myeloid hyperplasia.

A Brief Note About Bone Marrow Iron Studies

These involve assessment of iron stores (in bone marrow macrophages) and distribution of iron in the normoblasts. Iron stains up nicely with Perl's stain. Bear in mind that this is done on a separate smear, and always one is chosen with good particles since it is in the particles that most macrophages are found. It sometimes happens that out of all the smears submitted, only one has particles, and this must under most circumstances be used for morphology; the evidently contradictory report could thus emanate from the laboratory, giving a good report on the cellularity and morphology of the marrow, and then going on to say that iron stores could not be assessed due to the absence of particles! (As a general rule, it is essential that the laboratory not be taken for granted, and having an understanding of the type of practical problems that the laboratory faces leads to greater harmony, and more importantly to greater productivity).

Various patterns occur, and the laboratory report will usually give you the likeliest cause of the pattern.

To Return to the Interpretation of the FBC with Reference to the above

As a consequence of the foregoing, it must be seen that the evaluation of the FBC is not merely to look at the counts statically, but to attempt to **INFER WHAT IS HAPPENING IN THE MARROW AND THE TISSUES RESPONSIBLE FOR DISPOSAL,** that is to

say, to get an insight into the pathophysiology of the process. This process can be aided immeasurably where indicated by studying the marrow directly as well as looking at such measurements that are available that will suggest splenic function. It is clear that an understanding of (a small) number of pathophysiological principles is necessary.

Strictly speaking, the diagnostic process attempts to evaluate each of the compartments described above, both on their own and in relationship to one another; and without this being done, the interpretation of particularly the FBC degenerates into a static and mechanical algorithm-ridden exercise. There are tests available for evaluating most of these compartments. Some of these are very complex, expensive, and time consuming. Generally speaking, one can get by without them, relying on the FBC, a variety of fairly simple other blood tests, and quite frequently, bone marrow examination. However, the FBC remains the primary examination, and one that requires an understanding of some simple dynamics.

A Summary of Indications and Contra-Indications to Marrow Studies

With respect to **CONTRA-INDICATIONS**, there are only two, and these are generally speaking relative:

1. **SEVERE HEMOPHILIA** (but this problem can be overcome by the concurrent or subsequent administration of factor).
2. **SEPSIS.** One would be very chary indeed of causing osteomyelitis in the ilium or sternum. Fortunately, this situation very seldom crops up. (Bone marrow studies are generally of little value in the critically ill.)

Indications for bone marrow aspiration and/or trephine biopsy. (Adapted from EBMG database ebm00305/015.001.)

1. **THERE ARE A NUMBER OF CONDITIONS WHERE THE FULL DIAGNOSIS ABSOLUTELY DEPENDS ON BONE MARROW STUDIES**. These include the leukemias, the myelodysplastic syndromes, myelomatosis, macroglobulinemia, bone marrow metastases, and some storage diseases. Megaloblastic anemia is frequently included in this list; this is generally true but a case can be made out for avoiding marrow aspiration in an elderly patient with clinical and FBC features **FULLY** in keeping with

megaloblastosis, **AS WELL AS** indisputable megaloblasts in the peripheral blood **AND** significantly decreased vitamin B_{12} and/or red cell folate levels. Even in these cases, a trial of therapy is necessary; if unsuccessful, a marrow aspirate is mandatory.

2. **THERE ARE A NUMBER OF CONDITIONS WHERE MARROW ASPIRATION IS COMPLEMENTARY TO THEIR DIAGNOSIS**. These include hypersplenism and agranulocytosis. ITP is frequently included in this list; however, there is considerable dispute about this with respect to adults.

3. In addition, one **EVENTUALLY HAS OFTEN TO RESORT TO MARROW STUDIES** in the following conditions:

   a. Undefined anemia
   b. Undefined thrombocytopenia
   c. Undefined lymphadenopathy, splenomegaly, and/or hepatomegaly
   d. Follow-up of chemotherapy
   e. Local bone pain
   f. Lymphoma staging
   g. Pyrexia of unknown origin (as a very last resort).

   The motivation for aspiration is very often strengthened by the need for cytogenetic and/or flow cytometric studies. Indeed it is becoming standard practice to include these investigations in any case where a malignancy is suspected as well as in a few other conditions.

4. **TREPHINE BIOPSY** has become an outpatient procedure, and is done whenever there is a suggestion of malignancy. In addition, biopsy is essential in the following conditions:

   a. A "dry tap." Important causes of a dry tap include aplastic anemia, hairy cell leukemia, a marrow packed very tightly with other leukemic cells, and technical problems.
   b. Myelofibrosis, usually suspected on the basis of a patient with a massive splenomegaly plus characteristic appearances on the blood film.
   c. Bone marrow necrosis – see Chapter 2.
   d. Metabolic disease of bone – but usually an (open) wedge biopsy of bone is far preferable for diagnosis.

Know Your Limits!!! This book, aimed at the general reader, necessarily uses relatively straightforward and uncomplicated cases for teaching purposes. A minority of your patients will present atypically:

1. A rare or complex disorder may superficially resemble a well-known disorder. This can be very misleading and a potential danger to the patient. Careful observation of the clinical and/or laboratory features for features that do not fit will very often alert you to this possibility.

2. While most categories of disease can be classified very conveniently, in all of them presentations will be found that do not "fit" cleanly into one of the subdivisions, and these can be very problematical. This is quite common, and has been the subject of humorous "complaints" by the author to his patients, that "you don't get sick like the books say."

3. A number of blood diseases can have very nonspecific presentations, such as myelodysplasias, paroxysmal nocturnal hemoglobinuria, some hemolytic disorders, some strange bleeding tendencies, and so on.

4. Many hematological diseases are so rare that it would be foolhardy to try to sort them out at the general level.

In all these cases, it is the practitioner's responsibility to refer the patient to someone with the necessary expertise. In general terms, be prepared in these circumstances to say, with the doctor of physic in Macbeth: "This disease is beyond my practice."

Exercise 6.1

A Quick Self-Test (Answers below)

True	False	Questions
		1. If the RCC, MCV, Hb, WCC, and PC are normal, there is no need to look further at the FBC
		2. The general pathology causes of hematological diseases are identical to those in general medicine, i.e., vascular, infective, inflammatory, degenerative, and so on
		3. An increased prothrombin time can indicate defects in factors I, II, V, IX, and X
		4. The FBC can never provide the complete pathological diagnosis
		5. In chronic liver disease, almost any type of bleeding disorder may be found
		6. Suction pain during bone marrow aspiration always indicates pathology
		7. In bone marrow aspiration smears, one is only interested in the morphology of the cells
		8. Bone marrow aspiration is essential in all cases of hemolytic anemia
		9. Having good particles in a bone marrow aspiration specimen is critical for reliable diagnosis
		10. The normal M:E ratio in the bone marrow is 2:4
		11. A reported "normocellular" marrow implies a normal bone marrow

Exercise 6.2

Match the items in columns 1 and 2 (Answers below).

Column 1	Column 2
A. A platelet count from a citrate tube	1. Suggestive of either hemorrhage, hemolysis, hypoxia, or response to hematinic therapy
B. Diffuse basophilia	2. Classical causes are myelofibrosis and hairy cell leukemia
C. The diagnostic value of a PT and PTT on their own	3. Can by itself be a cause of a mildly raised ESR
D. A "dry tap" in a bone marrow aspiration	4. Is essential in all cases of isolated thrombocytopenia
E. Anemia	5. Is a strong relative contraindication to bone marrow aspiration or biopsy
F. Sepsis	6. Markedly and disproportionately less than used together

Answers

EXERCISE 6.1

1F; 2F; 3T; 4F; 5T; 6F; 7F; 8F; 9T; 10F; 11F.

EXERCISE 6.2

A4; B1; C6; D2; E3; F5.

Further Reading

Hoffbrand AV, Pettit JE (2001). Essential Haematology. 4th edn. Oxford: Blackwell Science.
Lewis SM, Bain B, Bates I (2006). Dacie and Lewis Practical Haematology. 10th edn. London: Churchill Livingstone.
Davis, BH (2001). Diagnostic advances in defining erythropoietic abnormalities and red blood cell diseases. Semin Hematol. 38:148.

Why so pale and wan, fond lover?
Prithee, why so pale?
Will, when looking well can't move her,
Looking ill prevail?

(John Suckling)

Preview *Anemia is undoubtedly the central abnormality and presentation in hematology and as such requires special consideration and emphasis. This chapter serves as a necessary introduction to the following three chapters that discuss the various types of anemia. A number of miscellaneous issues need clarification. This chapter also discusses various general features of anemia, regardless of the nature and cause of the anemia, in terms of their primary presentation, i.e., micro-, macro-, or normocytic. Topics discussed include*

1. *Anemia in relation to primary and secondary blood diseases.*
2. *The classification of the anemias.*
3. *The epidemiology of anemia.*
4. *Clinical diagnostic problems and presentations in anemia and the clinical examination in cases of suspected anemia. In particular, a few problematic and confusing issues are discussed:*

   a. *Assessing the severity of anemia*
   b. *Anemia and cyanosis*
   c. *Bone marrow failure and anemia*

5. *The laboratory diagnosis of anemia from the clinical point of view, with particular reference to red cell size, the RDW, and anisocytosis.*
6. *The physiological response to anemia and the effects on the FBC.*
7. *Introduction to the operating characteristics of tests in anemia, with particular reference to*

   a. *The diagnosis of anemia per se*
   b. *Screening for certain common hereditary blood diseases*
   c. *The characterization of the type of anemia*
   d. *The tests used to identify the specific cause of an anemia*

Chapters 8, 9, and 10 all deal with different types of one provisional first-stage diagnosis: anemia, and it is necessary to discuss general aspects of this topic separately. **"ANEMIA" IS BY FAR THE COMMONEST ABNORMALITY IN THE FBC AND REFLECTS A POTENTIALLY VAST NUMBER OF PATHOLOGICAL PROCESSES. NO ANEMIA THEREFORE IS TOO TRIVIAL TO INVESTIGATE. CLOSE TO 90% OF ALL HEMATOLOGICAL DISORDERS PRESENT WITH ANEMIA.** Very many non-hematological disorders have anemia as a complication or side effect. It follows that the causes and mechanisms of anemia are extremely diverse, and thus approaching anemia effectively is a far from trivial task. It can be difficult to decide

O.N. Beck, *Diagnostic Hematology*, DOI 10.1007/978-1-84800-295-1_7,
© Springer-Verlag London Limited 2009

if anemia represents, in a given patient, a primary blood disease or not.

A PRIMARY BLOOD DISEASE is very much more likely if the patient has, in addition to anemia, any one (and especially more than one) of the following:

1. Lymphadenopathy
2. Splenomegaly
3. Bone pain and tenderness to percussion (over the marrow-containing bones)
4. A bleeding tendency

ANEMIA SECONDARY TO DISEASE IN ANOTHER SYSTEM is usually easy to identify. Sometimes, however, the underlying primary disease can be occult, requiring a high index of suspicion.

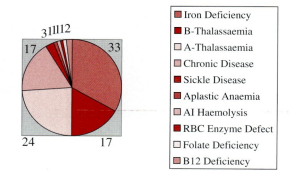

Fig. 7.1 Epidemiology of anemia

The Classification of the Anemias

Broadly there are two ways of classifying anemia:

1. **ETIOLOGICAL**. This is based on the supply and demand principle as discussed earlier. Thus there would be

   a. Defects of production, with all its sub-categories
   b. Loss or destruction of red cells in the circulation, again with all the sub-categories
   c. Abnormal destruction or sequestration in the reticulo-endothelial system (mainly the spleen), of various types

   This approach is the one generally taught to clinical students. It is nicely summarized in Fig. 7.1. However, there are problems with this method, mainly to do with overlap between the different classes. For example, thalassemia can be classified as

   a. An inherited disorder of hemoglobin synthesis,
   b. A disorder of decreased production,
   c. A disorder characterized by ineffective erythropoiesis,
   d. A chronic hemolytic disorder,
   e. An iron overload disorder,
   f. A hypercoagulable state,

   all of which are correct.
2. **MORPHOLOGICAL**. This is our preferred method and is based on the average size of the red cells (i.e., the MCV), thus resulting in **MICROCYTIC, MACROCYTIC, OR NORMOCYTIC** anemias. This approach is the one virtually universally in use with the FBC itself. Interestingly, however, it is very successful in

clinical work, as generations of students have assured the author, since, as an aide-memoire, it serves to focus the mind immediately and practically upon the possible causes of anemia and thence what features to ask about and look for. It can thus be used even if the FBC is not available. Besides, why learn two classifications of a set of disease processes when one will do? **IN GENERAL, THE ADVANTAGES OF THIS SCHEME ARE SEVERAL:**

a. **THE CLASSES THUS IDENTIFIED IMMEDIATELY SUGGEST THE NATURE OF THE UNDERLYING DEFECT** and hence the particular further investigations – clinical, laboratory, and often radiological – that would be most useful in confirming the diagnosis. In particular, the rest of the FBC, particularly the morphology, usually assists considerably.
b. **IT LENDS ITSELF TO A CONVENIENT WAY OF THINKING CLINICALLY OF THE CAUSES OF A CLINICALLY DIAGNOSED ANEMIA** and thence to what features to look for or ask about to more precisely identify the underlying pathological process.
c. **CHANGES IN AVERAGE RED CELL SIZE CAN OCCUR IN THE PRESENCE OF AN HB LEVEL WITHIN THE "NORMAL" RANGE.** These may thus suggest the nature of the underlying disorder early on, before the anemia has developed, or indicate a disorder where anemia does not develop or indeed may suggest that, while the Hb is within the normal range, it is abnormal for that patient.

However, rational treatment depends on knowing the specific causative pathology. Therefore, once the morphological diagnosis is made, the rest of the process – i.e., working out the general and specific pathology – is aimed at the etiological classification. This is presented in detail in the relevant chapters.

The Epidemiology of Anemia

If anemia can be regarded as a disease, there is no doubt that it is the commonest in the world – indeed iron-deficiency anemia is recognized as the commonest disease in the world. As such it is important to see how common the different causes of anemia are. Figure 7.1 shows the prevalence of the commonest causes of anemia on a worldwide basis.

These figures also thus contribute to the pre-test probabilities of an anemia, but depend very much on the geography: in a Norwegian town a microcytic anemia would in the first instance probably trigger a pre-test diagnosis of iron deficiency; in a town in Florida in the United States, with its high proportion of wealthy retired folk, anemia of chronic disorders (ACD) would probably equal iron deficiency as a pre-test probability; and in sub-Saharan Africa, α-thalassemia, ACD, and iron deficiency would all receive more or less equal weighting.

By reference to the pie-chart in Fig. 7.1 it will be seen that the microcytic anemias are by far the most common. It is very useful to realize that about 90% of **ALL** anemias are due to one or more of three causes – iron deficiency, anemia of chronic disease, and thalassemia (in very roughly equal proportions on a worldwide basis). All of these are characterized by **MICROCYTOSIS.** Thus, if the microcytic anemias and the operating characteristics of the relevant tests are known and understood thoroughly, the student will have made a good start in becoming effective in clinical hematology.

Note that, as mentioned previously, the operating characteristics of the various red cell measurements by themselves and on their own are of little value in identifying the specific causative disease – they only provide an extremely useful pointer as to what to do next.

Diagnostic Problems and Presentations in Anemia

The FBC (which usually is (or should be) used as a test of a clinical hypothesis) is nevertheless by necessity often also used to **DIAGNOSE THE PRESENCE OF ANEMIA**. However, even with this in mind, one does not want to order too many unnecessary FBCs. Yet it is important to establish the presence of anemia, since it very often is an independent adverse prognostic factor in many diseases, and if therapy is available, the overall outcome could sensibly be improved.

The optimal diagnosis of anemia involves a combination of probabilistic, morphological, physiological, and clinical approaches. Clinical features often have a significant impact on the interpretation of the FBC findings (see Tables 7.1 and 7.2 for the commonest examples).

The Clinical Examination in Cases of Suspected Anemia or Obvious Pallor

The clinical examination in cases of suspected anemia serves as the basis for collecting the data for identifying several issues:

1. The clinical diagnosis per se – essentially the pathological diagnosis, at least in terms of one or more hypotheses.
2. How severe the anemia is – essentially how soon and which therapeutic intervention is warranted.
3. What tests should be requested. Are they warranted? Are they likely to advance the diagnosis?

Figure 7.2 illustrates **SPECIFIC ASPECTS** of the examination of a patient in whom anemia is known or suspected; clearly it is part of the overall examination as is depicted in Fig. 5.4.

Table 7.1 The items in Tables 7.1 and 7.2 are perhaps the most important presentations involving anemia

Acute presentations	Cause/mechanism	Lab findings	Further studies
Sudden pallor, palpitations, queer feeling, especially with prior history of, e.g., GIT symptoms	Occult bleed	Thrombocytosis, neutrophilia, drop in Hb, reticulocytosis (all time-dependent)	Clinical, ? radiological
As above, but acutely ill, with jaundice, often splenomegaly, loin pain	Acute extravascular hemolysis, usually immune-mediated	Above, with unconjugated bilirubinemia, positive. Coombs, normocytic anemia. No bilirubinuria.	Numerous – see Chapter 10 for more details
Pallor, lassitude, purpura, sore throat, palpable spleen		Various, can be non-specific. Blasts in blood suggestive	Bone marrow aspiration, etc.

Table 7.2 The items in Tables 7.1 and 7.2 are perhaps the most important presentations involving anemia

Chronic presentations	Cause/mechanism	Lab findings	Further studies
Tiredness, malaise, dyspnea on effort, pale, ill, PLUS:	Anemia to be excluded		
1. Pica, koilonychia, dysphagia, sore tongue, bleeding source	Iron deficiency from chronic bleeding.	Hypochromic microcytic RBC, right shift of neutrophils, low ESR	Clinical, iron studies
2. Steatorrhea, allergies, previous iron deficiency responded to transfusion or IV iron	Malabsorption, typically adult-onset gluten enteropathy	As above plus dietary and stool history	As above
3. Poor diet (junk food, meat-free, bad teeth, poverty), especially females	Iron-deficient diet	As above plus dietary history	As above
4. An older patient, premature graying, jaundice, glossitis, neurological changes, no splenomegaly	Malabsorption of vitamin B_{12}	Macrocytic anemia, oval macrocytes, right shift, often pancytopenia, decreased B_{12} levels	Bone marrow aspiration, B_{12} levels
5. Multiple pregnancy or alcoholism, glossitis, no neurological features, often associated features of iron deficiency	Folate deficiency, often with associated iron deficiency	As above plus features of iron deficiency	Bone marrow aspiration, folate levels, iron studies
6. An elderly person living alone, features of both iron see item (1.) and folate deficiency	Combined iron and folate deficiency. Patient lives on toast and tea	As above	As above
7. Usually a young patient, jaundiced, pallor, splenomegaly, gall stones, family history of above	Chronic extravascular hemolysis due to red cell defects	Unconjugated bilirubinemia, negative Coombs. No bilirubin in urine. Often a classical blood picture	Osmotic fragility, RBC membrane and enzyme studies, electrophoresis
8. Chronically ill, such as rheumatoid disease or lymphoma, pale, ill	Iron malutilization	Positive activity tests, typical iron studies. Normo- or microcytic anemia	Clinical
9. Pale, sallow, enlarged spleen, perhaps frontal bossing, Mediterranean or Indian person	Defective Hb synthesis – thalassemia	Microcythemic picture	Hb electrophoresis, HbA_2, iron studies
10. Pale, sallow, pruritus, easy bleeding, hypertension	Defective EPO secretion from renal failure	Relevant biochemical studies. Normocytic	EPO levels, etc.
11. Pale, ill, bone pain, perhaps oliguria, renal failure, hyperviscosity syndrome	Myeloma	Normocytic anemia, rouleaux, raised ESR	Numerous
12. Severe bone pain with pallor. Evidence of malignancy of thyroid, prostate, lung, kidney	Metastases to bone	Leuko-erythroblastic blood picture	Bone marrow examination
13. Very large spleen, perhaps pallor, purpura	Chronic myelocytic leukemia or myelofibrosis	Typical blood picture	

Differentiating Clinical Features

Disorders presenting with anemia can be very vague; anemia covers such a wide multitude of possibilities that many people find it daunting. Especially in cases where there is no clear pointer to the diagnosis, either in the history (such as dysphagia or pica) or in the examination (such as koilonychia), it would be helpful to have at least some indication as how to proceed.

This is particularly so with the normocytic anemias, where the clearer pointers that are found in the micro- and macrocytic anemias are absent. There are,

however, some clinical features that can be of great assistance in at least pointing one in the right direction. These are

1. The size of the spleen
2. The presence of jaundice and its type
3. The presence of purpura
4. The presence of bone pain and tenderness
5. A number of rarer findings such as acrocyanosis

Because the significance of these features requires some preliminary discussion in the context of the anemias, they are discussed at different points in the chapters that follow.

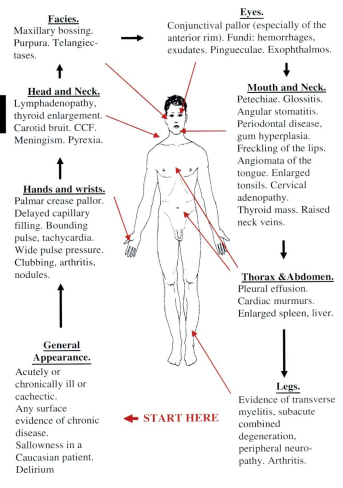

Facies.
Maxillary bossing. Purpura. Telangiectases.

Head and Neck.
Lymphadenopathy, thyroid enlargement. Carotid bruit. CCF. Meningism. Pyrexia.

Hands and wrists.
Palmar crease pallor. Delayed capillary filling. Bounding pulse, tachycardia. Wide pulse pressure. Clubbing, arthritis, nodules.

General Appearance.
Acutely or chronically ill or cachectic.
Any surface evidence of chronic disease.
Sallowness in a Caucasian patient.
Delirium

← **START HERE**

Eyes.
Conjunctival pallor (especially of the anterior rim). Fundi: hemorrhages, exudates. Pingueculae. Exophthalmos.

Mouth and Neck.
Petechiae. Glossitis. Angular stomatitis. Periodontal disease, gum hyperplasia. Freckling of the lips. Angiomata of the tongue. Enlarged tonsils. Cervical adenopathy. Thyroid mass. Raised neck veins.

Thorax &Abdomen.
Pleural effusion. Cardiac murmurs. Enlarged spleen, liver.

Legs.
Evidence of transverse myelitis, subacute combined degeneration, peripheral neuropathy. Arthritis.

Fig. 7.2 Examination: suspected anemia

The Assessment of the Severity of Anemia

This topic has already been alluded to, but perhaps in the light of what has been said in this chapter, the information given here might make this better understood. To summarize, once anemia is diagnosed or even strongly suspected, its severity must be assessed – it can be a medical emergency. It must be re-emphasized that the degree of anemia is a clinical decision, related to the patient's physiological reserves.

MODERATE ANEMIA can be defined as anemia of such severity that the blood is diverted to "vital" organs in order to sustain life. This level is usually found at an Hb level of around 8 g/dl. It can be clinically assessed with a fair degree of reliability by looking at the palmar creases – if they are as pale as the rest of the palm, the Hb is usually 8 or less (however, beware of the very fair thin female, as well as those with serious peripheral vascular disease).

SEVERE ANEMIA is diagnosed by the presence of a hyper-dynamic circulation – wide pulse pressure, harsh precordial flow murmurs, high output cardiac failure; in addition, two symptoms are of extreme importance:

1. DYSPNEA ON EFFORT, which differs from dyspnea due to cardiac disease by the fact that it is RELIEVED BY LYING DOWN. The rate of progression of anemia can also be assessed by the reduction of effort tolerance over a period of time.
2. ANGINA. The majority of patients over the age of 50 with severe anemia present with angina. Erroneous referral to cardiologists (in the first instance) is a common occurrence – often, subsequent angiography does not reveal EXTENSIVE atheromatosis in the coronary arteries.

Anemia, Hypoxia, and Cyanosis

Some students are confused by the relationship of anemia to cyanosis; some even think that severe anemia is accompanied by cyanosis. Cyanosis is further discussed in Chapter 17; for the moment, suffice it to say that true (central) cyanosis means an increased level of reduced Hb in the capillaries ($\pm$ 5 g/dl). Anemic patients do not show cyanosis even with a very low partial pressure of oxygen in the arterial circulation (Pao_2), unless there is an independent cause for cyanosis. Co-incidental anemia can complicate the clinical diagnosis of hypoxemia. By the same token, a patient with a normal Hb would not generate this amount of reduced Hb in the capillaries until oxygen saturation (Sao_2) reached a very low, perhaps life-threatening, figure. For example, consider two patients (at sea level – Table 7.3):

Table 7.3

Hb	Sao_2 % required for clinical cyanosis	Po_2
15 g/dl	77	45 mmHg
9 g/dl	64	35 mmHg

Bone Marrow Failure and Anemia

A very important and practical point must be made: THE VAST MAJORITY OF ANEMIAS HAVE UNDERLYING BONE MARROW FAILURE IN ONE FORM OR ANOTHER, SUCH AS

1. Damage, destruction, or loss of bone marrow itself. This may be due to aplasia, dysplasia, infiltration, necrosis, or malignant transformation.

2. Deficiencies in cytokines and other growth factors which render the marrow hypofunctional.

3. Deficiencies in one or more of the many essential nutrients, rendering the marrow dysfunctional.

Note that, associated with the above, the anemia is often accompanied by changes in the other cell lines.

THIS DOES NOT MEAN THAT A MARROW ASPIRATE SHOULD BE DONE IN ALL CASES OF ANEMIA! In Chapter 6 the indications for bone marrow examination were spelled out.

In the Optional Advanced Reading section, a new concept of bone marrow failure is presented.

Clinical Aspects of the Laboratory Diagnosis of Anemia

It has been stressed that the primary approach in the first instance to anemia is by reference to the MCV. **THERE IS ONE IMPORTANT WARNING WITH THE MCV.** It is a technical issue and should be thoroughly understood. A short description of how modern instruments count and size cells is necessary. These methods are based on the Coulter principle – see Fig. 7.3. Blood is sucked through an aperture in a glass tube on either side of which are electrodes. As a cell passes through the aperture, it causes a deflection in the current passing between the electrodes, and the size of the deflection is proportional to the size of the cell. The suction applied causes streamlines to develop in the onrushing blood; depending on how deformable the cell is, it will tend to elongate in the direction of flow – **AND IT IS IN THIS FORM THAT THE CELL IS MEASURED.**

Thus, in the case of the red cell, which is normally extremely deformable, it becomes an ellipse within the aperture, and it is this deformed cell that is sized (and counted at the same time).

In Fig. 7.3 observe how a normal red cell deforms as it approaches and passes through the aperture. Within the aperture the red cell width is measured; from this the volume is extrapolated and given as say 89 fl.

Iron-deficient cells (whether due to iron deficiency, anemia of chronic disorders, or thalassemia) all contain less Hb than normal. Hb is the major constituent of the red cell; a decrease in cellular Hb will make the cell smaller than normal, and therefore becomes even narrower in the aperture – besides, it may be elliptical to start off with.

It follows that cells with abnormally rigid membranes regardless of their Hb content (e.g., sickle cells) and spherocytes with a high Hb concentration will undergo less deformation and thus the MCV will be overestimated. Again this is seldom of practical significance unless the abnormality is very severe and/or the MCV is already high.

With cold agglutinins as found in certain immune hemolytic anemias, the agglutinated clumps of cells are **SIZED AND COUNTED AS SINGLE CELLS.** The MCV can thus be extremely high, well into levels that are impossible with pathological causes, e.g., 145 fl. Obviously the RCC is falsely low (see Fig. 7.4).

In Fig. 7.4 observe how a red cell agglutinate deforms minimally as it passes through the aperture. After extrapolation, the volume of the agglutinate as a whole could be given as say 200 fl. Of course, not all the red cells are necessarily agglutinated; some pass through singly and are sized correctly. On average, however, the MCV will be high – and its height depends mainly on how much autoagglutination there is.

The above applies to white cells as well. White cells are not much larger than red cells, but are far less deformable than red cells; as white cells pass through the aperture they deform much less, and **THEIR MEASURED SIZE** is considerably greater than that of the red cells (see Fig. 7.5). But since the number of white cells is normally very low with respect to the red cell count, this makes no **PRACTICAL** difference to the MCV. However, very high white cell counts (in the order of $300–400\times10^9$/l, as may be found in many

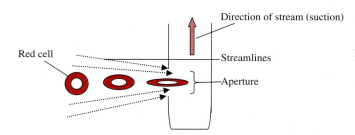

Fig. 7.3

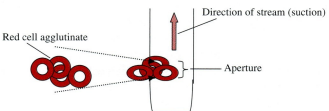

Fig. 7.4

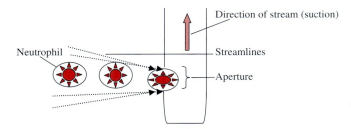

Direction of stream (suction)

Neutrophil

Streamlines

Aperture

Fig. 7.5

leukemias) **MAY PUSH THE MCV SPURIOUSLY INTO THE MACROCYTIC RANGE**, particularly if the MCV is already on the high side, typically due to relative folate depletion.

In Fig. 7.5 observe the minimal deformation the white cell undergoes as it passes through the aperture. Again the total volume is extrapolated and could be given as say 140 fl.

Using the Average Cell Size (i.e., MCV) Diagnostically

Clearly, when the MCV is above or below the reference ranges, there is no problem with labeling the picture macro- or microcytic and approaching them accordingly (as discussed in Chapters 8 and 9).

However, MCV's within the range, especially near the lower or upper end of it, may also be found in the conditions associated with measured macro- and microcytosis and should thus be approached in the same way. Identifying these cases is difficult. The issue is further discussed in the Optional Advanced Reading section, but as a brief guide, the following should be watched out for in cases with an apparently normocytic picture:

1. A very wide RDW (see the next section), especially where the MCV is close to the limits of the reference range
2. A report of "microcytes + or + +" or "macrocytes + or + +" (or both) by instruments capable of these flags
3. A morphological comment indicating hypochromia, anisochromia, microcytes, or macrocytes

Basically, one should simply be aware that the instruments report an average, and the outer limits of this average may comprise very abnormal cells, which should be picked up morphologically. A high index of suspicion is always advisable.

It is also clear that the sensitivity and specificity of the MCV near the reference ranges are not very high. This is further discussed later in the chapter.

And to reiterate a point made before – one cannot without further ado take any laboratory report as absolute.

Anisocytosis and the Raised RDW

Anisocytosis is such a common comment in FBC reports and has traditionally so seldom been associated with a particular disease process that there is a tendency to discount its importance. However, now that the degree of anisocytosis can be accurately measured (by the RDW), some valuable insights have emerged.

Anisocytosis, in principle, can be caused by any interference with red cell production, but with some exceptions. As such its sensitivity as a test is poor, and it serves only as a pointer to look further. Taken in conjunction with other measurements, however, its value for the interpretation of the FBC is enhanced considerably, in certain specific circumstances. To understand these it is necessary to look at some fundamentals.

The most convenient starting point in explicating the nature of the raised RDW is by looking at iron and folate deficiencies.[1] It is assumed that the RDW is normal (<14%) before the onset of deficiency.

The Effect of Developing Iron Deficiency on the RDW, MCV, and Hb

1. With the onset of iron deficiency the newest red cells produced will be microcytic (due to poor hemoglobinization of the cells – see Chapter 8 for a full explanation). There will now be a tiny "tail" of microcytic cells, and the RDW is slightly increased. The MCV is slightly decreased but the difference at this stage is hardly measurable.
2. With every day that passes, assuming iron deficiency persists, this "tail" and the RDW gets larger, the Hb also falls, and the MCV falls. . . .
3. Until practically **ALL** the cells are microcytic, whereupon the RDW decreases. The MCV is now at its lowest (around 55 fl).
4. Upon commencing treatment with iron (after the cause has been treated appropriately), the RDW (and Hb) once again increases. The "tail" is marginally smaller and the MCV marginally higher, every day.
5. Only when the majority of cells are once again normocytic does the RDW start to decrease.

Note that the same basic pattern occurs with developing anemia of chronic disorders (see Chapter 8), but in this case the ESR and other activity tests will be abnormal (the ESR is low or normal in pure iron deficiency).

With the other major cause of microcytosis – the thalassemias – the situation is, however, somewhat different. Uncomplicated thalassemia minor and intermedia (see Chapter 8) are characterized by defective α or β chains in all red cells; the red cells are smaller than normal de novo, and therefore the RDW is close to normal whilst the Hb and MCV are low. (The raised RDW in thalassemia major is due to other factors, associated with intramedullary breakdown, etc.)

The Effect of Developing Folate Deficiency on the RDW, MCV, and Hb

In principle, the same sequence of events follows as with iron deficiency, with the exception that the tendency is for the MCV to increase.

Other Causes of a Rise in RDW

Most disorders affecting red cell production will increase the RDW, prominent exceptions being polycythemia vera, Cushing syndrome and related conditions, the thalassemias unless in the major form, and aplastic anemia; with all of these the relation of the RDW to the MCV does not hold.

As stated, therefore, it is clear that the RDW has poor sensitivity and specificity for identifying the nature of an anemia. However, as a pointer to indicate that **SOMETHING** is wrong, its sensitivity is close to 100%. Consider the following case (Table 7.4).

CASE #13. EXAMINE TABLE 7.4

The only obvious abnormality is the considerably raised RDW. Subsequent morphological examination revealed numerous crenated and irregular red cells and some fragmentation. These features are commonly found in a malignant circulation. Further investigation of the patient revealed a fairly large ovarian carcinoma with implantation secondaries. The only other point of possible significance is the marginally raised eosinophil count, and it will be seen in Chapter 15 that this too can be a marker of malignancy.

Table 7.4

Patient	Age	Sex	Race	Altitude
Mrs J B	61 yrs	Female	White	Sea level

This lady complained of vague and non-specific symptoms. Systematic enquiry revealed no specific symptoms or possible contributory causes. She complained that she had gained a lot of weight recently. Examination revealed no obvious abnormality. The abdomen was very obese and possibly distended. As a first investigation the family practitioner decided to do only a FBC. He then referred the patient for an opinion, with the following FBC.

	Value	Units	Reference range Low	Reference range High	Permitted range Low	Permitted range High
Red cell count	4.56	$\times 10^{12}$/l	3.8	4.8	4.42	4.70
Hemoglobin (Hb)	13.1	g/dl	12	15	12.6	13.6
Hematocrit (Hct)	0.38	l/l	0.36	0.46	0.37	0.39
Mean cell volume	84	fl	80	99	82.3	85.7
Mean cell Hb	28.7	pg	27	31.5	28.2	29.3
Mean cell Hb conc.	34.2	g/dl	31.5	34.5	33.5	34.9
Red cell dist. width	20.2	%	11.6	14	18.2	18.2
Retic. count	0.66	%	0.25	0.75	0.6	0.7
Retic. absolute (abs.)	30.1	$\times 10^9$/l	30	100	29.2	31.0
White cell count	6.87	$\times 10^9$/l	4	10	6.35	7.39
Neutrophils abs.	3.50	$\times 10^9$/l	2	7	3.24	3.77
Band cells abs.	0.00		0	0		
Lymphocytes abs.	2.39	$\times 10^9$/l	1	3	2.21	2.57
Monocytes abs.	0.36	$\times 10^9$/l	0.2	1	0.34	0.39
Eosinophils abs.	**0.51**	$\times 10^9$/l	0.02	0.5	0.49	0.57
Basophils abs.	0.08	$\times 10^9$/l	0.02	0.1	0.08	0.09
Blasts		%	0	0		
Promyelocytes		%	0	0		
Myelocytes		%	0	0		
Metamyelocytes		%	0	0		
Normoblasts	0	/100 Wbc	0	0		
Platelet count	397.0	$\times 10^9$/l	150	400	357.3	436.7

THE ABOVE ISSUES ARE FURTHER DISCUSSED IN THE OPTIONAL ADVANCED READING SECTION OF THIS CHAPTER.

The Physiological Response to Anemia and the Effects on the Full Blood Count

THERE ARE FOUR SYSTEMS OR SUB-SYSTEMS THAT PLAY THE MAJOR ROLE IN ADAPTING TO ANEMIA. Here we are not discussing the cause or type of anemia, simply the response to anemia itself, and are assuming that the rest of the systems are anatomically and functionally normal. This is not just an academic exercise. **THERE ARE SIGNIFICANT**

IMPLICATIONS FOR THE INTERPRETATION OF THE FBC AND PARTICULARLY THE RETICULOCYTE COUNT. Note that in general the intensity of the response is dependent on the severity of the anemia and the rapidity with which it develops. Also, it will be seen that the severity of anemia is not primarily measured by reference to the level of Hb, but by the functional impairment caused – and this varies according to the reserves of the patient, notably correlated with age and the cardiovascular status, and thus with how gradually the anemia develops. For the sake of discussion we will use a gradually developing anemia and follow it as it becomes increasingly severe. **THE FOUR SUB-SYSTEMS ARE**

1. The vascular tree
2. The heart
3. The lungs
4. The bone marrow

The Response of the Micro-circulation to Anemia

There are three main mechanisms by which the tissues adapt to hypoxia:

1. Adaptations within the tissues and the red cells serve to increase the oxygen extraction from the red cells by the tissues.
2. Selective shunting of blood within the micro-circulation to the vulnerable areas.
3. **THE MAJOR EFFECT OF THE VASCULAR RESPONSE TO ANEMIA IS TO INCREASE THE LOCAL BLOOD FLOW.** The prime function of the red cells is the delivery of oxygen to the tissues. However, this depends on efficient vascular delivery of the blood. Even in health there is not enough blood to fill the whole of the vascular tree and only about 10% of the capillaries are open at any one time. To provide the required oxygen to the tissues that frequently have dynamically varying requirements, close and **RESPONSIVE** control of the micro-circulation is essential. Thus the capillary beds open and close all the time, sometimes for only seconds at a time. How does this come about?

Basically, the patency of micro-circulatory vessels at any one time is controlled by the tissues themselves, and primarily by the metabolic requirements of those tissues, as a direct feedback mechanism. The actual mechanism is uncertain: it used to be thought that the prime cause of compensatory vasodilatation was hypoxia; however,

there is no direct correlation between P_{O_2} and arteriolar diameter. However, tissue hypoxia will result in certain metabolites accumulating, and one or more of these is probably responsible for the vasodilatation and thus increased blood supply. These metabolites include

1. Nitric oxide (NO)
2. CO_2
3. Adenosine. In hypoxia there is a tendency to a decrease in ATP production, since this is oxygen dependent. This results in an accumulation of adenosine (a metabolite of ATP) which then diffuses out of the cells. It is an extremely powerful vasodilator (to say nothing of its profound pro- and anti-inflammatory functions).

A DECREASE IN CIRCULATING HEMOGLOBIN WILL BE MANIFEST IN THE TISSUES AS HYPOXIA. The effect of the many vasodilators enables more blood per unit cross-sectional area to reach the tissues, thus increasing the local blood supply.

In the early milder stages, the vasodilatation is confined to the so-called "vital" organs, whereas the skin and kidney, for example, will undergo vasoconstriction (controlled largely by the autonomic nervous system (ANS)). Consequently **A DROP IN HB WILL NOT NECESSARILY HAVE THE DELETERIOUS EFFECTS POSSIBLY EXPECTED BY REFERENCE TO THE HB LEVEL.**

However, as the anemia progresses, the ANS has to permit the degree of vasodilatation to become greater, and it eventually becomes the dominant clinical feature. The effects of this more or less parallel the degree of generalized vasodilatation and thus the degree of anemia.

THESE EFFECTS ARE THREEFOLD:

1. Decreased peripheral resistance with a drop in diastolic blood pressure.
2. Tendency to turbulent flow. This is potentially disadvantageous (for example, activation of the hemostatic system).
3. **VASOCONSTRICTION IN THE KIDNEY WILL LEAD TO INCREASED EPO PRODUCTION VERY EARLY.**

The Response of the Heart to Anemia

THE MAJOR EFFECT OF THE HEART'S RESPONSE TO ANEMIA IS TO INCREASE THE LOCAL BLOOD SUPPLY.

To cope with the demand for increased blood to the tissues, the circulation is speeded up, with tachycardia and increased stroke volume (thus increasing cardiac output), and consequently increased work of the heart. The results are as follows:

1. **AS THE ANEMIA WORSENS THE SYSTOLIC BLOOD PRESSURE INCREASES,** which together with the decreased diastolic pressure results in a widened pulse pressure, eventually with a water-hammer pulse, and other features of a hyper-dynamic circulation. It should be seen that the development of a hyper-dynamic circulation indicates that vasodilatation has become relatively generalized, implying a very significant anemia. **THE HB LEVEL AT WHICH A HYPER-DYNAMIC CIRCULATION DEVELOPS IS LARGELY DEPENDENT ON THE CARDIAC RESERVE – THUS THE HB LEVEL ON ITS OWN CANNOT BE USED AS AN ASSESSMENT OF THE SEVERITY OF THE ANEMIA.** There are other causes of a hyper-dynamic circulation (such as thyrotoxicosis), and it is obvious that **THE FBC, PARTICULARLY IN THOSE CASES WHERE THE CLINICAL FEATURES OF ANEMIA AS SUCH ARE NOT OBVIOUS, IS OF VITAL IMPORTANCE IN ASSESSING THE NATURE OF SUCH A HYPER-DYNAMIC CIRCULATION.**

2. **THE MYOCARDIUM IN THESE CIRCUMSTANCES USES A MASSIVE PERCENTAGE OF THE AVAILABLE OXYGEN,** and blood flow through the coronary arteries approaches the maximum. Any organic disease of the coronaries, in the presence of large oxygen demands, will tend to cause angina. The majority of people over 50 with severe anemia present with angina. With continued relative oxygen shortage, the myocardium dilates, with the following results:

   a. The valve rings do not dilate, producing a disparity between the diameter of the valves and the size of the chambers.
   b. There is increased turbulence of the flow of blood through the heart.
   c. The above two effects are responsible for widespread murmurs over the precordium.

   FINALLY, THE HEART TENDS TO FAIL, of the "forward failure" type. To return to the widened pulse pressure: the degree of this is more or less proportional to the degree of anemia, other things being equal; however, when the heart begins to fail, the **SYSTOLIC PRESSURE TENDS TO DECREASE** and the pre-load to increase results in a **TENDENCY FOR THE DIASTOLIC PRESSURE TO INCREASE.** It is thus critically important to realize that anemia in a patient with a more or less normal pulse pressure can be **SEVERE** (indeed extremely and dangerously severe). **IN THIS CASE THE INTERPRETATION OF THE HB CAN BE PARTICULARLY PROBLEMATICAL – ON THE ONE HAND IT ONCE AGAIN BECOMES VERY IMPORTANT IN THE ASSESSMENT OF THE DEGREE OF ANEMIA; ON THE OTHER, THE PRESENCE OF CARDIAC FAILURE AND OTHER CHANGES CAUSE FLUID SHIFTS WITH CHANGES IN PLASMA VOLUME AND THUS SPURIOUS HB LEVELS.**

The Response of the Lungs to Anemia

THE MAJOR EFFECT OF THE LUNGS' RESPONSE TO ANEMIA IS TO (ATTEMPT TO) INCREASE THE OXYGEN CONTENT OF THE BLOOD SUPPLY.

Other things being equal, severe hypoxemia (i.e., arterial $Po_2 < 4.5$ kPa, $\pm$ 35 mmHg) results in the tissue cells changing over to anerobic respiration, with severe metabolic disturbances, such as acidosis, etc., which has effects on the oxygen-dissociation curve among others, and thus affects the interpretation of the Hb level: this is a complex issue and is beyond the scope of a general primer.

THE REACTION OF THE LUNGS TO ANEMIA TAKES THE FORM OF TACHYPNEA AND HYPERPNEA, to maximize oxygen uptake. Note that these patients never have dyspnea at rest, only effort dyspnea more or less in proportion to the anemia. The dyspnea is also **IMPROVED** by recumbency (unlike, e.g., cardiac dyspnea).

The Response of the Bone Marrow to Anemia

THE MAJOR EFFECT OF THE MARROW'S RESPONSE TO ANEMIA IS TO INCREASE THE OXYGEN CONTENT OF THE LOCAL BLOOD SUPPLY BY INCREASING THE NUMBER OF RED CELLS.

ERYTHROPOIETIN (EPO) IS SECRETED, MAINLY BY THE KIDNEY, IN RESPONSE TO TISSUE ANOXIA. EPO ACTS ON THE ERYTHROID PRECURSORS, STIMULATING ERYTHROPOIESIS, WITH THE PRODUCTION FROM THE 4TH DAY ONWARD OF RETICULOCYTES. THE

RETICULOCYTE COUNT WILL CLIMB RAPIDLY WITHIN ANOTHER FEW DAYS (AND ASSUMING A NORMAL MARROW) TO A LEVEL DEPENDENT ON THE DEGREE OF ANEMIA. NORMALLY THE RETICULOCYTE COUNT RISES TO A LEVEL, WHICH, OTHER THINGS BEING EQUAL, WILL RESTORE THE HB TO NORMAL (FOR THAT PATIENT), WITHIN 3 WEEKS OR SO. THUS, THE GREATER THE DROP IN HB, THE HIGHER YOU EXPECT THE RETICULOCYTE COUNT TO BE.

You should try to assess whether the reticulocytosis is appropriate. An example will be of assistance: Mr A. F., an adult man, normally has a Hb of 15 g/dl, a RCC of 5.27×10^{12}/l, and retics of 0.8% (42×10^9/l). He develops an acute mild short-lived hemolysis and his Hb drops to 10 g/dl and his RCC to 3.55×10^{12}/l. From the 4th day onward, reticulocytes appear and rise to say 10% (345×10^9/l) by day 6. These will be sufficient to restore his Hb to 15 in 3 weeks or so. This response is depicted in Fig. 7.6.

In contrast, had his hemolytic episode been worse his Hb could have dropped to 5 g/dl and his RCC to 1.71×10^{12}/l, and here the normal reticulocyte response would be expected to be in the vicinity of 40% (740×10^9/l). This is depicted in Fig. 7.7. Note that in the latter case, not only reticulocytes but also normoblasts (red cell precursors) tend to appear. In this context the number of normoblasts should be seen functionally as retics. Once again his Hb is restored to pre-incident level in about 3 weeks. However, in this patient a retic of 10% would **NOT** be sufficient to restore the Hb in the expected time. This is a common error made by students (and many professionals!): the fact that an anemic patient has a reticulocytosis does **NOT** mean that the marrow is responding normally. In Fig. 7.8, this picture is presented; it will be seen that the patient takes more than 6 months to recover. Therefore there is, in addition, something wrong with his marrow.

Table 7.5 summarizes the responses to anemia. These only become measurable when the Hb drops to below 11 g/100 ml and are fairly linear if the decrease in Hb is slow and steady.

The work of the **NORMAL** heart remains more or less steady until the Hb drops below about 6 g/100 ml.

Fig. 7.6

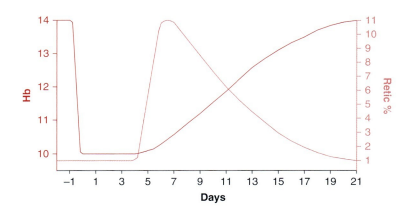

Fig. 7.7

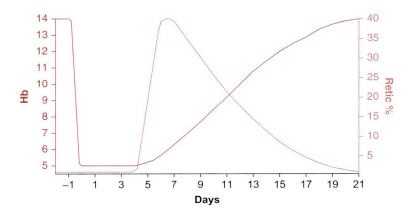

Fig. 7.8

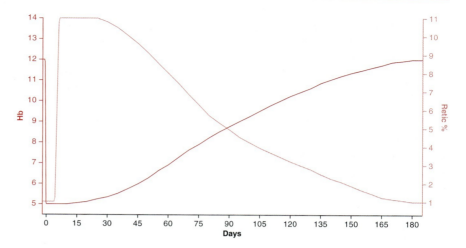

Table 7.5 The physiological responses to developing anemia

Quantities increasing	Quantities decreasing
Pulse rate	Diastolic blood pressure
Cardiac output	Circulation time
Heart size	Blood viscosity
Velocity of blood flow	Total blood volume
Pulmonary ventilation	A-V oxygen difference
Oxygen utilization	
Systolic blood pressure	

An Introduction to the Operating Characteristics of Tests in Patients with Anemia or Pallor

Clinical epidemiological aspects of specific presentations, i.e., the operating characteristics and related issues, are mentioned where relevant in the individual chapters. Our emphasis will be on when, how, and why to use blood tests in different clinical situations. (Unfortunately, hard data for most of these examples are not yet available). For example,

1. A patient with a history of hemorrhoids has a microcytic anemia. Are further investigations necessary and what should these be?
2. A man of 74 presents with clinical features typical of pernicious anemia and a blood picture highly suggestive of megaloblastic anemia. Is it necessary to do a marrow examination in the first instance?
3. A patient with "burnt-out" rheumatoid arthritis has a microcytic anemia. What further investigations, both clinical and laboratory, are necessary?
4. An Indian or Cypriot patient presents with microcytic anemia. Can one without further ado make a diagnosis of thalassemia?
5. A Rwandan patient has a microcytic anemia. What further investigations are warranted?

6. A pregnant patient has a normocytic anemia and a dimorphic blood picture. What further investigations are necessary; how reliable are they?
7. A patient has advanced bronchogenic carcinoma with cachexia and pallor, with pancytopenia. Is it warranted to do bone marrow examination?

In addition, in all cases one must also ask oneself if there are any other features to look for, either clinical or in the FBC or both, that would simplify this problem? It would be silly, for example, in an African patient of 11 years with microcytosis, to try to evaluate the significance of the microcytosis while ignoring an associated eosinophilia and characteristic clinical features strongly suggestive of hookworm infestation. Similarly, a raised RCC in the presence of microcytosis considerably narrows the possible causes.

In this chapter we discuss the operating characteristics of the diagnosis of anemia itself, including screening tests.

As has been stated before,

1. 90% of all hematological patients are anemic.
2. 90% of all anemias are microcytic.
3. A number of (potentially) serious hereditary blood diseases have an extremely high worldwide incidence. Screening for these, particularly among pregnant women, has a very high priority in endemic areas.

Operating characteristics relevant to the FBC tend mostly to concentrate on one or two measurements in the FBC, tending to cause a loss of overall perspective. Note that there is no complete agreement in the results of different researchers in their published operating characteristics.

The following section is included primarily as an introduction to the operating characteristics of confirmatory tests (such as ferritin) and to provide insight into the relative importance of some of the measurements in the FBC. Note that in this book we use a reasonable approximation of the results of various researchers, supported by our own data.

Note that most research into the operating characteristics of tests in hematology have been done in the diagnosis and investigation of the anemias. We shall discuss the operating characteristics of tests at different stages of diagnosis and from different perspectives:

1. The diagnosis of anemia per se
2. Screening for certain common hereditary blood diseases
3. The characterization of the type of anemia
4. The specific cause of the anemia

The Diagnosis of Anemia

Anemia unless severe is difficult to diagnose accurately. Yet requesting a FBC (or even just a Hb) merely to identify anemia as a routine is simply unacceptable. In any case, the problems in identifying anemia are most prominent in the borderline cases – nobody should have difficulty in diagnosing anemia in a patient with a Hb of 5 g/dl. This problem was extensively discussed in Chapter 3, with the following conclusions:

1. A value just below the lower reference range does not necessarily imply anemia.
2. Even assuming it does reflect anemia, it is not necessarily so that the anemia is a very mild one – the patient's "normal" Hb could be 18 g/dl
3. By the same token, even a Hb within the reference range could still imply anemia.

It is extremely difficult to provide sound guidelines as when to request a FBC to **DIAGNOSE THE PRESENCE OF ANEMIA.** (See Chapter 6 for a list of suggested indications to request a FBC.) It really is a matter of experience and nice judgment. Three clinical presentations suggestive of anemia have received some analytic attention – facial pallor, conjunctival pallor, and a dietary history:

1. **FACIAL PALLOR.** Only about 55% of people with anemia are pale. The positive and negative LR for facial pallor with a Hb of < 11 g/dl in females and < 13 g/dl in males is about 4 and 0.5, respectively. So, lack of facial pallor is not, on balance, a reliable sign to exclude anemia.
2. **CONJUNCTIVAL PALLOR.** A lot of research has confirmed the value of this sign. A major point to emerge is that it is not simply pallor of the whole palpebral conjunctiva, but of **THE ANTERIOR RIM**. The LR below a Hb value of 10 g/dl is poor, of the order of 5. But at the level of 11 g/dl, this rises to about 17. Thus if conjunctival pallor is noted (as defined above), the patient almost certainly has a Hb of < 11 g/dl. One important caveat, however: in these trials, a fair amount of time had to be spent in training the different observers just what conjunctival pallor was. It is thus very important that clinical tutors become involved in this.[2]
3. **A GOOD DIETARY HISTORY.** With respect to the differential diagnosis of microcytosis (Chapter 8), it has been found that a good, detailed dietary history has sensitivity of ± 70%, specificity of ± 80%, and negative predictive value of nearly 100% for the diagnosis of iron deficiency. It is clear that a good history can be of considerable assistance.

There are a number of other well-known clinical features that often are of assistance but data on their characteristics are not available:

1. **PALM CREASE PALLOR.** Normally the palm creases are pink. If they are pale the likelihood of the Hb being < 9 is very good. Of course, this sign is only of use in Caucasian skin. It is also of less validity in very fair females (i.e., this is a cause of decreased sensitivity of the test). We estimate that for the diagnosis of moderate to severe anemia in a Caucasian skin the sensitivity is to be in the order of 85% and the specificity about 90%.
2. **CAPILLARY REFILLING.** The features have already been described. We estimate that the sensitivity of this test for anemia is about 90% and the specificity about 75%.

The Characterization of the Type of Anemia

The tests and measurements used for identifying the general nature of an anemia are – in order of importance – MCV, MCH, RCC, RDW, and Hb, with the MCV bearing by far the major burden of identification:

1. **MICROCYTOSIS AND MICROCYTIC ANEMIA.** The sensitivity, specificity, and predictive values vary

quite a lot with different researchers. Many papers deal with the characteristics with respect to a specific proven cause of microcytosis. Thus, for example, one can see results of a MCV of <79, 78, 80, and 81 fl defining operating characteristics for iron deficiency, thalassemia, and ACD. Unless there is a very clear pre-test probability of one of these and a poor pre-test probability of the other two, this is hardly what we are looking for. We actually want to know if there is any assistance in the MCV in the discrimination of the three most common causes – and indeed there is not. To use the MCV as a screening test it must be done only with one purpose in mind – to **EXCLUDE FROM FURTHER STUDY** those people who almost certainly do **NOT** have the disease being screened for (such as thalassemia). So clearly we need to know what the specificity of the MCV for these diseases is. Since specificity at a level of <79 fl is high (about 93%), it is clearly valuable for this purpose. The point made is that one cannot expect to diagnose one of the three causes, only to exclude them.

Why, it may be asked, is the specificity not higher? There are two possible reasons:

a. There is a wide range of "normal" for the MCV. If a patient's normal MCV is unusually high, say 94 fl, then if it is now revealed as 81 fl, this represents quite a significant microcytosis for that patient.

b. Mild, perhaps unsuspected underlying liver or thyroid disease or folate deficiency could, because they are characterized by macrocytosis, cause the MFCV to be raised. This may be mild enough not to cause obvious morphological changes.

Note also that it is pointless to talk of likelihood ratios of a low MCV indicating any one of the causes without having a clear and strong pre-test probability – in which case one hardly needs the operating characteristics.

An interesting paper from Brazil tried a more pattern-orientated approach, specifically to see if the three major causes of microcytosis could be distinguished by reference to several measurements, i.e., the RCC, MCV, MCH, and the England–Fraser index (derived from the red cell measurements). It found that none of the indices allowed complete discrimination; also the raised RCC in thalassemia permitted better discrimination of thalassemia.[3]

2. **MACROCYTOSIS AND MACROCYTIC ANEMIA**. Much the same considerations apply to a raised MCV. Generally speaking a raised MCV without quantification is largely useless. Certain levels of increase, however, have been identified as related, with a good likelihood, as being suggestive of certain diseases. A raised MCV can also have a spurious cause, that of autoagglutination. Many workers have suggested using raised MCV as a screen for alcoholism; the sensitivity is too low to be of use, but the specificity is very high (± 95%). Thus a normal MCV is very likely to exclude alcoholism (so long as a cause of concomitant microcytosis can be excluded). The approach to macrocytosis is further discussed in Chapter 9.

3. **NORMOCYTIC ANEMIA**. With normocytosis the situation is very different and very difficult; after all we are dealing with a "normal" finding. **OPERATOR CHARACTERISTICS OF THE MCV ARE OF NO USE HERE**, and the approach must be logical, as described in Chapter 10.

Screening for Certain Common Hereditary Blood Diseases

Our major concern in this regard is with finding heterozygotes for: thalassemia, sickle disease, Hb-C disease, and hemochromatosis. The thalassemias are discussed in Chapter 8; sickle disease and Hb-C disease in chapter 10; and hemochromatosis in Chapter 20. At this stage we shall confine ourselves to screening for the thalassemia genes, to illustrate a number of points.

Screening for Thalassemia

In certain countries such as Cyprus and India this is a major problem. It is not feasible to thoroughly check the whole population, and thus a screening test (in this case a decreased MCV, since classically thalassemia is a microcytic disease), would be very valuable.

It will be seen that, all in all, operator characteristics of individual elements of the FBC in the diagnosis of the specific types of anemia are not good enough for routine use.

Confirmatory Tests in Cases of Anemia

These are discussed where relevant in the individual chapters. However, it should be noted that research has tended to concentrate on very few of these, such as ferritin levels.

Exercise 7.1

A quick self-test (Answers below)

True	False	Questions
		1. A mild anemia is of little clinical significance and need not be investigated
		2. The morphological approach to the classification of the anemias is probably the most practically useful
		3. The clinical examination of an anemic patient is generally of little value
		4. The severity of anemia is primarily a clinical decision
		5. A very high leukocyte count can cause a spuriously low MCV
		6. All patients with clinically significant anemia show peripheral and central cyanosis
		7. Because the sensitivity of the RDW as a test is so low, it is useless in the diagnostic enterprise
		8. Reticulocytosis becomes obvious about 24 h after a bleed
		9. A patient who develops any reticulocyte response in reaction to a bleed can be assumed to have a normally functioning marrow
		10. All patients with anemia are pale

Exercise 7.2

Match the items in columns 1 and 2 (Answers below)

Column 1	Column 2
A. An anemic patient with bone pain and tenderness	1. Controlled by the tissues themselves
B. Microcytic anemias	2. Account for 90% of all anemias
C. Dyspnea on effort relieved by lying flat	3. A tendency for turbulent flow. This can activate hemostasis
D. A high RDW in an otherwise normal FBC	4. Currently regarded as a reliable sign of anemia
E. Blood flow through the microcirculation	5. Is likely to be suffering from a primary blood disease
F. One of the effects on the microcirculation of significant anemia	6. Should alert one to the possibility of serious disease
G. Pallor of the anterior rim of the conjunctiva	7. A classical symptom of anemia

Answers

Exercise 7.1

1: False; 2: True; 3: False; 4: True; 5: False; 6: False; 7: False; 8: True; 9: False; 10: False

Exercise 7.2

A5; B2; C7; D6; E1; F3; G4

Optional Advanced Reading

Further Notes on the MCV, MCH, MCHC, RDW, and Anisocytosis

The MCV, MCH, and MCHC are fundamentally important measurements in the FBC. These three bear a close relationship to each other, and this is significant for interpretation, particularly in cases where you receive a report without a morphological assessment. We will first consider each individually. Their interrelationships will then follow.

The Mean Cell Volume (MCV)

The MCV is a critically important parameter for the interpretation of the FBC and, as has been emphasized, is the first parameter one looks at in the interpretation of an anemia.

The MCV as reported is not simply the average of the red cells measured, but is the result of a complex algorithm involving the MCV, MCH, and MCHC. Thus these measurements must also be more thoroughly discussed, a little later.

It is important to understand the mechanisms responsible for the variations in average red cell size that one sees. This variation can be analytical or pre-analytical.

Analytical Variation in the MCV. (Some of what follows is a recap of factors already mentioned in Chapter 3).

A FALSELY LOW MCV may result from any cause of cell shrinkage. This can occur if the EDTA tube is inadequately filled or there is marked increase in plasma osmolality, such as in hyperglycemia or hypernatremia.

COLD AGGLUTININS are a well-known cause of a falsely raised MCV, since the agglutinated clumps of cells are SIZED as single cells. The MCV can be extremely high, well into levels that are impossible with pathological causes, e.g., 145 fl. Note that the RCC is falsely low, since these clumps are COUNTED as single cells, and thus the effect on the Hct is much less, although it is still inaccurate. Again notice the importance of the morphological report, here of **AUTOAGGLUTINATION.**

CELLS WITH A REDUCED HB CONCENTRA-TION (MCHC) undergo more elongation whilst passing through the aperture, leading to underestimation of the MCV. Conversely, cells with abnormally rigid membranes (e.g., sickle cells) and spherocytes with a high Hb concentration will undergo less deformation and thus the MCV will be overestimated. Note that many of the new instruments attempt to get around this problem by sphering all the red cells before they pass through the aperture.

VERY HIGH WHITE CELL COUNTS, as found particularly in chronic leukemias, can cause a falsely elevated MCV. Normally the number of white cells (effectively larger than red cells because of less deformability) passing through the aperture is tiny compared with the huge number of red cells. As the white cell count rises much above around 200×10^9/l, a small but potentially significant rise in MCV generally occurs.

Pre-analytical Variation in the MCV

The average red cell size as measured electronically can vary for a number of pathophysiological reasons.

MATURATION OF THE NUCLEUS, PARTICU-LARLY THE RATE OF MATURATION. The longer the nucleus is in existence (remember that the nucleus is extruded just before the reticulocyte stage) then

1. The longer is the total time available (for that cell) for the DNA to be transcribed with ultimately the generation of more enzymes and structural proteins,
2. The longer is the time available to respond to external growth factors and thus more growth,
3. The longer the cell remains in the G1 phase.

thus the larger the cell ultimately becomes. Defects of DNA synthesis, such as Vitamin B_{12} and folate deficiencies, are the main causes of this delay in maturation. The mechanism in those myelodysplastic syndromes that show megaloblastoid change and thus macrocytosis is less well understood. In all these cases the macrocytes tend to be OVAL in form.

INCREASED RATE OF PROLIFERATION, as, e.g., under the influence of increased levels of erythropoietin, the more likely it is that a mitotic division will be skipped, resulting in a larger cell. (Under normal circumstances daughter cells have no time to "grow" and hence are smaller than the parent. There normally is a progressive decrease in size as maturation goes on). The macrocytes here tend to be ROUND in form.

HOW WELL THE CYTOPLASM IS HEMO-GLOBINIZED. Apart from some rare congenital disorders, the essential factor here is the incorporation of iron into hemoglobin. Deficient iron incorporation and/or utilization can be due to iron deficiency or defective transport of iron into the red cell, as in the anemia of chronic disorders and the thalassemias. In consequence the cytoplasm is less well formed and the cell is smaller than normal. The cells in all these conditions also have a tendency to be OVAL, sometimes extending to ELLIPTICAL. If severe the elliptocytosis can be so marked that the cells can be pencil-shaped.

THE LIPID CONSTITUENTS OF THE RED CELL MEMBRANE. Twenty-five percent of the red cell membrane consists of cholesterol that is in equilibrium with plasma cholesterol. Some causes of hypercholesterolemia such as hypothyroidism (but not all – e.g., not in diabetes), as well as some less well-defined disturbances in lipid metabolism such as found in liver disease, are associated with change in red cell membrane structure resulting in macrocytosis. The macrocytes are ROUND and in addition target cells and stomatocytes are often found, all part and parcel of the membrane disorder.

THE PRESENCE OF MORE THAN ONE POPULATION OF RED CELLS. Should there be, for example, a macrocytic plus a microcytic population present, the resultant MCV will be the average of these. If the populations are roughly equal in size and the variation from the norm of each population is about equal, then the MCV will be normocytic; if one population predominates or its change in size from the norm is very large (or both), then the MCV will be tipped one way or the other, reflecting the imbalance.

It should be realized that a decreased or increased MCV does not necessarily mean that **ALL** the red cells are smaller or larger than normal. The instrument print out (for laboratory use) in many modern instruments provides a graph of the size of the red cells. This issue is discussed below in relation to the RDW.

Mean Cell Hemoglobin (MCH)

There is a common misconception that a decreased MCH necessarily means hypochromia. It should not be interpreted without taking the MCV into account. This is explained later.

Mean Cell Hemoglobin Concentration (MCHC)

As stated before, this is a measure of how much Hb is packed into the RBC. In the days before electronic counters (and thus still a factor in level 1 laboratories), it was a valuable indicator of whether the red cells were hypo- (<32 g/l), normo- (32–36 g/l), or hyperchromic (>36 g/l). A hyperchromic MCHC is only found in spherocytosis. However, with automated counters, the MCHC as calculated is much less sensitive in this regard, for complex reasons, particularly with regard to iron deficiency. The MCHC can be artifactually raised where there is too little blood in relation to the anticoagulant in the tube.

The Red Cell Distribution Width (RDW)

THE RDW HAS EMERGED AS PROBABLY THE MOST VALUABLE "NEW-GENERATION" RED CELL PARAMETER. IT SHOULD BE INTERPRETED IN THE LIGHT OF THE MCV.

The RDW is the coefficient of variation of red cell volume distribution and is based on the ratio of standard deviation (of the mean red cell size) to the MCV. Because it is a reflection of the SD of cell size and the MCV, caution must be exercised in the interpretation of this measurement. A very heterogeneous cell population (i.e., with a high SD), but with a high MCV can give a normal RDW, whereas an almost normal distribution of size with a low MCV can give a raised RDW. It is clear that the morphology is extremely important.

The MCV, MCH, MCHC, and RDW Should Be Correlated and Interpreted Together

Having considered the MCV, MCH, RDW, and MCHC individually in your assessment, it is important to consider the four together before finally making up your mind. The MCH should always correlate with the MCV and the MCHC, and this is mainly of importance in the assessment of hypochromia:

1. If an anemia with decreased MCV (i.e., microcytic) is associated with a **PROPORTIONATE** decrease in MCH, then the MCHC is normal, i.e., the cells are NORMOCHROMIC; and the report is flagged as such. (**BUT PLEASE NOTE!!** This normochromia is only according to the instrument – examination of the smear may well show hypochromia; and other things being equal, it is usually wise to rely on the morphology rather than on the flags. The problem here is the experience of the technologist reviewing the smear.)

2. If, in an anemia, the decrease in MCH is disproportionately more than the decrease in MCV, then the cells are HYPOCHROMIC, and the report is flagged accordingly.

The laboratory version of the FBC printout in most cases displays the RDW in relation to the red cell size in a graphic fashion. It is unfortunate in many ways that it is scarcely feasible to include this graph in the final printed report, since it is very informative. If one looks at the graphical representation of the size and distribution of red cells, a **NORMAL PATTERN** is shown in Fig. 7.9.

It is with abnormal blood pictures that the real utility of this graph, as well as the relationship between these measurements, is manifest.

Consider some typical abnormalities. See Figs. 7.10, 7.11, 7.12, 7.13 and 7.14.

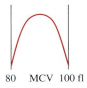

Fig. 7.9 The reported MCV is 90 fl and the RDW is 12, which is a measure of the scatter in red cell size (i.e., the degree of (in this case, normal) anisocytosis). This is a NORMOCYTIC picture. The morphology is unlikely to show any abnormalities.

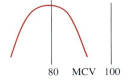

Fig. 7.10 The reported MCV is 75 fl and the RDW is 15, i.e., there is a degree of anisocytosis. It is clear that not all the cells are microcytic. Note too that the apex of the curve is just under 80, yet the MCV is 75 – this is the effect of a complex algorithm. Reported as MICROCYTOSIS. The likely morphological changes are described in the NOTE.

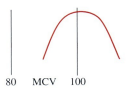

Fig. 7.11 The reported MCV is 121 fl, i.e., there is anisocytosis. Not all the cells are macrocytic. Reported as MACROCYTOSIS. The likely morphological changes are described in the NOTE.

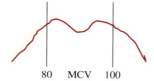

Fig. 7.12 Here the MCV is 89 fl (i.e., this is a NORMOCYTIC picture), but the RDW is given as 26.2 (i.e., there is marked anisocytosis). Likely morphological changes are described in the NOTE.

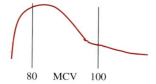

Fig. 7.13 The reported MCV is 82 fl (i.e., normocytic) and the RDW is 21.2, i.e., there is considerable anisocytosis. See the following NOTE.

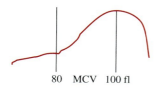

Fig. 7.14 The reported MCV is 102 fl (i.e., apparently macrocytic) and the RDW is 21.2, i.e., again there is considerable anisocytosis. See NOTE.

NOTE ON FIG. 7.10: The report will (or should) probably indicate one or more of the following: hypochromia, anisochromia, small oval cells, elliptocytes. Very occasionally very large numbers of fragmented cells can instead be responsible.

NOTE ON FIG. 7.11: As you have seen, there are numerous causes of macrocytosis, but in practice your major concern is to distinguish megaloblastosis from non-megaloblastic causes. Thus the report will (or should) probably indicate one or more of the following: oval macrocytes, tear-drop cells, and fragments (megaloblastic) OR round macrocytes, target cells, stomatocytes (liver disease, alcoholism, and hypothyroidism).

Observe the strange pattern in Fig. 7.12.

NOTE ON FIG. 7.12: The normocytic picture is the most difficult to interpret. The causes are numerous and not functionally related.

If you were to get a morphological comment on a FBC that said "There is a dimorphic red cell picture," it is this sort of thing that is being referred to in Fig. 7.12. Dimorphic pictures are discussed in Chapter 10.

Using the RDW

In most cases, after the MCV has been studied, the next thing is to look at the RDW. In general, the RDW has the following uses:

1. **TO EVALUATE THE HOMOGENEITY** of an apparently microcytic, normocytic, or macrocytic picture. For example, Figs. 7.12 and 7.13 both reflect a normocytic picture. If there were no morphological comment to indicate a dimorphic picture or other abnormalities in the red cells, you could be excused for not getting too alarmed about the FBC of the patient in Fig. 7.12. The markedly raised RDW, however, should alert you to the possibility that there is something very abnormal in that picture. You would be justified in demanding a proper morphological comment from the laboratory hematologist.

Many strange patterns are sometimes seen, such as a normocytic picture but with a tail of macrocytic cells, and so on. Examine Fig. 7.13.

NOTE ON FIG. 7.13: This is by definition a normocytic picture, but the distribution of the red cells is very odd. The bulk of the cells are hypochromic but with a distinct tail of macrocytic cells. There are many possible causes of this sort of picture. It frequently occurs in patients with chronic iron deficiency who then have a large acute bleed, resulting in considerable reticulocytosis – and reticulocytes are much larger than red cells. It can also be found in combined deficiencies of iron and vitamin B_{12} or folate but where the iron deficiency predominates. It may be found in patients with chronic liver disease and chronic bleeding as a result of portal hypertension.

The above picture is fundamentally different from that in Fig. 7.14.

NOTE ON FIG. 7.14: The picture in this figure is largely a macrocytic one but with a distinct microcytic tail. It can again be found in combined deficiencies of iron and vitamin B_{12} or folate but where the megaloblastic element predominates.

It is often difficult to work out precisely what is going on without reference to the RDW.

2. Occasionally it happens that the numerical results in a FBC are completely normal apart from an increased RDW. A morphological examination will usually show up an abnormality – e.g., a picture showing anisocytosis with numerous crenated cells, cells with odd projections, non-specifically deformed cells: this can indicate occult metastatic malignancy.

A Dynamic, Risk-Aware View of Blood Diseases, Primarily the Anemias

A recent paper[4] in the NEJM proposed a highly dynamic concept in the approach to heart failure. Prof. James Ker, of the Department of Medicine, University of Pretoria, and the author explored the possible application of the concepts presented in this part to bone marrow failure.

IN THE BROADEST TERMS, JESSUP AND BROZENA SUGGEST THAT HEART FAILURE SHOULD BE LOOKED AT IN TERMS OF A SERIES OF CLINICAL STAGES.

In **STAGE A**, the patient has significant risk factors for heart disease but no symptoms and no structural damage. The major structural change in stage B is myocardial remodeling, and thus the main thrust of treatment in stage A is the prevention of remodeling. The inclusion of a stage without heart failure in the schema of heart failure is very innovative, since it focuses the attention of the clinician on the importance of **PREVENTION** and thus the awareness of risk factors – the point being that progression to a further stage can mean permanent damage or great therapeutic difficulty in restoring the heart to normal.

STAGE B means structural heart disease without symptoms of heart failure, as found, for example, in previous myocardial infarction and valvular heart disease. Once again the attention is focused on prevention and therefore the careful clinical evaluation of a patient who does not present with symptoms, the implication being that all patients should at least be evaluated in terms of possible structural heart damage. It would be possible in many cases to restore cardiac structure to normal to varying degrees.

STAGE C represents patients with structural damage and current or previous symptoms of heart failure. This would be the "classical" stage of clinical heart failure as understood in traditional terms and would thus be classified as NYHA classes I, II, III, or IV. The chance of restoring these hearts to normal is very small.

STAGE D represents refractory heart failure despite maximal medical therapy.

Note that treatment at all stages becomes less reversible with progression along the stages.

Applying this concept to hematology seems promising, particularly the emphasis on being aware of, indeed looking for, risk factors before the development of overt disease. However, the parallels are by no means exact: most heart diseases if allowed to progress will end up with a permanently damaged myocardium, whereas much bone marrow pathology is potentially reversible. Marrow failure need not be primary; it is more commonly secondary to deficiency of nutrients, and so on, and there is a strong tendency to recovery with replacement of these nutrients. Thus marrow failure is seen in the broadest context – i.e., it includes the inability to produce blood cells both structurally and functionally normal.

Note also that it is not just the marrow that can fail but the liver and the endothelium, in terms of the hemostatic proteins.

THE FOLLOWING ARE SUGGESTED IN TERMS OF THE MARROW:

STAGE A. The patient is asymptomatic and has no structural damage to the marrow or the products of the marrow – the cells. The risk factors to consider are numerous, and only some will be mentioned, to illustrate the concept:

1. Diet, e.g., a vegetarian diet
2. Exposure to radiation, chloramphenical, co-trimoxazole, neomercazole, etc.
3. Family history of chronic hemolysis

Evaluation of stage A will involve not just history and physical examination but at least a FBC.

STAGE B. The patient has structural OR functional disease but without symptoms, such as a raised RCC, latent iron deficiency, or decreased MCV and very mild anemia in say a Greek patient (Thalassemia minor).

STAGE C. The patient has spherocytes in the blood, with a mildly enlarged spleen and episodes of jaundice. Alternatively he is pale with koilonychia and glossitis.

STAGE D. The patient has pancytopenia with aplasia of the marrow.

IN TERMS OF THE HEMOSTATIC SYSTEM, THE FOLLOWING ARE PROPOSED:

STAGE A. A family history of persistent bleeding in say a young boy.

STAGE B. A patient has a moderate decrease in factor VIII but no symptoms.

STAGE C. A patient has a moderate decrease in factor VIII with a target joint.

STAGE D. A patient has full-blown severe hemophilia.

Let us consider a man who is a heavy drinker. Early on (Stage A), there are no or minimal effects on the blood; he only has a serious risk factor for the development of blood disease (among others).

As his habit progresses, he enters stage B, with round macrocytes in the blood, very mild anemia, and a prolonged prothrombin time, but from the hematological point of view he is asymptomatic.

In stage C, he is quite significantly anemic and has a tendency to bleed excessively after trauma. The anemia is multifactorial, due partly to the liver disease per se, iron deficiency from bleeding (from the gut), and folate deficiency. His bleeding tendency is partly due to factor deficiency and partly to thrombocytopenia.

In stage D, his liver is irretrievably damaged, his marrow is becoming seriously hypoactive, and other complications such as hypersplenism are adding to the problem.

The value of the paradigm is that if this patient were seen earlier, steps could be taken to prevent the development of overt disease. This applies to any stage, but clearly the earlier the treatment is instituted the less likely permanent damage would ensue.

References

1. Dugdale AE (2006). Predicting iron and folate deficiency anemia from standard blood testing: the mechanism and implications for clinical medicine and public health in developing countries. Theor. Biol. Med. Model. 3: 34.
2. Sheth TS, Choudry NK, Bowes M, Detsky AS (1997). The relation of conjunctival pallor to the presence of anemia. J. Gen. Intern. Med. 12: 102.
3. Melo MR, et al. (2002). Rev. Assoc. Med. Bras. 48(3): 135–136.
4. Jessup M, Brozena S (2001). Heart failure. N. Engl. J. Med. 348: 2007–2017.

Further Reading

Lewis SM, Bain B, Bates I (2006). Dacie and Lewis Practical Haematology. 10th edn. Philadelphia: Churchill Livingstone.

Hoffbrand AV, Pettit JE (2001). Essential Haematology, 4th edn. Oxford: Blackwell Science.

Davis BH (2001). Diagnostic advances in defining erythropoietic abnormalities and red blood cell diseases. Sem. Hematol. 38: 148.

Defining Microcytosis

The first-stage diagnosis of "microcytosis" was reached by the recognition that the **AVERAGE** size of the red cells counted is below the reference range.

> **STEP 1:** "Where is the primary abnormality?" It lies in the MCV and therefore the size of the red cells.
>
> **STEP 2:** "What form does it take?" The MCV is decreased below the reference range.

Anemia need not be present. If there is an anemia, the anatomical diagnosis is "microcytic anemia"; otherwise, it is "a microcytic red cell picture."

> Microcytosis is by far the commonest first-stage finding in disorders of the red cells. Since it is so common, it can be expected that it frequently occurs in conjunction with other FBC abnormalities. In this chapter, however, we refer to microcytosis and microcytic anemias as *isolated disorders*. Complex conditions and combinations are discussed in several subsequent chapters.
>
> Please bear in mind the discussion in Chapter 6 with respect to normocytic pictures where the MCV is close to the lower limit of normal.
>
> In the same chapter, certain technical aspects of the measurement of the MCV and their relevance to the interpretation of the MCV were discussed; it is important to bear these in mind.

The General Pathology Causes of Microcytosis

AT THE GENERAL LEVEL THERE ARE ONLY TWO CAUSES:
1. **CERTAIN STRUCTURAL ABNORMALITIES OF THE RED CELL MEMBRANE, USUALLY HEREDITARY.** The most common of these is **HEREDITARY ELLIPTOCYTOSIS.** In the heterozygous form the red cells become elliptical soon after formation; since they enter the aperture longitudinally as a result of streamlines they are measured as smaller than normal. The MCV in these cases is usually around 75 fl. In the homozygous form (hereditary pyropoikilocytosis) and some other forms of physical damage to the red cell, very bizarre forms are seen. Physically broken red cells tend to reform in the circulation, in the process having lost a variable amount of Hb (due to the damage), and thus, when reformed are necessarily smaller than before. These cases are all hemolytic in nature, and are discussed in Chapter 10. **VERY OCCASIONALLY** the latter can cause a misleadingly and prominently decreased MCV.
2. **DEFECTIVE INCORPORATION OF IRON INTO THE RED CELL.** This results in a decreased amount of Hb in the cell, and therefore the cell is smaller than normal, since most of the cytoplasm consists of Hb. It is very important to subdivide the defective incorporation of iron as due to

   a) **DEFICIENCY OF IRON**
   b) **DEFECTIVE UPTAKE OF IRON** by the developing red cell (normoblast)

Be aware that there are a number of **SPURIOUS CAUSES OF A DECREASED MCV.** A falsely low MCV may result from any cause of cell shrinkage, as in an inadequately filled EDTA tube, or with marked increase in plasma osmolality, such as in hyperglycemia or hypernatremia.

Deficient Uptake of Iron into the Developing Normoblasts Required for the Formation of Heme

The development of normal Hb content of the developing red cell requires

1. **A NORMAL MECHANISM OF SYNTHESIS OF GLOBIN.** Note that this is dependent on the prior production of heme.
2. **A NORMAL MECHANISM OF SYNTHESIS OF HEME.** Heme synthesis requires prior synthesis of protoporphyrin, which, when Fe^{2+} is incorporated into it, becomes heme. When iron is absent, heme synthesis is defective and protoporphyrin levels increase. This in turn prevents proper hemoglobin synthesis, and therefore deficient O_2 carrying capacity. The reasons for deficient available iron are many, and have been discussed in Chapters 2 and 4.

The net effect of any of these deficiencies is the production of red cells containing less Hb than normal; since the bulk of the red cell consists of Hb, the cell is obviously going to be smaller than normal – hence "microcytic." We speak of the **HEMOGLOBINIZATION** of the red cells being defective.

THUS, IN SUMMARY: THERE ARE ONLY TWO FUNDAMENTAL POSSIBLE PATHOGENETIC PROCESSES THAT MAY BE RESPONSIBLE FOR MICROCYTOSIS AS A RESULT OF DEFECTIVE HEMOGLOBINIZATION:

a) A normal metabolic mechanism of heme synthesis but with lack of available iron
b) A sufficiency of available iron but a defective synthetic mechanism

FBC Features of Hb-Deficient Red Cells

1. **THE MCV IS BELOW NORMAL** for the patient, and morphologically the red cells appear microcytic. They also tend to show the formation of ovalocytes, elliptocytes, and target cells. A minor degree of fragmentation is not uncommon.
2. **THE MCH AND MCHC ARE BELOW NORMAL,** and morphologically the red cells generally appear hypochromic. A comment that quite commonly is seen in reports is **"ANISOCHROMIA."** In practice this terms can have two meanings:

    a) The color of the red cells or "chromicity" varies from normal to hypochromic. This usually indicates a developing or recovering iron deficiency.
    b) Two populations of red cells can be seen, one of which is hypochromic. This can have several causes; they are discussed in Chapter 7.

3. **THE RDW MAY OR MAY NOT BE SIGNIFICANTLY INCREASED.** A significant increase would be in favor of iron deficiency, anemia of chronic

disorders, or thalassemia major (in Chapter 7 we explained why thalassemia minor and intermedia could have a RDW close to normal).

Features in Other Laboratory Tests

1. Red cell protoporphyrin levels are increased.
2. Iron studies are very variable, depending on the cause of decreased iron uptake in the cell.

Common Clinical Features

There are no clinical features common to all types of defective iron incorporation. Fatigue, malaise, and so on are common, but these are relatively non-specific.

It seems clear that one way of identifying the specific cause would be the assessment of available iron. However, this neglects the other side of the equation: synthesis. Specific routine methods of assessing the synthetic mechanism are not available; however, there may be suggestive indications in the FBC itself of this.

Specific Causes of Microcytosis

There are three significant specific causes of microcytosis: **IRON DEFICIENCY, ANEMIA OF CHRONIC DISORDERS,** and **THALASSEMIA.**

1. **IRON DEFICIENCY.** Iron deficiency is in fact the commonest disease in the world; it is by no means confined even predominantly to the so-called Third World, and consequently deserves close study.
2. **ANEMIA OF CHRONIC DISORDERS (ACD).** This anemia is assuming more and more importance as people are living longer and acute diseases (mainly infections) are being brought more under control.
3. **THALASSEMIA.** This is extremely common in Third World countries, but with increasing travel and migration, more and more cases are being seen in First-World countries. As a hereditary condition it is clearly important to be able to identify the carriers, since the homozygous states can be lethal.

Microcytic anemia has profound epidemiological significance on a worldwide basis: very roughly speaking, the above three conditions are equal in incidence; but of course, in local terms, one or other may be far more common. In Cyprus, for example, a microcytic anemia is assumed to be β-thalassemia until proven otherwise – i.e., the pre-test probability is high. (It is illegal to marry there without each partner having been tested for thalassemia).

4. It is suggested that the general reader should at least have heard of two other conditions as causes (sometimes) of microcytosis: **LEAD POISONING** and **SIDEROBLASTIC ANEMIA.** These are also briefly mentioned in the Optional Advanced Reading section.

Iron Deficiency

There are only four general causes:

1. **CHRONIC BLEEDING.** This has been fully discussed in Chapter 4. In summary:

   a) Each milliliter of blood lost means a loss of 1 mg of iron.

   b) When you consider that the maximum amount of iron that can be absorbed is about 4–5 mg per day, it follows that a significant loss of blood will lead to iron deficiency once the stores are depleted.

   c) Iron stores vary considerably; it is usually a 6 months' supply in males but can be nil in females.

   d) With chronic bleeding on the one side and mildly increased absorption on the other (assuming a good diet), clearly the time taken for iron deficiency to manifest will vary a lot. In the typical case of bleeding hemorrhoids, for example, anemia will only occur after about 4 years, assuming a normal diet and an otherwise healthy marrow.

   e) It can be very difficult to find the source of bleeding. (In 10% of cases one struggles to find the source; sometimes it is never found). A distinction is made between **OCCULT** and **OBSCURE** bleeding:

      i. **OCCULT BLEEDING** refers to the presentation of iron-deficiency anemia without evidence of dietary or absorptive problems and no visible blood loss; it **MAY BE** accompanied by a positive test for occult blood in the feces.

      ii. **OBSCURE BLEEDING** refers to bleeding of unknown origin that persists or recurs after negative endoscopy.

2. **DIETARY FACTORS.** There are two broad aspects to these:

   a. **DIETARY INADEQUACY.** There are two forms of usable dietary iron:

      • **HEME IRON.** This is found in red meat and is very easily absorbed. It is already in the Fe^{2+} form and thus reducing agents, such as vitamin C or gastric acid, are not required. Gastric acid and pepsin ARE required, however, for the preliminary digestion of the food to release this heme iron.

      • **INORGANIC IRON.** This is the form found in most vegetables, dairy products, and iron tablets. Being generally in the Fe^{3+} form it does require reduction in the stomach. (Ascorbic acid has the additional role of enabling the formation of soluble iron chelates, facilitating the attachment of iron to the intestinal mucosa).

      In the "average" (I am not going to say "normal") Western diet, 80–90% of ingested iron is in the inorganic form but at least 50% of **ABSORBED** iron is heme iron, reflecting the much greater absorptive efficiency of the latter. In Third World countries and among the poor and the aged, the situation is very much worse, bearing in mind the price of red meat. There is another group where iron ingestion is very unsatisfactory – youngsters in their teens and early twenties, because of the large amount of junk food ingested. However, the metabolism in these people is different, and it is surprising how well they generally cope in terms of their iron status.

   b. **DIETARY COMPONENTS INTERFERING WITH ABSORPTION OF IRON.**
   The following is a brief list of dietary interferences:

      • Alkalis such as antacids (as well as excessive pancreatic secretion, e.g., due to fistulae)
      • Insoluble iron complexes formed from dietary phytates (e.g., as in spinach), tannates (e.g., as in tea and bran)
      • Many cereals
      • Drugs

A Note About Vegetarianism Despite the fact that our best source of iron is the heme in red meat, it is possible for vegetarians to avoid iron deficiency. A number of factors, however, play a very important role:

1. The diet should include pulses (peas, beans, and especially soybeans) as well as plenty of dairy products and salads (dark-green vegetables such as spinach should be avoided).
2. Substances that bind iron in the gut should be avoided. These include phytates (in dark-green vegetables), antacids, tetracycline, tea with meals, excessive intake of some cereals.

3. A very close watch should be kept on any untoward bleeding – the stores of iron may well be poor, with the result that overt iron deficiency could develop far more easily than otherwise.

3. **MALABSORPTION.** This has been discussed extensively in Chapter 4. To summarize the most important causes:

   a. **IMPAIRED DIGESTION.** There is a well-known aphorism that digestion starts in the mouth, and the truth of this statement is well exemplified by the nutritional anemias. Since iron is most effectively absorbed from red meat that needs to be properly digested, any interference with mastication will diminish such digestion. Thus ill-fitting dentures, the edentulous state and so on are significant causes of iron malabsorption. By the same token, achlorhydria and other diseases of the stomach, including certain operations, can also lead to poor iron absorption.

   b. **SMALL INTESTINAL MUCOSAL DISEASE.** There is a large list of possible causes. These are described in Chapter 5.

   Note, however, that one sometimes seeks in vain for a cause in many cases of proven iron malabsorption. It is estimated that malabsorption accounts for 8% of all cases of iron deficiency.

4. **INCREASED DEMAND.** A contributory factor to other causes is increased demand as in adolescence and particularly in pregnancy: the fetus acquires (from the mother) nearly 300 mg of iron, and the temporary expansion of the maternal red cell mass requires another 500 mg. Increased iron absorption throughout pregnancy and the cessation of menses is often not enough to offset these requirements.

The pathological conditions that can cause the above processes have been discussed extensively in Chapter 4.

The Characteristic Features of Established Iron Deficiency

1. FEATURES IN THE FBC.

a) Microcytic red cells, usually hypochromic as well – thus decreased MCV, MCH, MCHC
b) A variable degree of anemia

c) The presence of small oval cells, elliptocytes, pencil cells, and often some target cells
d) Raised RDW
e) Absent or minimal reticulocytosis (diffuse basophilia) unless there has also been an acute superimposed bleed
f) The neutrophils show a right shift

2. FEATURES IN OTHER LABORATORY TESTS.

a) Fasting serum iron decreased (morning specimen); this can be marked
b) Transferrin increased. This is an adaptive (physiological) response; it can also be marked
c) % Saturation therefore decreased, classically < 15%
d) Ferritin decreased
e) Serum transferrin receptor levels increased
f) ESR low, even 0 mm
g) Acute phase reactants normal
h) Bone marrow aspirate:

   • Cellularity varies from normal to increased
   • Stainable iron absent
   • Megakaryocytes and granulopoiesis normal, but minor dysplastic changes can be seen
   • Erythropoiesis increased until late, when it can decrease considerably
   • Sideroblasts (normoblasts with cytoplasm containing stainable iron granules) are absent

3. COMMON CLINICAL FEATURES AND ACCOMPANIMENTS.

If present, these are pretty specific for iron deficiency **IN THE PRESENCE OF AN ANEMIA:**

a) **KOILONYCHIA**
b) **PICA.** Typically, this is experienced as a craving for ice
c) **GLOSSITIS** (which differs from the glossitis of megaloblastosis in that the tongue is not the typical bright-red color)
d) **DYSPHAGIA,** sensed by the patient high up in the chest (due to esophageal webs)
e) **A SOURCE OF BLEEDING** (e.g., large uterine myomata)

The Characteristics of *Developing* Iron Deficiency

Iron deficiency frequently presents, or is incidentally discovered, **BEFORE** the established phase, as described above. Since it is so common, it is important to be able to recognize it if possible. For example, carcinoma of the cecum **PRESENTS** with iron deficiency; the earlier this disease can be recognized, the greater the chance of cure.

Clearly, as iron deficiency develops, it will go through various stages, each with its own pattern.

1. **IN THE EARLIEST STAGE,** iron is gradually being lost from the stores. The serum iron studies are still normal, the FBC appearance is normal. This is called **LATENT IRON DEFICIENCY,** and there is no specific clinical or laboratory feature to suspect it. It is only if a bone marrow aspirate were done – and clearly there would not normally be any indication for doing it – that one would see that stainable iron and sideroblasts are reduced, and ultimately absent. If one were really suspicious about the possibility of latent iron deficiency, one would still need considerable justification for submitting a patient to aspiration. However, red cell protoporphyrin levels (increased) are an acceptable substitute. Transferrin receptor levels are raised, and the RDW at this stage is still normal.

   As indicated above, this stage can last for a very variable time, depending on the balance between

   a) The rate of blood loss and
   b) The amount of dietary iron (and in what form), the efficacy of absorption, and the quality of the bone marrow

2. Once **IRON STORES ARE DEPLETED,** the following changes are seen:

   a) Serum iron decreases steadily.
   b) Transferrin increases steadily.
   c) % Saturation falls steadily.
   d) Stainable iron and sideroblasts are absent from the marrow.
   e) The RDW rises.
   f) A right shift of the neutrophils gradually develops.

3. It is only now that **IRON DEFICIENCY AS SUCH** is established:

   a) The % saturation is well below 15.
   b) The red cells become microcytic.
   c) The red cells start off by showing anisochromia then full-fledged hypochromia.
   d) The RDW tends to diminish.
   e) Plus the other changes as mentioned before.

Anemia of Chronic Disorders (ACD)

It was mentioned above that hemoglobinization of normoblast cytoplasm requires iron. This iron comes from the circulating iron and from the stores (all in a dynamic interchange), and is incorporated in the process of heme synthesis. The basic pathogenetic mechanism in ACD is that this incorporation of iron is blocked. Thus there is deficient iron in the normoblasts but plenty in the circulation and the stores – indeed, there is a tendency for the stores to become overloaded because while iron metabolism is otherwise (more or less) normal, iron is not being utilized.

The chronic disorders responsible can be any inflammatory or infiltrative condition, so long as it is of 6–8 weeks' duration or more. Since many of these conditions are occult, ACD can provide an important clinical clue to the presence of an underlying disease. Note that misdiagnosing ACD as iron deficiency will blind you to the possibilities; treating such an anemia with iron is not only blinding you to the possibilities, but you are doing the patient harm – she usually has more than enough iron!

The Characteristic Features of *Established* ACD

1. **FEATURES IN THE FBC.**

   a) **MICROCYTIC OR NORMOCYTIC RED CELLS** – this depends partly on the duration of the underlying disease (see below); they usually show hypochromia or anisochromia as well. Thus the MCV is decreased; however, the MCH and MCHC are often normal.
   b) **A VARIABLE DEGREE OF ANEMIA,** but the Hb is seldom below about 9 g/dl.
   c) **THE PRESENCE OF SMALL OVAL CELLS** and some contracted or crenated cells. Pencil and target cells are not characteristic.
   d) **THE RDW IS OFTEN NORMAL OR ONLY MILDLY RAISED,** unless the underlying disease is known to have a raised RDW associated, such as a malignant circulation, renal disease, and so on.
   e) **TRANSFERRIN RECEPTOR LEVELS** are normal.
   f) **THE NEUTROPHILS** do not show a right shift, unless the underlying disease is renal.
   g) **ROULEAUX** are often present, reflecting changes in plasma proteins, as a response to the underlying inflammatory or infiltrative process. Raised proteins may also cause a visible increase in background staining in the blood films.

2. **FEATURES IN OTHER LABORATORY TESTS.**

   a) **FASTING SERUM IRON DECREASED;** the decrease is never to the same extent as in iron-deficiency anemia **OF THE SAME DEGREE.**
   b) **TRANSFERRIN NORMAL OR DECREASED.** The latter is a negative acute phase response.
   c) **% SATURATION THEREFORE DECREASED,** classically > 15%
   d) **FERRITIN** normal or increased.

e) **ESR** generally raised.

f) **ACUTE PHASE REACTANTS** abnormal.

g) **BONE MARROW ASPIRATE:**

- Cellularity usually normal.
- Stainable iron normal or increased.
- Megakaryocytes and granulopoiesis normal, but minor dysplastic changes can be seen.
- Erythropoiesis may be increased.
- Sideroblasts: absent.

3. **COMMON CLINICAL FEATURES AND ACCOMPANIMENTS.** Typical features or iron deficiency are absent. The clinical features are those of the underlying disease.

The Characteristics of *Developing* ACD

As with iron deficiency, ACD has different hematological appearances depending on the stage of the causative disease. It is also a very frequent incidental discovery – the typical story is that the patient presents to the doctor with a variety of non-specific symptoms, such as loss of energy, malaise, etc. He requests an FBC and a microcytic picture is found; he proceeds to treat the patient with iron, to no avail.

The stages through which the FBC passes are not nearly as well established as with iron deficiency:

1. **ACD ALWAYS STARTS OUT AS NORMOCYTIC.** The serum iron studies are initially normal. The FBC appearance is normal unless it shows changes caused directly by the underlying disease. At this stage there is no specific clinical or laboratory feature to suspect it. However, as time passes, the MCV tends to fall slowly, and it takes anything up to 2 months for the MCV to fall below the lower limit of normal (if it ever does – see later); in the interim it may be observed that the MCV is lower than the patient's known MCV (and in a GP practice where patient records frequently go back for years, this may be apparent), and this should suggest to the doctor that the patient is tending toward microcytosis with all that it entails. If a bone marrow aspirate were done at this stage, it would be seen that stainable iron is at least normal and sideroblasts are reduced or absent. The problem here is that if one does the marrow too early, it may be impossible for the laboratory hematologist to be certain of the iron status. The same caveat applies to the serum iron studies. While the Hb and MCV fall, the serum iron studies gradually take on the characteristics of the classical ACD.

2. **EVENTUALLY THE MAJORITY OF CASES WILL BECOME MICROCYTIC.** There is no doubt, however, that a number of cases of ACD remain normocytic, even if the serum iron studies are quite characteristic.

Thalassemia

The mechanism of defective iron utilization in the developing normoblasts in the different thalassemia syndromes is due to a quantitative defect in globin synthesis. For heme to bind iron effectively, the heme itself must be bound to normal globin chains. Most of the circulating globins are a tetramer of two α-chains and two β-chains in the proper ratio. These two chains are coded separately on different chromosomes. Two broad types of genetic abnormalities produce:

1. The hemoglobinopathies, where the amino acid sequence is abnormal, i.e., a **QUALITATIVE** abnormality.

2. The **THALASSEMIAS,** where there is a **QUANTITATIVE** deficiency in the amount of the relevant chain produced. In the thalassemias there is thus a relative excess of one of the chains with a tendency to form crystals of the excess globin, having all sorts of deleterious effects:

a) Ineffective erythropoiesis due to intramedullary hemolysis.

b) A hemolytic tendency due to the red cell abnormalities (abnormal shapes, rigid cell membranes, and so on).

c) Because the globin chains are abnormal, iron cannot be incorporated into the heme moiety as efficiently. Thus the cells (not the patient) are iron deficient, and therefore microcytic and usually hypochromic.

It is very difficult to summarize the various changes that are found in the thalassemias, since there is such large variety of thalassemia syndromes. In regions where thalassemia is not endemic, only a set of general pointers will be given, to permit the suspicion of thalassemia, and hence to refer it. If the reader lives in an endemic area, it is suggested that the section in Optional Advanced Reading be read.

The Characteristic Features of Most Types of Thalassemia

1. **FEATURES IN THE FBC.**

a) The most characteristic feature is **MICROCYTHEMIA.** This refers to an increased number of red cells, but which are smaller than normal. Thus, the RCC is raised, and the MCV is decreased (i.e., microcytic); the MCH and MCHC also tend to be reduced.

b) Depending on the severity of the condition, the red cells show **ABNORMALLY SHAPED CELLS (POIKILOCYTOSIS),** which can include target cells, irregularly distorted cells, and, most typically, punctate basophilia (basophilic stippling of red cells). Consequently, the RDW can be increased.

c) Again, depending on the severity, there will be varying degrees of **ANEMIA** and diffuse basophilia (reticulocytosis).

2. FEATURES IN OTHER LABORATORY TESTS.

a) IRON STUDIES:

- Serum iron: normal to **INCREASED,** since iron absorption is **INCREASED.**
- Transferrin: levels are variable and complex in thalassemia:
  - Thalassemia minor and some cases of thalassemia intermedia: transferrin levels are normal.
  - Thalassemia major and many cases of thalassemia intermedia: transferrin levels drop.
- % Saturation: often increased.
- Ferritin: classically increased.

b) HEMOGLOBIN ANALYSIS:

- β-thalassemia: Hb electrophoresis abnormal, with HbA variably decreased, HbF variably increased, HbA$_2$ (by column chromatography) increased.
- α-thalassemia: Hb electrophoresis and HbA$_2$ are normal. Proof of α-thalassemia requires advanced PCR methodology.

c) UNCONJUGATED BILIRUBIN ("indirect") variably increased. This is because there is a hemolytic component in thalassemias. Conjugated ("direct") bilirubin may also be increased. Liver enzymes are usually normal.

3. COMMON CLINICAL ACCOMPANIMENTS.

These depend to a large degree on the genotype. Clinically, three presentations are recognized:

a) **THALASSEMIA MINOR.** The patient typically is asymptomatic; there is a microcythemia but very little in the way of poikilocytosis. The Hb is mildly decreased. Blood transfusions are never necessary.

b) **THALASSEMIA MAJOR.** The patient is seriously ill: he has usually been anemic since childhood, with growth disturbance; there typically is jaundice, skeletal changes as a result of expansion of many bones from increased intramedullary hemopoiesis (skull, maxillae, etc.), splenomegaly; regular transfusions (>2 per year) are needed. Without transfusion, the Hb is low – from 5 to 7 g/dl.

c) Thalassemia intermedia. As the name suggests, this is an intermediate stage. There is a microcythemia, some poikilocytosis, and the Hb is moderately low – around 9–10 g/dl. The patient requires no more than two transfusions per year.

Making the Diagnosis

As in all hematological disorders, it is very difficult to prescribe an approach to microcytosis, since so much depends on how the patient presents: clinical presentation is often decisive or bears a significant role in the diagnosis. On the other hand, frequently a patient will present only with vague symptoms and possibly pallor; a FBC will reveal microcytosis, which requires interpretation.

The following should be borne in mind:

1. Two or even three of these conditions could coexist.
2. Therapy of the three conditions is very different. Indeed, using the therapeutic regime of one for one of the others can be extremely deleterious. Iron therapy is indicated in iron deficiency but is contra-indicated in the other two; and iron is toxic – giving iron to someone who does not need it, particularly giving it parenterally, can lead to very serious problems.
3. Medico-legal considerations must of course always be remembered.

The clinical features are very often of considerable assistance. Even if the primary presentation is via a FBC, a proper clinical examination is essential, for various reasons (apart from the basic one of making professional and humane contact with the patient):

1. The clinical features may be so suggestive that certain possibly uncomfortable or expensive investigations may be avoided.
2. They may alert one to the possibility of combined defects, which may have an impact on therapy.

Figure 8.1 illustrates **SPECIFIC ASPECTS** of the examination of a patient in whom a microcytic blood picture is known or suspected; clearly it is part of the overall examination is as is depicted in Fig. 5.4.

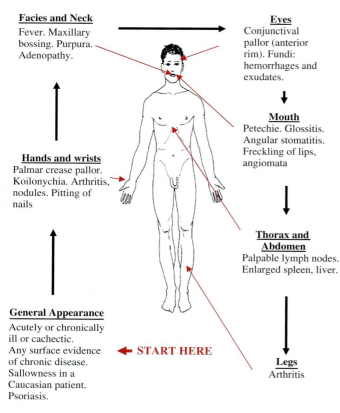

Facies and Neck
Fever. Maxillary
bossing. Purpura.
Adenopathy.

Eyes
Conjunctival
pallor (anterior
rim). Fundi:
hemorrhages and
exudates.

Mouth
Petechie. Glossitis.
Angular stomatitis.
Freckling of lips,
angiomata

Hands and wrists
Palmar crease pallor.
Koilonychia. Arthritis,
nodules. Pitting of
nails

**Thorax and
Abdomen**
Palpable lymph nodes.
Enlarged spleen, liver.

General Appearance
Acutely or chronically
ill or cachectic.
Any surface evidence
of chronic disease.
Sallowness in a
Caucasian patient.
Psoriasis.

◄ **START HERE**

Legs
Arthritis

Fig. 8.1 Examination: Microcytic Anemia

Clinically Obvious or Suggestive Cases

HERE THE BLOOD TESTS ARE ESSENTIALLY CONFIRMATORY:

1. **PROVISIONAL DIAGNOSIS OF IRON DEFICIENCY IS EASY** when one or particularly more than one of the following are present in a pale patient: pica, koilonychia, dysphagia, glossitis, blue sclerae, and a source of bleeding. The RCC, MCH, MCHC, and ESR if done are low; the microscopic features are typical with micro-ovalocytes, elliptocytes, and a right shift of the neutrophils; ferritin is decreased and iron saturation is below 15% (see Table 8.1).

Table 8.1 A Summary of the Common Patterns of Iron Studies

	Iron deficiency	ACD	Thalassemia
Serum iron	Decreased	Decreased	Normal to increased
Transferrin	Increased	Normal to decreased	Normal to decreased
% Saturation	Below 15%	Above 15%	Often raised
Ferritin	Decreased	Normal to increased	Increased

A clear history of recurrent bleeding obviously does not necessarily indicate iron deficiency, but is enough to warrant exclusion.

2. **PROVISIONAL DIAGNOSIS OF THALASSEMIA MAJOR** is usually easy: see Chapter 5 for clinical details.

3. **DIAGNOSIS OF THALASSEMIA INTERMEDIA AND MINOR.** These conditions are hardly diagnosable clinically unless there is a clear family and ethnic history. The RCC is raised, ferritin is normal or raised, saturation is over 15%. One would always suspect the possibility of thalassemia in a patient with a microcytic anemia if he is of certain heritage – Mediterranean or from the vicinity of the Black Sea (it will be remembered that the Attic and Ionian Greeks established trading colonies in these areas in ± 600 BC), Africa, the Far East. However, sporadic cases can occur in any population – some very rarely, and consequently often not thought of; and it is important that the possibility of thalassemia is always borne in mind when dealing with a microcytic anemia, because of the danger of administering iron to thalassemics.

4. **ACD** can encompass so many clinical presentations that it is not feasible to suggest any means of clinical diagnosis. The RCC and MCH are low, the ESR is raised.

In all other cases the diagnosis is exclusively by blood tests.

Clinically Undefined Cases

A COMMON MISCONCEPTION!!! Microcytosis does NOT, repeat NOT, equate to Iron Deficiency!!!!

THE FIRST AND MOST CRUCIAL DECISION TO BE MADE IS WHETHER THE MICROCYTOSIS IS CAUSED BY IRON DEFICIENCY OR NOT – AS STATED, TREATING A NON-IRON-DEFICIENCY MICROCYTIC PICTURE WITH IRON IS AT BEST A WASTE AND AT WORST SERIOUSLY DANGEROUS TO THE PATIENT.

The distinction between the three most common causes of microcytosis is generally quite straightforward using a combination of clinical skills, iron studies, activity tests, and Hb electrophoresis. The only significant problems arise when there are combinations present.

The differentiating features are essentially via the blood tests as described above. Bone marrow aspiration is seldom necessary; if done, the most valuable diagnostic features are the patterns of stainable iron in the stores and the sideroblasts. Iron deficiency will show absence of both; ACD will show normal to increased storage iron but decreased sideroblasts; and thalassemia will show increased storage iron and perhaps increased sideroblasts.

In all cases iron studies are mandatory, about which there are a few words of warning. Iron studies comprise serum iron and transferrin levels, with a percentage saturation, as well as ferritin levels. There can be no dispute about the diagnosis of iron deficiency if (see Table 8.1)

1. The serum iron is **LOW.**
2. The transferrin levels are **RAISED**
3. The percentage saturation is **BELOW 15.**
4. Ferritin levels are **LOW.**

However, a number of caveats should be noted:

1. The blood for iron studies should be drawn in the early morning after an overnight fast. A meal can lead to sufficient iron being absorbed (in the short term) so as to raise the serum iron level temporarily. Similarly, because serum iron levels follow a diurnal variation, drawing the blood at another time may also lead to a misleadingly normal serum iron. In both cases, it should be clear that the saturation can temporarily and misleadingly be over 15%.
2. Even if the iron studies do not unequivocally indicate iron deficiency, it can still be present. The operating characteristics particularly of serum iron and transferrin are not ideal. Ferritin is an acute phase reactant and any intercurrent infective, inflammatory, or infiltrative disorder (which may indeed be subclinical) can spuriously raise the ferritin levels into the normal range.
3. Associated other hematological disorders can be serious confounders, notably anemia of chronic disorders, thalassemia, folate deficiency, and vitamin B_{12} deficiency. These possible combinations will be discussed shortly.

> If the iron studies in a patient with a microcytic anemia are all typical of iron deficiency, you are in most cases obliged to further investigate the patient for the cause (the exception being in younger patients without evidence of bleeding, when it is permissible to administer iron *for a short period* (up to a month), with careful monitoring of the reticulocyte count and Hb). Unless there

> is something unusual, there is no justification in submitting the patient to further confirmatory tests (of iron deficiency).

> **A Note About Occult Blood Testing of Feces** There are two main techniques: biochemical and immunochemical. Measured operating characteristics vary considerably in different hands. Both methods appear to be of high specificity – in the order of 90%, but the sensitivity is fairly low. The tests are generally used to exclude a bleeding lesion in the GIT. But there are methodological problems, notably verification bias: it is unethical to submit a patient with a negative test to colonoscopy unless there are other suggestive features.
>
> In general, 5% of tests performed on standard-risk patients will be positive, and of these 75% will have no abnormality (Epstein 1996).
>
> Also, it is clear that most lesions do not bleed all the time, and some never bleed, including an estimated 20% of colonic carcinomas.
>
> The tests should be requested and interpreted with circumspection.

NOTES

1. Patients with ACD quite frequently have associated underlying iron deficiency. An important question is how far one should go in looking for this:

   a) The patient will benefit and possibly respond better to the treatment of the chronic condition if concomitant iron deficiency is corrected.

   b) Giving such a patient iron in any form is contraindicated unless a measure of iron deficiency co-exists.

      If there is any doubt at all, the simplest way to exclude iron deficiency is by serum transferrin receptor assay if available. If not, a bone marrow aspirate may be of assistance. Failing this, it is suggested that the chronic disorder be treated; as it responds and the Hb does not normalize, iron studies should be repeated.

2. In the case of thalassemia, confirmation may be

   a) **VERY EASY,** in the case of uncomplicated β-thalassemia:

      i. Iron studies show normal saturation and normal to raised ferritin levels.

ii. Hemoglobin electrophoresis shows a raised HbF and HbA$_2$.

b) **VERY DIFFICULT,** in the case of α-thalassemia, any thalassemia complicated by iron deficiency, or one of the rare genotypes:

  i. α-thalassemia:

  - Iron studies are as with uncomplicated β-thalassemia.
  - Hb electrophoresis is normal. Diagnosis is very complex.

  ii Thalassemia plus iron deficiency. This is discussed below.

  iii Rare genotypes. These can be extremely complex, and all require referral. The problem is to identify these cases as thalassemia in the first place.

Combined Iron Deficiency and Anemia of Chronic Disorders

It can readily be seen that this combination can occur in any chronic infiltrative or inflammatory disorder that also causes chronic bleeding. An example would be extensive and active Crohn disease, where the ileum is minimally involved.

It can also be found where the therapy of a chronic disorder has bleeding, usually gastro-intestinal, as a complication. The classical example here is in the therapy of rheumatoid arthritis with particularly some of the older forms of NSAIDS, or indeed with aspirin. Of course, the two conditions can occur independently.

The problem lies in the diagnosis of the microcytosis with which the patient has presented. **THE TYPICAL FEATURES IN THE LAB REPORTS ARE AS FOLLOWS:**

1. The Hb is typically lower than would be found with ACD alone.
2. The morphology may show the presence of rouleaux.
3. The iron studies are complicated, but often a fairly typical pattern is found:

   a) The serum iron is low.
   b) The transferrin is within the normal range.
   c) The % saturation is below 15%.
   d) The ferritin is normal or raised.

4. The acute phase proteins including the ESR will be raised – **THIS USUALLY IS THE KEY TO THE DIAGNOSIS** – i.e., an iron-deficient picture with a raised ESR or CRP. However, the picture can be confusing and one is tempted to order a bone marrow examination. This seldom gives an incontrovertible answer.

Combined Iron Deficiency and Thalassemia

There is no common causation, but patients with thalassemia are prone to all the usual causes of iron deficiency. The features of this combination can be very complex, but to simplify:

1. The Hb is seldom of much help in differentiation, nor are the MCV and RCC – the microcythemia persists.
2. The iron studies may be of assistance, in that the ferritin may be low or low normal, which in the face of a microcythemia is unexpected.
3. **THE MAJOR POINT HERE IS THAT HB ELECTROPHORESIS STUDIES CANNOT BE RELIED UPON** – iron deficiency will mask the typical electrophoretic pattern of thalassemia. Iron deficiency must be confirmed and corrected before repeating tests for thalassemia.

Combined Iron Deficiency and Folate or Vitamin B$_{12}$ Deficiency

This combination is by no means uncommon and usually produces a normocytic picture; as such the condition is discussed in Chapter 10. Sometimes the iron deficiency is the prominent feature, masking the effect of other deficiencies. What typically happens in these cases is that, once the cause of iron deficiency is located and treated, the Hb is seen to increase up to a sub-optimal point and then stop increasing. At this stage the morphological features of mild megaloblastosis may become obvious or assay of the relevant blood levels will show the deficiency. **IT IS NOT RECOMMENDED THAT ALL CASES OF IRON DEFICIENCY SHOULD BE INVESTIGATED FOR A MASKED DEFICIENCY OF FOLATE OR VITAMIN B$_{12}$.**

Features in Favor of Iron Deficiency

1. One or ideally more of pica, koilonychia, glossitis, dysphagia, and a source of bleeding or a poor diet or possible malabsorption.
2. Decreased MCV, MCH, MCHC, and RCC. A right shift of the neutrophils. No rouleaux. Normal or low ESR and CRP.

!

3. Decreased serum iron, raised transferrin, saturation below 15%, and a decreased ferritin.

Features in Favor of Anemia of Chronic Disorders

1. A recognizable chronic inflammatory or infiltrative condition of at least 4 weeks' standing.
2. Decreased MCV, MCH, MCHC, and RCC. The Hb is not below 9 g/dl. Rouleaux. No right shift of the neutrophils unless there is renal disease. Raised ESR and CRP.
3. Decreased serum iron, decreased or normal transferrin, saturation above 15%, and a normal or increased ferritin.

Features in Favor of a Thalassemia

1. Clinical features suggestive of thalassemia major: short stature, maxillary bossing, sallow complexion.
2. Pallor and sallowness in a patient currently or originally from an endemic area. Possibly a history of requiring transfusions chronically.
3. Decreased MCV and MCH, normal MCHC, and *raised RCC*. No rouleaux. No right shift of the neutrophils. Normal ESR and CRP.
4. Normal or increased serum iron, normal transferrin, saturation above 15%, and an increased ferritin. Hb electrophoresis may or may not be positive.

The Value of Splenomegaly in Microcytosis Unlike in many other anemias, splenomegaly does not play a large role in the differentiation of a microcytic anemia.

Mild splenomegaly may be found in chronic iron deficiency and in ACD (as part of the underlying pathology); and of course is typical of thalassemia major. Splenomegaly is, however, very much against the diagnosis of thalassemia minor and intermedia.

Massive splenomegaly in a case of microcytic anemia, if iron deficiency is proven, is likely to be due to chronic bleeding from varices due to portal hypertension. In a proven ACD, such a splenomegaly would strongly suggest an infiltrating lesion such as lymphoma.

Teaching Cases

CASE #14 (TABLES 8.2 AND 8.3)

Table 8.2

Patient	Age	Sex	Race	Altitude
Mr J v T	56 yrs	Male	White	5,000 ft

This patient was seen by an internist who found a microcytic anemia; iron deficiency was confirmed by iron studies. No cause for bleeding was found and there was nothing to suggest malabsorption or dietary inadequacy. Stools for occult blood were submitted and all found to be negative. The doctor felt that a trial of iron therapy was justified and repeated reticulocyte counts and Hb estimations failed to show any response. The patient was then referred.

			Reference range		Permitted range	
	Value	Units	Low	High	Low	High
Red cell count	**4.33**	× 10¹²/l	4.77	5.83	4.20	4.46
Hemoglobin (Hb)	**10**	g/dl	13.8	18.0	9.7	10.4
Hematocrit (Hct)	**0.32**	l/l	0.42	0.53	0.31	0.33
Mean cell volume	**74**	fl	80	99	68.8	79.2
Mean cell Hb	**23.1**	pg	27	31.5	22.6	23.6
Mean cell Hb conc.	**31.2**	g/dl	31.5	34.5	30.6	31.8
Red cell dist. width	**17.6**	%	11.6	14	17.6	17.6
Retic. count %	0.98	%	0.27	1.00	1.0	1.0
Retic. absolute (abs.)	42.4	× 10⁹/l	30	100	41.2	43.7
White cell count	6.68	× 10⁹/l	4	10	6.18	7.18
Neutrophils abs.	**3.81**	× 10⁹/l	2	7	3.52	4.09
Band cells abs.	0		0	0	0	0
Lymphocytes abs.	1.76	× 10⁹/l	1	3	1.63	1.89
Monocytes abs.	0.74	× 10⁹/l	0.2	1	0.69	0.80
Eosinophils abs.	0.30	× 10⁹/l	0.02	0.5	0.28	0.32
Basophils abs.	0.07	× 10⁹/l	0.02	0.1	0.07	0.08
Normoblasts	0	/100 WBC	0	0		
Platelet count	304.0	× 10⁹/l	150	400	281.2	326.8
Sedimentation	1	mm/h	0	10	1	1

Table 8.3

	Value	Units	Low	High
S-Ferritin male	**8.9**	μg/l	20.0	250.0
S-Iron	**7.9**	μmol/l	11.6	31.3
S-Transferrin	**3.61**	g/l	2.12	3.60
S-Fe saturation	**8.1**	%	20.0	50.0

DISCUSSION

1. There can be no doubt that the diagnosis of iron deficiency is correct.
2. The normal reticulocyte, platelet, and neutrophil counts suggest that there is no significant active bleeding.
3. The low ESR also is in keeping with iron deficiency.

FURTHER EXAMINATION

On examination no abnormalities apart from mild pallor were found. A very careful history elicited a pattern of vaguely alternating diarrhea and constipation. The patient was submitted to colonoscopy, and a large fungating carcinoma was found near the hepatic flexure.

Comment

1. Even though the various tests on feces for detection of occult bleeding have fair specificity, they are by no means infallible. It should be remembered that of all the special investigations available to find the source of occult bleeding, colonoscopy has by far the highest yield, although this does depend on the experience of the operator; barium enema with double contrast can have the same degree of yield, but again this depends on the operator.

2. The common practice of approaching occult iron deficiency by trial of therapy can only be justified in a young patient. Even then, it should not continue for more than a month if the response is sub-optimal – "optimal" being

   a) A significant reticulocyte response, i.e., well above $100 \times 10^9/l$
   b) A steadily rising MCV and Hb
   c) Restoration of normal Hb within at the latest 2 months

3. Treating an *undefined* microcytic anemia in this way is absolutely contra-indicated.

CASE #15 (EXAMINE TABLES 8.4 AND 8.5)

DISCUSSION

1. The major question is – can one be justified in ascribing the iron deficiency to her diet? She is only one of

---

Table 8.4

Patient	Age	Sex	Race	Altitude
Miss J O	20 yrs	Female	White	5,000 ft

The patient is a 3rd year medical student. Self-testing in a laboratory class showed a Hb of 9 g/dl. She was then referred by the student health service. The patient lives in a student commune and has a very good socio-economic background. Her only complaint is tiredness, which she puts down to pressures of work (and play). On systematic questioning she reveals that she subsists almost exclusively on vegetarian pizza and soft drinks; this appears to be a standard diet for all the residents. Physical examination is non-contributory.

	Value	Units	Reference range Low	Reference range High	Permitted range Low	Permitted range High
Red cell count	**4.01**	$\times 10^{12}/l$	4.03	5.09	3.89	4.13
Hemoglobin (Hb)	**10.8**	g/dl	12.7	15.9	10.4	11.2
Hematocrit (Hct)	**0.31**	l/l	0.38	0.49	0.30	0.32
Mean cell volume	**77.2**	fl	80	99	75.7	78.7
Mean cell Hb	**26.9**	pg	27	31.5	26.4	27.5
Mean cell Hb conc.	**34.9**	g/dl	31.5	34.5	34.2	35.6
Red cell dist. width	**16.4**	%	11.6	14	16.4	16.4
Retic. count %	1.14				1.1	1.2
Retic. absolute (abs.)	45.7	$\times 10^9/l$	30.0	100	44.3	47.1
White cell count	8.43	$\times 10^9/l$	4	10	7.80	9.06
Neutrophils abs.	4.42	$\times 10^9/l$	2	7	4.09	4.75
Band cells abs.	0.00		0	0.00	0.00	0.00
Lymphocytes abs.	2.96	$\times 10^9/l$	1	3	2.74	3.18
Monocytes abs.	0.68	$\times 10^9/l$	0.2	1	0.63	0.73
Eosinophils abs.	0.28	$\times 10^9/l$	0.02	0.5	0.26	0.30
Basophils abs.	0.09	$\times 10^9/l$	0.02	0.1	0.09	0.10
Normoblasts	0	/100 WBC	0	0		
Platelet count	259.0	$\times 10^9/l$	150	400	233.1	284.9
Sedimentation	2	mm/h	0	20	2	2
Morphology	The red cells are microcytic and show moderate anisocytosis and anisochromia, with a number of small ovalocytes. Iron studies are indicated.					

Table 8.5

			Low	High
S-Ferritin	**11.4**	µg/l	14.0	233.1
S-Iron	**9.91**	µmol/l	11.6	31.3
S-Transferrin	3.55	g/l	2.12	3.60
S-Fe saturation	**12.1**	%	15.0	35.0

---

many partaking of the same diet, so either they are all mildly iron deficient or there is an additional source of bleeding or malabsorption in this patient or there is something idiosyncratic about her metabolism. At our urging, she got the other members of her commune to be tested for Hb (although in view of the disparity between the results of the hemoglobinometer and the electronic counter, the results were perhaps doubtful – see later). Predictably, all the male students had normal levels; the other females too also appeared normal. Some of the latter were concerned, however, and had themselves tested at the hematology department: while the results showed differences from the hemoglobinometer, they were nevertheless just within the reference ranges. It was not considered ethical to suggest bone marrow studies, although these would have provided interesting information on their iron status.

Subsequent further questioning of the patient revealed that the economic status of the family had not always been good, and that she had experienced her menarche at the age of 10, suggesting that her iron stores had always been poor.

2. It is noteworthy how few youngsters subsisting on junk food develop nutritional deficiencies, at least of clinical significance. Why some develop these and not others is not known.

3. Outpatient hemoglobinometers need very careful operation as well as constant calibration to be reliable. Generally their use is falling away.

PROGRESS

On consideration it was decided to treat her as a dietary deficiency (relative to the state of her stores). She was prescribed a proper diet as well as an iron maltose preparation, and the reticulocyte count, Hb, and MCV monitored regularly. She responded very satisfactorily.

Note that she was enjoined to continue with the iron preparation for 6 months after her FBC had normalized.

!

Comment It is very important that the treatment of any iron deficiency does nor stop once the FBC has achieved normality. Treatment should continue for at least 6 months, to replenish the iron stores.

CASE #16 (EXAMINE TABLE 8.6)

This FBC is quite typical of iron deficiency, and iron studies confirmed this.

DISCUSSION

1. Clinically, one could have strongly suspected iron deficiency, because of pallor, koilonychia, and alternating diarrhea and constipation (in its turn suggesting a lesion in the colon).

Table 8.6

Patient	Age	Sex	Race	Altitude
Mr J K	84 yrs	Male	White	5,000 ft

The patient had been found to be weak, pale, and in mild cardiac failure. He was admitted to a general ward. The initial history was not contributory. He complained of marked constipation with episodes of diarrhea. He was found to be pale, ill, and somewhat underweight, with koilonychia. There were no features suggestive of a bleeding lesion. He said his diet was satisfactory. He lives in an old-age home. His FBC follows:

	Value	Units	Reference range Low	Reference range High	Permitted range Low	Permitted range High
Red cell count	3.51	× 10¹²/l	4.77	5.83	3.40	3.62
Hemoglobin (Hb)	9.4	g/dl	13.8	18.0	9.1	9.7
Hematocrit (Hct)	0.25	l/l	0.42	0.53	0.25	0.26
Mean cell volume	72.1	fl	80	99	67.1	77.1
Mean cell Hb	26.8	pg	27	31.5	26.2	27.3
Mean cell Hb conc.	37.1	g/dl	31.5	34.5	36.4	37.9
Red cell dist. width	16.3	%	11.6	14	16.3	16.3
Retic. count %	0.91	%	0.27	1.00	0.9	0.9
Retic. absolute (abs.)	31.9	× 10⁹/l	30	100	31.0	32.9
White cell count	8.65	× 10⁹/l	4	10	8.00	9.30
Neutrophils abs.	4.24	× 10⁹/l	2	7	3.92	4.56
Band cells abs.	0.00		0	0	0	0
Lymphocytes abs.	2.93	× 10⁹/l	1	3	2.71	3.15
Monocytes abs.	0.96	× 10⁹/l	0.2	1	0.89	1.03
Eosinophils abs.	0.44	× 10⁹/l	0.02	0.5	0.41	0.47
Basophils abs.	0.08	× 10⁹/l	0.02	0.1	0.07	0.08
Normoblasts	0	/100 WBC	0	0		
Platelet count	209.0	× 10⁹/l	150	400	193.3	224.7
Sedimentation	4	mm/h	0	10	4	4
Morphology	The red cells are hypochromic and microcytic and show considerable anisocytosis with oval and elliptical poikilocytes. The neutrophils show a right shift.					

2. In the lab tests there is no doubt that the patient had an iron deficiency.

3. There are a number of very instructive points so far:

   a) In patients of this age one must be very careful, since malignancy is always high on the cards. The history of constipation evidently with episodes of diarrhea is alarming.

   b) The fact that he resides in an old-age home could lead one to think that his diet is satisfactory. This unfortunately is not always true. Apart from the inherent problems of institutional cooking, specific individual problems of feeding, boredom, and so on can lead to sub-optimal nutrition. These diets are also frequently poor in roughage.

4. While a right shift undoubtedly is a feature of iron deficiency, it can also indicate associated folate or

vitamin B$_{12}$ deficiency, or renal disease, all of which are possible in this patient.

FURTHER INVESTIGATIONS

1. Renal function was evaluated and found to be satisfactory for his age.
2. Vitamin B$_{12}$ and folate levels were found to be satisfactory.
3. His bowel was prepared for gastro- and colonoscopy. It was noted at the time that his colon was almost impacted with feces. Both gastroscopy and colonoscopy revealed no pathology.
4. A dietitian's assessment was now sought. The report, in brief, was that his diet was satisfactory in red meat, vegetables, and salads, but very poor in fiber.
5. The patient's pathology now had become a conundrum.

The solution came about fortuitously. While on a teaching round, the consultant noted that the patient's false teeth were in a glass next to the bed. Upon being asked why, the patient said that his teeth hurt him. An examination of the mouth revealed numerous infected ulcers. A subsequent dental consultation confirmed that the teeth were very ill fitting. When the patient was asked again about his meat intake, it having been noted by the dietician that he had red meat five times a week, he said that indeed he started eating his food and then after a mouthful of two, had to remove his teeth and eat only soft food.

FOLLOW-UP

His prostheses were corrected, and the mouth ulcers treated. It was then confirmed that he could chew properly. The patient recovered well. Note that the history of constipation was related to fecal impaction, with overflow diarrhea.

CASE #17 (EXAMINE TABLES 8.7 AND 8.8)

DISCUSSION

1. The diagnosis of iron deficiency is doubtful, mainly because of the iron saturation and the ESR. Note that the lack of response to oral iron is **NOT** in itself a cause for this doubt.
2. Serum transferrin receptors were not at the time available, and the patient was submitted to bone marrow examination, which showed, in brief:

   a) Mildly hyperplastic erythropoiesis but normal granulopoiesis and megakaryopoiesis. Lymphocytes were slightly prominent at 24%, but morphologically normal.

Table 8.7

Patient	Age	Sex	Race	Altitude
Mrs T V	31 yrs	Female	White	2,500 ft

The patient was referred with a FBC that had been interpreted by the clinician as that of iron deficiency. The patient had not responded to iron therapy. Her history was unproductive. She was a businesswoman with a busy social life, and had lately felt run down and lacking her usual verve. She was of Dutch origin, making thalassemia unlikely. On examination there was nothing to suggest iron deficiency or chronic disease. She presented with the following FBC and iron studies:

	Value	Units	Reference range Low	Reference range High
Red cell count	3.58	× 10^{12}/l	3.91	4.94
Hemoglobin (Hb)	10.1	g/dl	12.4	15.5
Hematocrit (Hct)	0.28	l/l	0.37	0.47
Mean cell volume	77.1	fl	80	99
Mean cell Hb	28.2	pg	27	31.5
Mean cell Hb conc.	36.6	g/dl	31.5	34.5
Red cell dist. width	16.5	%	11.6	14
White cell count	6.98	× 10^9/l	4	10
Neutrophils abs.	2.99	× 10^9/l	2	7
Band cells abs.	0.00		0	0
Lymphocytes abs.	2.99	× 10^9/l	1	3
Monocytes abs.	0.64	× 10^9/l	0.2	1
Eosinophils abs.	0.29	× 10^9/l	0.02	0.5
Basophils abs.	0.08	× 10^9/l	0.02	0.1
Normoblasts	0	/100 WBC	0	0
Platelet count	387.0	× 10^9/l	150	400
Sedimentation	21	mm/h	0	20

Table 8.8

			Low	High
S-Ferritin	159.2	µg/l	14.0	233.1
S-Iron	9.01	µmol/l	11.6	31.3
S-Transferrin	2.29	g/l	2.12	3.60
S-Fe saturation	15.1	%	25.0	35.0

b) Iron stores were graded as normal but sideroblasts were absent, strongly in favor of ACD.

FOLLOW-UP

The patient was re-examined very carefully. The only positive feature was very mild tenderness to percussion over the right loin posteriorly. Abdominal sonography revealed a hydronephrosis on the right side. CT examination confirmed this and showed the presence of an infiltrating tumor around and compressing the right ureter. Subsequent investigation by a urologist showed the mass to be a small cell lymphoma, confirmed by immunophenotyping. The patient responded extremely well to chemotherapy, and the anemia disappeared. Points to note:

1. The lymphocyte count in the peripheral blood is relatively high – there is almost a reversal of the neutrophil:lymphocyte ratio. Subsequent morphological examination of the blood smear showed only some non-specific atypia of the lymphocytes. Of interest was that no right shift of the neutrophils was observed, despite the hydronephrosis; this too was against the diagnosis of iron deficiency.

2. The ESR is also relatively high – indeed, if one were to look at the permitted range of this ESR, one could see that this was 19–21; the ESR could thus undoubtedly have been abnormal. It was in any case far too high to be compatible with iron deficiency.

CASE #18 (TABLES 8.9 AND 8.10)

Table 8.9

Patient	Age	Sex	Race	Altitude
Mr Y F	31 years	Male	Burmese	5,000 ft

The patient is a Buddhist monk. On a visit to a local family doctor he was found to have a microcytic anemia. He was seen by a physician who found no cause for iron deficiency or ACD, and no evidence of thalassemia. The patient was referred. Communication was a major problem, and indeed no helpful history was forthcoming. He appeared well, and physical examination was quite normal. Evidently he had required a blood transfusion on three occasions before, and had on occasion been given iron.

	Value	Units	Reference range Low	High	Permitted range Low	High
Red cell count	**5.97**	$\times 10^{12}$/l	4.77	5.83	5.79	6.15
Hemoglobin (Hb)	**12.5**	g/dl	13.8	18.0	12.1	12.9
Hematocrit (Hct)	0.46	l/l	0.42	0.53	0.45	0.47
Mean cell volume	**77.1**	fl	80	99	71.7	82.5
Mean cell Hb	**20.9**	pg	27	31.5	20.5	21.4
Mean cell Hb conc.	**27.2**	g/dl	31.5	34.5	26.6	27.7
Red cell dist. width	**14.2**	%	11.6	14	14.2	14.2
Retic. count %	**1.91**	%	0.27	1.00	0.0	0.0
Retic. absolute (abs.)	**114.4**	$\times 10^9$/l	30	100	0.0	0.0
White cell count	7.65	$\times 10^9$/l	4	10	7.08	8.22
Neutrophils abs.	4.38	$\times 10^9$/l	2	7	4.05	4.70
Band cells abs.	0		0	0	0	0
Lymphocytes abs.	2.01	$\times 10^9$/l	1	3	1.86	2.16
Monocytes abs.	0.73	$\times 10^9$/l	0.2	1	0.68	0.79
Eosinophils abs.	0.47	$\times 10^9$/l	0.02	0.5	0.43	0.50
Basophils abs.	0.06	$\times 10^9$/l	0.02	0.1	0.06	0.07
Normoblasts	0	/100 WBC	0	0		
Platelet count	357.0	$\times 10^9$/l	150	400	330.2	383.8
Sedimentation	4	mm/h	0	10	4	4
Morphology			There is a microcythemia. The red cells are mildly hypochromic. The reticulocyte preparation shows no morphological abnormality.			

Table 8.10

			Low	High
S-Ferritin male	**287.3**	μg/l	20.0	250.0
S-Iron	13.6	μmol/l	11.6	31.3
S-Transferrin	2.65	g/l	2.12	3.60
S-Fe saturation male	22	%	20.0	50.0

DISCUSSION

1. The FBC picture was very suspicious of thalassemia (microcythemia, nearly normal RDW).

2. The racial background raised suspicions of **ALPHA**-thalassemia or possibly HbE disease or trait.

3. Both of these were supported by the raised ferritin levels (it will be remembered that iron absorption is increased in thalassemia; in addition the patient had evidently had blood transfusions previously.

4. Hemoglobin electrophoresis showed no abnormalities whatsoever. At the time, confirmatory tests for α-thalassemia were not easily available, Nevertheless, one felt confident in making the diagnosis.

CASE #19 (TABLES 8.11 AND 8.12)

Table 8.11

Patient	Age	Sex	Race	Altitude
Mr J McA	57 yrs	Male	White	5,000 ft

This patient had presented to his family doctor with fatigue and loss of vigor. He was found to be pale but no other features were observed. There was no history of dysphagia, glossitis, or bleeding. He was of Scottish origin. Stools were regular and normal in appearance. There were no hemorrhoids. The GP requested the following FBC. He followed this up with iron studies, feces for occult blood, and a CRP (to exclude significant chronic disease).

	Value	Units	Reference range Low	High	Permitted range Low	High
Red cell count	**4.55**	$\times 10^{12}$/l	4.77	5.83	4.41	4.69
Hemoglobin (Hb)	**10.3**	g/dl	13.8	18.0	9.9	10.7
Hematocrit (Hct)	**0.34**	l/l	0.42	0.53	0.33	0.35
Mean cell volume	**69.1**	fl	80	99	61.8	75.2
Mean cell Hb	**22.6**	pg	27	31.5	22.2	23.1
Mean cell Hb conc.	**30.6**	g/dl	31.5	34.5	30.0	31.2
Red cell dist. width	**16.4**	%	11.6	14	16.4	16.4
Retic. count %	**0.22**	%	0.27	1.00	0.2	0.2
Retic. absolute (abs.)	**10.0**	$\times 10^9$/l	30	100	9.7	10.3
White cell count	**4.12**	$\times 10^9$/l	4	10	3.81	4.43
Neutrophils abs.	**2.02**	$\times 10^9$/l	2	7	1.87	2.17
Band cells abs.	0.00		0	0	0	0
Lymphocytes abs.	1.45	$\times 10^9$/l	1	3	1.34	1.56

Table 8.11 (continued)

	Value	Units	Low	High	Low	High
Monocytes abs.	0.35	× 10⁹/l	0.2	1	0.33	0.38
Eosinophils abs.	0.25	× 10⁹/l	0.02	0.5	0.23	0.27
Basophils abs.	0.05	× 10⁹/l	0.02	0.1	0.04	0.05
Normoblasts	0	/100 WBC	0	0		
Platelet count	**156.1**	× 10⁹/l	150	400	144.3	167.7
Sedimentation	**1**	mm/h	0	10	1	1

No morphological
report was given.

Table 8.12

	Value	Units	Low	High
C-reactive protein	**5.2**	mg/l	0.0	10.0
S-Ferritin male	**5.1**	µg/l	20.0	250.0
S-Iron	**5.51**	µmol/l	11.6	31.3
S-Transferrin	**3.74**	g/l	2.12	3.60
S-Fe saturation male	**5.8**	%	20.0	50.0

A stool specimen for occult blood was negative

DISCUSSION

1. The diagnosis of iron deficiency is not in doubt.
2. A single specimen for occult blood analysis is not sufficient – it is recommended that at least three be submitted on separate days.
3. Further investigation of (or referral for investigation of) such a patient is necessary, in view of the patient's age.
4. Note the relatively low neutrophil and platelet counts. This is sometimes found in chronic iron deficiency, which can even cause pancytopenia. See Table 8.13 for follow-up.

FURTHER DISCUSSION

1. Angiodysplasia confined to the small bowel is not uncommon, and poses a specific diagnostic challenge.

Table 8.13

Follow up:
1. The clinical findings were confirmed. There was no suggestion of malabsorption and it was felt that thalassemia was very unlikely, partly because of the late onset of disease, the low RCC, and the race.
2. Gastroscopy with duodenal biopsy and colonoscopy were performed and no lesions were discovered.
3. The patient was referred for radio-nuclide scanning for blood loss and the results were ambiguous. Enteroscopy was eventually managed and numerous angiodysplastic lesions were discovered in the jejunum. These were cauterized. The patient subsequently did very well and his iron deficiency responded to oral iron therapy.

2. Diagnosis by enteroscopy is always preferable since cautery is possible – indeed, no other treatment is possible unless the lesion is very localized.

Comment There are several reasons for iron-deficiency anemia not to respond to iron therapy:

1. The diagnosis is wrong – the patient has a microcytic anemia due to another cause.
2. If oral iron therapy is used, the patient may have malabsorption.
3. The patient is actively losing blood, such that the marrow cannot catch up, even with plentiful iron.
4. The patient is not complying with treatment. Some iron preparations may cause considerable discomfort, with nausea, vomiting, abdominal pain.
5. The patient is ingesting iron-chelating medicines or foods, drinking tea with the iron preparation, or taking certain other drugs.

Exercise Cases

CASE #20 (TABLE 8.14)

Table 8.14

Patient	Age	Sex	Race	Altitude
Mr J B	55 yrs	Male	White	5,000 ft

The patient is a storekeeper. His history is long and unusual. He states that about 10 years previously he had become weak and tired, and had eventually been diagnosed with iron deficiency anemia (the reports were available and were satisfactory). No source for bleeding had been found, and he had always been a strong meat-eater. He does complain, however, of vague gastro-intestinal upset from time to time, but denies any vomiting or hematemesis or melena. Eventually it had been decided to transfuse him with three units of packed cells. He immediately felt better, and thought no further about his problem. About 4 years later he again became symptomatic and once again iron deficiency was diagnosed and investigated. Once again no cause could be found, he was once again transfused, and once again responded well. Now, 4 years later, he has again been diagnosed with iron deficiency. Because of the AIDS scare he is now loth to have further transfusions, and was referred for an opinion. His latest blood count follows:

	Value	Units	Reference range Low	Reference range High	Permitted range Low	Permitted range High
Red cell count	4.41	$\times 10^{12}$/l	4.64	5.67	4.28	4.54
Hemoglobin (Hb)	10.61	g/dl	13.4	17.5	10.2	11.0
Hematocrit (Hct)	0.34	l/l	0.41	0.52	0.33	0.35
Mean cell volume	76.2	fl	80	99	74.7	77.7
Mean cell Hb	24.1	pg	27	31.5	23.6	24.5
Mean cell Hb conc.	31.6	g/dl	31.5	34.5	30.9	32.2
Red cell dist. width	15.8	%	11.6	14	15.3	16.3
Retic. count %	0.68	%	0.26	0.77	0.7	0.7
Retic. absolute (abs.)	30.0	$\times 10^9$/l	30	100	27.7	32.2
White cell count	8.15	$\times 10^9$/l	4	10	7.54	8.76
Neutrophils abs.	4.99	$\times 10^9$/l	2	7	4.61	5.36
Band cells abs.	0.00		0	0	0	0
Lymphocytes abs.	2.09	$\times 10^9$/l	1	3	1.93	2.24
Monocytes abs.	0.67	$\times 10^9$/l	0.2	1	0.62	0.72
Eosinophils abs.	0.32	$\times 10^9$/l	0.02	0.5	0.29	0.34
Basophils abs.	0.09	$\times 10^9$/l	0.02	0.1	0.08	0.10
Normoblasts	0	/100 WBC	0	0		
Platelet count	287.0	$\times 10^9$/l	150	400	265.5	308.5
Sedimentation	1	mm/h	0	10	1	1

Questions

1. Before looking at the FBC, what do you make of the clinical features? There is one very strong clue, supported by a weak one, as to the nature of the diagnosis. What do think these are?

2. What is the first-stage diagnosis?

3. In view of the patient's history, do you think it is necessary to confirm iron deficiency or do you think there is an alternative explanation for the microcytic anemia?

4. If so, what would you think of, and how would you proceed to investigate this?

5. In view of the above, what tests should be requested, and what would the results be if your suspicion is correct?

Answers

1. The clinical features are in fact very suggestive. It is unusual for an anemia to require transfusion only every 4 years: this effectively rules out thalassemia major, aplastic anemia, myelodysplasia, any of the malignancies except perhaps CLL, and so on. Possibilities are thalassemia intermedia, a very low-grade or intermittent folate or vitamin B_{12} deficiency, chronic hemolytic states, and of course the condition suffered by this patient.
2. Microcytic anemia.
3. It is probably not necessary to confirm the iron deficiency, but this depends on the reputation of the laboratories that did the previous investigations. Nevertheless a chronic recurrent microcytic anemia without any evidence of bleeding or dietary insufficiency is suspicious – iron deficiency may be complicating another disease.
4. The history is far too long for this to have been a sideroblastic anemia. Lead poisoning and copper deficiency are possibilities, as is an atypical presentation of a thalassemic syndrome. None of these appear likely on the basis or racial origin, absence of heavy metal exposure, and so on. (Hb electrophoretic studies were done for completeness and were found to be completely normal – although it was borne in mind that this did not exclude α-thalassemia or indeed even β-thalassemia if there was co-existent iron deficiency).
5. Iron absorption studies. These were performed on the patient, and the results follow (Tables 8.15 and 8.16).

Table 8.15 Fasting iron studies

S-Ferritin	4.1	µg/l	20.0	250.0
S-Iron	5.2	µmol/l	11.6	31.3
S-Transferrin	3.91	g/l	2.12	3.60
S-Fe saturation	0.1	%	20.0	50.0
MCV	72	fl	80	99

Serum iron results post-dosage with 10 ml iron maltose syrup, containing 5 mg Fe^{2+}:

Table 8.16

15 min	5.3
30 min	4.2
60 min	5.0
120 min	4.2

COMMENT ON TABLE 8.16. Very poor iron absorption, in keeping with an iron-deficient individual with malabsorption.

FOLLOW-UP AND DISCUSSION

The diagnosis of iron malabsorption seems established. The patient was referred for gastroscopy and duodenal biopsy. The result of the histology was unequivocally that of celiac disease. The final diagnosis was thus made of adult-onset gluten enteropathy. Of interest was that malabsorption of no other dietary elements, such as folate, was found. Anti-gliadin antibodies were strongly positive.

The patient's diet was adjusted, and the iron deficiency was treated with intravenous iron maltose preparation. His FBC normalized within 3 months, with a marked reticulocyte response.

Iron malabsorption and its investigation are fully discussed in Chapter 4.

CASE #21 (EXAMINE TABLE 8.17)

Questions

1. There is no doubt that she has a microcytic anemia. Do you think there could be more than one cause operating? If so, why?

2. If this were the case, would this complicate the diagnosis? How?

3. Since she is still marginally anemic, why is the reticulocyte count so low? What further question would you ask to possibly explain this?

Table 8.17

Patient	Age	Sex	Race	Altitude
Mrs J M	63 yrs	Female	White	5,000 ft

The patient was referred because of enlarged lymph nodes in the axillae and a massive splenomegaly. She has several complaints. She has been in a state of emotional turmoil for a year since her husband died. She has had several episodes of hematemesis and melena, which have been proven to be due to duodenal ulcers, and for which she has received triple therapy. She has lost a considerable amount of weight recently, which she has put down to poor appetite plus dyspepsia. There is no history of night sweats. She was told on a recent occasion that she was anemic, but states that she has always been anemic, and that many members of her family have had the same problem. On further enquiry she states that she is of French origin, and that the family came from Marseilles. On examination lymphadenopathy and splenomegaly were confirmed. She was somewhat pale and sallow, but no other abnormalities were found. CT scanning of the abdomen revealed significantly enlarged para-aortic lymph nodes, measuring from 1 to 3.4 cm in diameter.

	Value	Units	Reference range Low	Reference range High	Permitted range Low	Permitted range High
Red cell count	4.16	× 10^{12}/l	4.03	5.09	4.04	4.28
Hemoglobin (Hb)	**11.32**	g/dl	12.7	15.9	11.1	11.9
Hematocrit (Hct)	**0.33**	l/l	0.38	0.49	0.32	0.34
Mean cell volume	**79.1**	fl	80	99	77.5	80.7
Mean cell Hb	27.7	pg	27	31.5	27.1	28.2
Mean cell Hb conc.	35.0	g/dl	31.5	34.5	34.3	35.7
Red cell dist. width	**16.1**	%	11.6	14	16.1	16.1
Retic. count %	0.5		0.1	0.8	0.4	0.6
Retic. absolute (abs.)	20.8	× 10^9/l	30	100	20.2	21.4
White cell count	8.51	× 10^9/l	4	10	7.87	9.15
Neutrophils abs.	3.88	× 10^9/l	2	7	3.59	4.17
Band cells abs.	0.00		0	0	0	0
Lymphocytes abs.	3.25	× 10^9/l	1	3	3.01	3.49
Monocytes abs.	0.88	× 10^9/l	0.2	1	0.81	0.94
Eosinophils abs.	0.43	× 10^9/l	0.02	0.5	0.40	0.47
Basophils abs.	0.07	× 10^9/l	0.02	0.1	0.06	0.07
Normoblasts	0	/100 WBC	0	0		
Platelet count	421.0	× 10^9/l	150	400	378.9	463.1
Sedimentation	26	mm/h	0	20	25	27

Answers

1. There is a clear history of chronic bleeding, potentially causing iron deficiency; and she has a chronic infiltrative or inflammatory disease of some sort, potentially causing ACD. There is also a history plus family history of chronic anemia, which may indicate a hereditary blood disease; the family's origin in Marseilles makes a strong case for β-thalassemia (Massilia was one of the many colonies established by Ionian Greeks in about 600 BC).

2. The presence of iron deficiency makes the diagnosis of thalassemia by electrophoresis very difficult. The iron deficiency must be corrected before requesting electrophoretic studies. Co-existence of iron deficiency and ACD can be a very difficult diagnosis to make.

3. There is always the possibility that she has very recently undergone an aplastic crisis. Far more likely, however, is that she may have had a transfusion recently (this tends to dampen a reticulocyte count). Thus the important question to ask is how recently she has had a transfusion. In this case the answer was 2 weeks ago, sufficient to explain the decreased reticulocyte count. The effect of the recent transfusion also makes the diagnosis of the underlying condition/s very difficult.

FOLLOW-UP AND DISCUSSION

Iron studies in this patient were in fact completely ambiguous as were tests for thalassemia. The priority was the diagnosis of the lymphadenopathy; biopsy revealed a non-Hodgkin lymphoma (these are discussed in Chapter 22). She responded well to therapy but the Hb and MCV did not improve, although the RCC gradually rose. Once in remission, tests were repeated and β-thalassemia was confirmed. The iron deficiency had responded well to oral iron therapy.

Comment This case illustrates the importance of a good history. When it comes to blood diseases, especially deficiency diseases and possible infections, this is critical. The history should always include details of diet, family origin, and recent travel.

CASE #22 (EXAMINE TABLES 8.18 AND 8.19)

Questions

1. The diagnosis of iron deficiency seems clear and yet the ferritin level is within the normal range, albeit on the low side. Does this negate the diagnosis of iron deficiency in this case?

_____

_____

2. Is there any clinical suggestion as to the nature of the pathology?

_____

_____

Table 8.18

Patient	Age	Sex	Race	Altitude
Mrs B P	24 yrs	Female	White	2,500 ft

This patient developed overt iron deficiency at the age of 17 years. There was no menorrhagia. She lived on a farm and her diet was very good. The only possible contributory factor was frequent nosebleeds. She had been treated with iron preparations with only moderate success. For want of a diagnosis, Little's areas on both sides were cauterized. The anemia persisted and slowly got worse, eventually necessitating transfusions. Barium meal and enema studies revealed no pathology. A bone marrow aspirate showed the picture classical of iron deficiency only. Two years ago she commenced with severe classical migraine attacks, and recently she started getting occasional grand mal seizures. She was referred.

A detailed history was completely non-contributory. She did mention though that a few small "birth marks" on her face had been "burnt off."

Examination revealed a pale woman. The only other positive feature was numerous small angioma-like lesions on the hard palate and tongue and a few telangiectatic lesions on the neck and chest. The conjunctivae were clear albeit pale and there were no cerebellar signs. Her last transfusion (two units) was 2 months ago – the consultant had stipulated that she should if possible not be transfused for that period prior to consultation.

	Value	Units	Reference range Low	Reference range High	Permitted range Low	Permitted range High
Red cell count	3.87	$\times 10^{12}$/l	3.91	4.94	3.75	3.99
Hemoglobin (Hb)	9.15	g/dl	12.4	15.5	8.8	9.5
Hematocrit (Hct)	0.29	l/l	0.37	0.47	0.28	0.30
Mean cell volume	75.1	fl	80	99	73.6	76.6
Mean cell Hb	23.6	pg	27	31.5	23.2	24.1
Mean cell Hb conc.	31.5	g/dl	31.5	34.5	30.9	32.1
Red cell dist. width	17.1	%	11.6	14	17.1	17.1
Retic. count %	3.15	%	0.25	0.75	3.1	3.2
Retic. absolute (abs.)	121.9	$\times 10^9$/l	30	100	118.2	125.6
White cell count	5.65	$\times 10^9$/l	4	10	5.23	6.07
Corrected WCC	5.49	$\times 10^9$/l				
Neutrophils abs.	3.46	$\times 10^9$/l	2	7	3.20	3.72
Band cells abs.	0.00		0	0	0	0
Lymphocytes abs.	1.37	$\times 10^9$/l	1	3	1.27	1.48
Monocytes abs.	0.46	$\times 10^9$/l	0.2	1	0.43	0.50
Eosinophils abs.	0.29	$\times 10^9$/l	0.02	0.5	0.27	0.32
Basophils abs.	0.06	$\times 10^9$/l	0.02	0.1	0.06	0.07
Normoblasts	3	/100 WBC	0	0		
Platelet count	415.0	$\times 10^9$/l	150	400	373.5	456.5
Sedimentation	3	mm/h	0	20	3	3

Table 8.19

	Value	Units	Low	High
S-Ferritin female	16.2	µg/l	14.0	233.1
S-Iron	9.25	µmol/l	11.6	31.3
S-Transferrin	3.61	g/l	2.12	3.60
S-Fe saturation	10.1	%	15.0	35.0

3. What would you suggest is a good way to confirm this possibility?

_____

_____

_____

4. What do you infer from the raised reticulocyte count and platelet count?

_____

_____

5. Would you reach the same conclusion if only the platelet count were raised?

_____

Answers

1. There are two possibilities for the ferritin to be within the reference range with the other iron studies suggesting iron deficiency:

   a) There is an associated chronic disease (causing ACD) or thalassemia.
   b) The patient has been frequently transfused. If she is not bleeding regularly (assuming that to be the cause), a transfusion of two units would have provided her with ± 500 mg iron and hence ferritin. Thus, no, the ferritin level does not negate the diagnosis of iron deficiency.

2. The numerous angioma-like lesions suggest the possibility of hereditary hemorrhagic telangiectasia.

3. First, confirm that the lesions blanch on pressure – if they do not they are not angiomata. Second, look further for lesions, especially in the GIT and vagina.

4. That the patient had a recent fairly substantial bleed, at least 24 h ago.

5. No. A raised platelet count alone in such a patient could indicate continuing, perhaps intermittent, low levels of bleeding – or of course it could be incidental to many other causes – see Chapter 12.

   For follow-up details, see Table 8.20.

Further Questions

1. Do you think there is enough evidence for the diagnosis? Is it possible to confirm this?

   _____

   _____

Table 8.20

Case #22: Follow-up and further developments
1. Despite the ferritin level, it was decided not to investigate for chronic disease, at any rate not for the time being.
2. Specialist ENT consultation revealed numerous pinhead-sized angiomata in the nasopharynx. Gastroscopy revealed similar lesions in the esophagus and stomach. (One of the major advantages of endoscopy over barium studies is the visualization of tiny lesions). Note that it is important that the anemia be corrected before endoscopic investigation: pinhead hemangiomata are difficult to see in an anemic patient.
3. The diagnosis was made of hereditary hemorrhagic telangiectasia. The patient's iron stores were repleted with a ferro-maltose intravenous preparation.

2. What do you think of the neurological features?

_____

3. If this is a hereditary condition, why does it manifest so relatively late?

_____

_____

Answers

1. The clinical evidence is very strong. The Curaçao criteria[1] were applied. A minimum of two out of four of the following should be present:

   a) **EPISTAXIS** – spontaneous and recurrent
   b) **MULTIPLE TELANGIECTASES** at characteristic sites (lips, oral cavity, fingers, nose)
   c) **VISCERAL LESIONS,** such as GI telangiectases, or pulmonary, hepatic, cerebral, and spinal AV abnormalities
   d) **A FIRST-DEGREE RELATIVE** with this condition. It can be seen that three of the criteria are present. As far as genetic confirmation is concerned, this was not available at the time. Three HHT gene loci have been isolated

2. These can well be complications of the disease. Migraine and seizures are well-recognized complications. They are due to AV malformations in the brain or lungs (the latter responsible for repeated paradoxical embolization of products of coagulation).

3. It is not unusual for hereditary conditions only to manifest in later life. Nevertheless HHT can present very late indeed, even at age 40. One point to make: it has often been thought that the condition is worse in

females, on the grounds that the lesions are aggravated by estrogens.

Extensive angiographic studies were undertaken. A number of AV malformations in the lungs and liver were demonstrated. The patient was referred to the relevant specialists.

Comments

1. *To repeat*: Microcytosis does not equate to iron deficiency.
2. With the exception of the young patient, all patients with proven iron deficiency must be investigated for the cause. In young people without evidence of bleeding (and do not forget hemorrhoids), it is permissible to give a trial of an oral iron preparation with weekly monitoring of the reticulocyte count. This means that a baseline reticulocyte count must be done before starting treatment. If the reticulocyte count is not showing a steady rise, the patient must be further investigated.
3. Occult blood testing while fairly specific is not good enough to exclude colonic pathology particularly in the patient at risk.
4. The diagnostic test with by far the best yield is colonoscopy. Colonoscopy can only be omitted (in cases of obscure iron deficiency) if

   a) There is clear clinical evidence of Peutz–Jegher syndrome or hereditary hemorrhagic telangiectasia
   b) A prior gastroscopy has revealed a bleeding lesion or there is unquestionable evidence of portal hypertension with varices

5. Confirming iron deficiency requires iron studies: these must be drawn fasting in the morning. A decreased ferritin level is the sine qua non of iron deficiency. Sometimes the iron saturation will be below 15% (the diagnostic cutoff point) with a ferritin level in the normal range. This requires further investigation since you may be dealing with a patient with iron deficiency combined with something else; if this is say thalassemia iron therapy can be perilous and the case requires expert assessment.

To repeat: it is dangerous or futile to prescribe iron to any patient who does not have proven iron deficiency. Intravenous iron in particular can be hazardous with the wrong indications.

OPTIONAL ADVANCED READING

Rarer Causes of a Microcytic or Hypochromic Red Cell Picture

1. **HEMOGLOBIN E TRAIT OR DISEASE.** HbE is the second most common Hb variant. The gene is common in Southeast Asia, but can occur sporadically elsewhere. In addition to causing a structural Hb variant, it can be regarded as a β^+-thalassemia. Heterozygotes show a microcytosis without anemia, whereas homozygotes show microcytosis, hypochromia, and target cell formation but, surprisingly, little or even no anemia. The various clinical pictures will be discussed under thalassemias below.
2. **COPPER DEFICIENCY.**
3. **LEAD POISONING.** Lead interferes with heme synthesis. This results in a normochromic normocytic anemia that eventually tends to evolve into microcytosis and hypochromia. It is characteristically accompanied by punctate basophilia of the red cells. Strictly speaking, one needs to see 11% of red cells with punctate basophilia to suggest the diagnosis (there are numerous other causes of punctate basophilia). Lead poisoning must be confirmed biochemically.
4. **SIDEROBLASTIC ANEMIAS.** These are a group of diverse diseases associated with abnormal iron metabolism, and characterized by

   a. An **INCREASE** in total body iron
   b. Ringed sideroblasts in the marrow
   c. (Usually) hypochromic anemia

5. **PAROXYSMAL NOCTURNAL HEMOGLOBINURIA.** This rare condition can present in many different ways; only one of which is classical hemoglobinuria. This is sometimes so severe as to lead to iron deficiency. The condition is very briefly discussed in Chapter 23.
6. **PULMONARY HEMOSIDEROSIS AND GOODPASTURE SYNDROME.**

Classification of the Sideroblastic Anemias

1. **HEREDITARY,** which may be of two forms, X-linked and autosomal recessive. Note that these typically present in the teenage years.
2. **ACQUIRED.**

   a. **PRIMARY SIDEROBLASTIC ANEMIA** (or refractory anemia with ringed sideroblasts). This is one of the myelodysplastic syndromes.
   b. **ASSOCIATED WITH HEMATOLOGICAL MALIGNANCIES,** such as leukemia, lymphomas,

myelomas. In the case of leukemia, it is sometimes difficult to decide which came first. It may also appear apparently for the first time **AFTER** treatment of hematological malignancies; this is a very poor prognostic sign – these cases almost always terminate in acute leukemia.

  c. **SECONDARY TO DRUGS AND TOXINS,** such as

    i. Chemotherapeutic drugs
    ii. Anti-tuberculosis drugs
    iii. Alcohol
    iv. Lead. Note, however, that the anemia of lead poisoning is a complex process. The most important factor is defective heme synthesis, due to mitochondrial poisoning by the lead. However, the life span of the red cells is considerably reduced as well. Note that it is now recognized that lead poisoning per se does not cause a hypochromic microcytic anemia, but is typically normocytic. If a microcytic anemia is present, this is now thought most likely to be due to associated iron deficiency or α-thalassemia trait. Co-existent iron deficiency is common and extremely serious, since absorption of lead is even higher in the presence of iron deficiency.

The Anemia of Chronic Disorders Revisited

This is a condition characterized by a chronic mild anemia and defective iron metabolism, in association with any chronic disease. Its main features are

1. Occurring in association with any chronic inflammatory or infiltrative disorder
2. Developing within 2 months after the appearance of the primary disorder. It can occasionally occur as early as 2 weeks after the appearance of the disease (This varying time may be related to the time of diagnosis)
3. Presenting with an Hb of 9–11 g, with the severity of the anemia being roughly proportional to that of the underlying condition
4. Usually normochromic and normocytic but often hypochromic
5. Associated with decreased serum iron and decreased to normal transferrin, resulting in a decreased % saturation but usually above 15%.
6. Increased iron stores in the marrow with virtually absent sideroblasts
7. Normal to increased ferritin levels, the interpretation of which is complicated by the fact that ferritin is an acute phase reactant

Pathogenesis

This is not fully understood, but there are several facts known which throw some light on this, and the importance of some of these facts have been questioned:

1. **DECREASED LIFE SPAN OF THE RBC** – it is known to be 80–90 days instead of the usual 120
2. **RETICULOCYTES ARE NOT INCREASED IN PROPORTION** to the anemia, indicating an element of marrow insufficiency
3. **DEFECTIVE IRON METABOLISM.** Note that normal erythropoiesis requires about 800 μg of iron per day, almost all from breakdown of senescent red cells:

  a. The total body iron absorption is normal but the transfer of iron from the intestinal mucosa to the plasma is reduced.
  b. A block in the release of iron from the RE stores. Evidence for this is conflicting – some studies show that release is in fact normal but that the iron is unavailable to the precursors that would result in an increase of RBC free protoporphyrin, which in fact is demonstrable.
  c. Ferrokinetic studies are in fact unremarkable.
  d. Inadequate erythropoietin (EPO) response to anemia – this is no longer supported.
  e. Defective marrow response to EPO – probably insignificant.
  f. Abnormal erythroid colony growth. These experiments have shown that in SLE, RA, and juvenile arthritis, in some cases a humoral factor inhibits erythropoiesis. Indeed plasmapheresis helped considerably in two of these cases in one series.

Advanced Notes on the Thalassemias[2]

This is a very complex topic, and what follows is a brief and somewhat simplified explanation. It is primarily intended for students and doctors working in endemic areas, although specialists in training may also find it valuable.

β-Thalassemia Mutations

These are found with high frequency in a broad subtropical region from Southern Europe to Southeast Asia. There is strong epidemiological association with endemic falciparum malaria but the biological basis has not properly been defined.

Well over 100 mutations have been characterized. Many of these produce more-or-less identical clinical pictures, but occasionally apparently identical molecular defects can present with different clinical pictures. In addition, some of the "typical" thalassemia presentations have been shown to occur in some hemoglobinopathies, e.g., Hb Lepore and HbE.

THREE GENERAL TYPES OF MUTATION ARE DESCRIBED:

1. **MUTATION CAUSING LOSS** of all or part of the β-globin gene cluster.

    a. Loss only of the β-globin gene itself, resulting in one form of β-thalassemia
    b. More extensive loss involving others in the cluster, resulting in various $\delta\beta$-thalassemia syndromes

2. **POINT MUTATIONS** or insertions or deletions of a small number of nucleotides in critical sites:

    a. Among the most important point mutations are nonsense mutations that create termination codons within the normal sequence. The effect is an abnormally shortened and non-functional chain. Since there is no gene product, this is termed a β^0-thalassemia mutation. The site of the nonsense mutation can be at different places and is often found at the same place in different populations.
    b. Insertion or deletion mutations in exon regions are known as frame-shift mutations and produce changes in the actual reading frame. These also produce β^0-thalassemias.
    c. Defects in RNA splicing. These are of two broad groups:

        i. Where the mutation is in or near the invariant boundary sequence between exon and intron. The effect depends on exactly where the mutation occurs:

            • If occurring in the sequence itself, no functional RNA will be formed, producing the β^0 phenotype.
            • If occurring immediately adjacent, the sequences are substantially preserved, producing the β^+ phenotype.

        ii. Where the mutation is within an exon or intron and creates a splicing sequence. Usually these produce a β^+ phenotype, but β^0 can occur.

3. **MUTATIONS IN THE PROMOTER REGION:**

    a. These generally result in a 70–80% reduction in the amount of β-globin synthesized, thus producing a β^+-thalassemia.

    b. Uncommonly, they may lead to increased γ-chain production, resulting in the HPHF (hereditary persistence of hemoglobin F) phenotype.

SO, TO SUMMARIZE

1. β^0-thalassemia means lack of any gene product, due to absence of the gene or functionally defective gene. It can be produced by

    a. Loss of the β-hemoglobin gene itself
    b. Nonsense point mutations causing inappropriate termination codons
    c. Frame-shift mutations due to insertion or deletion
    d. Defective RNA splicing due to point mutation in the boundary sequence between intron and exon
    e. Occasionally due to a mutation in the exon producing a splicing sequence – if close enough to the boundary

2. β^+-thalassemia means a reduction in the amount of gene product:

    a. Mutations in the promoter region
    b. A point mutation in the intron or exon themselves causing a splicing sequence

Note that many individual mechanisms described above are very much more prevalent in certain geographical regions than others, with the result that there appear to be clear racial differences in the way of presentation.

The Pathophysiology of β-Thalassemia

In summary several processes can be described:

A. **DECREASE IN THE FORMATION OF HBA** results in poor hemoglobinization and thence anemia. "Compensatory" increases in HbF and HbA$_2$ are inadequate.

B. **ACCUMULATION OF EXCESS,** unused α-chains. The net effect is to cause a hemolytic aspect to the disease, since the α-chains are very unstable and become oxidized and damage the red cell membrane:

1. **THEY EASILY ARE CHANGED INTO METHEMOGLOBIN,** in the process generating free radicals. These cause severe damage:

    a. Formation of additional methemoglobin
    b. Membrane lipid peroxidation. This results in

        i. Increased rigidity
        ii. Increased antigenicity, with increased recognition of the altered red cells. The effect of both contributes to the hemolytic element of this disease.

c. Oxidative damage to both globin and membrane proteins

2. **THE PRODUCTION OF HEMICHROMES.** Soluble and reversible in the early stages, later they are insoluble and visible with special staining as Heinz bodies. They are later broken down to heme, denatured globin, and iron, which are all deposited on the red cell membrane. One of the effects is also to change the antigenicity of the membrane and increase the binding of immuno-globulins, thus further aggravating the hemolytic process.

Hemichromes tend to aggregate with protein 3, and hence to interfere with the binding of spectrin and ankyrin, and possibly directly, to interfere with the binding of spectrin and actin.

C. **INEFFECTIVE ERYTHROPOIESIS,** adding to the hemolytic component. The large number of abnormal cells being formed in the marrow leads to the destruction in the marrow of these precursors, primarily of nucleated forms – thus ineffective erythropoiesis.

The anemia plus the accumulation of products of hemolysis produces an intense EPO response, with marked erythropoietic hyperplasia: this has its own complications.

D. **IRON OVERLOAD.** This is due to two general causes:

1. Transfusion. Depending on the severity of the disease, the transfusion requirements may be substantial, particularly with so-called hypertransfusion regimens (to reduce the EPO drive). In heavily transfusion-dependent cases, even optimal chelation therapy will not be enough to prevent iron accumulation.
2. Increased absorption. The mechanism/s are not understood. The increased absorption appears to parallel the increased red cell production rate.

The α-Chain Group

These are the α-chain itself and the ζ-chain (embryonic). The α-globin genes are normally duplicated, with therefore a normal diploid complement of four α-globin genes. Consequently from one to four genes may be abnormal, with a wide spectrum of effects. Normally we indicate the structure of the four α-genes as follows: [αα/αα], i.e., normal. Thus a single gene deletion would be indicated as say [αα/-α], and so on. The structure of each of the four genes is very similar to that of the β-gene. Of significance, however, is the presence of a number of pseudogenes lying between

the ζ-gene and the α1- and α2-genes; another pseudo-gene lies outside the α2-gene.

α-Globin Mutations

Virtually all the types of single-base substitutions described above for the β-globin genes have been found in α-thalassemia. However, these account for relatively few cases, most of the forms resulting from **GENE DELETIONS.**

Deletions have varying effects, depending on which segments of the total cluster are missing. It is suggested that most of these deletions occur as a result of mispairing during a crossing-over recombination in meiosis, resulting in a single α-globin locus plus a chromosome with three loci. The single α-globin locus will be either a fusion product of parts of the α1-globin and of the α2-globin genes, or an intact α1-gene with deletion of the α2-gene. Various other deletions result in a total or partial loss of both of the α-globin genes, with consequent lack of gene product.

The different genetic patterns in α-thalassemia are as follows:

1. α^+ trait: one of the four missing or dysfunctional, e.g., [α-/αα]
2. Homozygous α^+: "homologous" genes on both chromosomes missing or dysfunctional, e.g., [-α/-α]
3. α^0 trait: both genes on one chromosome absent or dysfunctional, e.g., [–/αα]
4. HbH disease: three of the four genes absent or dysfunctional, e.g., [–/α–]
5. Hydrops fetalis: all four genes missing or dysfunctional, i.e., [–/–].

Uncommon α-Thalassemia Syndromes

1. Mutation in the translation termination codon, producing longer than normal α-chains; the classical example here is Hb Constant Spring.
2. Structurally abnormal hemoglobins, such as

   a. The synthesis of very unstable α-chains which undergo rapid proteolysis in the red cell, e.g., Hb Quong Sze
   b. HbG Philadelphia: the gene for this hemoglobin exists on a single α-locus chromosome

Clinical Presentations of the Thalassemia Syndromes

The traditional classification into thalassemia minor, intermedia, and major is still very useful, as long it is realized that it is no longer as cut-and-dried as it used to be, particularly from the etiopathogenetic point of view. Both the β- and the α-thalassemias can be accommodated without too much violence, as well as many of the hemoglobinopathy/thalassemia double heterozygotes that may be found.

It is perhaps an idea to make another category, thalassemia minima, to cater for those cases where the hematological changes are so mild as usually to be ignored: the MCV on the low side and the red cell count on the high side of normal. These patients are rarely investigated and their incidence is not known; it is probably significant in "endemic" areas. Common causes of this picture would be single gene deletions of α-thalassemia (the so-called "silent carrier"), and some of the β^+-thalassemias. Their clinical importance lies in the fact that when they procreate, their partner may also have a mild form of the disease but the offspring can be disastrously affected.

Double Heterozygosity

Another factor influencing the varying clinical pictures of the thalassemia syndromes is co-inheritance of another defect of the same or the other globin chain. The clinical effects of the particular combination cannot be predicted from the effects of each on its own.

Thalassemia Minor

These patients are characterized by generally satisfactory health, usually symptom-free except in periods of stress (notably pregnancy) when the anemia can deteriorate fairly suddenly and even severely. They commonly have a mild anemia, but occasionally in the normal range. However, the characteristic blood picture is a microcythemia accompanied by a low MCH. There is a more-or-less normal morphology, sometimes with a slight reticulocytosis. The bone marrow shows mild to moderate erythropoietic hyperplasia with normal to possibly mildly increased stores especially in older patients, and decreased sideroblasts.

Genotypes That May Present with Thalassemia Minor

Essentially these are all heterozygous forms, with synthesis of only one chain reduced; there is an exception: where both an α-thalassemia and a β-

thalassemia coexist (as a double heterozygote), one or both in a form that would otherwise cause more severe disease, the clinical presentation is much milder, since much of the pathophysiology of thalassemia is due to the unbalanced production of globin chains – here both are reduced (Note that all the α-thalassemias causing this appearance have normal HbA_2 and HbF – indeed the β-thalassemias all characteristically have raised HbF and HbA_2, apart from hereditary persistence of hemoglobin F, Hb Lepore, and HbE.):

1. Heterozygous hereditary persistence of HbF: HbF 5–20%, HbA_2 normal or low
2. Heterozygous Hb Lepore [HbA 80–90%, Hb Lepore 10%, HbA_2 decreased]
3. Heterozygous HbE; HbE 45–60%, HbA most of the balance
4. Heterozygous β^0 [β/-;$\alpha\alpha$/$\alpha\alpha$]
5. Heterozygous β^+ [β*/β;$\alpha\alpha$/$\alpha\alpha$]
6. Heterozygous $\delta\beta$ and related syndromes
7. Heterozygous α^0: [–/$\alpha\alpha$]
8. Heterozygous α^+: [-α/$\alpha\alpha$], (usually thalassemia "minima")
9. Occasionally as mentioned before, double heterozygote α- and β-thalassemia which could otherwise cause severer disease

Thalassemia Intermedia

These patients have a moderate anemia, marked microcythemia, and are basically not transfusion dependent. However, there is a lot of variation within these limits, and the separation from thalassemia major especially can be a problem. Bone deformities can occur, extramedullary hemopoiesis is fairly common, and iron overload is a problem. A commonly used criterion is the degree of transfusion dependency – we consider more than two transfusions a year to put the patient into the major category.

Genotypes That May Present with Thalassemia Intermedia

This really is a mixed bag, and often one can find no reason why two patients with the same genotype can vary so much clinically:

1. Mild forms of β-thalassemia

   a. Homozygous mild β^+-thalassemias
   b. Double heterozygous genotype of two different β^+-genes

2. Double heterozygous α- and β- thalassemia of certain types

   a. Notably β^+ with α^0 [$-/\alpha\alpha$] or $\alpha+$
   b. β-Thalassemia plus HbH disease.

3. β-Thalassemia plus a miscellany of other alleles as double heterozygotes:

   a. HPFH
   b. HbE
   c. $\delta\beta$ variants

4. So-called dominant heterozygous β-thalassemia.

A Note About the Manifestations of HbE

1. While the gene has high prevalence in SE Asia, sporadic cases in Caucasians do occur.
2. α-Thalassemia is common also in SE Asia, and co-inheritance of this condition with HbE will cause the MCV to be even lower than with each on its own.
3. β-Thalassemia also is common in the area. The HbE/β-thalassemia double heterozygote has remarkably variable clinical presentations, from thalassemia minor to thalassemia major. The Hb pattern usually consists of HbE and HbF in the 10–50% range. Occasionally HbA is found if there is an interacting β^+-thalassemia determinant. The severity of the condition is not explained, since homozygous HbE is a mild condition.

Further Reading

Lewis SM, Bain B, Bates I (2006). Dacie and Lewis Practical Haematology. 10th edn. Churchill Livingstone.

Hoffbrand AV, Pettit JE (2001). Essential Haematology. 4th edn. Oxford, Blackwell Science.

Andreoli TE, Bennett JC, Carpenter CCJ, Plum F (eds) (1997). Cecil Essentials of Medicine. 4th edn. Philadelphia: WB Saunders Company.

Epstein RJ (1996). Medicine for Examinations. 3rd edn. Churchill Livingstone.

References

1. Plauchu H, de Chadarevian JP, Bideau A, Robert JM (1989). Age-related clinical profile of hereditary hemorrhagic telangiectasia in an epidemiologically recruited population. Am. J. Med. Genet. 32: 291–297.
2. Weatherall DJ (1994). The thalassaemias. In Stamatoyannopoulos GA, Menhuis AW, Majerus PW, Varmus HE (eds). The Molecular Basis of Blood Diseases. 2nd edn, Saunders, Philadelphia.

Defining Macrocytosis

The first-stage diagnosis of "Macrocytosis" was reached by the recognition that that the **AVERAGE** size of the red cells counted is above the reference range.

> **STEP 1:** "Where is the primary abnormality?" It lies in the MCV and therefore the size of the red cells.
>
> **STEP 2:** "What form does it take?" The MCV is increased above the reference range.

Anemia need not be present. If there is an anemia, the anatomical diagnosis is "macrocytic anemia"; otherwise, it is "a macrocytic red cell picture."

The General Pathology Causes of Macrocytosis

AT THE GENERAL LEVEL THERE ARE ONLY FOUR GROUPS OF CAUSES:

1. **MEGALOBLASTIC ERYTHROPOIESIS CAUSED BY DEFECTS IN DNA SYNTHESIS**
2. **DISORDERS OF THE LIPID ELEMENTS IN THE RED CELL MEMBRANE**
3. **HYPERSTIMULATED ERYTHROPOIESIS WITH SKIPPING OF MATURATION STEPS**
4. **RETICULOCYTOSIS**

In addition, three uncommon causes should be mentioned:

1. **THE ACQUIRED MYELODYSPLASTIC CONDITIONS** are frequently characterized by macrocytic red cells. The bone marrow typically shows the so-called megaloblastoid change, apart from other evidence of myelodysplasia.

2. **AUTOAGGLUTINATION**. Here masses of agglutinated red cells pass through the aperture of the instrument and are measured as very large cells – note that **THIS IS A SPURIOUS, ARTEFACTUAL MACROCYTOSIS.**

3. **CERTAIN DRUGS**, notably many chemotherapeutic agents, are known to be associated with macrocytosis (and indeed macrocytosis is used as a measure of compliance with treatment). The major pathogenetic mechanism is probably interference with folate metabolism.

There are no specific clinical or laboratory findings (except for a raised MCV) that are common to all causes.

Specific Causes of Macrocytosis

1. **MEGALOBLASTIC ERYTHROPOIESIS**. The specific causes fall into two groups.

   a. **VITAMIN B$_{12}$ DEFICIENCY**. This is most commonly due to pernicious anemia but can be found post-gastrectomy, in Crohn disease and those subsisting on a vegan diet.

      i. **PERNICIOUS ANEMIA**. The basic pathology is an autoimmune destruction of gastric parietal cells resulting in absent intrinsic factor. Thus, ingested vitamin B$_{12}$ cannot be absorbed in the ileum. Normally, the hepatic stores of the vitamin are sufficient for 4 years; thus the clinical features take a long time to develop.

      ii. **OTHER DISEASE OF THE STOMACH.** Other forms of gastropathy very rarely cause deficiency of Intrinsic Factor. It is sometimes thought that a partial gastrectomy should not cause vitamin B_{12} deficiency since the body of the stomach (where the Intrinsic Factor-producing parietal cells are) is not resected. However, secondary atrophy of the rest of the stomach mucosa often follows a partial gastrectomy; this may have a vascular element but most likely is due to chronic gastritis from biliary reflux. Formerly, it was most unlikely for a total gastrectomy to lead to vitamin B_{12} deficiency: with few exceptions, total gastrectomy was (and is) done for carcinoma of the stomach, whose average survival post-operatively was 6 months; and since the normal vitamin B_{12} stores last for an average of 4 **YEARS**, there was simply no time for it to develop. Modern advances, however, have considerably improved survival and deficiency can occur. Note that this consideration does not apply to iron – its stores at the best of times last only 6 months, and gastrectomy patients may well have bled considerably before and during their operation, depleting their stores.

   iii. **CROHN DISEASE**. This and other disease or surgery of the distal ileum can cause defective absorption of the vitamin B_{12} bound to intrinsic factor reaching it. Two other factors may aggravate vitamin B_{12} deficiency in Crohn disease:

     – Bacterial overgrowth
     – Fistula formation

Note that, by the time the patient develops anemia, the diagnosis is obvious anyway – Crohn disease will never **PRESENT** with megaloblastic anemia. Also the deficiency in Crohn disease is never as severe as in pernicious anemia.

  b. **FOLATE DEFICIENCY**. Note that since the stores of folate are very limited, folate deficiency, unlike that of vitamin B_{12}, develops very rapidly once a cause is operative.

    i. **PREGNANCY**. The developing fetus naturally has an enormous rate of DNA synthesis, thus, as with iron, huge amounts of folate are transferred to the fetus.

    ii. **ALCOHOLISM** and various forms or malnutrition including malabsorption. Development of folate deficiency in malabsorption is particularly rapid since there is an enterohepatic circulation of folate.

    iii. **CERTAIN DRUGS**, as mentioned before.

2. **DISORDERS OF THE LIPID ELEMENTS IN THE RED CELL MEMBRANE.** The most important causes are

  a. Chronic liver disease and alcoholism (note thus two possible pathogenetic mechanisms of macrocytosis in alcoholism)

  b. Hypothyroidism.

3. **HYPERSTIMULATED   ERYTHROPOIESIS WITH SKIPPING OF MATURATION STEPS.** The most important cause here is aplastic anemia.

4. **RETICULOCYTOSIS**. Reticulocytes are normally significantly larger than mature red cells. The greater the number of reticulocytes the more the average MCV will be increased.

Making the Diagnosis

The approach to macrocytosis is much simpler than with the microcytic pictures. Nevertheless, much depends on how the patient presents: clinical presentation is only occasionally decisive. Generally, a patient will present with vague symptoms and possibly pallor; a FBC will reveal macrocytosis, which requires interpretation.

    The clinical features are however very often of considerable **SECONDARY** assistance, i.e., as an aid to

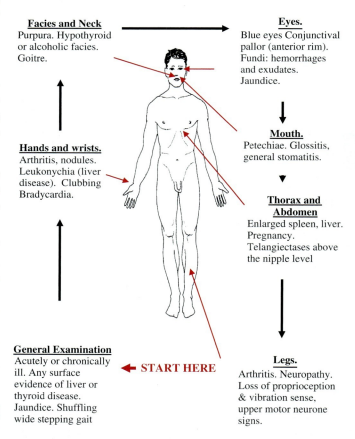

Facies and Neck
Purpura. Hypothyroid or alcoholic facies. Goitre.

Eyes.
Blue eyes Conjunctival pallor (anterior rim). Fundi: hemorrhages and exudates. Jaundice.

Mouth.
Petechiae. Glossitis, general stomatitis.

Hands and wrists.
Arthritis, nodules. Leukonychia (liver disease). Clubbing Bradycardia.

Thorax and Abdomen
Enlarged spleen, liver. Pregnancy. Telangiectases above the nipple level

General Examination
Acutely or chronically ill. Any surface evidence of liver or thyroid disease. Jaundice. Shuffling wide stepping gait

← **START HERE**

Legs.
Arthritis. Neuropathy. Loss of proprioception & vibration sense, upper motor neurone signs.

Fig. 9.1 Examination: The macrocytic anemias

interpretation of the raised MCV. Thus, in all cases, a proper clinical examination is essential.

Figure 9.1 illustrates **SPECIFIC ASPECTS** of the examination of a patient in whom a macrocytic blood picture is known or suspected; clearly, it is part of the overall examination as depicted in Fig. 5.4.

> **A COMMON MISCONCEPTION!!!** Macrocytosis does NOT, repeat NOT, equate to Megaloblastic Anemia!!!!

The clinical presentation is occasionally decisive or at least highly suggestive. In cases where the clinical features are insubstantial or ambiguous, a purely algorithmic approach to the FBC is necessary.

Clinically Obvious or Suggestive Cases

Pernicious anemia is the only macrocytic anemia that can (sometimes) permit a clinical diagnosis.

PERNICIOUS ANEMIA. Diagnosis is relatively easy in a patient with pallor and lemon-yellow jaundice, with diarrhea, premature graying of the hair, blue eyes, marked glossitis and stomatitis, and a with shuffling wide-stepping gait associated with demonstrable features of subacute combined degeneration of the cord.

Clinically Undefined Cases

DIFFICULTIES ARISE WHEN the patient presents with pregnancy or features of liver disease, alcoholism, or hypothyroidism. The presence of purpura may cause further difficulties. In these cases one is lost without a FBC. Many approaches to a raised MCV have been described, but generally they tend to neglect the clinical features. As a first step, we describe the backbone of our algorithm, using the degree of increase in the MCV. The complete approach is presented on page 249):

1. MCV over ±128: consider autoagglutination.
2. MCV over ±118: consider autoagglutination, megaloblastosis.
3. MCV between ±118 and ±108: consider autoagglutination, megaloblastosis, liver disease, alcoholism, and hypothyroidism.
4. MCV below ±108: consider all the above, plus reticulocytosis and aplasia.

COMMENTS ABOUT THE ABOVE APPROACH

1. Too often, hard-and-fast criteria are laid down. For example, one author says that the diagnosis of a megaloblastic anemia requires a MCV of > 115 fl. This is hardly practical in the case of early megaloblastic disease, where the MCV may be only mildly raised. Would this author therefore exclude from consideration as a possible case of folate deficiency a patient with an MCV of 114 fl? This reflects a common problem with numeric criteria; it is far better to see the possible diagnosis in terms of a spectrum of alteration of a particular result. Thus, one big advantage of this approach is flexibility.
2. It will exclude from consideration all causes with an MCV below the given level. Thus, with an MCV of 112 fl, one can confidently exclude aplastic anemia and reticulocytosis, thus saving time, money, and possible discomfort.

(Spurious) Macrocytosis Caused by Autoagglutination

CLINICAL FEATURES: These are, when present, the features of a (cold antibody) type of immune hemolytic anemia, and are discussed in Chapter 10. Note that the autoagglutination and hence the clinical features can be mild and ambiguous.

FBC FEATURES: There is usually anemia. Morphology will report autoagglutination and usually spherocytes.

FEATURES IN OTHER TESTS: The Coombs test will be positive for IgG and complement.

Bear in mind that certain chronic types of immune hemolysis may develop a true secondary folate deficiency, due to increased demand.

The Megaloblastic Blood Picture

FBC FEATURES

There may be a pancytopenia. This aspect is discussed further in Chapter 13.

RED CELLS: The typical appearance is as follows:

1. The anemia can be very severe.
2. The MCV is raised but seldom above ± 125 fl, as is the RDW.
3. The MCH is normal to raised and the MCHC is normal.

4. The morphology of the red cells is striking: moderate to marked anisocytosis, normochromia. The macrocytes are **OVAL** and there are numerous tear-drop poikilocytes and some fragmented cells. Unusual morphological features are sometimes reported, such as punctate basophilia and Cabot rings. Rouleaux formation is sometimes noted. The ESR is almost always moderately raised, unlike the situation in iron deficiency.

WHITE CELLS: Apart from the frequent accompanying neutropenia, the characteristic finding is a marked right shift. It will be remembered that the causes of a right shift in general are megaloblastosis, iron deficiency, renal failure, and congenital.

PLATELETS: Thrombocytopenia may be noted.

FEATURES IN OTHER TESTS

The most obvious changes are as follows:

1. A **MARKEDLY** raised LDH – levels over 2,000 IU are not uncommon. This reflects the marked intramedullary hemolysis (i.e., ineffective erythropoiesis).
2. The serum potassium level tends to be on the high side of normal. This should be interpreted with caution – the issue is discussed in Case #23. The practical point is that in patients with co-existing renal disease, the potassium may be falsely raised, prompting alarm.
3. The bone marrow aspirate will show classical features of megaloblastosis, and will also serve to identify any other cause for marrow hyperactivity with consequent folate depletion, such as some forms of leukemia or compensatory hypercellularity.

Bone Marrow Aspiration It is generally accepted that bone marrow aspiration should be done in all cases of suspected, even probable, megaloblastic anemia. Practice varies, however, and a case can be made out to avoid this procedure if

1. Normoblasts in the peripheral blood show indisputable megaloblastic features AND the clinical and FBC features are compatible.
2. It is sometimes held that in the elderly patient with a macrocytic anemia where the FBC features are fully compatible with megaloblastosis, it is permissible to avoid aspiration, treat the patient with vitamin B_{12} and folate, and watch for a reticulocyte response.
3. Occasionally the clinical and FBC features are so convincing that treatment can commence without prior aspiration – see Case #23.

The Treatment of Megaloblastic Anemia Treatment of a megaloblastic anemia should, if possible, never begin without biochemical diagnosis – i.e., whether it is folate of vitamin B_{12} responsible. Should it not be possible, *never ever* use folate as the first line of therapy – if the deficiency is of vitamin B_{12} you will precipitate extremely severe neurological damage by giving folate alone. Always start with a dose of vitamin B_{12} and then follow with folate.

The Non-megaloblastic Macrocytic Blood Picture

THE MOST IMPORTANT CAUSES HERE ARE CHRONIC LIVER DISEASE, ALCOHOLISM, AND HYPOTHYROIDISM.

FBC FEATURES

There may be a pancytopenia with chronic liver disease, since it is often associated with portal hypertension, splenomegaly, and hypersplenism, the features of which will be added to the total picture. These aspects are discussed further in Chapter 13.

RED CELLS: The typical appearance is as follows:

1. The anemia can be very severe. Note that in all these cases the pathogenesis of anemia may be complex, and may include elements of iron deficiency, chronic disease, hemolysis, bone marrow depression, and indeed folate deficiency. In this chapter we shall discuss only the most typical blood picture.
2. The MCV is raised but seldom above ± 115 fl, as is the RDW.
3. The MCH and the MCHC are normal.
4. The morphology of the red cells is striking: moderate to marked anisocytosis, normochromia. The macrocytes are **ROUND** and there are numerous target cells and often stomatocytes. Rouleaux formation is sometimes noted. The ESR is almost always moderately raised.

WHITE CELLS AND PLATELETS: No specific changes are typical. Toxic granulation of neutrophils may be present.

FEATURES IN OTHER TESTS

These depend on the underlying cause, and the features should be known. Importantly, the LDH is never **MARKEDLY** raised, even with severe liver disease.

The Blood Pictures of Aplasia and Reticulocytosis

These can be summarized very briefly, since they are discussed elsewhere. Aplastic anemia typically presents as a pancytopenia and mild round macrocytosis without target cells, tear-drop poikilocytes, fragmentation, or stomatocytes.

Reticulocytosis will show increased diffuse basophilia and often features reflecting the underlying anemia. Note that reticulocytosis purely as a response to hypoxia is seldom more than 3 or 4%, thus hardly likely to significantly raise the MCV.

The Complete Brief Pseudoalgorithmic Approach to Macrocytosis

The following approach has been found to work in the vast majority of cases. It cannot, however, cater for multiple pathologies and for the occasional atypical case:

1. **IS THERE PANCYTOPENIA**? There are three possibilities: megaloblastosis, myelodysplasia and aplastic anemia.

    a. **ARE THE MORPHOLOGICAL FEATURES SUGGESTIVE OF MEGALOBLASTOSIS**? See box below. If yes, see confirmatory test box.

    b. **ARE THE MORPHOLOGICAL FEATURES SUGGESTIVE OF CHRONIC LIVER DISEASE**? See box below.

    c. **ARE THE MORPHOLOGICAL FEATURES,** particularly of the red cells, **UNREMARKABLE**? If so, the probable diagnosis is aplastic anemia; proceed as described in Chapter 13.

    IF THERE IS NOT A PANCYTOPENIA,

2. **IS THE MCV > ± 128 FL**? Probable **IMMUNE HEMOLYSIS**. If so, proceed as described in Chapter 10 (but see case #26).

3. **IS THE MCV BETWEEN ± 115 AND ± 128 FL**? Are the morphological features suggestive of **MEGALO-BLASTOSIS**? If so, see box. Otherwise, are the morphological features suggestive of **IMMUNE HEMOLYSIS** (see box)? If so, proceed as described in Chapter 10.

4. **IS THE MCV BETWEEN ± 108 AND ± 115 FL**? Possibilities are **IMMUNE HEMOLYSIS, MEGALOBLASTOSIS** or **LIVER DISEASE,** **ALCOHOLISM OR HYPOTHYROIDISM.** For morphological features of the latter, see box.

5. **IS THE MCV < 108 FL**? Possibilities are **ANY OF THE FOUR GROUPS OF CONDITIONS** described. See boxes, including that for reticulocytosis.

Morphological Features Strongly Suggestive of Megaloblastosis

1. Oval macrocytes, tear-drop poikilocytes, sometimes fragmentation, punctate basophilia, or Cabot rings.
2. A marked right shift of the neutrophils.
3. If normoblasts are present, do they have megaloblastic features.

Confirmatory Tests of Megaloblastosis

1. Markedly raised LDH
2. Bone marrow appearance

Note that, once megaloblastosis is confirmed, further tests to identify the cause are necessary:

1. Serum vitamin B_{12} and folate levels, and red cell folate levels.
2. If the latter are ambiguous, examine the drugs the patient is on.
3. It may be necessary in cases of doubt to request further tests – Schilling test, deoxyuridine suppression test and methylmalonic acid level and excretion – consult your laboratory.

Morphological Features Strongly Suggesting Immune Hemolysis

1. Agglutinated red cells
2. Spherocytes
3. Sometimes fragmented red cells
4. No macrocytes

For associated and confirmatory tests, see Chapter 9.

Morphological Features of Non-megaloblastic Macrocytoses

1. Round macrocytes, target cells, sometimes stomatocytes, particularly with liver disease.
2. No right shift of neutrophils.
3. In the case of chronic liver disease, the features of hypersplenism may be superadded. See Chapter 9.

Morphological Features of Reticulocytosis

1. Diffuse basophilia (reflecting a raised reticulocyte count)
2. The features of the underlying condition that led to the reticulocytosis

The Value of Splenomegaly in Macrocytosis

Splenomegaly can be of considerable assistance in the differentiation of a macrocytic anemia.

1. Splenomegaly is very much against most types and causes of megaloblastosis, the only significant exception being when it is due to bone marrow infiltration that is also affecting the spleen. In these cases, the megaloblastosis is almost always due to (relative) folate deficiency.
2. Splenomegaly is common in liver disease but is not a feature of thyroid disease.
3. In macrocytosis due to reticulocytosis, splenomegaly would reflect an underlying hemolytic state in most cases.
4. Splenomegaly is not a feature of aplastic anemia.

Teaching Cases

CASE #23 (TABLES 9.1 AND 9.2)

Table 9.1

Patient	Age	Sex	Race	Altitude
Mrs B H	58 yrs	Female	White	5,000 ft

Before a history was taken, it was observed that as the patient walked into the office, her gait was peculiar: combined shuffling and wide-stepping. She had numerous complaints: tiredness, malaise, marked dyspnea on effort, recurrent diarrhea, a very sore mouth, tendency to fall and weakness in the arms and legs, and marked tingling in the lower legs. Up to 1 year ago she had been in good health, and had been very active running a farm with her husband. On examination she looked ill, very pale, with completely gray hair and with a tinge of jaundice. The BP was 106/60 and the PR was 96/min and fibrillating. The JVP was raised 3 cm, and there was a trace of ankle edema. There was no purpura or lymphadenopathy. The mouth and tongue were very red and atrophic. She was in moderate cardiac failure with a harsh murmur across the precordium. The cranial nerves and fundi were intact. There were numerous patches of vitiligo. There was no splenomegaly. Examination of the long tracts revealed severely impaired proprioception with absence of vibration sense; upper motor weakness was present mainly in the legs, with a positive Babinski sign.

	Value	Units	Reference range Low	High	Permitted range Low	High
Red cell count	2.22	$\times 10^{12}$/l	4.03	5.09	2.15	2.29
Hemoglobin (Hb)	7.61	g/dl	12.7	15.9	7.3	7.9
Hematocrit (Hct)	0.25	l/l	0.38	0.49	0.24	0.26
Mean cell volume	112	fl	80	99	109.8	114.2
Mean cell Hb	32.5	pg	27	31.5	31.8	33.1
Mean cell Hb conc.	29.0	g/dl	31.5	34.5	28.4	29.6
Red cell dist. width	18.1	%	11.6	14	18.1	18.1
Retic count %	0.5				0.5	0.5
Retic absolute (abs.)	11.1	$\times 10^9$/l	50	100	10.8	11.4
White cell count	4.21	$\times 10^9$/l	4	10	3.89	4.53
Corrected WCC	3.97	$\times 10^9$/l				
Neutrophils abs.	2.53	$\times 10^9$/l	2	7	2.34	2.72
Band cells abs.	0.00		0	0	0	0
Lymphocytes abs.	1.17	$\times 10^9$/l	1	3	1.09	1.26
Monocytes abs.	0.34	$\times 10^9$/l	0.2	1	0.32	0.37
Eosinophils abs.	0.12	$\times 10^9$/l	0.02	0.5	0.11	0.13
Basophils abs.	0.04	$\times 10^9$/l	0.02	0.1	0.04	0.04
Normoblasts	6	/100 WBC	0	0		
Platelet count	121.0	$\times 10^9$/l	150	400	108.9	133.1
Sedimentation	54	mm/h	0	20	51	57
Morphology	There is a pancytopenia. The red cells are normochromic and macrocytic with marked anisocytosis. The macrocytes are largely oval, and there are numerous tear-drop poikilocytes. The normoblasts show megaloblastic change.					

Table 9.2

(Case #23 cont.)			Reference range	
	Value	Units	Low	High
S-Urea	6.9	mmol/l	2.1	7.1
S-Creatinine	86	mmol/l	62	115
S-Sodium	141	mmol/l	136	145
S-Potassium	5.2	mmol/l	3.5	5.1
S-Chloride	101.0	mmol/l	98	108
S-Total CO_2	23	mmol/l	22	28
S-Anion gap	22.2	mmol/l	5	14
S-Bilirubin (total)	44.9	μmol/l	6.8	34.2
S-Bilirubin (direct)	7.1	μmol/l	1.7	8.6
S-Bilirubin (indirect)	37.8	μmol/l	5.1	25.6
S-LDH	2,684	IU/l	90	180
S-Vitamin B_{12}	93	pg/ml	193	982
S-Folate	7.1	ng/ml	3.0	17.0
RBC-Folate	90.4	ng/ml	93.0	641.0

For completeness' sake two final confirmatory tests were done (Table 9.3)

Table 9.3

	Value	Units	Low	High
S-Gastrin	921.3	ng/ml	10.0	100.0
Anti-parietal cell ab	+ + +		–	–

DISCUSSION

1. **THE CLINICAL FEATURES** are very typical indeed of pernicious anemia. Indeed the diagnosis of PA was confidently made before the results of the FBC or other tests were available. The positive features **FOR MEGALOBLASTIC ANEMIA** were

   a. **THE SYMPTOMS** of diarrhea, sore mouth and malaise
   b. **THE SIGNS** of pallor with a tinge of jaundice, glossitis and stomatitis and absence of splenomegaly

   The features specific for PA were

   a. **SKIN CHANGES**. Vitiligo is a prominent pointer to PA; the gray hair could have been explained by her age.
   b. The clinical features of **SUBACUTE COMBINED DEGENERATION OF THE CORD**. (This condition is extremely rare in folate deficiency). The features of peripheral neuritis were of less specificity.

2. **THE PATIENT WAS IN CARDIAC FAILURE**, clearly at least in part as a result of the anemia: the marked pallor, the wide pulse pressure, and harsh murmur over the precordium were convincing. The patient was urgently admitted to hospital; the management is detailed later. By the time the patient was admitted the blood results were available.

3. **THE FBC** shows numerous highly significant findings. The features are absolutely typical of **MEGALOBLASTIC ANEMIA**. In addition, the comment that the normoblasts showed megaloblastic features was extremely strong confirmatory evidence. Some practitioners maintain that this appearance obviates the need for a bone marrow aspirate. In this case, an immediate aspirate was not contemplated.

4. **THE BIOCHEMICAL TESTS** too are very informative. The markedly raised LDH is typical, as are the bilirubin results. The decreased vitamin B_{12} levels are fully compatible with PA; the slightly decreased RBC-folate levels are not to be construed as necessarily being due to associated folate deficiency – this is a common finding in vitamin B_{12} deficiency. The marginally raised potassium level is not necessarily a reflection of renal disease; this will be discussed below. Raised serum gastrin levels reflect the achlorhydria caused by autoimmune damage.

5. **ECG FINDINGS** confirmed the fibrillation. There was also a mild right axis deviation and non-specific ST segment changes.

6. **MANAGEMENT**:

   a. The first decision that had to be made was, why was the patient in cardiac failure, and what should be done about it? It is unusual for a Hb level of 7.71 g/dl to result in cardiac failure in a patient of this age, and with her evident good and physically active previous health. It was possible that underlying cardiac disease had emerged, but eventually it was felt that the atrial fibrillation was sufficient to tip the balance into failure. As a general principle, it is dangerous (and indeed unnecessary in most cases) to transfuse a patient with severe megaloblastic anemia: she already has a hemolytic state; and blood volume is high and adding to it with blood may be lethal.

   b. The patient was given a loading dose of vitamin B_{12} and furosemide plus regular high doses of a potassium preparation, as well as a moderate dose of digoxin for 2 days. The potassium level was monitored twice daily, and in addition ECGs were done twice daily to monitor for the development of hypokalemia. The reticulocyte count was repeated daily. Table 9.4 shows composite follow-up results.

Table 9.4

Day #	AM K+	PM K+	Retic %
1	5.3	3.5	0.6
2	3.3	3.0	0.7
3	3.0	3.1	0.6
4	3.4	3.3	5.1
5	3.5	3.7	9.2

The strong reticulocyte response can be seen. The dramatic hypokalemia should be noted. The cause of this is that as the vitamin B_{12} corrects the DNA synthesis, cell membrane function is restored and potassium is driven into the cells, much as insulin does in diabetic hyperkalemia. Although the low levels were worrying, on none of the days did the ECG show the changes of hypokalemia.

FOLLOW-UP

The patient made a rapid and uneventful recovery. Her cardiac failure disappeared and she has remained free of illness or disability since – with one exception: the damage to the cord is permanent, although over the next 2 years she did subjectively experience some gradual improvement.

CASE #24 (TABLE 9.5)

Table 9.5

Patient	Age	Sex	Race	Altitude
Mr J M	59 yrs	Male	Black	5,000 ft

The patient was referred by a urologist who had admitted the patient for the repair of a severe urethral stricture. He noticed that the patient was looking ill and underweight. A FBC (plus some other tests) were ordered, after which a consultation was arranged.

	Value	Units	Reference range Low	Reference range High	Permitted range Low	Permitted range High
Red cell count	3.46	$\times 10^{12}$/l	4.77	5.83	3.36	3.56
Hemoglobin (Hb)	10.8	g/dl	13.8	18.0	10.4	11.2
Hematocrit (Hct)	0.38	l/l	0.42	0.53	0.37	0.39
Mean cell volume	110	fl	80	99	107.8	112.2
Mean cell Hb	31.2	pg	27	31.5	30.6	31.8
Mean cell Hb conc.	28.4	g/dl	31.5	34.5	27.8	28.9
Red cell dist. width	15.9	%	11.6	14	14.7	17.1
Retic count	1.21	%	0.27	0.80	1.1	1.3
Retic absolute (abs.)	41.9	$\times 10^9$/l	30	100	38.7	45.0
White cell count	3.51	$\times 10^9$/l	3.5	10	3.25	3.77
Neutrophils abs.	1.52	$\times 10^9$/l	1.5	7	1.40	1.63
Lymphocytes abs.	1.40	$\times 10^9$/l	1	3	1.29	1.50
Monocytes abs.	0.38	$\times 10^9$/l	0.2	1	0.35	0.41
Eosinophils abs.	0.17	$\times 10^9$/l	0.02	0.5	0.16	0.18
Basophils abs.	0.04	$\times 10^9$/l	0.02	0.1	0.04	0.05
Normoblasts	0	/100 WBC	0		0	
Platelet count	187.0	$\times 10^9$/l	150	400	168.3	205.7
Sedimentation	29	mm/h	0	10	28	30

DISCUSSION

1. In the absence of morphology, all that one can say is that there is a mild to moderate macrocytic anemia. Two processes were followed – clinical evaluation of the patient (Table 9.6), and doing a morphological assessment of the film (Table 9.7).

Table 9.6

Clinical evaluation

The patient complained of chronic fatigue but no specific symptoms were forthcoming. He gives a history of substantial previous alcoholic intake and pipe smoking, but not for the last 3 years. On examination he appears thin without clinical anemia, jaundice, cyanosis, or purpura. The cardiovascular and respiratory systems were clinically normal. His abdomen revealed a 3 cm enlarged liver, firm and with a rounded edge. The spleen was not enlarged to palpation and there was no ascites.

Table 9.7

Morphology	The red cells are normochromic and macrocytic; the macrocytes are round and there is moderate anisocytosis.

2. Observe that the clinical features in this case are of considerable help in identifying the nature of the illness – i.e., alcoholic liver disease. However, this does not help much in suggesting the probable FBC findings: chronic liver disease can have very numerous hematological complications, including microcytic, macrocytic, and normocytic anemia. Without a FBC one is usually lost, unless there were other clinical features, such as koilonychia.

3. Although splenomegaly was not clinically detectable, the normal size of the spleen was confirmed sonographically.

4. A hemostatic screen was performed. The prothrombin time was found to be mildly prolonged – see Chapter 18.

Comment Chronic liver disease has multiple possible effects on the first-line tests. These were more fully discussed in Chapter 3.

Three short cases are now presented to illustrate a few more problems. Only the significant elements of the cases are presented.

CASE #25 (TABLE 9.8)

Table 9.8

Patient	Age	Sex	Race	Altitude
Miss Y K	19 yrs	Female	White	2,500 ft

This patient had been diagnosed with grand mal epilepsy at the age of 10. She had been reasonably well controlled on phenytoin and phenobarbitone. On a routine follow-up visit, her doctor noticed that she was pale and that the gums were markedly hypertrophied. He requested a FBC at his local lab, and on seeing the result and fearing leukemia, he referred the patient.

She had no specific symptoms. She had a maximum of two seizures a year. Recently, she had been feeling very tired and "fluey" and had noticed that her gums were swollen.

	Value	Units	Reference range Low	High	Permitted range Low	High
Red cell count	3.21	$\times 10^{12}$/l	3.91	4.94	3.11	3.31
Hemoglobin (Hb)	11.2	g / dl	12.4	15.5	10.8	11.6
Hematocrit (Hct)	0.35	1 / 1	0.37	0.47	0.34	0.36
Mean cell volume	109	fl	80	99	106.8	111.2
Mean cell Hb	34.9	pg	27	31.5	34.2	35.6
Mean cell Hb conc.	32.0	g/dl	31.5	34.5	31.4	32.7
White cell count	12.3	$\times 10^9$/l	4	10	11.38	13.22
Neutrophils abs.	4.43	$\times 10^9$/l	2	7	4.10	4.76
Band cells abs.	0.25		0	0.00	0.22	0.27
Lymphocytes abs.	6.40	$\times 10^9$/l	1	3	5.92	6.88
Monocytes abs.	0.62	$\times 10^9$/l	0.2	1	0.57	0.66
Eosinophils abs.	0.49	$\times 10^9$/l	0.02	0.5	0.46	0.53
Basophils abs.	0.12	$\times 10^9$/l	0.02	0.1	0.11	0.13
Normoblasts	0	/100 WBC	0	0		
Platelet count	103.0	$\times 10^9$/l	150	400	92.7	113.3
Sedimentation	35	mm/h	0	20	33	37
Morphology	Macrocytosis + Thrombocytopenia + Lymphocytosis + Atypical lymphocytes noted.					

DISCUSSION

1. One can understand the doctor's concern since gum hyperplasia occurs in acute monocytic or myelomonocytic leukemia (due to tissue infiltration). The FBC too is very worrying. There clearly is an anemia, lymphocytosis, and mild thrombocytopenia. Is it possible that this is a leukemia? It is clear that the morphology report consisted mainly of "flags"; it frequently occurs in country towns that there is a dearth of expert morphologists; thus this report must be taken seriously.

2. Once again it was the clinical features and detailed morphological examination that provided the answer.

3. Morphological reassessment confirmed macrocytosis, consisting of oval macrocytes, with some tear-drop cells; the lymphocytes while atypical showed no disquieting features. The impression was more that of a mild megaloblastic anemia plus a probable recent infection.

4. Clinically, the patient was suffering from a viral infection, probably with some secondary bacterial infection. The gum hyperplasia was obvious.

5. It was provisionally decided that the diagnosis was folate deficiency secondary to phenytoin (aggravated by phenobarbitone). Folate estimations showed a moderate decrease. It was felt that bone marrow examination could be postponed depending on her response.

6. The anti-epileptic medication was changed, and she was given large doses of folate. She responded fairly slowly with a significant reticulocytosis and the gums gradually came back to normal.

Exercise Case

CASE #26 (TABLE 9.9)

Table 9.9

Patient	Age	Sex	Race	Altitude
Mr J D	63 yrs	Male	White	5,000 ft

The patient is a hobo, living on the streets, and is possibly mildly retarded. Although he denies this, he almost certainly drinks a great deal of alcohol. He has been attending hematology clinic irregularly for many years. He had been diagnosed with chronic cold agglutinin disease (an uncommon form of immune hemolytic anemia). He has always suffered considerably in winter. Extensive search for underlying lymphoma had been planned, but the patient invariably refused hospital treatment after a few days. He was advised about keeping warm and prescribed folate, but compliance was very poor. On his latest visit was (after not having been seen for 2 years) he said he had deteriorated, feeling very poorly and complaining of diarrhea. It was noted that he had a tinge of jaundice and was paler than usual. We present first an FBC of several years ago when he was in a stable condition.

	Value	Units	Reference range Low	High	Permitted range Low	High
Red cell count	3.59	$\times 10^{12}$/l	4.77	5.83	3.48	3.70
Hemoglobin (Hb)	11.9	g/dl	13.8	18.0	11.5	12.3
Hematocrit (Hct)	0.39	l/l	0.42	0.53	0.38	0.40
Mean cell volume	110	fl	80	99	101.4	116.6
Mean cell Hb	33.1	pg	27	31.5	32.5	33.8
Mean cell Hb conc.	30.4	g/dl	31.5	34.5	29.8	31.0
Red cell dist. width	17.2	%	11.6	14	17.2	17.2
Retic count	3.1	%	0.27	1.00	3.0	3.2
Retic absolute (abs.)	111.3	$\times 10^9$/l	30	100	108.0	114.6
White cell count	5.98	$\times 10^9$/l	4	10	5.53	6.43
Corrected WCC	5.86	$\times 10^9$/l				
Neutrophils abs.	3.37	$\times 10^9$/l	2	7	3.11	3.62
Lymphocytes abs.	1.87	$\times 10^9$/l	1	3	1.73	2.01
Monocytes abs.	0.48	$\times 10^9$/l	0.2	1	0.45	0.52
Eosinophils abs.	0.21	$\times 10^9$/l	0.02	0.5	0.19	0.22
Basophils abs.	0.05	$\times 10^9$/l	0.02	0.1	0.04	0.05
Normoblasts	2	/100 WBC	0	0		
Platelet count	321.0	$\times 10^9$/l	150	400	296.9	345.1
Sedimentation	26	mm/h	0	10	25	27
Morphology	The red cells are normochromic and normocytic, and show some autoagglutination and spherocytes.					

Questions

1. What is the first-stage diagnosis? What features make you doubt the accuracy of this conclusion?

   _____

   _____

   _____

2. What do you think of the hematocrit and red cell count?

   _____

   _____

3 What are the possible general pathology diagnoses?

   _____

4 Do you think that there could be more than one cause for the macrocytosis? Which ones?

   _____

5 Do you think that the raised ESR necessarily signifies some form of infection or infiltration?

   _____

6. Why was the patient prescribed folate?

   _____

7. Why are his symptoms worse in winter? What would these symptoms be?

   _____

Answers

1. Macrocytic anemia. Autoagglutination is a potent source of spurious macrocytosis. It is important to note that if autoagglutination is mild it may cause only a mild rise in the MCV.
2. They are most probably inaccurate, since they depend on counting and sizing of individual red cells. Agglutinates are counted as single cells.
3. Reticulocytosis, megaloblastosis, chronic liver disease/alcoholism/ hypothyroidism, autoagglutination.
4. It is likely that three causes may be present: autoagglutination, reticulocytosis, and alcoholism.
5. The ESR measures the rate of fall of a column of red cells in plasma. One of the factors influencing the rate of fall is the weight of the red cells. Agglutinated red cells are slightly heavier than normal.
6. Chronic hemolysis results in a hyperactive marrow (compensatory) and thus requires more folate than normal.

7. The agglutination gets worse with cold. The agglutinins tend to clog the small peripheral vessels in the cold. The fingers tend to be particularly affected, becoming white, then blue, and recovery red. This condition is known as acrocyanosis, and is often misnamed Raynaud's phenomenon.

Table 9.10 shows the current FBC.

Table 9.10

Case #26 cont.	Value	Units	Reference range Low	Reference range High	Permitted range Low	Permitted range High
Red cell count	3.22	× 10¹²/l	4.77	5.83	3.12	3.32
Hemoglobin (Hb)	9.94	g/dl	13.8	18.0	9.6	10.3
Hematocrit (Hct)	0.37	l/l	0.42	0.53	0.36	0.38
Mean cell volume	116	fl	80	99	107.9	124.1
Mean cell Hb	30.9	pg	27	31.5	30.3	31.5
Mean cell Hb conc.	26.6	g/dl	31.5	34.5	26.1	27.1
Red cell dist. width	21.8	%	11.6	14	19.1	19.1
Retic count	0.9	%	0.27	1.00	0.9	0.9
Retic absolute (abs.)	29.0	× 10⁹/l	30	100	28.1	29.8
White cell count	3.25	× 10⁹/l	4	10	3.01	3.49
Corrected WCC	3.04	× 10⁹/l				
Neutrophils abs.	1.34	× 10⁹/l	2	7	1.24	1.44
Band cells abs.	0		0	0	0	0
Lymphocytes abs.	1.52	× 10⁹/l	1	3	1.41	1.64
Monocytes abs.	0.19	× 10⁹/l	0.2	1	0.18	0.21
Eosinophils abs.	0.16	× 10⁹/l	0.02	0.5	0.15	0.17
Basophils abs.	0.03	× 10⁹/l	0.02	0.1	0.03	0.03
Normoblasts	7	/100 WBC	0	0		
Platelet count	91.0	× 10⁹/l	150	400	84.2	97.8
Sedimentation	49	mm/h	0	10	47	51
Morphology	There is a pancytopenia. The red cells show anisochromia and anisocytosis. They are largely macrocytic; the macrocytes are both round, with some target cell formation, as well as oval, with numerous teardrops and some fragmentation. A small population of microcytic cells is seen, including small ovalocytes. The neutrophils show a prominent right shift					

Questions

1. What do you think has happened, to account for the deterioration in his blood picture?

   _____

   _____

   _____

   _____

2. What do you think of the small population of micro-cytic hypochromic cells and small oval cells?

_____

_____

3. What has happened to the previously high reticulocyte count?

_____

_____

Answers

1. The patient has not taken any folate for years, eventually resulting in a megaloblastic element to the anemia (the features of megaloblastic anemia should by now be well known). This aggravated by alcohol as well as the underlying autoagglutination has contributed to raising the MCV considerably.
2. These suggest either mild or developing iron deficiency or ACD. Poor diet and alcoholic gastritis would be potent causes of iron deficiency. It is not the major abnormality, the picture being overshadowed by the folate deficiency.
3. Megaloblastic anemia is frequently associated with a low reticulocyte count, since there is a metabolic block in red cell formation.

Comment It should be clear that unraveling a complex picture such as Case #26 requires insightful interpretation of the FBC; however, the answers would not easily be forthcoming without considerable clinical experience. Getting the answers to all the complexities of this patient's disease via blood tests would be very expensive indeed, and would still not provide the complete answer.

Comment

1. It is critically important to differentiate megaloblastic from non-megaloblastic causes of macrocytosis. The best way of doing this is by bone marrow aspiration if the clinical and FBC features are ambiguous.
2. The shape of the macrocytes (plus accompanying changes as described) is extremely valuable in differentiation. If you receive a report with a raised MCV without morphological comment, insist that it be done.
3. Once megaloblastosis is diagnosed, biochemical estimations are needed for the specific diagnosis.
4. However, biochemical tests can be confusing. A slightly decreased folate (and you should rely only on RBC-folate, not serum folate) frequently occurs in a primary vitamin B_{12} deficiency; treating the vitamin B_{12} deficiency results in the folate normalizing by itself.
5. In Chapter 2 we discussed the effect a ward diet can have on certain deficiency anemias. The sooner these patients are investigated the better.
6. Do not be misled by strict diagnostic "cutoff" points. For example, a patient with a MCV of 105 fl can have **any** of the causes of macrocytosis listed.

Further Reading

Andreoli TE, Bennett JC, Carpenter CCJ, Plum F (eds) (1997). Cecil Essentials of Medicine. 4th edn. Philadelphia: WB Saunders Company.

Epstein RJ (1996). Medicine for Examinations. 3rd edn. Churchill Livingstone.

Hoffbrand AV, Pettit JE (2001). Essential Haematology. 4th edn. Oxford: Blackwell Science.

Lewis SM, Bain B, Bates I (2006). Dacie and Lewis Practical Haematology. 10th edn. Churchill Livingstone.

Defining Normocytosis

To refresh your memory, "normocytic" means that the MCV lies between 80 and 98 fl. It does NOT mean that the morphology of the red cells is normal. Note that a first-stage diagnosis of "normocytosis" is pointless – after all, a normal FBC also is "normocytic." "Normocytosis" as a first-stage diagnosis is only of relevance if there is anemia. The stage 1 diagnosis must therefore start with **ANEMIA**:

> **STEP 1:** "Where is the primary abnormality?" **IT LIES IN THE HB**. The Hb is decreased. Therefore there is **ANEMIA**.
>
> **STEP 2:** "What form does it take?" The MCV is within the reference range. Therefore it is a **NORMOCYTIC ANEMIA**.

The normocytic anemias are the most difficult to interpret for a number of reasons:

1. They are the result of a large group of disparate causes; there are no unifying themes, as there are with the micro- and macrocytic anemias.
2. With macro- and microcytic pictures one can talk of macrocytosis and microcytosis respectively without anemia being present. As indicated, this is not possible with the normocytic anemias. Of course, absence of an anemia does not exclude any of the causes we shall be discussing if mild enough or compensated.

The essential pathogenesis of each cause must be understood.

The General Pathology Causes of a Normocytic Anemia

!

AT THE GENERAL LEVEL THERE ARE EIGHT CAUSES:
1. Certain endocrine deficiencies
2. Renal insufficiency
3. Post-hemorrhagic anemia
4. Anemia of chronic disorders (ACD)
5. Combinations of megaloblastic anemia with iron deficiency or ACD
6. Bone marrow infiltration or replacement
7. Hemolytic anemias
8. Hypersplenism

Before we can discuss the specific causes, it will be very helpful to understand the physiological basis of how the Hb level comes to be what it is

1. If all the known stimuli for erythropoiesis were theoretically removed, the "basal" Hb in an adult would probably be around 5–6 g/dl.
2. The influence of erythropoietin (EPO) more or less doubles this to say 11 g/dl.
3. The difference between this and the **FEMALE**'s normal Hb of say 13 would be due to hormonal influences, notably cortisol, thyroxine, estrogen, and small amount of testosterone.
4. In the case of a **MALE** with a normal Hb of say 15, the difference from the female level would be largely due to the effect of testosterone.

It can thus be expected that endocrine deficiencies and renal anemia would be characterized by anemia. Since these hormones have little or no direct effect on **QUALITATIVE** red cell formation, the cells are more or less normal in size, color, and shape.

The Specific Causes of a Normocytic Anemia

Endocrine Deficiencies

Anemia is a common finding in many endocrine deficiencies, and with one exception, they are all normocytic – the exception being hypothyroidism, which is frequently macrocytic, and sometimes as a result of some of its complications, microcytic. We are primarily concerned here with

1. Hypopituitarism
2. Addison disease
3. Hypogonadism

THESE ENDOCRINE DEFICIENCIES ARE CHARACTERIZED BY

1. FEATURES IN THE FBC.

    a. The anemia is mild – seldom below about 11 g/dl in a female and about 12 g/dl in a male.

    b. The red cells are normal in shape and size; the RDW is thus normal.

    c. There is no diffuse basophilia and the reticulocyte count is characteristically low.

    d. The white cells and platelets are normal, with one exception – the mild eosinophilia of established Addison disease (the eosinophil count varies inversely with the cortisol level – see Chapter 4).

2. FEATURES IN OTHER LABORATORY TESTS.

    These depend very much on the underlying endocrine disorder. If the primary disorder is central (i.e., in the pituitary or hypothalamus), all the hormone levels of the affected axis will be decreased. For example in Cushing disease (i.e., a pituitary adenoma), ACTH, cortisol, and adrenal androgen levels will be low, whereas in Cushing syndrome (primary adrenal disease), cortisol and adrenal androgens (and mineralocorticoids, which are independent of pituitary control) will be raised, but the ACTH will be decreased. Many of these conditions have characteristic secondary effects on electrolytes, etc.

3. COMMON CLINICAL ACCOMPANIMENTS.

    These are very variable, depending on the underlying disorder, and are outside the scope of this book. Some features will be presented in the cases.

Renal Anemia

There are many possible causes of anemia in the patient with renal insufficiency, such as anemia of chronic disorders, shortened life span, blood loss; the major cause, however, is due to EPO deficiency (the mechanism has been explained above).

RENAL ANEMIA DUE TO EPO DEFICIENCY IS CHARACTERIZED BY

1. FEATURES IN THE FBC.

    a. The degree of the anemia due to EPO deficiency more or less parallels the creatinine clearance. The Hb only reaches its nadir with a clearance of <20 ml/min.

    b. The relatively minor morphological abnormalities are largely due to secondary vascular and toxic influences on the red cell; the RDW is mildly, occasionally moderately raised.

    c. Diffuse basophilia is normally absent and the reticulocyte count is low.

    d. The white cell count is normal and the neutrophils characteristically show a right shift.

    e. The platelet count is generally normal, but note that platelet function is abnormal (due to uremic toxicity), tending to cause a purpuric bleeding disorder. This is discussed in Chapter 18; an integrated view of the hematology of renal disease is presented in Chapter 5.

2. FEATURES IN OTHER LABORATORY TESTS.

    The biochemical changes in renal insufficiency should be well known. The bleeding time is characteristically prolonged; this is due to platelet dysfunction.

3. COMMON CLINICAL ACCOMPANIMENTS.

    The clinical features of renal disease are beyond the scope of this book.

Post-hemorrhagic Anemia

The blood volume after acute blood loss is corrected either by withdrawal of fluid from the tissues or by treatment with crystalloid. This leaves in effect a deficiency of (normal) red cells, i.e., anemia.

POST-HEMORRHAGIC ANEMIA IS CHARACTERIZED BY

1. FEATURES IN THE FBC (the hematological changes following acute hemorrhage have been extensively discussed in Chapter 4; what follows is a brief summary):

    a. The Hb level depends on how much blood was lost and how much fluid was replaced.

    b. The red cells are normocytic and normochromic, unless there have been repeated episodes of acute hemorrhage, in which case, without replacement of red cells, microcytosis and hypochromia may already have developed.

    c. There may be increased diffuse basophilia (and a reticulocytosis) if the bone marrow response has already started. In this case the RDW is likely to be mildly increased.

    d. There may be a neutrophilia and thrombocytosis (reactive).

2. FEATURES IN OTHER LABORATORY TESTS.

    These are non-specific or are the result of the underlying lesion causing the hemorrhage.

3. **COMMON CLINICAL FEATURES.**

These have been discussed at length in Chapter 4.

Anemia of Chronic Disorders (ACD)

The pathogenesis of this condition was explained in Chapter 8, as were the laboratory and clinical features. The only point to reiterate here is that it always starts as a normocytic anemia and only later tends to become microcytic.

Combinations of Megaloblastic Anemia with Iron Deficiency or ACD

The point has repeatedly been made – the MCV as measured by electronic counters is an average of very many cells. Thus where a microcytic and a macrocytic anemia coexist, the MCV represents a mixture of the two. There are many causes of this picture: important ones at the general level are the toast-and-tea syndrome, Crohn disease, pregnancy, and chronic liver disease/alcoholism.

THIS PICTURE IS CHARACTERIZED BY

1. **FEATURES IN THE FBC.**

   a. The Hb is variable, depending on the severity of the two processes – one tending to microcytosis and the other to macrocytosis.
   b. The MCV lies anywhere between 80 and 98 fl. Where exactly it lies suggests which of the two processes is dominant. As was discussed in Chapters 8 and 9, a microcytic or macrocytic anemia could also have associated mild megaloblastosis or iron deficiency, respectively, which would only be recognized by morphological examination of the smear, and the MCV in either case would be affected by the other process.
   c. The RDW is characteristically very high.
   d. Diffuse basophilia is typically absent and the retic count is low.
   e. Cell morphology generally shows two populations of cells, one being microcytic and hypochromic and with small oval or even elliptical cells, and the other macrocytic with large oval cells, tear-drop poikilocytes, and fragmentation. In the case of ACD, rouleaux may be present.
   f. The neutrophils show a right shift.

2. **FEATURES IN OTHER LABORATORY TESTS.**

   This depends to an extent on the cause, but the LDH is typically raised, and the ESR is raised, often

moderately. The iron studies again are rather complex, reflecting the mixture of processes.

3. **FEATURES IN THE BONE MARROW EXAMINATION.**

   In view of the complexity of the other results, it is frequently thought valuable to do a bone marrow aspirate. This will show features of both processes, and the report will establish this.

4. **COMMON CLINICAL FEATURES.**

   This very much depends on the underlying condition. Clinical features of both megaloblastosis and iron deficiency or ACD will be present.

Bone Marrow Infiltration or Replacement

In this condition, since the bone marrow milieu is very abnormal due to the infiltration, the red cells can also be deformed; but generally speaking the average size is normal, but typically with a raised RDW.

An isolated normocytic anemia is only one of many presentations of bone marrow infiltration. These are discussed fully in the Chapter 13. In summary, they are

1. Pancytopenia and bicytopenia
2. Thrombocytopenia
3. Leukocytosis, varying from general increase in cells with or without normoblasts (leuko-erythroblastic picture), to neutrophilia, to leukemic blasts, to lymphoma and plasma cells
4. Thrombocytosis

Hemolytic Anemias

This is a vast and difficult subject and has been adequately explored in Chapters 2, 4, and 5. While most of these anemias are normocytic, exceptions do exist, such as in hereditary elliptocytosis. It has already been explained that hemolysis may be intravascular or extravascular. In intravascular hemolysis the red cells are damaged or destroyed within the circulation. Extravascular hemolysis is an accentuation of the normal splenic breakdown of red cells and is due to primary abnormalities of the red cells. Consequently the RDW is usually raised and the shape is often abnormal, and they may show **FRAGMENTATION, AUTOAGGLUTINATION**, or specific morphological changes indicating the cause of premature breakdown.

The hemolytic-uremic syndrome is a complex disorder and is discussed in Chapter 23.

Hypersplenism

This is a condition where the spleen is enlarged for any reason and causes various cytopenias. Note that the blood cells are **NORMAL**. The formal criteria for the diagnosis are detailed later.

The Distinction Between Hypersplenism and Hemolysis

A great deal of confusion still exists in certain quarters about the distinction between hypersplenism and hemolysis. For many people these are virtually synonymous. In fact they are both pathologically and clinically entirely different. The differences were implicitly touched on in Chapter 2; more formally, the following are the essential points of difference:

1. In hemolysis the red cells are primarily abnormal, and the **NORMAL** spleen enlarges to cope with the increased breakdown; in hypersplenism the spleen is **PRIMARILY ABNORMAL** (almost always enlarged as a result) and the blood cells passing through are **NORMAL**.
2. In hemolysis only the red cells are involved (except for rare occasions in immune hemolysis where the antibodies have specificity against other blood cells); in hypersplenism any or all of the three cell lines may be affected.
3. In hemolysis the marrow is hypercellular as a compensatory mechanism, there is a reticulocytosis, and the red cell survival is demonstrably shortened; in hypersplenism the situation is complex and ill-understood:

    a. The marrow is seldom hypercellular – but it is never hypocellular (of relevance when we discuss pancytopenia in Chapter 13).
    b. There is seldom a significant reticulocytosis – and if there is it is never appropriate to the degree of anemia.
    c. Red cell (and platelet and white cell) survival is not often demonstrably shortened.

4. In hemolysis the major pathology is red cell destruction; in hypersplenism the major pathology, in the majority of cases, appears to be sequestration of cell within the spleen (and not their destruction).

For those interested, there are two other rare causes of a normocytic anemia:

1. **PURE RED CELL APLASIA**. Instead of, as in aplastic anemia all the cell lines being affected, only the red cell series are affected. There is an association with thymoma.

2. **SYNDROME OF INAPPROPRIATE SECRETION OF ADH**. Multiple general conditions can cause this. It results in water retention, which can amount to 5 l in total. This may effectively cause a dilutional anemia if the patient's pre-existing Hb was on the low side of normal. The anemia is clearly spurious and must not in itself be treated.

Making the Diagnosis

From the hematologist's point of view, one is faced with a patient who is anemic and whose MCV is within the reference range. But in fact in clinical practice one is faced with a sick patient, perhaps pale, in whom we **THEN** discover a **NORMOCYTIC** anemia. This can be a bewildering finding unless a logical, clinically orientated approach is adopted, since so much depends on the clinical features.

There are four practical issues in the diagnostic approach:

1. The problem for the clinical instructor is that the clinical conditions associated with a normocytic anemia cover a wide spectrum of general clinical medicine, and it is not feasible in a book such as this to go into all of these extensively. The cases presented have been selected to illustrate some representative presentations as well as some more unusual ones that are valuable from a teaching point of view.
2. Anemia is only sometimes the primary focus. Most commonly it is a secondary consideration in a case that presents with features of disease in other systems, such as renal failure, Simmond disease, and so on, and the primary focus is on these.
3. The FBC findings are decisive or at least highly suggestive in only a few of these conditions. The blood cell morphology is as important in the normocytic anemias as in other anemias, yet ironically they tend to be the least likely to be studied morphologically, probably because the micro- and macrocytic anemias are far more on the forefront of thinking (and perhaps subconsciously the normocytic features are regarded as "normal"). It is advisable to insist on a morphological assessment for **ALL** your anemias.
4. In all the conditions the clinical input is critical – indeed, of all hematological presentations, the normocytic anemias are the most requiring of broad-based clinical assessment.

Figure 10.1 illustrates **SPECIFIC ASPECTS** of the examination of a patient in whom a normocytic anemia is found; clearly it is part of the overall examination as is depicted in Fig. 5.4.

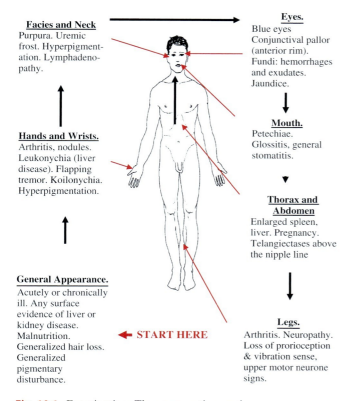

Facies and Neck. Purpura. Uremic frost. Hyperpigmentation. Lymphadenopathy.

Hands and Wrists. Arthritis, nodules. Leukonychia (liver disease). Flapping tremor. Koilonychia. Hyperpigmentation.

General Appearance. Acutely or chronically ill. Any surface evidence of liver or kidney disease. Malnutrition. Generalized hair loss. Generalized pigmentary disturbance.

← **START HERE**

Eyes. Blue eyes Conjunctival pallor (anterior rim). Fundi: hemorrhages and exudates. Jaundice.

Mouth. Petechiae. Glossitis, general stomatitis.

Thorax and Abdomen Enlarged spleen, liver. Pregnancy. Telangiectases above the nipple line

Legs. Arthritis. Neuropathy. Loss of proriception & vibration sense, upper motor neurone signs.

Fig. 10.1 Examination: The normocytic anemias

Once again we will divide our discussion into those cases that **CAN** present in a clinically obvious way, and the others.

Clinically Obvious or Suggestive Cases

The following disorders are often clinically obvious or can at least have highly suggestive features:

1. **RENAL FAILURE.** Suggestion of uremia – uremic frost, hypertension, dehydration, bleeding tendency, confusion, leukonychia.
2. **HYPOPITUITARISM, HYPOADRENALISM, HYPOGONADISM.** The clinical features should be known.
3. **GENERAL CHRONIC DISEASE,** particularly chronic arthritides (often with acute exacerbations), and malignancies.
4. **LIVER DISEASE AND OTHER CAUSES OF HYPERSPLENISM.**
   NOTE THE FORMAL CRITERIA FOR THE DIAGNOSIS OF HYPERSPLENISM:

   a. An enlarged spleen (perhaps only radiologically demonstrated)

b. A peripheral cytopenia
c. Bone marrow is never hypocellular
d. Splenectomy permanently and completely cures the condition

5. **NUTRITIONAL DEFICIENCY.** The most important nutritional disorders here are iron, folate, and vitamin B$_{12}$ deficiency. See Chapters 5, 8, and 9. The clinical features of both iron deficiency and megaloblastosis may be present.
6. **A RECENT BLEED.** This is usually clinically obvious, but can be occult – see under The Physiological Response to Acute Hemorrhage and the Effects on the FBC in Chapter 2.
7. **HEMOLYSIS.** The clinical features are very variable, but some broad generalizations can be made:

   a. Acutely developing pallor or anemia in the absence of serious bleeding.
   b. A patient such as in (a) above but also with high fever, chills, sweating, mental confusion, and perhaps even severe hemoglobinuria would be suspicious of hemolysis due to infection, such as malaria or DIC.
   c. A patient such as (b) above but without the high fever, but with loin pain, may be indicative of acute immune hemolysis (autoimmune, post-transfusion, etc.).
   d. Chronic anemia with a tinge of jaundice, absence of bilirubin in the urine, splenomegaly, and perhaps gallstones or leg ulcers, which can be a feature of chronic hemolytic states.
   e. Chronic anemia with jaundice, acute severe bone, abdominal and chest pains, leg ulcers and absence of a spleen, usually in a Black patient, would be suggestive of sickle disease.

Clinically Undefined Cases

DIFFICULTIES ARISE WHEN the patient presents with ambiguous symptoms and signs; a FBC is done and a normocytic anemia is found. Figure 10.1 is particularly valuable here. In these cases, **THE DEGREE OF ANEMIA IS OF ASSISTANCE:**

1. If the Hb is below ± 7 g/dl, the following can probably be eliminated, at least in the first instance:

   a. Hypersplenism
   b. Anemia of chronic disorders
   c. Endocrine deficiencies

2. If the Hb is > ± 7 g/dl, the above causes become possible (although ACD seldom produces a Hb of

< 9 g/dl). Of course, milder cases of the other causes listed may also be responsible.

In addition, certain specific or associated clinical features may be of great assistance: splenomegaly, lymphadenopathy, and bone tenderness. Splenomegaly in particular is usually of great assistance in differentiation. This is further discussed after the case presentations.

AN INTEGRATED CLINICAL/LABORATORY ASSESSMENT IS OF MAJOR IMPORTANCE IN THESE CASES. THE FBC ALONE WILL SELDOM PROVIDE THE SPECIFIC DIAGNOSIS ALTHOUGH IT CAN PROVIDE VERY HELPFUL POINTERS.

Teaching Cases

CASE #27 (EXAMINE TABLE 10.1)

NOTE

1. Only the red cells show changes. These are not very severe. The red cells are normochromic and normocytic; the normal RDW suggests that morphology is likely to be normal.
2. There is no history of recent bleeding, no neutrophilia, no thrombocytosis, and no reticulocytosis. The history is long. All this is very much against a recent bleed. In fact the reticulocytes are decreased, suggesting a decreased production. Decreased production may be due to

   a. **PRIMARY MARROW FAILURE** (aplastic anemia). This presents with pancytopenia.
   b. **DEFECTIVE RELEASE AS IN MEGALOBLASTOSIS**, which presents typically with pancytopenia and a macrocytic anemia, or myelodysplastic syndrome: this also typically presents with cytopenia involving more than one cell line, is often macro- or microcytic, and shows lots of anisocytosis. Although very unlikely, in the absence of a morphological comment this possibility must be borne in mind.
   c. **BONE MARROW INFILTRATION OR REPLACEMENT**. The neutrophils do not show a left shift, there are no normoblasts, and no evident poikilocytosis of the red cells, arguing strongly against this.

3. The ESR is mildly raised. This may be due to the anemia alone. However, an inflammatory or

Table 10.1

Patient	Age	Sex	Race	Altitude
Mrs J K	35 yrs	Female	Black	2,500 ft

This patient presented with an 18-month history of progressive tiredness, effort dyspnea, amenorrhea, and loss of libido. She was pale, with loss of head as well as secondary sexual hair. Her skin showed blotchy changes in pigmentation. She looked considerably older than her years.

	Value	Units	Reference range Low	High	Permitted range Low	High
Red cell count	3.71	× 10^{12}/l	3.91	4.94	3.60	3.82
Hemoglobin (Hb)	10.6	g/dl	12.4	15.5	10.2	11.0
Hematocrit (Hct)	0.32	l/l	0.37	0.47	0.31	0.33
Mean cell volume	86	fl	80	99	84.3	87.7
Mean cell Hb	28.6	pg	27	31.5	28.0	29.1
Mean cell Hb conc.	33.2	g/dl	31.5	34.5	32.6	33.9
Red cell dist. width	13.5	%	11.6	14	13.5	13.5
Retic. count %	0.11	%	0.25	0.75	0.1	0.1
Retic. absolute	4.1	× 10^9/l	30	100	3.7	4.5
White cell count	5.56	× 10^9/l	3.5	10	5.14	5.98
Neutrophils %	61.0	%			61.0	61.0
Band cells %	0.0	%	0		0.0	0.0
Lymphocytes %	23.0	%			23.0	23.0
Monocytes %	7.0	%			7.0	7.0
Eosinophils %	8.0	%			8.0	8.0
Basophils %	1.0	%			1.0	1.0
Neutrophils abs.	3.39	× 10^9/l	1.5	7	3.14	3.65
Band cells abs.	0.00		0	0	0	0
Lymphocytes abs.	1.28	× 10^9/l	1	3	1.18	1.37
Monocytes abs.	0.39	× 10^9/l	0.2	1	0.36	0.42
Eosinophils abs.	0.44	× 10^9/l	0.02	0.5	0.41	0.48
Basophils abs.	0.06	× 10^9/l	0.02	0.1	0.05	0.06
Normoblasts	0	/100 WBC	0	0		
Platelet count	231.0	× 10^9/l	150	400	207.9	254.1
Sedimentation	28	mm/h	0	20	27	29

infiltrative process cannot be excluded, and should thus be borne in mind. Unfortunately there is no comment on the presence of a left shift, or of rouleaux, which would have helped considerably.

4. Mild renal insufficiency is a possibility. Comment on the presence of burr cells, fragments, or a right shift in the neutrophils would have helped.

Table 10.2

Case #27 cont.			Reference range	
	Value	Units	Low	High
S-Urea	2.7	mmol/l	2.1	7.1
S-Creatinine	71	mmol/l	62	115
S-Urea:creatinine	38.0			
S-Calcium (total)	2.35	mmol/l	2.2	2.55
S-Magnesium	0.94	mmol/l	0.66	1.07
S-Phosphate	0.99	mmol/l	0.87	1.45
S-Albumin	39	g/l	34	48
S-Bilirubin (total)	19.4	µmol/l	6.8	34.2
S-Bilirubin (direct)	5.1	µmol/l	1.7	8.6
S-Bilirubin (indirect)	14.3	µmol/l	5.1	25.6
C-reactive protein	2.9	mg/l	0.0	10.0
S-Ferritin female	109.1	µg/l	14.0	233.1
S-Iron	19.1	µmol/l	11.6	31.3
S-Transferrin	2.98	g/l	2.12	3.60
S-Fe saturation female	30.3	%	15.0	35.0
S-Vitamin B_{12}	501	pg/ml	193	982
RBC-folate	428	ng/ml	93.0	641.0
S-Erythropoietin	41.1	ng/ml	10	55
S-ACTH	0.9	ng/l	0.0	46.0
S-Cortisol	6.1	nmol/l	38	690
S-T4	5.5	pmol/l	9.1	23.8
S-TSH	0.31	mIU/l	0.49	4.67
S-FSH	3.6	IU/l		
S-LH	2.9	IU/l		
S-Estradiol	5.6			
S-Progesterone	1.1			
S-Prolactin	1	ng/ml	1	25

5. The clinical features, however, are very suggestive.

A number of further investigations were done (Table 10.2).

In the various tests, there is nothing to suggest renal insufficiency, iron deficiency, megaloblastosis, hemolysis, or hypersplenism. There is clear evidence of hypopituitarism. Reviewing her history revealed that she had had a child after a very difficult delivery 4 years before. The diagnosis of Sheehan syndrome was finally made. She was placed on replacement therapy of corticosteroids, thyroxine, and female sex hormones; she quite rapidly started improving and within a year was normal. The Hb recovered without specific hematinic therapy.

Comment Anemia or pallor would clearly not in practice be the major clinical focus in the above type of case.

CASE #28 (TABLES 10.3 AND 10.4)

Table 10.3

Patient	Age	Sex	Race	Altitude
Mr A R	33 yrs	Male	White	2,500 ft

The patient has lived all his life in a country town. He and others have noticed that he usually has shown a tinge of jaundice since childhood. Otherwise he has felt reasonably well. Recently he made application for a life insurance policy. His local doctor found an enlarged spleen, which led to his proposal being postponed pending a specialist report.

Systematic history is entirely non-contributory, except for episodes of vague upper abdominal pain with nausea. His urine is normal in color. He has had no abdominal pain. He can supply no clear details of his family history. His son is healthy, not jaundiced. He can remember no episodes suggesting hepatitis, and does not take more than occasional social alcohol. On examination he had a mild lemon-yellow jaundice. The spleen was enlarged 5 cm below the costal margin. The liver and lymph nodes were normal. Urinalysis show no bilirubin but 2+ urobilin.

	Value	Units	Reference range Low	Reference range High	Permitted range Low	Permitted range High
Red cell count	4.15	$\times 10^{12}$/l	4.64	5.67	4.03	4.27
Hemoglobin (Hb)	11.7	g/dl	13.4	17.5	11.3	12.1
Hematocrit (Hct)	0.36	l/l	0.41	0.52	0.35	0.37
Mean cell volume	87	fl	80	99	85.3	88.7
Mean cell Hb	28.2	pg	27	31.5	27.6	28.8
Mean cell Hb conc.	32.4	g/dl	31.5	34.5	31.8	33.1
Red cell dist. width	16.1	%	11.6	14	14.9	17.3
Retic. count %	3.11	%	0.26	0.77	2.9	3.3
Retic. absolute (abs.)	129.1	$\times 10^9$/l	50	100	119.4	138.7
White cell count	5.97	$\times 10^9$/l	4	10	5.52	6.42
Corrected WCC	5.85	$\times 10^9$/l				
Neutrophils abs.	3.65	$\times 10^9$/l	2	7	3.37	3.92
Lymphocytes abs.	1.50	$\times 10^9$/l	1	3	1.39	1.61
Monocytes abs.	0.47	$\times 10^9$/l	0.2	1	0.43	0.50
Eosinophils abs.	0.30	$\times 10^9$/l	0.02	0.5	0.28	0.33
Basophils abs.	0.05	$\times 10^9$/l	0.02	0.1	0.05	0.06
Normoblasts	2	/100 WBC	0	0		
Platelet count	289.0	$\times 10^9$/l	150	400	260.1	317.9
Morphology	The red cells show anisocytosis with large numbers of target cells and occasional cells showing condensed hemoglobin. There is increased diffuse basophilia.					

Table 10.4

Case #28 cont.			Reference range	
	Value	Units	Low	High
S-Bilirubin (total)	58.2	µmol/l	6.8	34.2
S-Bilirubin (direct)	11.1	µmol/l	1.7	8.6
S-Bilirubin (indirect)	47.1	µmol/l	5.1	25.6
S-LDH	316	IU/l	90	180
S-Folate	6.3	ng/ml	3.0	17.0
RBC-folate	101.6	ng/ml	93.0	641.0
S-Haptoglobin	0.03	g/l	0.16	2
U-Bilirubin	Absent	"+"		
U-Urobilin	++	"+"		

DISCUSSION

1. The first-stage diagnosis is clearly that of normocytic anemia.

2. The general pathology diagnosis is almost certainly chronic extravascular hemolysis: it is difficult to see an alternative diagnosis in the light of chronic acholuric jaundice and splenomegaly, even without a family history being available. Indeed, in practice this general diagnosis was made clinically, before the FBC and other tests were available.

3. The FBC confirms this hypothesis in the light of a normocytic anemia, reticulocytosis, and no abnormalities in the other cell lines.

4. The chemical tests confirm the features of a hemolytic state: raised indirect bilirubin, decreased haptoglobin, and urobilin in the urine.

5. The specific diagnosis in these cases always involves laboratory investigation, sometimes very elaborate. However, the large numbers of target cells and condensed Hb suggested the possibility of HbC disease.

6. The next step was ordering Hb electrophoresis. This revealed homozygous HbCC disease. The hemoglobin C gene is particularly prevalent – indeed apparently originated – in West Africa. This case show that sporadic cases can occur in other racial groups.

7. Why was this not suspected to be hypersplenism? There are numerous factors against this possibility:

   a. The jaundice (although jaundice can occur in association with hypersplenism in cases where the enlarged spleen is due to portal hypertension – in these cases the raised bilirubin is direct as well as indirect)
   b. The reticulocytosis
   c. The long history

8. HbC trait and disease are rare except in endemic areas. By far the most common specific cause of this general presentation is hereditary spherocytosis.

9. The vague upper gastro-intestinal symptoms prompted sonography of the abdomen; numerous gallstones were demonstrated. Later, at operation these turned out to be the classical pigment stones of chronic hemolysis.

10. His son was tested and he turned out, as expected to have the HbC trait. He need expect no problems but must make very sure that a prospective wife is screened for a hemoglobinopathy or thalassemia.

Comment The above presentation is typical in almost all cases of extravascular hemolysis. Severity both of the clinical features and laboratory changes depends largely on the zygosity. The most common of these disorders is hereditary spherocytosis.

The only significant exception is sickle disease, whose clinical features can include many other symptoms and signs. It is a rather complex disorder and is discussed in Chapter 22.

Observe that red cell morphology can make a very significant contribution to the diagnosis, potentially saving a great deal of time and money.

CASE #29 (TABLES 10.5 AND 10.6)

Table 10.5

Patient	Age	Sex	Race	Altitude
Mr J T	37 yrs	Male	Black	2,500 ft

The patient is a manual laborer in a subtropical region. He has been feeling fatigued for some years but about 2 years ago this worsened considerably. He attended a rural clinic and was then referred to a tertiary center. He says he is constantly tired and lacks energy; he has a good appetite but feels satiated very soon; he has lost a lot of weight. He denies excessive alcohol. On examination he is underweight and ill looking. There is no jaundice but he is possibly pale. He has an enlarged spleen extending to 8 cm below the costal margin. The liver is quite hard, extending 2 cm below the costal margin. An early caput medusae was observed. No other relevant clinical features were found.

	Value	Units	Reference range Low	Reference range High	Permitted range Low	Permitted range High
Red cell count	3.51	× 10¹²/l	4.64	5.67	3.40	3.62
Hemoglobin (Hb)	10.6	g/dl	13.4	17.5	10.2	11.0
Hematocrit (Hct)	0.31	l/l	0.41	0.52	0.30	0.32
Mean cell volume	88	fl	80	99	86.2	89.8
Mean cell Hb	30.2	pg	27	31.5	29.6	30.8
Mean cell Hb conc.	34.3	g/dl	31.5	34.5	33.6	35.0
Red cell dist. width	15.1	%	11.6	14	14.0	16.2
Retic. count %	0.89	%	0.26	0.77	0.9	0.9
Retic. absolute (abs.)	31.2	× 10⁹/l	30	100	30.3	32.2
White cell count	2.91	× 10⁹/l	3.5	10	2.69	3.13
Neutrophils abs.	1.27	× 10⁹/l	1.5	7	1.18	1.37
Lymphocytes abs.	1.19	× 10⁹/l	1	3	1.10	1.28
Monocytes abs.	0.24	× 10⁹/l	0.2	1	0.22	0.25
Eosinophils abs.	0.18	× 10⁹/l	0.02	0.5	0.16	0.19
Basophils abs.	0.03	× 10⁹/l	0.02	0.1	0.03	0.03
Normoblasts	0	/100 WBC	0	0		
Platelet count	101.0	× 10⁹/l	150	400	90.9	111.1
Morphology	There is a mild pancytopenia. The red cells are normochromic and normocytic. No abnormal forms are seen.					

Table 10.6

Case #29 cont.			Reference range	
	Value	Units	Low	High
S-Bilirubin (total)	31.5	µmol/l	6.8	34.2
S-Bilirubin (direct)	7.8	µmol/l	1.7	8.6
S-Bilirubin (indirect)	23.7	µmol/l	5.1	25.6
S-ALP	**173**	IU/l	53	128
S-gGT	**48**	IU/l	8	37
S-ALT	37	IU/l	19	40
S-AST	**34**	IU/l	13	32
S-LDH	**191**	IU/l	90	180
S-Haptoglobin 60 yrs	0.99	g/l	0.35	1.75
U-Urobilin	+	" + "		

DISCUSSION

1. From the clinical point of view there are suggestions of some form of tropical disease. It was known that schistosomiasis is endemic in the area and this was an early consideration.

2. The caput medusae was extremely suggestive of portal hypertension, which, in the context of the rest of the clinical features and the FBC features, permitted the hypothesis to be made of hypersplenism.

3. Purely from the FBC point of view, the first-stage diagnosis is a mild pancytopenia with a normocytic picture.

4. In view of his native environment and the knowledge of disease prevalences in the area, the possibility of hypersplenism as a result of schistosomiasis was entertained. Certainly the other laboratory features are not contradictory.

5. Various investigations were undertaken:

   a. A barium swallow and meal confirmed fairly large esophageal varices.

   b. Serological tests revealed fairly high titers of specific bilharzial antibodies.

   c. Liver biopsy revealed classical granulomata of schistosomiasis, some of which were surrounding ova of **S. MANSONI**, and the typical pipe-stem fibrosis.

   d. Doppler studies revealed significant portal hypertension.

6. As a matter of interest, the early satiety was provisionally ascribed to pressure on the stomach of the large spleen. This was confirmed after splenectomy and porto-caval shunting.

CASE #30 (EXAMINE TABLE 10.7)

The results of selected tests are shown in Table 10.8 to illustrate some differences from the cases we have hitherto seen.

Table 10.7

Patient	Age	Sex	Race	Altitude
Mr J T	52 yrs	Male	White	Sea level

The patient was referred after having been found by his doctor to have a very large spleen and a peculiar FBC, which had been reported without morphology or comment. He complained of mild but increasing fatigue and ill health and a sense of fullness in his abdomen. Systemic history was quite non-contributory. On examination he looked mildly chronically ill. His color was normal and there was no purpura. The only positive feature was the very large spleen. The liver was not palpably enlarged. No lymphadenopathy or bony tenderness was demonstrable.

	Value	Units	Reference range Low	High	Permitted range Low	High
Red cell count	**3.84**	× 10^{12}/l	4.5	5.5	3.72	3.96
Hemoglobin (Hb)	**10.8**	g/dl	13	17	10.4	11.2
Hematocrit (Hct)	0.33	l/l	0.4	0.5	0.32	0.34
Mean cell volume	86	fl	80	99	84.3	87.7
Mean cell Hb	28.1	pg	27	31.5	27.6	28.7
Mean cell Hb conc.	32.7	g/dl	31.5	34.5	32.0	33.4
Red cell dist. width	**17**	%	11.6	14	16.5	17.5
Retic. count %	**0.94**	%	0.25	0.75	0.9	1.0
Retic. absolute (abs.)	36.1	× 10^9/l	30	100	35.0	37.2
White cell count	**13.1**	× 10^9/l	4	10	12.12	14.08
Corrected WCC	**12.24**	× 10^9/l				
Neutrophils abs.	**7.79**	× 10^9/l	2	7	7.21	8.38
Lymphocytes abs.	2.84	× 10^9/l	1	3	2.63	3.06
Monocytes abs.	0.80	× 10^9/l	0.2	1	0.74	0.86
Eosinophils abs.	**0.60**	× 10^9/l	0.02	0.5	0.56	0.65
Basophils abs.	**0.28**	× 10^9/l	0.02	0.1	0.25	0.30
Blasts %	0	%	0	0		
Promyelocytes %	0	%	0	0		
Myelocytes %	**3**	%	0	0		
Metamyelocytes %	**3**	%	0	0		
Normoblasts	**7**	/100 WBC	0	0		
Platelet count	**141.2**	× 10^9/l	150	400	130.6	151.8
Morphology	There is a leukoerythroblastic reaction. The red cells are normochromic and show considerable anisocytosis, with numerous tear-drop poikilocytes and fragments.					

Other values have been included to show that the patient most probably does not have liver disease or hemolysis.

DISCUSSION

1. This is a complex FBC and the case will be discussed more fully in Chapter 23. It is presented briefly here for didactic reasons, i.e., to demonstrate one of the types of changes the FBC can show secondary to bone marrow infiltration, and which are normally characterized by a normocytic anemia.

2. There is a normocytic anemia with an increased RDW, as well as changes in morphology and in the other cell

Table 10.8

Case #30 cont.			Reference range	
	Value	Units	Low	High
S-Uric Acid	**0.43**	mmol/l	0.21	0.42
S-Protein (total)	78	g/l	64	83
S-Albumin	41	g/l	34	48
S-Globulin	37	g/l	30	35
S-Bilirubin (total)	25.9	μmol/l	6.8	34.2
S-Bilirubin (direct)	5.2	μmol/l	1.7	8.6
S-Bilirubin (indirect)	20.7	μmol/l	5.1	25.6
S-ALP	121	IU/l	53	128
S-gGT	31	IU/l	8	37
S-ALT	32	IU/l	19	40
S-AST	26	IU/l	13	32
S-LDH	**212**	IU/l	90	180
S-Haptoglobin 60 yrs	1.11	g/l	0.35	1.75
U-Bilirubin	-	" + "		
U-Urobilin	+	" + "		

lines. In Chapter 16 it will be seen how many of the abnormalities strongly suggest a general pathology diagnosis. Suffice it to say, for the present, that we are dealing with a chronic myeloproliferative disease with replacement of marrow by fibrous tissue, called primary myelofibrosis. The very large spleen is characteristic.

CASE #31 (EXAMINE TABLE 10.9)

Liver functions at the time again confirmed only a mild bilirubinemia, mainly indirect, with normal enzymes.

DISCUSSION

1. It is true that strictly speaking this is a normocytic anemia. However, not only is the MCV very close to the top of the range, and the permitted range includes a frankly macrocytic possibility, but the morphological examination reveals some large oval cells. Doubtlessly this then was the motivation for the marrow aspirate done before, although the enlarged spleen would strongly be against megaloblastosis.
2. The jaundice would thus require a different explanation, and the possibility of hemolysis is very strong.
3. Here then was a patient with what looked very much like a chronic hemolytic anemia. Where should one go from here?
4. Suspicion was raised by certain features of the FBC:

   a. On review, the eosinophilic inclusions in occasional red cells resembled Shüffner's dots, which are pathognomonic of ovale and vivax malaria.

Table 10.9

Patient	Age	Sex	Race	Altitude
Mr J K	41 yrs	Male	Black	5,000 ft

About 1 year ago he had felt poorly and been to his doctor, who discovered splenomegaly and anemia. No firm diagnosis had been reached on the FBC, which showed only a mild normocytic anemia, with a tendency to oval macrocytes. A bone marrow examination at the time revealed no evidence of megaloblastosis; folate and vitamin B$_{12}$ levels were normal. Liver functions at the time showed only mildly raised bilirubin levels, but normal enzymes.

The patient recovered reasonably well from this episode but he was lacking in energy. Repeated visits to the doctor revealed that the splenomegaly and anemia were persistent. A course of antibiotics caused some relief and he went back to work, only to relapse again, sometimes with episodes of fever. Despite the fact that spherocytes were not observed, eventually, probably due to desperation, osmotic fragility studies were done and these had demonstrated increased fragility of the red cells. The question now arose as to some form of hereditary hemolytic state. The patient was referred, with a view to splenectomy.

His history including family history at this stage was entirely non-contributory. On examination he was pale with a very mild tinge of jaundice. The spleen was enlarged 4 cm below the costal margin and was a little tender. He was apyrexial. No other relevant clinical features were found.

	Value	Units	Reference range		Permitted range	
			Low	High	Low	High
Red cell count	**4.11**	× 10^{12}/l	4.77	5.83	3.99	4.23
Hemoglobin (Hb)	**12.3**	g/dl	13.8	18.0	11.9	12.7
Hematocrit (Hct)	**0.4**	l/l	0.42	0.53	0.39	0.42
Mean cell volume	98.5	fl	80	99	96.5	100.5
Mean cell Hb	29.9	pg	27	31.5	29.3	30.5
Mean cell Hb conc.	30.4	g/dl	31.5	34.5	29.8	31.1
Red cell dist. width	**16.9**	%	11.6	14	15.3	17.9
Retic. count %	**1.35**	%	0.27	0.80	1.2	1.5
Retic. absolute (abs.)	55.5	× 10^9/l	30	100	51.3	59.6
White cell count	**3.11**	× 10^9/l	3.5	10	2.88	3.34
Neutrophils %	46.8	%				
Lymphocytes %	31.4	%				
Monocytes %	**16.1**	%				
Eosinophils %	4.9	%				
Basophils %	0.8	%				
Neutrophils abs.	**1.46**	× 10^9/l	1.5	7	1.35	1.56
Lymphocytes abs.	**0.98**	× 10^9/l	1	3	0.90	1.05
Monocytes abs.	0.50	× 10^9/l	0.2	1	0.46	0.54
Eosinophils abs.	0.15	× 10^9/l	0.02	0.5	0.14	0.16
Basophils abs.	0.02	×10^9/l	0.02	0.1	0.02	0.03
Normoblasts	0	/100 WBC	0	0		
Platelet count	**111.0**	× 10^9/l	150	400	105.1	122.9
Morphology	There is a very mild pancytopenia. The red cells are large and rather pale; many are oval in form. There is a suspicion of eosinophilic inclusions in the occasional red cell. No tear-drop poikilocytes or fragments were observed. There was no right shift of the neutrophils.					

b. The large pale oval red cells were also consistent with vivax malaria.

c. Thrombocytopenia is classical of all forms of malaria. Note that the leukopenia is very marginal.

d. The relative monocytosis also is a feature of malaria.

5. The problem is, however, that vivax malaria is not endemic at this altitude. The past history was eventually further gone into. About 5 years ago he had come down with severe typical "flu-like" illness, with headache, muscle pain, and nausea. This subsided but recurred. Since this was in the middle of an influenza epidemic, and this pattern of recurrence was occurring frequently, little importance was attached to this. Eventually his illness settled down, and he felt moderately well, except that he had lacked energy, and was in danger of losing his job. In addition he stated that he had never left his current place of residence and never visited a tropical area.

6. The final clue, however, came when he volunteered that he worked as a baggage handler at the local international airport. It is well known that infected anopheline mosquitoes can be carried by aircraft from endemic areas.

7. It was very difficult to establish the diagnosis. Numerous thick and thin smears were examined until very occasional ring forms and gametocytes were observed.

8. The treatment of chronic vivax malaria requires the use of primaquine phosphate. This drug is dangerous and contra-indicated in severe G6PD-deficient patients and must be used with caution in mild cases. This patient was tested and found to be normal. Primaquine therapy was therefore instituted, with excellent results.

Comment As has been stated, malaria is the commonest cause of hemolysis in the world, and taking into account mass travel it should always be considered in the differential diagnosis of any hemolytic state.

Malaria is the commonest disease facing travelers (0.8% of travelers from developed countries being infected annually. 10,000 cases of malaria are imported into Europe every year).

1. When presenting as chronic hemolytic states, the usual causes are vivax, ovale, and malariae malaria.

2. When presenting as acute hemolytic states, falciparum malaria is by far the most dangerous, but vivax malaria can also be very acute.

3. Falciparum malaria is characterized by severe hemolysis with mental confusion, even seizures. There may be associated gross hemoglobinuria ("blackwater fever") and renal failure. It is a medical emergency, and the percentage of infected cells is critical to management.

4. Malaria causes severe damage to red cells, both infected and non-infected, such as damage to the membrane manifested by increased osmotic fragility, and decreased deformability, with a tendency to sludging in capillaries.

5. Massive splenomegaly may occur, as a result of disordered immune complex production.

6. The bone marrow in cases of malaria shows prominent dyserythropoiesis.

Splenomegaly It is in the normocytic anemias that splenomegaly plays the most valuable differentiating role:

1. An enlarged spleen effectively eliminates as causes:

   a. Endocrine deficiencies
   b. Post-hemorrhagic anemia
   c. Combined iron deficiency and megaloblastic anemia
   d. Renal anemia except in unusual cases such as amyloidosis

2. An enlarged spleen is or can be found in all the others.

3. Splenomegaly is particularly valuable in distinguishing extravascular hemolysis from megaloblastic anemia (otherwise they clinically resemble each other).

Exercise Cases

CASE #32 (TABLE 10.10)

Table 10.10

Patient		Age	Sex	Race	Altitude
Mrs J S		91 yrs	Female	White	5,000 ft

The patient was noticed by a family member to be very pale and complaining of marked tiredness. She was brought to the clinic. As she walked in she was seen to be a sprightly old lady but very pale, with a normal gait. She complained of a very sore mouth and difficulty in swallowing. She denied any abnormal bleeding or pica.

On examination she was not jaundiced. Her weight was within the 9th percentile of normal for her age and sex. The BP was 120/60, and the pulse rate at rest was 84/min. On being asked to get up and walk about the room for a while, her pulse rate rose to 108/min; upon resting the rate fell back to 86 within 2 min. The JVP was marginally raised. The heart was not enlarged but she had a grade 4/6 rather harsh murmur across the precordium. Her whole mouth was bright red and the tongue smooth. There was striking koilonychia affecting practically all the fingers. The abdomen was soft and there was no splenomegaly.

	Value	Units	Reference range Low	Reference range High	Permitted range Low	Permitted range High
Red cell count	**2.71**	$\times 10^{12}/l$	4.03	5.09	2.63	2.79
Hemoglobin (Hb)	**7.49**	g/dl	12.7	15.9	7.2	7.8
Hematocrit (Hct)	**0.24**	l/l	0.38	0.49	0.23	0.25
Mean cell volume	88	fl	80	99	86.2	89.8
Mean cell Hb	27.6	pg	27	31.5	27.1	28.2
Mean cell Hb conc.	31.4	g/dl	31.5	34.5	30.8	32.0
Red cell dist. width	**21.1**	%	11.6	14	21.1	21.1
Retic. count %	**0.3**	%	0.5	0.9	0.3	0.3
Retic. absolute (abs.)	**8.1**	$\times 10^9/l$	30	100	7.9	8.4
White cell count	4.11	$\times 10^9/l$	4	10	3.80	4.42
Neutrophils abs.	**1.94**	$\times 10^9/l$	2	7	1.79	2.09
Lymphocytes abs.	1.53	$\times 10^9/l$	1	3	1.42	1.65
Monocytes abs.	0.37	$\times 10^9/l$	0.2	1	0.35	0.40
Eosinophils abs.	0.23	$\times 10^9/l$	0.02	0.5	0.21	0.24
Basophils abs.	0.04	$\times 10^9/l$	0.02	0.1	0.03	0.04
Normoblasts	0	/100 WBC	0	0		
Platelet count	**148.0**	$\times 10^9/l$	150	400	97.2	118.8
Sedimentation	**41**	mm/h	0	20	39	43

Questions

1. What is the first-stage diagnosis?

   _____

2. What possibilities do the clinical features suggest?

   _____

   _____

3. What do the FBC features suggest in the light of the above? What single measurement in the FBC is critically important and sheds light on the likely pathology?

   _____

   _____

4. What important part of the FBC is missing, in the light of your answer? How would this help?

   _____

   _____

Answers

1. Normocytic anemia.
2. Some features suggest megaloblastic anemia: the stomatitis and glossitis. Against this was the absence of jaundice, as well as some of the other clinical features, which were in favor of another pathology. Other features suggest iron deficiency: the koilonychia and dysphagia.
3. On their own the FBC features are not very informative. The very high RDW is extremely suggestive: one possible cause of this is that there are two populations of cells, each suggesting a different pathology.
4. The morphological appearances. They would be of great value in possibly identifying the nature of the wide RDW.

The morphological report was purposely omitted for didactic purposes. It is shown in Table 10.11.

Table 10.11

FBC Morphology of Case #32
There are two populations of red cells. One is macrocytic with numerous oval macrocytes and tear-drop poikilocytes; the other is microcytic and hypochromic with small oval cells and elliptocytes. The neutrophils show a marked right shift. The features suggest a combined deficiency of iron and folate or vitamin B_{12}.

Further Questions

5. What would the biochemical tests typically show? Do you think that these would be easy to interpret without the clinical and FBC background?

   _____

   _____

6. What essential part of the clinical history was purposely omitted? What single question was asked that explained her pathology?

   _____

   _____

7. What do you think is the cause of the dysphagia? What diagnostic methods are used for diagnosis?

_____

8. The patient was evidently in cardiac failure – i.e., a severe anemia. Is this not somewhat surprising with a Hb of 7.48 g/dl?

_____

_____

Answers

5. The results are displayed in Table 10.12.

These results are on the face of it somewhat ambiguous. The iron saturation clearly indicates iron deficiency, yet the ferritin is within the reference range. This pattern is not uncommon. See the comment box. The interpretation of the results is certainly very much facilitated by reference to the clinical and FBC features.

The mildly raised indirect bilirubin is compatible with the megaloblastic aspect of the disease. It is well known that minor degrees of jaundice ("biochemical jaundice") are not perceivable clinically.

6. The dietary history also was purposely omitted. The single question asked to the old lady that answered this and other questions was "Where do you live?" The answer was "By myself in a room." From this her diet could be inferred, and this was later corroborated. This patient has a classical toast-and-tea syndrome. It is also clear that there was a strong social problem here with an element of neglect. This had to be addressed apart from specific replacement therapy. However, the patient resolutely refused to go into an old-age home.

7. One strong possibility is of course the Plummer–Vinson syndrome – i.e., post-cricoid webs due to iron deficiency. However, it was decided to defer specific investigation pending response to treatment. With adequate dietary support by social services plus iron and folate supplementation, the dysphagia disappeared within 2 weeks; this suggested that the dysphagia had been due to the stomatitis and not webs. Normally esophageal webs are diagnosed by barium swallow but using very thick barium.

8. The development of cardiac failure due to anemia is dependent upon the cardiac reserve. In a patient of 90 years, this is always likely to be restricted.

Comment Dimorphic red cell pictures (i.e., the presence of two populations of red cells) are quite commonly reported. There are a few important causes:

1. Combined iron deficiency and megaloblastosis.
2. An iron-deficient patient who has been transfused. The red cells may show minor degrees of agglutination due to slight, insignificant incompatibility.
3. Other combinations of any of the microcytic anemias with any of the macrocytic anemias.
4. Sideroblastic anemia and sometimes other myelodysplastic syndromes may also show a dimorphic picture.

Comment Iron-deficient saturation studies accompanied by a ferritin level in the reference range are not uncommon. There are several causes. They all involve iron deficiency in combination with:

1. Chronic disease. Ferritin is an acute (and chronic) phase reactant and can be raised independently of the iron status
2. Thalassemia
3. Megaloblastic disease
4. Recent transfusion

Table 10.12

Case #32 cont.	Value	Units	Low	High
S-Bilirubin (total)	36.9	μmol/l	6.8	34.2
S-Bilirubin (direct)	8.4	μmol/l	1.7	8.6
S-Bilirubin (indirect)	28.5	μmol/l	5.1	25.6
S-Ferritin female	31.2	μg/l	14.0	233.1
S-Iron	7.1	μmol/l	11.6	31.3
S-Transferrin	3.12	g/l	2.12	3.60
S-Fe saturation female	5.6	%	15.0	35.0
S-Vitamin B$_{12}$	389	pg/ml	193	982
S-Folate	2.1	ng/ml	3.0	17.0
RBC-folate	72.1	ng/ml	93.0	641.0

CASE #33 (TABLE 10.13)

Table 10.13

Patient	Age	Sex	Race	Altitude
Mrs S v S	26 yrs	Female	White	2,500 ft

This patient, from a small country town had complained of recurrent sharp pains in her abdomen, chest and legs since the age of 9 years. Repeated examinations both clinical and radiological had revealed no pathology, and she had been treated symptomatically. There had been a tendency to ascribe the problem to psychological causes, since she had shown signs of maladjustment for many years. On examination she was an obese, pale, and depressed-looking young woman with a tinge of jaundice; otherwise no abnormal findings were obtained. There was no splenomegaly. The history was quite non-contributory, although she did say that the pains had come on very severely

Questions

1. On the basis of the clinical features alone, have you any suspicions as to the diagnosis?

2. What do you find surprising about this possible diagnosis?

3. What do you want to see now?

Answers

1. The features of pallor and jaundice could be ascribed to hemolysis or megaloblastosis, with the latter being most likely since there is no splenomegaly. The recurrent sharp pains in different regions of the body could possibly be crises as found in sickle disease; this would explain the absence of splenomegaly in a hemolytic disorder.
2. Sickle disease would be extremely unusual in a white person.
3. A FBC.

The FBC is shown in Table 10.14

Questions

1. How has this FBC report helped you?

2. What else would you like to see?

Table 10.14
FBC report of Case #33

	Value	Units	Reference range Low	High	Permitted range Low	High
Red cell count	3.05	× 10¹²/l	3.91	4.94	2.96	3.14
Hemoglobin (Hb)	10.4	g/dl	12.4	15.5	10.0	10.8
Hematocrit (Hct)	0.30	l/l	0.37	0.47	0.29	0.31
Mean cell volume	99	fl	80	99	97.0	101.0
Mean cell Hb	34.1	pg	27	31.5	33.4	34.8
Mean cell Hb conc.	34.4	g/dl	31.5	34.5	33.8	35.1
Red cell dist. width	16.2	%	11.6	14	16.2	16.2
Retic. count %	3.98	%	0.25	0.75	3.9	4.1
Retic. absolute (abs.)	121.4	× 10⁹/l	30	100	117.7	125.0
White cell count	8.25	× 10⁹/l	4	10	7.63	8.87
Neutrophils abs.	5.63	× 10⁹/l	2	7	5.20	6.05
Band cells abs.	0.00		0	0	0.00	0.00
Lymphocytes abs.	1.66	× 10⁹/l	1	3	1.53	1.78
Monocytes abs.	0.64	× 10⁹/l	0.2	1	0.60	0.69
Eosinophils abs.	0.26	× 10⁹/l	0.02	0.5	0.24	0.27
Basophils abs.	0.07	× 10⁹/l	0.02	0.1	0.06	0.07
Normoblasts	0	/100 WBC	0	0		
Platelet count	222.0	× 10⁹/l	150	400	199.8	244.2
Sedimentation	18	mm/h	0	20	17	19

Answers

1. It supports the diagnosis of hemolysis more than that of megaloblastosis.
2. The morphology of the cells.

The morphology is shown in Table 10.15

Table 10.15
FBC morphology of Case #33 (Table 10.13)

The red cells are normochromic and normocytic, with moderate anisocytosis. A small number of sickle-shaped cells are seen as well as numerous target cells, some of which showing condensed Hb crystals. The neutrophils show a mild right shift.

Questions

1. How has the morphology helped you?

2. What do you think is the likely diagnosis?

3. How would you confirm this diagnosis?

4. Why do you think there is a right shift of the neutrophils?

Answers

1. On the one hand the sickle cells tend to confirm the diagnosis of sickle disease. The target cells and condensed Hb suggest HbC disease.
2. The likely diagnosis is a double heterozygous HbSC disease.
3. A sickle preparation and Hb electrophoresis.
4. The right shift might indicate renal damage, such as papillary necrosis which is known to occur with sickle disease; or it may be due to mild folate deficiency as a result of the hyperactive marrow.

Comments

1. Electrophoresis did indeed confirm HbSC disease.

2. The parents' blood was tested; the mother was HbSA and the father HbCA. It is emphasized that it is most unusual to find these genes in a white person.
3. Renal function was shown to be normal. The right shift responded to folate therapy.

Further Reading

Andreoli TE, Bennett JC, Carpenter CCJ, Plum F (eds) (1997). Cecil Essentials of Medicine. 4th edn. Philadelphia: WB Saunders Company.

Epstein RJ (1996). Medicine for Examinations. 3rd edn. Churchill Livingstone.

Hoffbrand AV, Pettit JE (2001) Essential Haematology. 4th edn. Oxford: Blackwell Science.

Lewis SM, Bain B, Bates I (2006) Dacie and Lewis Practical Haematology. 10th edn. Churchill Livingstone.

Thrombocytopenia

11

Defining Thrombocytopenia

Thrombocytopenia may occur in association with numerous other FBC changes. In this chapter we are concerned primarily with **ISOLATED** thrombocytopenia. Thrombocytopenia found in association with other conditions is presented either as part and parcel of those disorders or as part of complex conditions to be discussed in Chapter 23. Aspects of their general pathology are, however, discussed in this chapter, to provide a context. Also, there is considerable overlap with the bleeding disorders, which are discussed in Chapter 18, and where clinical aspects of thrombocytopenia are discussed more comprehensively.

The first-stage diagnosis of "thrombocytopenia" was thus reached by the recognition that the platelet count was below the reference range:

> **STEP 1.** "Where is the primary abnormality?" It lies in the platelet count (PC).
> **STEP 2.** "What form does it take?" The PC is decreased below the reference range.

The General Pathology Causes of Thrombocytopenia

All forms of thrombocytopenia are due to one (or more) of five groups of general causes. It is useful to redisplay the diagrammatic outline of the pathology of the blood system (Fig. 11.1). It is particularly relevant to thrombocytopenia.

Hence, the general causes of thrombocytopenia are

1. **DEFECTIVE PRODUCTION BY THE MARROW**
2. **DEFECTIVE RELEASE FROM THE MARROW**
3. **PERIPHERAL DESTRUCTION**

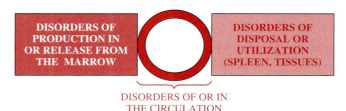

Fig. 11.1 Basic diagram of the hematological system

4. **PERIPHERAL SEQUESTRATION**
5. **SPURIOUS THROMBOCYTOPENIA**

Specific Causes of Isolated Thrombocytopenia

1. **SPURIOUS THROMBOCYTOPENIA ("PSEUDO-THROMBOCYTOPENIA").** This is by no means uncommon. It is mentioned first because it is so potent a source of misdirection. A typical case has been presented in detail in Chapter 6. There are several causes for platelets to appear decreased in a FBC:

   a. **PLATELET SATELLITISM.** See the case in Chapter 6.
   b. **PLATELET CLUMPING.** Generally this is due either to the effect of EDTA or heparin on the platelets or to mild platelet activation, as may occur, for example, with poor venesection technique.

2. **DEFECTIVE PRODUCTION BY THE MARROW SUCH AS IN MEGAKARYOCYTIC HYPOPLASIA.** This is a rare cause of **ISOLATED** thrombocytopenia, with two exceptions:

O.N. Beck, *Diagnostic Hematology*, DOI 10.1007/978-1-84800-295-1_11,
© Springer-Verlag London Limited 2009

a. In various stages of **APLASTIC ANEMIA** – either very early, before the leukopenia and anemia have had a chance to manifest (since the normal survival of platelets is so much shorter than the others), or in the recovery stage – it is known that the platelets usually take the longest to recover, and sometimes never do completely recover.

b. Some **THROMBOCYTOPENIAS DUE TO INFECTION** appear to be due to damage to the megakaryocytes, unlike the common scenario where the circulating platelets are destroyed. Examples are measles, dengue and CMV, disseminated tuberculosis.

c. **THROMBOCYTOPENIA IS A FAIRLY COMMON COMPLICATION OF ALCOHOLISM** and is probably due to direct toxic damage of the marrow, but platelet survival may also be decreased. The spleen is usually not enlarged in these patients. It is reversible after alcohol withdrawal and is followed by a rebound thrombocytosis (see Chapter 14).

d. Note that **SOME DRUGS** are known to selectively suppress the megakaryocyte, the most important of which are chlorothiazide and ethanol.

3. **DEFECTIVE RELEASE FROM THE MARROW.** This is a very rare cause of **ISOLATED** thrombocytopenia. It may occur in the early stages of the **MYELODYSPLASTIC SYNDROMES.**

4. **PERIPHERAL SEQUESTRATION.** The most important site for sequestration is the spleen (as, for example, in hypersplenism). Endothelial adherence of platelets occurs in many infections including sepsis, some vascular diseases, cirrhotic nodules, and in certain forms of abnormal circulation. Giant hemangiomata, >5 cm in diameter, can sequester platelets – this is known as the Kasabach–Merritt syndrome and is found particularly in small children.

5. **PERIPHERAL DESTRUCTION.** This is by far the commonest general cause of thrombocytopenia. It can be classified into **IMMUNE-MEDIATED** and **NON-IMMUNE-MEDIATED.** In either of these the process may occur **IN THE CIRCULATION** or **IN THE SPLEEN.** These causes are all discussed separately.

a. **NON-IMMUNE-MEDIATED.** There are five main causes:

i. **DISSEMINATED INTRAVASCULAR COAGULATION.**
ii. **PROSTHETIC INTRAVASCULAR DEVICES.**
iii. **EXTRACORPOREAL CIRCULATION** (heart–lung machine, dialysis membrane).

iv. **THROMBOTIC THROMBOCYTOPENIC PURPURA, HEMOLYTIC-UREMIC SYNDROME** (TTP and HUS, respectively) and the **HELLP SYNDROME.** These complex conditions are discussed in Chapter 23.
v. **OTHER FORMS OF MICRO-VASCULAR DISEASE.**

b. **IMMUNE-MEDIATED.** There are three groups of conditions:

i. **DRUG-INDUCED THROMBOCYTOPENIA**
ii. **INFECTIONS**
iii. **ALLOIMMUNE THROMBOCYTOPENIA**
iv. **AUTOIMMUNE THROMBOCYTOPENIA**

Disseminated Intravascular Coagulation

The pathology and pathogenesis of this condition have already been discussed. It is seldom a cause of isolated thrombocytopenia. Mild cases of DIC, particularly when caused by viruses, may be well compensated from the Hb and WCC point of view, and frequently all one sees is the thrombocytopenia (plus, of course, suggestive changes in red cell morphology).

Prosthetic Intravascular Devices

By far the most important of these is artificial heart valves and intra-aortic balloons. As the blood passes through the valve, the cells are physically damaged; red cells show mild fragmentation and the thrombocytopenia is usually mild and does not lead to abnormal bleeding. While the condition is most common with metal prostheses, it can also be found with tissue valves.

Extracorporeal Circulation

Adhesion of platelets to the various components of heart–lung and dialysis machines is frequently a major problem and does not seem to be helped significantly by any anticoagulants.

Micro-vascular Disease

There is a tendency for platelets to adhere to injured or diseased endothelium, and this is found in many conditions: DIC, TTP/HUS, chronic myeloproliferative diseases such as essential thrombocythemia and poly-cythemia vera, diabetes mellitus, antiphospholipid syndrome, SLE, pre-eclampsia, etc. Platelets also become more sticky in hypothermia.

Drug-Induced Thrombocytopenia

Over 100 drugs have been implicated as causing thrombocytopenia. The best known are

1. Quinine and quinidine
2. Gold
3. Sulphonamides
4. Cephalosporins
5. Heparin

As far as is known, the mechanisms are all immune-mediated, and there are two forms: dose dependent and idiosyncratic.

HEPARIN-INDUCED THROMBOCYTOPENIA (HIT) requires special mention, since heparin is used so frequently. There are two forms:

1. **TYPE I.** This is the commonest, occurs within a week of exposure to heparin, and is due to platelet aggregation due to heparin itself. It is not necessary to stop the heparin therapy.
2. **TYPE II.** This usually starts 10–20 days after exposure to heparin **BUT MAY OCCUR SOONER IF THERE WAS PREVIOUS EXPOSURE TO HEPARIN.** Although the platelet count rarely falls below 60×10^9/l, there is a high associated risk of arterial or venous thrombosis in this condition, especially myocardial infarcts, strokes, pulmonary embolism, and large artery thromboses; this occurs because antibodies bind to a heparin/platelet 4 complex, and this induces intravascular platelet activation. It is not dose dependent. Early recognition is critical.

Note that the incidence of HIT with the fractionated heparins is about one tenth that with unfractionated heparin.

Thrombocytopenia Due to Infections

Infections are a prominent source of thrombocytopenia, including sepsis from any cause. Two mechanisms are common:

1. **DIC OR PLATELET ADHESION** to damaged endothelium or both. There is a wide variety of different organisms that may be responsible, from bacteria and fungi (particularly in the critically ill), to rickettsiae (e.g., Rocky Mountain spotted fever), and occasionally to viruses (e.g., arboviruses).
2. **IMMUNE-MEDIATED.** Immune destruction may also occur in bacterial and fungal infections, but is most prominent in viral infections, the most important ones being EBV, hepatitis, rubella, CMV, and HIV. There is also the clinical association between any viral illness and ITP, including the cases of sudden falls in PC in a patient with ITP.
3. Uncommonly due to decreased production, as discussed above.
4. Thrombocytopenia is known to occur in numerous disparate conditions, notably in malaria (almost always), babesiosis, and infectious mononucleosis.

Alloimmune Thrombocytopenia

About 2% of the population is negative for the platelet-specific antigen Pl^{A1}. If such a patient has previously been sensitized to this antigen (typically therefore in multiparous women) and then receives blood from a positive donor, a profound thrombocytopenia develops in 7–10 days. This is a life-threatening condition.

Neonatal alloimmune thrombocytopenia has a mechanism analogous to hemolytic disease of the newborn.

Autoimmune Thrombocytopenia

This is commonly known as immune thrombocytopenic purpura (ITP). The formal definition of the condition is "An acquired disease of children or adults characterized by an isolated thrombocytopenia with no clinically apparent or other causes of a low platelet count." This is all very well as a definition but is not very useful in practice. In particular, how far must one go in excluding underlying known secondary causes? For example, it is known that ITP can manifest in a patient with sub-clinical SLE (and even predate it). Must one then automatically test for SLE in every case?

In children the disease is acute with rapid onset and almost always resolves within 6 months. In adults, however, it tends to be insidious, usually in patients over 50 years, with a tendency to chronicity, and is more frequent among females.

There are a number of conditions that may be associated with thrombocytopenia:

1. Immune hemolysis (Evan's syndrome)
2. Immune neutropenia
3. Antiphospholipid syndrome (see Chapter 21)
4. SLE and lymphoproliferative disease

Thrombocytopenia in Pregnancy Thrombocytopenia in pregnancy represents a particular clinical problem. The different types and causes have been detailed in Chapter 4. All the general causes mentioned may of course be found in pregnancy. However, some particular disorders are unique to pregnancy:

1. *Gestational thrombocytopenia.* This is a common condition of uncertain pathogenesis and with minimal obstetric or hematological significance or danger to the neonate. It is found in 10% of pregnancies, usually incidentally. The platelet count is seldom below 80×10^9/l, but can occasionally be as low as 65.
2. *ITP* has the same incidence in pregnancy as otherwise. It has serious implications:

   a. Obstetrical, notably peripartum hemorrhage
   b. Hematological: other bleeding problems
   c. Neonatal: serious thrombocytopenic bleeding

3. *Pre-eclampsia.* Thrombocytopenia is regularly found in PET. Its mechanism is unknown.
4. The *HELLP syndrome* (*h*emolysis, *e*levated *l*iver enzymes, *l*ow *p*latelets) is probably a subgroup of PET and is potentially fatal.
5. *TTP* typically occurs before the 24th week. It is discussed in Chapter 22.
6. *HUS* typically occurs within 48 h of delivery. It is also discussed in Chapter 22.

Making the Diagnosis

The knee-jerk reaction with very many students and practitioners is, upon encountering a patient with an isolated thrombocytopenia, to label it as ITP. It should be obvious from what has been said that this is a potent source of possibly missing another serious condition.

In days gone by, the approach to a patient with thrombocytopenia was very simple: one immediately did a marrow aspirate. Intensive studies have considerably altered this algorithm. There were several reasons for this:

1. The recognition that there were many reasons for isolated thrombocytopenia and bone marrow examination showed megakaryocytic hyperplasia in **ALL** causes of peripheral destruction.
2. There is nothing specific in the bone marrow morphology to indicate the actual cause. The only value is to exclude primary bone marrow pathologies as the cause, and these are the distinct minority.
3. Epidemiological studies have shown that a marrow examination is warranted in patients over the age of ± 50 years, unless of course there is clear independent evidence of primary marrow disease or a relapse after complete remission or if one is considering a splenectomy.

The point must be emphasized: the diagnosis of the cause of thrombocytopenia is actually difficult, unless the history and examination are positive.

Before proceeding we need to outline various possible therapeutic modalities:

1. *Platelet transfusions. If the thrombocytopenia is due to ITP, the transfused platelets will not last long – 30–60 min; in fact this can sometimes be used as a diagnostic test for ITP if all else fails. If the bleeding does stop, one has at least bought some time to make a definitive diagnosis; also one is more convinced that one is not dealing with ITP.*
2. *High-dose (intravenous) steroids.* This is only justified in two sets of conditions:

   a. ITP
   b. Thrombocytopenia secondary to acute leukemias and high-grade lymphomas, and then only as an interim measure
      Note that steroids will not act quickly enough in the ITP patient who is actively bleeding, but it is probably advisable to start them anyway.

3. *High-dose immunosuppressants,* such as cyclophosphamide. This is only justified in ITP and TTP.
4. *High-dose gammaglobulin.* Again this is only going to be effective in ITP, and without a firm diagnosis one is chary about prescribing

this course of action in view of the enormous cost of the gammaglobulin. Nevertheless, one sometimes has no choice but to use transfusions plus gammaglobulin in cases of emergency.

5. *Urgent splenectomy.* This is sometimes unavoidable.

THE FOLLOWING APPROACH IS SUGGESTED:
A. THE NON-PREGNANT PATIENT.

1. **IS THERE EVIDENCE OF BLEEDING, AND IF SO, HOW SEVERE?** Severe bleeding needs urgent attention. It is important to exclude sepsis and drugs as a cause and treat these aggressively. Generally speaking, without a firm diagnosis the choice of therapy can be very difficult. It is always worthwhile to check the PC in a FBC done from a citrate tube – the bleeding may be due to something other than thrombocytopenia.

   It is clear that ITP must be diagnosed as soon as possible. Since we have no specific reliable positive test for ITP, we must make do with the bone marrow appearances: generally speaking, if there is megakaryocytic hyperplasia and no other marrow abnormalities, we are justified in assuming that the case is one of ITP. The only possible exception to this rule is in the ICU in a patient who is obviously septic: this is a very difficult and complex problem and should be referred.

   Note that in cases where no causal diagnosis has been made, it is extremely important to draw bloods for the FBC, platelet antibodies (for what they are worth), and a bone marrow aspirate before treatment is begun. At least a FBC with good morphology should be done.

2. **IF THE BLEEDING IS MILD OR ABSENT,** one can proceed more systematically. The main task is to look for a credible possible clinical cause:

   a. Does the FBC done from a citrate tube still show the thrombocytopenia? If not, we are probably dealing with a spurious case.
   b. Has the patient had (or is having) cardiac or vascular surgery?
   c. Has the patient had a recent transfusion?
   d. What drugs are the patient being exposed to? Heparin in particular should be excluded.
   e. Does the patient have a known history of aplastic anemia or other primary blood disease?
   f. Are there clinical and/or FBC features suggesting an infection, especially viral infection?
   g. Is there an enlarged spleen? This may be related to an infection but may have an independent pathology.
   h. Are there any features suggesting vascular malformations, especially large hemangiomata?
   i. Are there any features suggesting micro-vascular disease, notably TTP and HUS? One must look for neurological disorders in TTP and renal involvement in HUS. These conditions are further discussed in Chapter 23.
   j. It is very important to exclude SLE insofar as this is possible. In all these cases, the primary disease must be addressed. Specific treatment of the thrombocytopenia is only necessary if the patient starts bleeding or the PC is below about 10; in the latter case, should the thrombocytopenia become refractory and chronic, one is sometimes forced to stop treatment, either because of the cost or the danger of side effects.

3. **RECOURSE TO BONE MARROW EXAMINATION IS USUALLY NECESSARY:**

   a. If the above considerations do not lead to an answer
   b. If there is no satisfactory response to steroids or gammaglobulins
      The reasons are that one must then exclude conditions such as MDS, malignancy, and the like.

B. **THE PREGNANT PATIENT.**
   Because of the potential for disastrous effects on the fetus and neonate, the above-mentioned approach must be adapted. The major concern is to distinguish gestational thrombocytopenia from the others, since this is a benign condition.

   A good starting point is to evaluate the platelet count in the context of the patient's clinical condition: if she is ill, hypertensive, or shows hemolytic features or evidence of neurological damage, the platelet count may well be part of a serious disorder; if she is bleeding it is essential to try to establish that it is purpuric in nature, since there are many non-hematological causes of bleeding, which, thankfully, are outside the scope of this book.

   If she is not ill and shows purpuric bleeding (see Chapter 18) and the platelet count is below 20 or $30 \times 10^9/l$, it can be assumed that she has ITP and this must be treated extremely aggressively – if possible delivery should be induced, since the danger to the neonate is very great.

   If she is not ill and is not bleeding and the platelet count is above 65, one can assume that one is dealing with gestational thrombocytopenia, which does not require therapy.

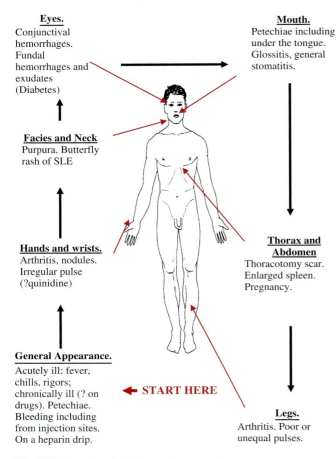

Eyes.
Conjunctival hemorrhages.
Fundal hemorrhages and exudates (Diabetes)

Mouth.
Petechiae including under the tongue. Glossitis, general stomatitis.

Facies and Neck
Purpura. Butterfly rash of SLE

Hands and wrists.
Arthritis, nodules. Irregular pulse (?quinidine)

Thorax and Abdomen
Thoracotomy scar. Enlarged spleen. Pregnancy.

General Appearance.
Acutely ill: fever, chills, rigors; chronically ill (? on drugs). Petechiae. Bleeding including from injection sites. On a heparin drip.

← **START HERE**

Legs.
Arthritis. Poor or unequal pulses.

Fig. 11.2 Examination: Thrombocytopenia

In all patients, clinical examination must be directed at finding a known cause. Figure 11.2 illustrates **SPECIFIC ASPECTS** of the examination of a patient in whom thrombocytopenia is known or suspected; clearly it is part of the overall examination as depicted in Fig. 5.4.

Apart from evidence of bleeding, the major things to look for are

1. Features of infection or sepsis.
2. An enlarged spleen. Note that the spleen is enlarged on only 3% of cases of ITP – and then it is almost always only just palpable.
3. Arterial and micro-vascular disease.

It is clear that the diagnosis of ITP is one of exclusion. Once known secondary causes of thrombocytopenia are excluded, many people will then consider platelet-associated antibody titers, in an attempt at confirmation.

Platelet-Associated Antibody Testing

This test has limited usefulness. Its sensitivity is between 50 and 65%, in different hands and the specificity about 85%. The positive predictive value is only about 80%. It is clear therefore that a negative result does not rule out ITP; it cannot also distinguish primary from secondary immune thrombocytopenias and cannot predict which patients will have a chronic course.

By and large, therefore, these assays are not regarded as important in the diagnosis of ITP.

Diagnosis and Principles of Management of ITP

These are discussed together since in ITP confirmation of the diagnosis is sometimes made in retrospect by reviewing the response to various treatment modalities.

The response to IV gammaglobulin is regarded by many as the single best **DIAGNOSTIC** test. There are particular problems associated with IV gammaglobulins, however, and these are discussed shortly. It will be seen that it is probably preferable to confirm the diagnosis as far as possible by other means and to see the response to high-dose steroids (1 mg/kg prednisone/day). Only if there is no good response **WITHIN 2 WEEKS (MAXIMUM)** can one then consider the next step. It is at this stage that controversy exists:

1. If a marrow aspirate has not yet been done, some practitioners will now proceed to this, and there is some merit to this – for example, an acute lymphoblastic leukemia occasionally presents as an isolated thrombocytopenia, and high-dose steroids can induce a temporary remission in the leukemia, giving a false sense of certainty.
2. Others will proceed to immune suppressants, such as azathioprine or cyclophosphamide.
3. Others will proceed to IV gammaglobulin. However, very high doses have to be given over a period of several days. It is also extremely expensive. Only if this fails will other options be explored, such as splenectomy. The problem here is that there is some evidence that response to splenectomy in such patients is worse than in those in whom splenectomy was done first.
4. Others will proceed directly to splenectomy (while others again will wait for 3–6 months to offer this); ± $2/3$ of patients will respond completely or partially to splenectomy. While around 40% of such patients will have a PC $< 50 \times 10^9/l$, the count in about half of these cases is usually $> 20 \times 10^9/l$, which in practical terms means that bleeding tendency in these cases is minimal, given adequate precautions against physical injury. Note, however, that there are specific issues around splenectomy:
   a. If at all possible, splenectomy should not be undertaken without first having given the patient

pneumococcal vaccine, since post-splenectomy patients are particularly prone to pneumococcal infections. Hemophilus vaccines are often also prescribed. Note that vaccines imply a wait of at least 2 weeks, preferably 1 month, before the splenectomy is undertaken – it is relatively ineffective if given post-splenectomy.

b. Splenectomy must be avoided if the patient is resident in a malarial area.

5. In cases where splenectomy does not result in a PC > $20–30\times10^9$/l, other options are considered. One of these is high-dose IV gammaglobulin. However, very high doses have to be given over a period of several days, in hospital, since the patient has to be carefully monitored.

It can be seen that there is considerable controversy in this matter. It is probable that the following consensus will emerge: once the diagnosis of ITP is made as certainly as possible and there is no significant response within 2 weeks to high-dose steroids, splenectomy is the most effective option.

Note that it is probably good practice to administer at least the pneumococcal vaccine as soon as the diagnosis is made, regardless of expected response to therapy.

Note also that there are many experimental new therapies being tested, for two major reasons:

1. The refractory cases
2. The side-effect profile of many existing therapies

These include apheresis.

Teaching Cases

CASE #34 (EXAMINE TABLE 11.1)

DISCUSSION

1. It may be argued that the patient does not have an isolated thrombocytopenia, since the red cells show abnormalities. However, there is good independent reason for these changes – the recent trauma and bleeding.
2. The positive platelet-associated antibody titer and the bone marrow report are suggestive but not conclusive of ITP. It may be argued that his poor response to steroids was against ITP. First, not all (by any means) ITP patients respond to steroids. Second, the dose was suboptimal and the length of treatment far too short. The dosage should be 1 mg/kg/prednisone/day for about 2 weeks, then tapering off very slowly, over a period of **2 YEARS** (unless of course the effect on the PC is suboptimal, pending a decision on what to do next, in which case tapering is very much quicker. Sub-optimal in this context usually means a PC of $< \pm 80\times10^9$/l.)

Table 11.1

Patient	Age	Sex	Race	Altitude
A v D	13 yrs	Male	White	2500 ft

This boy had been diagnosed in his hometown with ITP 18 months before. A bone marrow aspirate done at the time had shown the typical megakaryocytic hyperplasia. Platelet-associated antibodies had been positive. He had been placed on prednisone orally, with a dosage of $\pm$ 0.5 mg/kg. The platelet count had responded but poorly. A few days ago he had injured himself playing rugby and was oozing constantly from a skull laceration, which had been sutured. He was referred.

On examination the boy was pale with scattered purpuric spots across the chest, thighs, and on the palate. No other positive features were found on examination. He acknowledged that he had played rugby against express prohibition by his doctor.

	Value	Units	Reference range Low	Reference range High	Permitted range Low	Permitted range High
Red cell count	**4.53**	$\times10^{12}$/l	4.64	5.67	4.39	4.67
Hemoglobin (Hb)	**12.1**	g/dl	13.4	17.5	11.7	12.5
Hematocrit (Hct)	**0.37**	l/l	0.41	0.52	0.36	0.38
Mean cell volume	81	fl	80	99	79.4	82.6
Mean cell Hb	**26.7**	pg	27	31.5	26.2	27.2
Mean cell Hb conc.	33.0	g/dl	31.5	34.5	32.3	33.6
Red cell dist. width	**15.6**	%	11.6	14	15.1	16.1
Retic. count	**2.11**	%	0.26	0.77	2.0	2.2
Retic. absolute (abs)	95.6	$\times10^9$/l	30	100	88.4	102.8
White cell count	9.54	$\times10^9$/l	4	10	8.82	10.26
Neutrophils abs.	6.03	$\times10^9$/l	2	7	5.58	6.48
Lymphocytes abs.	2.35	$\times10^9$/l	1	3	2.17	2.52
Monocytes abs.	0.68	$\times10^9$/l	0.2	1	0.63	0.73
Eosinophils abs.	0.40	$\times10^9$/l	0.02	0.5	0.37	0.43
Basophils abs.	0.09	$\times10^9$/l	0.02	0.1	0.08	0.09
Normoblasts	0	/100 WBC	0	0		
Platelet count	**13.1**	$\times10^9$/l	150	400	12.1	14.1
Morphology	The red cells show mild anisocytosis and anisochromia. The white cells are normal in distribution and appearance. There is a severe thrombocytopenia. Numerous giant platelets are seen.					

3. It is most unusual for childhood ITP to become chronic.
4. Subsequent progress is detailed in Table 11.2.

Table 11.2

Case #34 cont. Subsequent Progress

The patient was put on high doses of prednisone and monitored. The platelet count rose to 121×10^9/l; however, when the dose was tapered off very slowly, as soon as the dose reached 25 mg/day, the platelet count plummeted. Splenectomy was then suggested to the parents; permission was refused. The patient was then given a 5-day course of IV gammaglobulin. The count rose dramatically, but once the course was over, it started falling. Splenectomy still being refused, the patient was given 2 mg vincristine IV weekly for 4 weeks. The platelet count eventually settled down at $30–40\times10^9$/l.

As indicated before, chronicity in such a young patient is most unusual.

CASE #35 (TABLE 11.3)

Table 11.3

Patient	Age	Sex	Race	Altitude
Mrs C G	47 yrs	Female	White	5000 ft

This lady had been diagnosed some years before with SLE and mild to moderate renal insufficiency that left her with a mild normocytic anemia. Recently a FBC showed the development of a moderately severe thrombocytopenia (a report sent with the patient showed a platelet count at the time of 13×10^9/l). A bone marrow examination was arranged. She was placed on high doses of prednisone and referred for assessment.

She complained of chronic tiredness and dyspnea on effort – this had not significantly deteriorated over the last few years. She developed a rash on exposing herself to the sun. She experienced aching pains in many joints, both large and small, with swelling of the knee joints, and there was significant morning stiffness, lasting for at least 30 minutes. There were no mouth ulcers but recently had noticed blackish blebs in her mouth.

On examination she was an obese lady. The BP was 130/90 in both arms; the pulse rate was 64/min and regular, and all pulses were present. Numerous bruises were seen in the soft palate, pharynx, arms, and legs, but no clear purpura. There was no evidence of psoriasis or pitting of the nails. The heart sounds were normal. No pericardial or pleural rubs were detected. The liver and spleen were not clinically enlarged. No neurological signs were present, and there was no evidence of vasculitis. The knee joints were not clinically swollen but were painful on movement; the left knee joint displayed crepitus. None of her joints were swollen. She said that the diagnosis of SLE had been made "with a blood test." Extensive investigations were undertaken to establish the diagnosis.

.	Value	Units	Reference range Low	Reference range High	Permitted range Low	Permitted range High
Red cell count	3.41	$\times 10^{12}$/l	4.03	5.09	3.31	3.51
Hemoglobin (Hb)	9.21	g/dl	12.7	15.9	8.9	9.5
Hematocrit (Hct)	0.30	l/l	0.38	0.49	0.29	0.31
Mean cell volume	87.2	fl	80	99	85.5	88.9
Mean cell Hb	27.0	pg	27	31.5	26.5	27.5
Mean cell Hb conc.	31.0	g/dl	31.5	34.5	30.4	31.6
Red cell dist. width	15.1	%	11.6	14	15.1	15.1
Retic. count	0.3	%	0.5	0.9	0.3	0.3
Retic. absolute (abs)	10.2	$\times 10^9$/l	30	100	9.9	10.5
White cell count	12.97	$\times 10^9$/l	4	10	12.0	13.94
Neutrophils abs.	8.52	$\times 10^9$/l	2	7	7.88	9.16
Lymphocytes abs.	3.64	$\times 10^9$/l	1	3	3.57	3.92
Monocytes abs.	0.49	$\times 10^9$/l	0.2	1	0.46	0.53
Eosinophils abs.	0.25	$\times 10^9$/l	0.02	0.5	0.23	0.26
Basophils abs.	0.06	$\times 10^9$/l	0.02	0.1	0.06	0.07
Platelet count	15.9	$\times 10^9$/l	150	400	14.3	17.5
Sedimentation	47	mm/h	0	20	45	49
Morphology	The red cells are normochromic and normocytic, with some rouleaux formation. The neutrophils show a prominent right shift. There is a mild neutrophilia, most likely the effect of steroid administration. There is a severe thrombocytopenia. There is no platelet sludging or satellitism.					

This case while rather complex is shown because of the significant and extremely important clinical association between SLE and thrombocytopenia. There are also several general instructive features.

The accompanying bone marrow report read, in summary, as follows:

1. Erythropoiesis and granulopoiesis were normal.
2. Lymphocytes, plasma cells, and reticulum cells were normal.
3. Megakaryocytes were **DECREASED.**
4. Iron staining showed normal stores but decreased sideroblasts.

My comments

1. The iron staining pattern is typical of anemia of chronic disease.
2. The decreased megakaryocytes were puzzling – it was very much against the diagnosis of ITP. However, bone marrow aspirates quite commonly show this picture. In this case, however, it was critical, since genuinely decreased megakaryocytes could mean another diagnosis, and the possible therapeutic options for the condition would have to be reconsidered. Accordingly, a bone marrow biopsy was arranged: this showed normal megakaryocyte numbers.

The immune markers of SLE were repeated. See Table 11.4

Table 11.4

Case #35 cont.	Value	Low	High
Antinuclear antibody	160 (titer)	0	40
Anti-double stranded DNA	< 2.5 IU/ml	0.0	15.0
Anti-SM	Negative		
Anti-RNP	Negative		
Anti-SSA (Ro)	Negative		
Anti-SSB (La)	Negative		
Comment	ANA shows a speckled pattern, mitotic chromosome negative.		

Extended biochemical investigations were performed. See Table 11.5

SONOGRAPHY of the abdomen showed normal liver and spleen. The kidneys were within normal limits for size but the cortex was thinner than the average. **CHEST X-RAY** was normal.

DISCUSSION

1. It may be claimed that the above case does not represent an isolated thrombocytopenia. While it is true that there are changes in the other cell lines, there are

Table 11.5

	Value	Units	Reference range Low	Reference range High
S-Urea	**14.2**	mmol/l	2.1	7.1
S-Creatinine	**151**	mmol/l	62	115
S-Urea:creatinine	94.0			
S-Sodium	136	mmol/l	136	145
S-Potassium	4.4	mmol/l	3.5	5.1
S-Chloride	103.00	mmol/l	98	108
S-Total CO_2	27.2	mmol/l	22	28
S-Anion gap	10.2	mmol/l	5	14
S-Osmolarity	276	mmol/l	275	295
S-Uric acid	**0.51**	mmol/l	0.21	0.42
S-Protein (total)	72	g/l	64	83
S-Albumin	41	g/l	34	48
S-Globulin	31.0	g/l	30	35
S-α1-Globulin	**6.0**	g/l	2.6	5.1
S-α2-Globulin	**7.4**	g/l	3.4	7.1
S-β-Globulin	9.4	g/l	5.5	9.4
S-γ-Globulin	10.1	g/l	5.3	14.3
S-Immunoglobulin G	6.9	g/l	2.5	12
S-Immunoglobulin M	2.06	g/l	0.19	1.93
S-Immunoglobulin A	0.88	g/l	0.07	0.94
S-Bilirubin (total)	7.6	μmol/l	6.8	34.2
S-Bilirubin (direct)	2.1	μmol/l	1.7	8.6
S-Bilirubin (indirect)	5.5	μmol/l	5.1	25.6
S-ALP	77	IU/l	53	128
S-gGT	**75**	IU/l	8	37
S-ALT	**63**	IU/l	19	40
S-AST	29	IU/l	13	32
S-LDH	**421**	IU/l	90	180
C-reactive protein	6.7	mg/l	0.0	10.0
S-Ferritin female	**453.6**	μg/l	14.0	233.1
S-Iron	**10.1**	μmol/l	11.6	31.3
S-Transferrin	2.54	g/l	2.12	3.60
S-Fe saturation female	**15.1**	%	20.0	35.0
U-Volume (24 h)	1800	ml		
U-Creatinine	4.8	mmol/l	1	20
U-Protein	97	mg/l	10	140
U-Protein excretion	**175**	mg/24 h	0	100
Creatinine clearance	**38.6**	ml/min	90	130
Protein electrophoresis	The pattern was that of an acute inflammatory response.			

known independent causes for these – renal insufficiency in the case of the red cells and steroid use in the case of the white cells; the thrombocytopenia is something new and is not related to these causes. It is fair therefore to approach the thrombocytopenia as an isolated one. It is also a true thrombocytopenia, with reference to the morphological report.

2. There is a close causal relationship between SLE and thrombocytopenia. It is essential therefore to verify this diagnosis. The evidence for the original diagnosis is not convincing. The ANA of 160 is not diagnostic. Clinically the features are those of a sero-negative spondyloarthropathy. The swelling of the knees appears to be due to

osteoarthritis – this was later confirmed radiologically. The photosensitive rash was not typical of SLE and was later confirmed to be due to porphyria variegata.

3. Several blood tests confirm the presence of active chronic disease: the protein electrophoretic pattern, the iron studies, and the raised ESR – this despite the normal CRP.

4. The raised LDH was cause for concern. A Coombs test was performed to exclude immune hemolysis (since she may already have an autoimmune disease). This was negative. This, however, did not exclude hemolysis from another cause, although it was unlikely, given the low bilirubin levels and no evidence of red cell abnormality morphologically. In the interim it was decided that the LDH was probably due to the renal disease, and investigation for a hemolytic disorder could be deferred.

5. The nature of the renal pathology required a biopsy but this was not possible in view of the thrombocytopenia. The response to high-dose steroids was very poor, and there was no doubt that on tapering down her PC would once again enter the danger zone. It was decided to do a splenectomy. This was done endoscopically. At operation, as soon as the splenic artery was clamped she was given one mega unit of platelets; 18 h after the surgery, the PC was 224×10^9/l. Eventually this rose to 756, and then over a period of weeks settled down at 171.

Comment Systemic lupus erythematosus has a distinct relationship with thrombocytopenia, particularly in females. The thrombocytopenia can occur at any stage of the disease and can predate its clinical onset by years. Its first occurrence once the SLE is clinically manifest is a poor prognostic sign.

It is acceptable practice that all female patients presenting with thrombocytopenia be tested for SLE; however, this diagnosis can be very difficult, and one can be seriously misled, as the above case demonstrates.

"Safe" Platelet Counts One is sometimes asked what a safe platelet count is for various procedures to be carried out without untoward bleeding. As a general rule, and assuming there is no functional platelet defect, the following can be suggested (in counts $\times10^9$/l):

1. Ordinary dentistry: 10
2. Extractions: > 30
3. Mandibular block: > 30
4. Minor surgery: > 50

5. Major surgery: > 80
6. Epidural block, lumbar puncture: >80
7. Retrobulbar block: >80

Aspects of thrombocytopenia are further discussed in Chapter 18.

Further Reading

Andreoli TE, Bennett JC, Carpenter CCJ, Plum F (eds) (1997). Cecil Essentials of Medicine. 4th edn. Philadelphia: WB Saunders.

Epstein RJ (1996). Medicine for Examinations. 3rd edn. London: Churchill Livingstone.

Hoffbrand AV, Pettit JE (2001). Essential Haematology. 4th edn. Oxford: Blackwell Science.

Lewis SM, Bain B, Bates I (2006). Dacie and Lewis Practical Haematology. 10th edn. London: Churchill Livingstone.

Leukopenia – a decrease in one or more of the components of the white cell count – involves a complex discussion, because of the many different cell types that can be affected and because each of the different cell types can be reduced for different reasons. Leukopenia is also seen as a form of immune insufficiency, hence there is overlap with the subject matter of Chapter 22.

Defining Leukopenia

The following patterns can occur:

1. **LEUKOPENIA.** Here all the white cell types are reduced.
2. **NEUTROPENIA**. This is by far the commonest. The term **GRANULOCYTOPENIA** means a decrease in all the granulocytes, sometimes including the monocytes, but with normal lymphocyte counts.
3. **LYMPHOPENIA.** This is discussed in greater detail in Chapter 22.
4. **EOSINOPENIA, MONOCYTOPENIA, AND BASOPENIA WILL NOT BE DISCUSSED.**

Generalized Leukopenia

As stated, this implies a reduction in all the white cell series and is relatively uncommon. It occurs almost always as part of severe bone marrow destruction or suppression, in which case the red cells and the platelets are also usually affected. These are discussed in Chapter 13: "Pancytopenia and the Bicytopenias." Even in these cases, the lymphocyte series is often not involved or less seriously affected, since the peripheral lymphocyte count is only partly dependent on bone marrow function.

Neutropenia

One problem with discussing neutropenia is that there are many congenital causes, some of which can present in adult medicine. Generally they are rare and will only briefly be mentioned, apart from one or two practical exceptions.

General Pathology Causes of Neutropenia

The most convenient way of presenting these is to look at the way neutropenia is classified. The problem is that there are several ways of classifying neutropenia: formal, pathophysiological, and clinical.

The Formal (Pathological) Classification of Neutropenia

As with thrombocytopenia, it is useful to redisplay the diagrammatic outline of the pathology of the blood system. See Fig. 12.1.

The causes of neutropenia are

1. **DEFECTIVE PRODUCTION BY THE MARROW**
2. **NEUTROPENIA AS A RESULT OF DAMAGE OR SEQUESTRATION IN THE CIRCULATION**
3. **DISORDERS OF PERIPHERAL UTILIZATION**

This classification does not, however, emphasize the peculiar dynamics of the granulocytes. There are two important issues:

1. **MARGINATION**: As indicated in Chapter 2, at any one time (in the resting state) about half of the granulocytes are loosely adherent to the endothelium, with the result that the actual count of white cells in the

O.N. Beck, *Diagnostic Hematology*, DOI 10.1007/978-1-84800-295-1_12,
© Springer-Verlag London Limited 2009

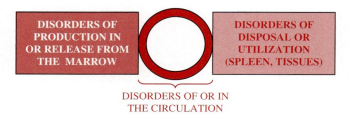

Fig. 12.1 Basic diagram of the hematological system

circulation is markedly underreported. While these can be mobilized (by adrenaline, corticosteroids, etc.), in the process markedly increasing the evident WCC, this adherence can also be **INCREASED** due to endothelial activation, as occurs in infections, sepsis, immune complex deposition, etc. The latter may occur as a prior step to actual invasion of the tissues to combat infection (which in fact is the biological function of the neutrophils) or as part of a vasculitis.

2. The short normal intravascular life span of the neutrophils (hours). Their destiny is the tissues, whether or not there is an infection.

Thus two further reasons for neutropenia will be

1. Causes that increase margination followed by invasion of the tissues; naturally this is usually compensated for by increased release of neutrophils from the marrow pool and increased production.
2. Exhaustion of the marrow pool. Hence we can also classify neutropenia as follows.

The Pathophysiological Classification of Neutropenia

1. **DEFECTIVE PRODUCTION BY OR RELEASE FROM THE MARROW.**
2. **DAMAGE TO OR SEQUESTRATION IN THE CIRCULATION.**
3. **INCREASED MARGINATION AND ADHERENCE TO ENDOTHELIUM.**
4. **INCREASED EGRESS TO THE TISSUES.** This occurs in infections. Neutropenia only supervenes once the marrow is exhausted.

The above classification is far more meaningful. Nevertheless it fails to address one specific practical diagnostic (and prognostic) factor.

The Clinical Classification of Neutropenia

The most practical classification is in terms of the likely effects of neutropenia. The only significant effect of neutropenia is the tendency to recurrent, even fatal, bacterial

and fungal infections. But there is something odd about this tendency to infection with neutropenia. To explain: When we consider the dysfunctional effects of anemia – i.e., tissue hypoxia – there is no relationship between the degree of tissue hypoxia at any given Hb and the **CAUSE** of the anemia. Similarly with the platelets, given normal function, the tendency to bleed with low platelet counts is dependent on the level and not on the cause.

In the case of the neutrophils the above concept does not apply:

1. If a neutropenia is due to **DECREASED PRODUCTION**, the tendency to develop infections is directly related to the **DEGREE** of neutropenia.
2. If a neutropenia is due to **INCREASED MARGINATION OR PERIPHERAL DESTRUCTION** from any cause, this relationship does not hold. Very many such patients with a neutrophil count of $< 500 \times 10^9$/l appear to live quite normal lives. They typically have a monocytosis. The reason for this phenomenon is (currently) a mystery. It is possible that the (relative) monocytosis is one factor preventing serious infections. Certainly, where neutropenia is accompanied by monocytopenia, as in aplastic anemia and cytotoxic therapy, there is a far greater predisposition to infection and from a broader spectrum of infectious agents.

The practical implications are very significant, particularly since treatment with G-CSF or GM-CSF is extremely expensive, and may be unnecessary.

In adult medicine isolated neutropenia is most commonly due to infection and drugs (as with thrombocytopenia but with the addition in the latter of ITP).

There tend to be fundamental differences in the bone marrow appearances between the acquired and congenital causes.

Bone Marrow Appearances in Acquired Neutropenia The bone marrow in acquired cases depends on two factors: whether there is a primary bone marrow disease responsible for the neutropenia (such as bone marrow necrosis, leukemia, myelodysplasia, etc.) – in which case the appearances will be of these changes plus of course evidence of diminution or absence of neutrophil precursors – and in the case of peripheral causes, whether the marrow shows any signs of regenerating the granulocyte series.

The bone marrow appearances in the congenital causes can show highly suggestive changes; these will be discussed later.

Specific Causes of Neutropenia

Neutropenia Due to Infection

There are several established mechanisms by which infections cause neutropenia:

1. **DIRECT INFECTION OF THE GRANULOPOIE-TIC CELLS IN THE MARROW**. Viral infections are predominantly responsible here, notably EB virus, HIV, Kawasaki disease, hepatitis, parvovirus, CMV, and rubella (rubella should never be forgotten – in adults it may be very evanescent and non-specific). In a large clinical laboratory practice, it was concluded that by far the commonest cause of neutropenia was viral infections (Niemann, personal communication).

    FBC FEATURES: The neutropenia may be profound; it is often accompanied by monocytosis, lymphocytosis, and atypical "viral" lymphocytes. Neutrophil precursors (i.e., a left shift) may be seen in the recovery phase.

    BONE MARROW APPEARANCES: These will typically show lack of granulocytic precursors and at a later stage will show evidence of regeneration.

    CLINICAL FEATURES: The patient very often feels awful, and there may be muscle pains and pharyngitis but seldom anything worse. Lymphadenopathy is unremarkable.

2. **INCREASED ADHERENCE OF NEUTROPHILS TO ENDOTHELIUM** (as the first stage in a developing vasculitis). Many organisms have been associated with this: Babesia, rickettsiae, dengue, and measles.

3. In **SEPTICEMIA**, neutropenia is due to both increased endothelial adherence and increased utilization in the tissues. In general, bacterial infections cause neutropenia only if they are so severe and prolonged as to overwhelm the marrow stores and productive capacity. (Note that with septic lesions in enclosed spaces, pus formation in the presence of neutropenia is very poor – at best a seropurulent exudate is found).

4. **IN INFECTIONS CAUSING SPLENOMEGALY**, such as brucellosis, typhoid, etc., neutropenia may be caused both by splenic sequestration and marrow suppression.

Drug-Induced Neutropenia

As with all drug-induced cytopenias, there are three ways of looking at this:

1. **THE PRIMARY SITE OF THE PATHOLOGY**. This is either direct suppression of the marrow (most common) or by peripheral destruction.

2. **THE MECHANISM**. This is either toxic or immunological. In the latter case, there are a number of well-documented pathophysiologies:

    a. Antineutrophil antibodies.
    b. Cytotoxic T-cells.
    c. Haptens.
    d. Autoimmune mechanisms.
    e. Oxidative modifications of drugs.

3. **THE PROCESS**. One of two processes is predominant:

    a. **DOSE DEPENDENT.** This process almost always affects marrow production. It is due to interference with protein synthesis, DNA synthesis (folate inhibitors), or cell replication. Important drugs here include the cytotoxic chemotherapeutic agents, phenothiazines, the antithyroid drugs, and chloramphenicol.

        FBC FEATURES: Many pictures can be found. A marked left shift is very common, with toxic granulation, despite the neutropenia. Normocytic anemia is common. If the disease process has proceeded to DIC, the characteristic features of this may be superimposed.

        FEATURES IN OTHER LABORATORY TESTS: Opportunistic infections due to organisms such as pseudomonas and fungi are common. Activity tests are often positive.

        CLINICAL FEATURES: Infective complications may be very severe.

    b. **IDIOSYNCRATIC.** This process is found with an even larger group of drugs, including many antibiotics. Typically the neutropenic response is sudden and occurs on re-exposure to the drug (and the patient may not even remember the previous exposure).

        FBC FEATURES: Apart from the neutropenia and often a monocytosis, there may be very little to see.

        CLINICAL FEATURES: Severe infections are uncommon.

BONE MARROW APPEARANCES OF DRUG-INDUCED NEUTROPENIA: These are as described for neutropenia due to infection.

Please note:

1. Chloramphenicol can act by the idiosyncratic mechanism as well.

2. Some drugs tend to cause neutropenia in the presence of immune deficiency from other causes.

3. Drugs have many other effects on the immune system as a whole. These are discussed in Chapter 22.

Agranulocytosis

In days gone by, agranulocytosis was effectively the name of a clinical presentation. Cases presenting with the classical description are still occasionally seen. It is essentially an acute severe neutropenia, usually due to drugs, and used to be almost uniformly fatal.

Usually it manifests itself 2 or 3 weeks after the patient has started taking the drug; on subsequent exposure to the drug it will occur with dramatic suddenness. The patient is extremely ill with a very sore throat, fever, and rigors. The FBC will show an extremely low neutrophil count. The bone marrow appearances depend very much on when the aspiration is done: if done at the time of the first presentation the marrow will show virtually no neutrophil precursors; with every day that passes (assuming the patient survives), one starts seeing more and more precursors appearing in the marrow and then, after a day or two, in the blood. The precursors will start with the earliest and progress through to the later forms.

Neutropenia Due to Immune Mechanisms

The mechanisms of these **CHRONIC NEUTROPENIAS** are most conveniently classified as follows[1]:

1. **NEUTROPHIL-SPECIFIC ALLOANTIBODIES.** Mainly neonatal and rare.
2. **NEUTROPHIL-SPECIFIC AUTOANTIBODIES** These are found in a condition called autoimmune neutropenia. This is a **CHRONIC NEUTROPENIA**, usually with a neutrophil count of around 0.25×10^9/l and often with compensatory monocytosis and eosinophilia, and although associated with recurrent infections (mostly of the skin and oropharynx), these are not severe, and treatment is of the infection only. Prophylactic co-trimoxazole seems to be a common form of prevention. The condition may be primary (which is rare and transient) or secondary (associated with other autoimmune disease, typically occurring in the 40- to 60-year age group).

   FBC FEATURES: Essentially an isolated neutropenia, perhaps with a monocytosis and precursors in the recovery phase (should there be recovery).
   BONE MARROW APPEARANCES: These will typically show lack of granulocytic precursors, and at a later stage will show evidence of regeneration.
   CLINICAL FEATURES: These are very variable, ranging from minimal and non-specific to recurrent mild infections and, only occasionally, severe and life-threatening infections.

3. **CIRCULATING IMMUNE COMPLEXES.** This is thought to be the mechanism in certain immune neutropenias, notably those associated with SLE and rheumatoid arthritis (Felty syndrome):

   a. **SYSTEMIC LUPUS ERYTHEMATOSUS (SLE).** The development of autoimmune neutropenia is often regarded as a poor prognostic sign – for the SLE, but not for infections (infections when they do occur are usually due to steroid therapy). A factor complicating the understanding of neutropenia in SLE is that, in addition, marrow suppression or dysfunction is common.

   b. **FELTY SYNDROME.** This is a (usually) isolated neutropenia associated with a large spleen (which can be massive) in a patient with chronic, often burnt-out, rheumatoid arthritis and features of ulceration, nodules, and vasculitis. There is no correlation between the size of the spleen and the degree of neutropenia. It is interesting that it has been shown that there is increased margination in this disease, suggesting that a part of the neutropenia is relative and not absolute and also suggesting some sort of endothelial activation.

   The neutrophils that are present are also functionally defective: impaired bactericidal activity, decreased chemotaxis, and abnormal migration. There is a 20-fold increase in bacterial infections but they tend not to be very severe in most cases. There is also an increased risk of developing malignancies, especially non-Hodgkin lymphoma. Felty syndrome is often distinguished from LGL neutropenia (see below), but many consider them to be different manifestations of the same disease. Spontaneous remission occurs but is uncommon.

   Note that only 1% of rheumatoid arthritis patients develop Felty syndrome or LGL (see below).

   FBC FEATURES: Primarily an isolated neutropenia. Occasionally there are decreases affecting the other two cell lines.
   FEATURES IN OTHER LABORATORY TESTS: 95% of patients are HLA-DR4 positive. FBC features of rheumatoid arthritis may be superimposed, i.e., ACD, iron-deficiency anemia, folate deficiency, thrombocytopenia.

4. **LARGE GRANULAR LYMPHOCYTOSIS** (LGL) with neutropenia. The autoimmune status of this condition is not clear.

   CLINICAL FEATURES: Many of the features are similar to those of Felty syndrome. The course is usually benign but there is increased susceptibility to infection.

FBC FEATURES: Apart from the neutropenia numerous large granular lymphocytes (mostly NK cells) are seen (the count must be $> 2000 \times 10^9/l$ for the diagnosis to be entertained) but they may only be seen in the marrow ($>23\%$). Immunophenotyping shows these cells to have CD3 + clonality with T-cell receptor rearrangements.

Miscellaneous Causes of Neutropenia

This section includes conditions either whose immune etiology is not clear, that are features of marrow dysfunction, or that are rare congenital neutropenias:

1. **NEUTROPENIA SECONDARY TO BONE MARROW INFILTRATION**, such as lymphoma, myeloma, leukemia, or **APLASIA**.
2. **CHRONIC ACQUIRED IDIOPATHIC NEUTROPENIA**. The spleen is usually not enlarged. Bone marrow appearances are of three types:

   a. **NORMOCELLULAR**,
   b. **NEUTROPHIL HYPOPLASIA**,
   c. **MATURATION ARREST**, usually at the myelocyte stage.

3. **PRIMARY SPLENIC NEUTROPENIA**. This is found where the enlarged spleen is due to sarcoidosis, lymphoma, tuberculosis, malaria, kala-azar, or Gaucher disease. It is probably a form of hypersplenism.
4. **MYELOKATHEXIS**. The neutrophils show pyknotic nuclei with bizarre hypersegmentation, and the marrow shows neutrophil hyperplasia.
5. **CYCLIC NEUTROPENIA**. In this autosomal dominant condition, the peripheral neutrophil count oscillates between 0.1 and $1.5 \times 10^9/l$, regularly every 3–6 weeks. The neutropenia lasts for 5 or 6 days and during this time the patient will have fever, malaise, lymphadenopathy, and mouth ulcers. Fatalities often are associated with clostridial infections. Some patients also show a large granular cell proliferation. Of interest is that the reticulocytes, platelets, and the other white cells also oscillate but in a mirror-image fashion. The neutrophil precursors in the marrow will parallel the peripheral blood count.
6. **OTHER CONGENITAL NEUTROPENIAS**. There is a very large group of rare congenital neutropenias found mostly in children.

The Bone Marrow Examination in Congenital Neutropenia Bone marrow appearances in congenital neutropenias can sometimes be very informative. This short description is included since,

although these conditions are uncommon and found mainly in children, with the continuing advances in therapy, more and more of these cases are surviving to adulthood. The appearances may resemble those found in acquired forms, in which case they do not in themselves assist in the differential diagnosis. Sometimes, however, the appearances are in themselves so suggestive, particularly in conjunction with the clinical features, that differentiation from acquired causes is relatively straightforward. Basically there are three types of appearance (the disorders in each type are only listed):

1. *Normal marrow appearances.* That is, the morphology is normal, but its activity is not sufficient to compensate for the peripheral neutropenia. This appearance is found in one type of chronic idiopathic neutropenia, in the Schwachman–Diamond syndrome (where one also often sees dysplasia), and in glycogen storage type Ib disease (which is also accompanied by neutropenia).
2. *Hypoplastic marrow.* This is found in the cartilage-hair syndrome, reticular dysgenesis, and hypogammaglobulinemia with high IgM and IgA.
3. *Myelodysplastic features.* This is found in myelokathexis and chronic dysgranulopoiesis.
4. *Hyperactive with ineffective granulopoiesis.* This is found in the Kostmann syndrome and the other type of chronic idiopathic neutropenia.
5. *Increase in large granular lymphocytes.* This is found in large granular lymphocytosis with neutropenia.
6. *Maturation arrest.* This is characteristic of the Kostmann syndrome.
7. *Megaloblastic picture.* This is found in transcobalamin II deficiency (and which typically is associated with neutropenia).

Making the Diagnosis in a Case of Neutropenia

One would suspect the possibility of an immune deficiency of some sort in any patient with recurrent infections for no obvious cause. However, neutropenia is only one of these causes, and in practice the diagnosis of neutropenia is made initially from the FBC.

The first consideration is to decide on the acuteness and severity of the clinical presentation; clearly this would impact on the need for urgent intervention. Thus, effectively, we need to distinguish between the acutely, usually seriously ill, and the chronic case.

THE PATIENT'S HISTORY IS EXTREMELY IMPORTANT:

1. **RAPID ONSET**, the presence of rigors, possibly mental confusion and delirium. Here one thinks first of septicemia, agranulocytosis, other forms of neutropenia due to drugs, neutropenia secondary to bone marrow infiltration, or aplasia.

   By contrast, many causes are **LESS LIKELY TO PRESENT IN THIS WAY** (although exceptions occur in all cases):

   a. Viral infections. These do tend, however, to cause severe prostration and chills.
   b. Autoimmune neutropenia.
   c. Systemic lupus erythematosus (SLE).
   d. Felty syndrome.
   e. Large granular lymphocytosis (LGL) with neutropenia.
   f. Chronic acquired idiopathic neutropenia.
   g. Primary splenic neutropenia.
   h. Myelokathexis.

2. **CONSTITUTIONAL SYMPTOMS SUCH AS PROSTRATION, SEVERE MALAISE**. Viral neutropenias very often present in this way.
3. **RECURRENT INFECTIONS OF THE SKIN AND OROPHARYNX**. One particular clinical presentation deserves special mention – **THE SORE THROAT**. This is a very common complaint and is frequently underestimated; it can be the indicator of serious disease. There are seven "danger signs" that may occur in patients with sore throats, any of which should prompt search for soft tissue space infection, abscess, angina, or **NEUTROPENIA**:

   a. Persistence of symptoms for longer than 1 week without improvement,
   b. Respiratory difficulty, particularly stridor,
   c. Difficulty in handling secretions,
   d. Difficulty in swallowing,
   e. Severe pain in the absence of erythema,
   f. A palpable mass,
   g. Blood in the pharynx or ear.

4. **A CYCLIC PATTERN**. If one is aware of the disorder, a cyclic pattern is usually easy to discover: malaise, perhaps fever and chills, sore throat, etc., every 3–6 weeks, lasting for 5 or 6 days. This condition is commoner than one would think:

   a. Cyclic patterns are very common, both in health and disease; doctors are aware of this and may tend to ascribe recurrent mild infections to being "normal."
   b. Very often a patient with cyclic neutropenia will consult a doctor after the cycle is more or less over, by which time the FBC will be completely or nearly normal.
   c. This disorder tends not to be thought of, in any case, as being regarded as very rare.

5. **DRUGS**. A large number of drugs can be responsible for neutropenia. The commoner ones are listed in Appendix A.
6. **BONE PAIN**. This may suggest bone marrow infiltration by leukemia or myeloma.
7. **OTHER AUTOIMMUNE DISEASE**. Very often, even with negative antineutrophil antibodies being found, this can be the clue to the etiology. Rheumatoid arthritis, SLE, ulcerative colitis, etc., must all be considered.
8. **FAMILY HISTORY**. A positive family history may point to one of the congenital forms of neutropenia.
9. **THE DISCOVERY OF NEUTROPENIA IN A FBC IN A PATIENT WITH OR WITHOUT SYMPTOMS.**

The Clinical Examination

Figure 12.2 offers suggestions on **SPECIFIC ASPECTS** of the examination of a patient in whom neutropenia is

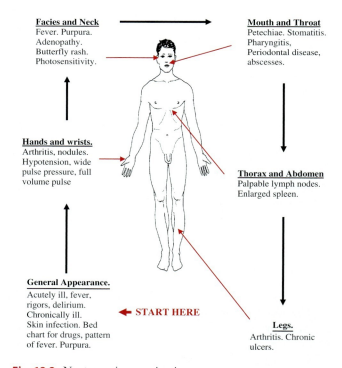

Facies and Neck
Fever. Purpura.
Adenopathy.
Butterfly rash.
Photosensitivity.

Mouth and Throat
Petechiae. Stomatitis.
Pharyngitis,
Periodontal disease,
abscesses.

Hands and wrists.
Arthritis, nodules.
Hypotension, wide
pulse pressure, full
volume pulse

Thorax and Abdomen
Palpable lymph nodes.
Enlarged spleen.

General Appearance.
Acutely ill, fever,
rigors, delirium.
Chronically ill.
Skin infection. Bed
chart for drugs, pattern
of fever. Purpura.

◄ **START HERE**

Legs.
Arthritis. Chronic
ulcers.

Fig. 12.2 Neutropenia: examination

known or suspected; clearly it is part of the overall examination as depicted in Fig. 5.4.

The subsequent investigation depends to a considerable extent on the clinical findings. Our major task is to exclude known causes that are clinically apparent, such as drugs, the presence of other autoimmune disease, a cyclic pattern, or infection prior to the development of neutropenia. This requires active searching and judgment. Of great value are

1. The severity of infection
2. The presence of splenomegaly with or without lymphadenopathy
3. Many other conditions whose major and commonest features are summarized in the boxes below

The Differential Diagnosis of Splenomegaly and Neutropenia

1. *Amyloidosis*. See Chapter 22.
2. *Lymphoma*. See Chapter 22.
3. *Drugs*.
4. *Sarcoidosis*. Diagnosis is ultimately by biopsy.
5. *Chronic infections*, e.g., tuberculosis
6. *Systemic lupus erythematosu*
7. *Felty syndrome*.
8. *Large granular lymphocytosis*.
9. *Sjögren syndrome*.
10. *Myelofibrosis*.
11. *Leukemia and lymphoma*.
12. *Storage diseases* such as Gaucher disease.

Features Suggesting an Autoimmune Neutropenia

1. *Associated autoimmune disease*: rheumatoid arthritis, SLE, ulcerative colitis.
2. *Infective complications typically not severe*, only involving skin and oropharynx if present.
3. *Antineutrophil antibodies* – but see box.

Features Suggesting an Acquired Neutropenia

1. *Acute onset*, particularly after early childhood
2. *Splenomegaly*
3. Evidence of *primary hematological disease*
4. Evidence of *other autoimmune disease*
5. Recent *drug* ingestion
6. *Significant infection*

Features Suggesting a Congenital Neutropenia

1. *Chronic neutropenia*
2. *Onset at a young age*
3. *Clinically less severe infections*, if any
4. *Monocytosis*
5. *No evidence of autoimmune disease or drug ingestion*

Features Suggesting Primary Bone Marrow Disease

1. *Splenomegaly* especially if accompanied by hepatomegaly and/or lymphadenopathy
2. *Bone pain and tenderness*
3. *Precursors* and abnormal cells in the blood

Features Suggesting Neutropenia of Viral Origin

1. Acute onset, chills, muscle pain, headache, dyspnea, cough, nausea, vomiting, diarrhea, prostration.
2. Lymphocytosis with viral lymphocytes.
3. Generally few toxic changes in the neutrophils.
4. Activity tests are normal or at most only moderately raised.

Features Suggesting Neutropenia of Bacterial or Fungal Origin

1. *Septicemic presentation*, often with DIC.
2. Often a *left shift and toxic change* despite neutropenia.
3. Localized infections show very *poor pus formation*.
4. *Activity tests* are markedly raised.

Antineutrophil Antibodies It may be thought that antineutrophil cytoplasmic antibodies (ANCA) would be of great value in the identification of autoimmune neutropenia. Unfortunately this is not so. Tests for these antibodies are most useful in the vasculitides and are particularly associated with Wegener's granulomatosis and idiopathic crescentic glomerulonephritis. We do not, in routine use, have a satisfactory test for antibodies in autoimmune neutropenia per se, where the sensitivity and specificity of ANCA are low.

Special Investigations in Neutropenia The selection of further tests depends on the clinical features and, within that context, on whether you want to confirm or exclude a diagnosis.

1. *Suspicion of an autoimmune cause*:

   a. Rheumatoid factor and antinuclear antibodies are very specific in confirming clinically diagnosed rheumatoid arthritis and systemic lupus erythematosus, respectively. Negative tests are very specific in excluding active disease.
   b. ANCA – see box above.
   c. Other autoantibodies may be suggestive of an autoimmune cause of the neutropenia.
   d. HLA-DR4. Since this is positive in 95% of cases of Felty syndrome and LGL-associated neutropenia, it serves as an excellent marker of these disorders.
   e. HLA-B27 is positive in most cases of ankylosing spondylitis and ulcerative colitis with arthropathy.

2. *Suspicion of primary bone marrow disease*. Depending very much on what the disease is, the peripheral blood may be very indicative:

   a. Plasma cells and malignant lymphocytes would point to myeloma and lymphoma, respectively.
   b. A leukoerythroblastic picture would suggest some form of bone marrow infiltration.

      Ultimately bone marrow aspiration and biopsy are the only routine means of making a diagnosis.

3. *Suspicion of a viral cause*. If the clinical features suggest a particular type of virus, virus studies can clinch the diagnosis. Too often, however, this is not feasible, and one is reliant on a combination of clinical exclusion and activity tests, such as the ESR and CRP – which may be normal or, if raised, seldom more than moderately.

4. *Suspicion of a bacterial or fungal infective cause*. The clinical features are usually convincing. Confirmatory tests include radiology, CRP and ESR (typically higher than in viral infections), gallium scanning, etc.

5. *Suspicion of a congenital cause*. Age of onset, family history, and the clinical features may be very suggestive. Generally speaking, bone marrow examination is necessary to complete the picture. In addition, neutrophil function tests are also abnormal in many of them.

6. *Cyclic features*. Serial FBCs are necessary. See Case #39.

Indications for Bone Marrow Examination in Neutropenia

1. Clinical and/or FBC features suggesting that the neutropenia is due to primary bone marrow disease
2. Clinical and/or FBC features suggesting a congenital neutropenia
3. Any neutropenia diagnosed and treated on clinical grounds that does not respond to therapy
4. Any obscure neutropenia

Lymphopenia

Lymphopenia is closely associated with immune deficiencies, and as such is the subject matter of Chapter 22. However, the primary immune disorders associated with lymphopenia are too complex for a book of this kind. Very briefly, lymphopenia may be associated with several of the primary immune deficiencies (which are mainly pediatric), such as severe combined immune deficiency (SCID) and the Wiskott–Aldrich syndrome. It will be remembered that there are two major groups of T-cells – T helper (T_H) and T suppressor (T_S), or CD4+ and CD8+, respectively. The T_H:T_S ratio in these conditions is normal despite the lymphopenia, in sharp contradistinction to what is found in many of the secondary causes. This is really one of the major features to assist in the diagnosis.

Secondary Lymphopenia

As a brief introduction, it should be recalled that the peripheral blood lymphocyte count represents only 2% of the total body lymphocytes, and that there is extremely active trafficking of the lymphocytes between the lymphoid tissues and the blood. Many causes of secondary lymphopenia are due not to a deficiency in the cells but to temporary retention of lymphocytes by the lymphoid tissues. This is classically demonstrated by the effect of corticosteroid therapy, which causes a temporary lymphopenia on commencement of therapy, but normalizes within 2 days. Only the commonest causes will be mentioned:

1. Infections, notably influenza
2. Effect of therapy: steroids, radiation, cytotoxics
3. Advanced malignant disease
4. Loss of lymphocytes: intestinal lymphangiectasia, severe right-sided heart failure
5. SLE and chronic graft-versus-host disease

Unlike the case with neutropenia, lymphopenia is not going to be the presenting feature with any of these disorders; the clinical focus will be on the major diseases. It is thus considered unnecessary to include cases for study.

Teaching Cases

CASE #36 (EXAMINE TABLE 12.1)

DISCUSSION

1. The neutropenia is very severe. Apart from a possible very mild thrombocytopenia (see the range of permitted values), this is an isolated neutropenia.
2. Despite the marked neutropenia the infective complications do not appear very serious (note the normal ESR). This may to some extent be due to the high relative monocyte count, but this is also characteristic of early viral neutropenia.
3. The presence of atypical lymphocytes reinforces the suggestion of a viral cause. However, it seems clear that the slide was not reviewed by a hematologist, and the atypical lymphocytes mentioned may have a more sinister implication, such as LGL (despite the absence of splenomegaly). A blood smear was reviewed and the atypical lymphocytes were considered to be typical of a viral infection. The neutrophils showed no toxic change. The CRP was normal. The patient was treated symptomatically

Table 12.1

Patient	Age	Sex	Race	Altitude
Mr J M	26 yrs	Male	Black	2500 ft

The patient is an artisan. He complained to his doctor that he had been feeling "fluey" for a few days, but woke up that morning feeling "like I'm going to die." The doctor found a mild pharyngitis and otitis but was concerned at the marked prostration demonstrated by the patient. He ordered a FBC, whereupon the patient was referred. On examination, his blood pressure was normal, his chest clear, and the heart sounds closed. The abdomen was soft with no masses or organomegaly.

	Value	Units	Reference range Low	High	Permitted range Low	High
Red cell count	5.11	×10^{12}/l	4.64	5.67	4.96	5.26
Hemoglobin (Hb)	14.9	g/dl	13.4	17.5	14.4	15.4
Hematocrit (Hct)	0.47	l/l	0.41	0.52	0.45	0.48
Mean cell volume	91.6	fl	80	99	89.8	93.4
Mean cell Hb	29.2	pg	27	31.5	28.6	29.7
Mean cell Hb conc.	31.8	g/dl	31.5	34.5	31.2	32.5
Red cell dist. width	14.6	%	11.6	14	13.5	15.7
White cell count	2.91	×10^9/l	3.5	10	2.69	3.13
Neutrophils	14.2	%				
Band cells	0	%	0	0		
Lymphocytes	53.4	%				
Monocytes	26.1	%				
Eosinophils	5.5	%				
Basophils	0.8	%				
Neutrophils abs.	0.41	×10^9/l	1.5	7	0.38	0.44
Band cells abs.	0		0	0	0	0
Lymphocytes abs.	1.55	×10^9/l	1	3	1.44	1.67
Monocytes abs.	0.76	×10^9/l	0.2	1	0.70	0.82
Eosinophils abs.	0.16	×10^9/l	0.02	0.5	0.15	0.17
Basophils abs.	0.02	×10^9/l	0.02	0.1	0.02	0.03
Platelet count	131.1	×10^9/l	150	400	120.0	142.2
Sedimentation	8	mm/h	0	10	8	8
Morphology	Neutropenia + + atypical lymphocytes					

and monitored. He recovered completely. Bone marrow studies were thus avoided.

CASE #37 (EXAMINE TABLE 12.2)

DISCUSSION

1. The patient undoubtedly has a severe neutropenia. Of all the general causes, only one – autoimmune neutropenia – appears to have some substance. Accordingly, antineutrophil cytoplasmic antibodies (ANCA) were ordered and these, on two occasions, were positive but in rather low titers. There were two problems with this result:

Table 12.2

Patient	Age	Sex	Race	Altitude
Miss C M	21 yrs	Female	White	5000 ft

The patient was a national swimming champion and has been very fit for years except for complaints of chronic intermittent diarrhea and vague abdominal pains. Recently she started experiencing recurrent sore throats with mouth ulcers, progressing recently to bronchopneumonia, during which a FBC revealed severe neutropenia. On examination she is a well-built athletic-looking young woman. She has been receiving intensive antibiotic treatment and the acute symptoms had subsided. Nevertheless, she appeared chronically ill. A detailed history failed to reveal any drug usage except for therapeutic antibiotics. There was no suggestion of arthropathy or a previous serious viral infection. There was no suggestion of periodicity in the infective episodes. Her problems had commenced in her later teens; before that she had been very well and fit. She admitted to being extremely competitive and there was a background of considerable family conflict. Systemic examination revealed no enlarged organs, normal skin and no joint involvement, and only very vague abdominal tenderness. Quite severe periodontal disease was found. Stools contained mucus but no blood.

	Value	Units	Reference range Low	Reference range High	Permitted range Low	Permitted range High
Red cell count	4.66	$\times 10^{12}$/l	4.03	5.09	4.52	4.80
Hemoglobin (Hb)	12.8	g/dl	12.7	15.9	12.4	13.2
Hematocrit (Hct)	0.37	l/l	0.38	0.49	0.36	0.38
Mean cell volume	80	fl	80	99	78.4	81.6
Mean cell Hb	27.5	pg	27	31.5	26.9	28.0
Mean Cell Hb Conc.	34.3	g/dl	31.5	34.5	33.6	35.0
Red cell dist. width	15.9	%	11.6	14	15.9	15.9
White cell count	2.8	$\times 10^9$/l	4	10	2.59	3.01
Corrected WCC	2.67	$\times 10^9$/l				
Neutrophils	11.9	%			11.9	11.9
Band cells	5.0	%	0	0		
Lymphocytes	58.5	%			58.5	58.5
Monocytes	14.2	%			14.2	14.2
Eosinophils	5.1	%			5.1	5.1
Basophils	1.3	%			1.3	1.3
Neutrophils abs.	0.33	$\times 10^9$/l	2	7	0.31	0.36
Band cells abs.	0.14		0	0	0.13	0.15
Lymphocytes abs.	1.64	$\times 10^9$/l	1	3	1.52	1.76
Monocytes abs.	0.40	$\times 10^9$/l	0.2	1	0.37	0.43
Eosinophils abs.	0.14	$\times 10^9$/l	0.02	0.5	0.13	0.15
Basophils abs.	0.04	$\times 10^9$/l	0.02	0.1	0.03	0.04
Blasts		%	0	0		
Promyelocytes	1	%	0	0		
Myelocytes		%	0	0		
Metamyelocytes	3	%	0	0		
Normoblasts	0	/100 WBC	0	0		
Platelet count	161.3	$\times 10^9$/l	150	400	145.2	177.4
Sedimentation	33	mm/h	0	20	31	35

a. ANCA is not by any means specific for neutrophil antibodies, being more significantly associated with vasculitis of various kinds, of which there was no clinical evidence.

b. There are many causes of false-positive ANCA, one of these being ulcerative colitis (UC), especially if it is complicated by sclerosing cholangitis (SC). There was no evidence of SC, either clinically or biochemically, but UC was a possibility in this case.

2. UC was investigated by colonoscopy, and several biopsies confirmed the diagnosis. Several stool specimens revealed no pus cells or organisms, but fair amounts of mucus. Consequently, it was decided that the neutropenia was autoimmune in origin. The patient was placed on high doses of steroids and immunosuppressants, and eventually the neutrophil count rose to around 1.0×10^9/l, which was considered acceptable to prevent infections. The patient's infections did indeed resolve, and she remains in fair health albeit severely Cushingoid.

3. Of interest also is that the MCV and Hb both rose, and the ESR fell as she responded to therapy, indicating almost certainly that there had been an element of ACD. Serum that had been stored by the lab was retrieved and tested for iron studies – these confirmed mild ACD during active illness.

CASE #38 (EXAMINE TABLE 12.3)

DISCUSSION

1. The first-stage diagnosis – isolated neutropenia – is clear. However, some might be tempted into another conclusion:

   a. The apparently high **MONOCYTE COUNT** may cause one to think of a more complex presentation. It is important to remember that the absolute counts are primarily important. This is not to say that the relative monocytosis should be ignored – as indicated in the text, this may well be part of the reason that severe neutropenia does not necessarily lead to severe infections. Certainly patients, for example, receiving chemotherapy with a neutrophil count of this level almost invariably are direly ill.

   b. That the picture is that of a **REVERSAL OF THE NEUTROPHIL:LYMPHOCYTE RATIO** (see Chapter 15). Such a conclusion would certainly lead one down the wrong path – a reversal can only be diagnosed if the two counts are both within their reference ranges.

Table 12.3

Patient	Age	Sex	Race	Altitude
Mrs J S	57 yrs	Female	White	5000 ft

This lady was referred because she was convinced she had leukemia and was "going to die." She had been told that she had a "blood disease." The FBC accompanying the patient is shown below. She states that she was treated for "arthritis" for years. The disease had eventually regressed to a large extent and she had no more joint pain, although there was a fair amount of disability. On examination she was a drawn- and depressed-looking woman, rather pale. There was no jaundice. The vital signs were all reasonably normal except for an irregular pulse. The hands showed arthritis deformans and there were a few nodules above the right elbow. There was a small chronic ulcer over the right lateral malleolus. The most prominent feature was a massive splenomegaly, extending 15 cm below the costal margin. It was non-tender.

	Value	Units	Reference range Low	Reference range High	Permitted range Low	Permitted range High
Red cell count	4.09	$\times 10^{12}$/l	4.03	5.09	3.97	4.21
Hemoglobin (Hb)	12.8	g/dl	12.7	15.9	12.4	13.2
Hematocrit (Hct)	0.36	l/l	0.38	0.49	0.35	0.37
Mean cell volume	88	fl	80	99	86.2	89.8
Mean cell Hb	31.3	pg	27	31.5	30.7	31.9
Mean cell Hb conc.	35.6	g/dl	31.5	34.5	34.9	36.3
Red cell dist. width	12.6	%	11.6	14	12.6	12.6
Retic. count	0.8	%	0.3	1.2	0.8	0.8
Retic. absolute (abs)	32.7	$\times 10^9$/l	30	100	31.7	33.7
White cell count	**2.91**	$\times 10^9$/l	4	10	2.69	3.13
Neutrophils	17.5	%			17.4	17.4
Lymphocytes	**52.5**	%			65.6	65.6
Monocytes	**21.9**	%			9.9	9.9
Eosinophils	7.1	%			6.1	6.1
Basophils	1.0	%			1.0	1.0
Neutrophils abs.	**0.51**	$\times 10^9$/l	2	7	0.47	0.55
Band cells abs.	0.0		0	0	0	0
Lymphocytes abs.	1.53	$\times 10^9$/l	1	3	1.41	1.64
Monocytes abs.	0.64	$\times 10^9$/l	0.2	1	0.59	0.64
Eosinophils abs.	0.21	$\times 10^9$/l	0.02	0.5	0.19	0.22
Basophils abs.	0.03	$\times 10^9$/l	0.02	0.1	0.03	0.03
Blasts		%	0	0		
Promyelocytes		%	0	0		
Myelocytes		%	0	0		
Metamyelocytes		%	0	0		
Normoblasts	0	/100 WBC	0	0		
Platelet count	201.3	$\times 10^9$/l	150	400	181.2	221.4
Sedimentation	11	mm/h	0	20	10	12
Morphology	The red cells are normocytic and normochromic. There is a profound neutropenia. The lymphocytes are normal in appearance. Bone marrow aspiration may be indicated.					

Table 12.4

	Value	Low	High
Rheumatoid factor	80	0	40
Antinuclear factor	Absent		
Anti-dsDNA	Absent		
HLA-DR4	Positive		

2. A very low count involving any of the white cells is frequently alarming, probably because of the well-merited fear of the strange ways that leukemia can sometimes present.

3. The clinical features are in fact highly suggestive of Felty syndrome. All that remains is how to prove it and how to treat it.

4. The following tests were done (Table 12.4):

    In addition, the smear was reviewed and a careful differential count was made. Large granular cells were assessed at 960×10^9/l. These results were fully in keeping with Felty syndrome.

5. The next decision was whether a bone marrow aspirate was necessary. One can be confident of the diagnosis of Felty syndrome but can never be 100% sure. Nevertheless, it was decided to postpone the aspirate pending response to treatment. To be on the safe side a buffy coat preparation revealed no primitive or indeed precursor cells in the peripheral blood. (A buffy coat preparation is a smear made from the coat of mostly white cells that can be produced by differential centrifugation.) The patient was placed on methotrexate 15 mg weekly as a single dose. Over a period of 6 months the neutrophil count and the spleen returned to normal. Note that splenectomy is only curative in about half the cases.

Exercise Case

CASE #39 (TABLE 12.5)

Table 12.5

Patient	Age	Sex	Race	Altitude
Mrs J W	28 yrs	Female	White	5000 ft

This lady had seen her family doctor often over the last several years, complaining of periodic weakness, malaise, sore throat, and mouth ulcers, occurring monthly and coinciding with her menses, dating she thinks from her last pregnancy. She suffered from quite severe post-partum depression after this pregnancy. Various investigations had been undertaken, including hormonal studies, as well as radiological and bacteriological investigations. Nothing specific had been found. Recently she was placed on the pill – this regulated her flow and only alleviated her other symptoms for a few months, whereupon they returned. It was recently decided to do a laparoscopy and D&C. She decided to seek a second opinion. On examination nothing specific had been found apart from quite severe chronic periodontal disease. A careful history was more productive: the cycles were not really co-terminous with the menses, starting always a few days later; secondly there was a distinct history of increasingly severe symptoms recently. FBCs done at various times in the past were evidently interpreted as suggesting a recurrent viral or other infection. A FBC done at the present consultation showed no abnormality. The last episode of illness was 3 weeks ago.

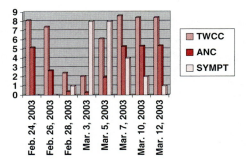

Fig. 12.3

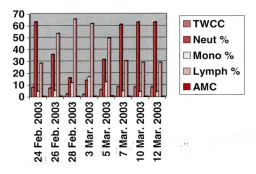

Fig. 12.4

Questions

1. The FBC on presentation is normal. Are you justified, in view of the history, to leave it at that?

2. If not, what are your reasons? Specifically, what part/s of the clinical presentation are cause for concern?

3. What possibilities occur to you?

4. How would you proceed to investigate this?

Answers

1. In our opinion, no.

2. The cyclic pattern of disease is striking. It is easy to see how the thought arose that the picture is possibly related to her menstrual cycle, and that a conclusion could be reached that a strong psychosomatic element is present. However, the clinical features of the infective episodes are very suggestive, as is the chronic periodontitis.

3. The possibility of cyclic neutropenia is a strong one and should be excluded.

4. Serial FBCs, three times a week for 4–6 weeks.

Figures 12.3 and 12.4 show the results of the first 2 weeks of FBCs.

Figure 12.3 shows the symptoms appearing as the absolute neutrophil count (ANC) falls, and slowly disappearing as it corrects. Figure 12.4 shows the monocytes and lymphocytes apparently increasing in a fashion reciprocal to the neutrophil count; this pattern has been stated as a feature of the disease. While it is true that the absolute lymphocyte count on one occasion exceeded the reference range, basically all these other counts stay within the reference range as far as their absolute values are concerned.

Comment Cyclic neutropenia is under-diagnosed, partly because it is widely considered to be very rare and partly because the clinical features very often are very mild and are not investigated until, as happened in this case, they became serious. A further reason for the diagnosis to be missed is that, by the time the patient gets to see the doctor, the cycle is over and the neutrophil count is normal. The author's own records suggest that nearly 8% of all cases of neutropenia are due to cyclic neutropenia. However, isolated neutropenia is very uncommon except for viral causes, and wider studies are necessary. In addition a clinical hematologist is necessarily going to see a very selected (i.e., skewed) sample of cases.

Reference

1. Palmblad JEW, von dem Borne AEG (2002). Severe Congenital Neutropenia. Semin. Hematol. 39: 113–120.

Further Reading

Andreoli TE, Bennett JC, Carpenter CCJ, Plum F (eds) (1997). Cecil Essentials of Medicine. 4th edn. Philadelphia: WB Saunders.

Epstein RJ (1996). Medicine for Examinations. 3rd edn. London: Churchill Livingstone.

Hoffbrand AV, Pettit JE (2001). Essential Haematology. 4th edn. Oxford: Blackwell Science.

Lewis SM, Bain B, Bates I (2006). Dacie and Lewis Practical Haematology. 10th edn. London: Churchill Livingstone.

Broadly speaking, pancytopenia refers to a decrease in all three cell lines, while bicytopenia refers to decrease in any two of the three cell lines. Bicytopenia is commonly the result of two pathologies or represents a stage in a developing pancytopenia. Consequently, our major discussion is on pancytopenia.

Defining Pancytopenia

Strictly speaking, pancytopenia means a decrease below their reference ranges of the red cell count (RCC), the white cell count (WCC), and the platelets (PC). There is some controversy, however, with regard to two issues:

1. In the presence of a decreased WCC and PC, it is possible for the hematocrit and/or Hb to be decreased below reference, whilst the RCC is within the normal range.
2. In the presence of a decreased RCC (or Hct or Hb) and PC, it is possible for the lymphocyte count to be high enough in the face of a decreased number of granulocytes and monocytes to edge the total WCC into the normal range.

It is suggested that in both these cases, the provisional diagnosis of pancytopenia be made and approached accordingly.

THE FIRST-STAGE DIAGNOSIS is thus straightforward. When it comes to the general pathology causes of pancytopenia, it is important to understand that pancytopenia has multiple, often unrelated causes, and **ALWAYS** requires further investigation, almost always including bone marrow examination. To understand this, it is advisable to review the section in Chapter 6, pages 192–194, which discusses the relation between bone marrow cellularity and morphology, and the cellularity of the peripheral blood. Essentially, we relate the concentrations of **EACH**

CELL LINE to marrow production. The essential questions in cases of pancytopenia are

1. **DOES THE MARROW ACTIVITY REFLECT THE PERIPHERAL COUNT**?
2. **IS THE MARROW ACTIVITY DECREASED**? This suggests that the cause for the decreased peripheral counts is due to marrow failure. It is also sometimes seen in the condition known as hemophagocytosis (see below).
3. **IS MARROW CELLULARITY NORMAL**? This is particularly problematical, and a very thorough search of the marrow smears must be made to find any possible pathology that does not affect the cellularity. Important in this regard are hypersplenism and hemophagocytosis (mentioned in Chapter 2). Phagocytosis of blood cells and their precursors in the marrow can be due to many, usually unrelated causes, and is discussed shortly.
4. **IS THE MARROW CELLULARITY GREATER THAN THE PERIPHERAL COUNT WOULD SUGGEST**? This would in turn suggest one of three processes:
   a. **PERIPHERAL DESTRUCTION OF CELLS** with attempt at compensation by the marrow. One would expect to see an increase in the relevant precursors in the marrow. This is the picture one finds in conditions where the blood cells are being broken down or sequestered in the periphery. This is rare when all three lines are involved (remember that hypersplenism is usually accompanied by a normocellular marrow).
   b. **DESTRUCTION OF BLOOD CELL PRECURSORS**, usually the later ones, within the marrow – i.e., an ineffective erythropoiesis. This is the typical picture seen in megaloblastic anemia and often in the myelodysplasias, and occasionally in conditions associated with hemophagocytosis.

O.N. Beck, *Diagnostic Hematology*, DOI 10.1007/978-1-84800-295-1_13,
© Springer-Verlag London Limited 2009

Table 13.1

Marrow cellularity	Marrow characteristics	Peripheral blood counts
Normocellular	Normal	Normal
	Infiltrated by non-hemopoietic cells	Decreased (typical); normal; increased (rare)
	Infiltrated by abnormal hemopoietic cells	Increased (typical); normal; decreased
Hypercellular	Otherwise normal	Normal: marrow compensating fully Decreased: marrow not compensating adequately
	Abnormal	Decreased: either poor release of cells or replacement of hemopoietic tissues Increased: myeloproliferative disorders
Hypocellular	Otherwise normal	Decreased (aplastic anemia)
	Abnormal	Decreased: hypoplastic myelodysplasia, hypoplastic leukemia
		Increased: e.g., myelofibrosis

c. **THE MARROW IS INFILTRATED BY ABNORMAL CELLS**, displacing the blood cell precursors.

One can see how important the morphology of the marrow is in these cases.

IT MAY BE OF ASSISTANCE TO SUMMARIZE THE POSSIBLE RELATIONSHIPS BETWEEN MARROW CELLULARITY AND THE PERIPHERAL COUNTS. SEE TABLE 13.1.

TO SUMMARIZE, A DECREASED PERIPHERAL COUNT MAY BE FOUND IN ASSOCIATION WITH

1. **A HYPOCELLULAR MARROW**, such as aplasia, etc.
2. **A NORMOCELLULAR MARROW** due to infiltration
3. **A HYPERCELLULAR MARROW**, due to abnormal release of cells, such as megaloblastosis, or inadequate compensation for peripheral loss, or bone marrow infiltration.

General Causes of Pancytopenia

1. **PERIPHERAL DESTRUCTION (OR SEQUESTRATION) OF ALL THE BLOOD CELLS**. The features vary somewhat with the specific cause.
2. **DESTRUCTION OF BLOOD CELLS IN THE MARROW,** prior to release into the circulation. The features of these are very variable depending on the

specific causes. The commonest causes are **MEGALOBLASTIC ANEMIA, MYELODYSPLASIA,** and **HEMOPHAGOCYTIC SYNDROME**.

3. **DECREASED PRODUCTION BY THE MARROW.** Two major subsections exist:

   a. **APLASIA OR HYPOPLASIA OF THE MARROW**. There are numerous specific causes.
   b. **INFILTRATION OF THE MARROW**, by a large variety of pathologies.

Note: a combination of pathological processes may lead to pancytopenia where each of the cell lines is *independently* affected, by different processes. This is particularly a problem in septic shock with DIC. Here platelets and red cells are damaged and/or consumed; and severe infection has led to exhaustion of granulopoiesis, resulting in neutropenia. While this is strictly speaking a pancytopenia, it is of a fundamentally different nature, requiring a different approach. The problem is to suspect the truth of what is going on. It is a very difficult diagnostic problem, made worse by the fact that one does not want to do marrow aspiration in a septic patient, not only because of the danger of osteomyelitis but because the marrow morphology is not, in practice, of much help. This problem should primarily be handled clinically. It is important however that this possibility, i.e., multiple independent causation, be recognized.

Specific Causes of Pancytopenia

It is convenient to discuss these within the context of the pathogenesis:

1. **PERIPHERAL DESTRUCTION (OR SEQUESTRATION) OF ALL THE BLOOD CELLS**. The only condition that is at all common is **HYPERSPLENISM**.

   CLINICAL FEATURES OF HYPERSPLENISM: The only constant and common feature here would be an enlarged spleen. However, since most splenomegaly is due to portal hypertension, the features of chronic liver disease, liver failure or chronic alcoholism, as well of course of the features of portal hypertension per se may be seen.

   FBC FEATURES: In most cases, the morphology of the blood cells is more or less normal. Note that the pancytopenia is typically not severe, unlike with many other causes.

BONE MARROW FEATURES: The marrow is at least normocellular, with normal hematopoiesis, and no abnormal cells visible.

2. **DESTRUCTION OF BLOOD CELLS IN THE MARROW**, prior to their release into the circulation.

MEGALOBLASTOSIS:

THE CLINICAL, FBC, AND BONE MARROW FEATURES HAVE BEEN DESCRIBED.

The cardinal feature is a hypercellular marrow with megaloblastic hematopoiesis.

MYELODYSPLASTIC SYNDROMES (MDS):

FBC FEATURES: The morphology gives the major clue to the diagnosis. The white cells are the most obviously affected, with dysplastic changes both in the nuclei and the cytoplasmic granules. The platelets may show bizarre forms. The red cells picture is variable, from very little to serious abnormality; one quite common appearance is elliptocytosis, which can be confusing since elliptocytes are seen in hereditary elliptocytosis and iron deficiency. **THE DIAGNOSIS OF MYELODYSPLASIA CANNOT BE MADE ON THE FBC**.

CLINICAL FEATURES: Many cases are diagnosed from a FBC done for other reasons. The others present with the features of one or more of anemia, recurrent infection, and bleeding.

BONE MARROW FEATURES: The bone marrow is definitive in most cases, with well-defined dysplastic changes reported in usually all three cell lines.

OTHER TESTS: The bone marrow aspiration properly includes a specimen for cytogenetic studies and immunophenotyping.

THE HEMOPHAGOCYTIC SYNDROMES.

The pathology and general causes have been described in Chapter 2.

CLINICAL FEATURES: The patient is ill with fever and jaundice. There may be evidence of coagulopathy.

FBC FEATURES: The pancytopenia is often very profound. The white blood cells and the platelets are usually morphologically normal. The red cells may show considerable anisopoikilocytosis.

FEATURES IN OTHER TESTS: Liver functions are generally very abnormal.

BONE MARROW FEATURES: The marrow cellularity is variable, hematopoiesis may be normal or abnormal, and phagocytosis of cells can be seen.

3. **DECREASED PRODUCTION BY THE MARROW**

a. **APLASIA OR HYPOPLASIA OF THE MARROW**. The most common disease here is aplastic anemia, but there are two occasional causes: hypoplastic acute leukemia and hypoplastic myelodysplasia. There is also a hereditary form known as Fanconi anemia.

APLASTIC ANEMIA: There are numerous causes, but the majority of cases are idiopathic. Other causes include radiation and drugs. In Chapter 2, brief mention was made of paroxysmal nocturnal hemoglobinuria (PNH); one feature of this complex disorder is that it frequently ends up as aplastic anemia – conversely aplastic anemia can transform into PNH.

CLINICAL FEATURES: Onset is typically gradual, with the patient becoming more and more anemic, sometimes with purpura and infections. Since the disease develops so slowly (months), if the patient does not have a bleeding disorder or an infection, the Hb can be very low (typically around 8 g/dl) by the time the condition is diagnosed (physiological adaptations to slowly developing anemia have been discussed in Chapter 7). Splenomegaly is against the diagnosis.

FBC FEATURES: There is characteristically a mild (round) macrocytosis and very little else to see. If there is significant anisocytosis, you are almost certainly not dealing with an aplastic anemia.

BONE MARROW FEATURES: Classically, the bone marrow is very hypocellular, with all cell line precursors involved.

FANCONI ANEMIA: Although this is a hereditary condition, it frequently comes under the purview of the adult physician. It is due to increased chromosomal fragility.

CLINICAL FEATURES: Typically, the condition presents in childhood with progressive anemia. Very often some typical associated findings are present, such as café-au-lait spots, short stature, and abnormalities of the radii and/or thumbs. In a male child at puberty, there is typically a short-lived improvement in the condition as a result of the testosterone secreted. The condition is sometimes considerably improved by the administration of androgens.

FBC FEATURES: Generally, the patient has a pancytopenia with no significant morphological changes.

b. **INFILTRATION OF THE MARROW**. This ranges from primary blood disease such as myeloma, leukemia, and myelofibrosis to bone disease such as osteopetrosis, to proliferation of macrophages due to storage diseases such as Gaucher disease, to secondary malignancies, most commonly from the breast, the thyroid, the kidneys, and the prostate. The effect is that normal hemopoietic elements are displaced.

CLINICAL FEATURES: These are very variable, depending on the cause.

FBC FEATURES: The morphology is almost always abnormal. A common picture is pancytopenia with the red cells showing prominent tear-drop poikilocytes. Alternatively, there may be a leukoerythroblastic reaction. In addition, the infiltrating lesion (e.g., leukemia) may also appear in the peripheral blood.

BONE MARROW FEATURES: The marrow morphology will always be abnormal, and it will indeed usually give the final diagnosis. There is also a subset of cases where one can find both a hypoplastic marrow plus abnormal cells.

Making the Diagnosis

As with the vast majority of our disease processes in hematology, a great deal depends on how the patient presents and whether clinical features are suggestive enough to start along a specific pathway.

Clinically Suggestive Presentations

Pancytopenia differs from first-stage diagnoses already described in that pancytopenia is very seldom suspected clinically, regardless of the features. Typically one has diagnosed pancytopenia on the FBC; at this stage, the clinical features may suggest the general cause. The following appearances will be very suggestive:

1. The typical features of pernicious anemia, or folate deficiency in alcoholism, chronic liver disease or pregnancy (see Chapter 9).
2. Any patient with an enlarged spleen – possibilities are hypersplenism, a storage disease such as Gaucher disease, hemophagocytosis, or a chronic infection also involving the marrow, such as kala-azar.
3. The patient is ill with fever and jaundice – possibilities here are hemophagocytosis, sepsis, and even megaloblastic anemia.
4. A patient with a clinical suspicion of cancer of the breast, thyroid, kidney or prostate, or who has had mastectomy, thyroidectomy, etc.
5. A patient who gives a history of exposure to radiation or certain drugs such as chloramphenicol.
6. A patient with the stigmata of Fanconi disease.

7. A patient with overt hemoglobinuria with or without stigmata of iron deficiency.

Note that marrow aspiration and biopsy will be required for final diagnosis in almost every case. Certainly in cases without any clinical pointers or suggestive changes on the FBC, this would be mandatory.

Teaching Cases

CASE #40 (TABLE 13.2)

Table 13.2

Patient	Age	Sex	Race	Altitude
Mr D K	63 yrs	Male	White	5,000 ft

This patient was conducting a tour. While in a seaside city, he discovered numerous blue-black spots on the skin. He was seen locally; a marrow aspirate was performed and the diagnosis of ITP was made. He was placed on high doses of steroids. On his return 3 weeks later, he came for a second opinion. The purpura had not improved very much. His general condition was fairly good except for considerable obesity and mild hypertension, but he felt unusually tired. There was no splenomegaly, tissue infiltration, or bony tenderness.

	Value	Units	Reference range Low	High	Permitted range Low	High
Red cell count	4.63	× 10^{12}/l	4.77	5.83	4.49	4.77
Hemoglobin (Hb)	12.9	g/dl	13.8	18.0	12.4	13.4
Hematocrit (Hct)	0.40	l/l	0.42	0.53	0.39	0.41
Mean cell volume	107	fl	80	99	80.9	93.1
Mean cell Hb	27.9	pg	27	31.5	27.3	28.4
Mean cell Hb conc.	32.0	g/dl	31.5	34.5	31.4	32.7
Red cell dist. width	14.9	%	11.6	14	14.9	14.9
Retic count %	0.11	%	0.27	1.00	0.1	0.1
Retic absolute	5.1	× 10^9/l	30	100	4.9	5.2
White cell count	4.54	× 10^9/l	4	10	4.20	4.88
Neutrophils	36.1	%				
Lymphocytes	52.4	%				
Monocytes	9.9	%				
Eosinophils	1.1	%				
Basophils	0.5	%				
Neutrophils abs.	1.64	× 10^9/l	2	7	1.52	1.76
Band cells abs.	0.00		0	0	0	0
Lymphocytes abs.	2.38	× 10^9/l	1	3	2.20	2.56
Monocytes abs.	0.45	× 10^9/l	0.2	1	0.42	0.48
Eosinophils abs.	0.05	× 10^9/l	0.02	0.5	0.05	0.05
Basophils abs.	0.02	× 10^9/l	0.02	0.1	0.02	0.02
Blasts		%	0	0		
Promyelocytes		%	0	0		
Myelocytes		%	0	0		
Metamyelocytes		%	0	0		
Normoblasts	0	/100 WBC	0	0		
Platelet count	16.6	× 10^9/l	150	400	24.6	28.6
Sedimentation	14	mm/h	0	10	13	15
Morphology	There is a pancytopenia with a relative lymphocytosis. The red cells are normochromic and normocytic					

DISCUSSION:

1. The comment that there is a pancytopenia reflects the controversy mentioned in the discussion on nomenclature in chapter 1. Indeed the relative lymphocytosis could, unless the FBC as a whole were looked at, (mis)lead to one approaching this case either as a neutropenia or a reversal of the neutrophil: lymphocyte ratio. There is unquestionably a neutropenia but accompanied by anemia and thrombocytopenia; these cell lines are all primarily marrow dependent, whereas the lymphocytes are not. The diagnosis of pancytopenia is thus correct, or at least justified.

2. The pancytopenia is not severe. The absence of splenomegaly rules out hypersplenism and there is nothing to suggest megaloblastosis or myelodysplasia. Possibilities include aplastic anemia, myelodysplasia, hemophagocytosis (although he is probably too well for this) and bone marrow infiltration. Accordingly bone marrow studies were undertaken. Marrow was aspirated with ease from the posterior iliac crest. Suction pain was present. Marrow particles were very scanty. A 2 cm core for histology was obtained. See Tables 13.3 and 13.4

3. The diagnosis is so far very clear. Note that the aplasia is of very recent origin (at most about 8 weeks), since the RCC and Hb are only mildly decreased, reflecting the much longer survival of red cells compared with platelets and granulocytes. At the time of his first visit to a doctor at the seaside city, the red cell indices would still have been normal and the white cells only slightly decreased if at all, thus mimicking an isolated thrombocytopenia.

SUBSEQUENT INVESTIGATIONS AND PROGRESS:

4. Several investigations were done in an attempt to identify a possible etiological factor. Viral studies for Parvovirus B19, hepatitis, Epstein–Barr, and CMV were negative. There was no history of exposure to radiation or drugs. Indeed the patient had enjoyed unusually good health until this episode.

5. Although his age was against him, transplantation was suggested as a possibility–this the patient refused. The steroid therapy was stopped and the FBC monitored. As expected, the Hb and RCC dropped steadily over the next 6 weeks. The patient was supported with transfusions. Fortunately, he developed no infective complications and, of interest, his purpura largely disappeared.

6. Approximately a year later he presented in a very serious state, with swinging pyrexia and shock. He was urgently admitted in septic shock. There was quite extensive purpura. A central venous line was inserted and he was given a great deal of IV fluid and broad-spectrum antibiotics, which were then adapted once the results of blood cultures became available.

Table 13.5 shows the FBC at this time.

Table 13.3

Case # 40 cont. Bone marrow cytology on Mr D K (abridged).
The few marrow particles present were very hypocellular as were the cell trails. Megakaryocytes were not seen. Such hemopoietic elements that were present were morphologically normal. No abnormal cells were seen, and there was no evidence of hemophagocytosis. The features are strongly in favor of a developing aplastic anemia.

Table 13.4

Case # 40 cont. Bone marrow histology on Mr D K (summarized).
Microscopic examination of this marrow specimen revealed a severely hypocellular marrow without evidence of abnormal cell morphology or infiltration. Conclusion: Aplastic anemia.

Table 13.5

	Value	Units	Reference range Low	Reference range High	Permitted range Low	Permitted range High
Red cell count	3.24	$\times 10^{12}$/l	4.77	5.83	3.14	3.34
Hemoglobin (Hb)	9.5	g/dl	13.8	18.0	9.2	9.8
Hematocrit (Hct)	0.28	l/l	0.42	0.53	0.27	0.29
Mean cell volume	86	fl	80	99	80.0	92.0
Mean cell Hb	29.3	pg	27	31.5	28.7	29.9
Mean cell Hb conc.	34.1	g/dl	31.5	34.5	33.4	34.8
Red cell dist. width	14.2	%	11.6	14	14.2	14.2
Retic count %	2.21	%	0.27	1.00	2.1	2.3
Retic absolute (abs.)	71.6	$\times 10^9$/l	30	100	69.5	73.8
White cell count	2.98	$\times 10^9$/l	4	10	2.76	3.20
Neutrophils abs.	0.33	$\times 10^9$/l	2	7	0.31	0.36
Band cells abs.	0.11	$\times 10^9$/l	0	0	0	0
Lymphocytes abs.	2.02	$\times 10^9$/l	1	3	1.87	2.17
Monocytes abs.	0.29	$\times 10^9$/l	0.2	1	0.27	0.31
Eosinophils abs.	0.02	$\times 10^9$/l	0.02	0.5	0.02	0.02
Basophils abs.	0.01	$\times 10^9$/l	0.02	0.1	0.01	0.01
Blasts		%	0	0		
Promyelocytes		%	0	0		
Myelocytes	3	%	0	0		
Metamyelocytes	4	%	0	0		
Normoblasts	3	/100 WBC	0	0		
Platelet count	11.2	$\times 10^9$/l	150	400	10.4	12.0
Sedimentation	74	mm/h	0	10	70	78
Morphology	There is a severe pancytopenia. The red cells are normochromic and normocytic with some diffuse basophilia. The neutrophils show a significant left shift and there is considerable toxic granulation.					

Table 13.6

	Value	Units	Low	High
Bleeding time	**11**	min	3	5
INR	1.11	ratio	0.9	1.2
Partial thromboplastin time	33	s	25	35
D-dimers	280	ng/ml		<250
Thrombin–antithrombin complexes (TAT)	Normal			

Table 13.7

Bone marrow cytology on Mr D K (abridged)
Marrow particles were present and mildly hypercellular. Megakaryocytes were markedly decreased. The ME ratio was 1:1 with relative erythroid hyperplasia. All cells were morphologically normal.

DISCUSSION:

1. The WCC and PC are relatively speaking very much lower than the RCC. This is because the patient had been transfused relatively recently.
2. CRP, procalcitonin and neutrophil elastase levels were markedly raised, suggesting sepsis.
3. A major difficulty was to decide whether the patient had developed DIC or whether the purpura could be ascribed purely to the aplasia. There was no evidence of fragmentation of red cells (a cardinal feature of DIC). Nevertheless further tests to investigate this were undertaken. See Table 13.6
4. One of the criteria for the diagnosis of DIC is a decreased platelet count. It is clear that in the type of case demonstrated by this patient (with aplastic anemia), the platelet count cannot be utilized for the diagnosis of DIC (this is one of the many issues that make diagnosis of blood diseases in the ICU so complex). The slightly raised dimers are of little clinical significance (see Chapter 21). These results and the normal TAT levels were convincing evidence that the patient did not have overt DIC.
5. Note the normal reticulocyte count – this is markedly different from the first count. It provided a clue to what was going on, and this will be discussed later.
6. The patient had a very difficult time of it, and responded poorly to therapy. Eventually funding for filgastrim (GM-CSF) was obtained; this was administered and the results were very gratifying. Ultimately the patient could be discharged after transfusion but was told to return after convalescence for further investigation.
7. Upon his return, he was found to be in reasonable health. A repeat FBC showed some improvement in the WCC but otherwise the indices were much as before. A major difference though was the appearance of an absolute reticulocyte count of 111×10^9/l. This raised a suspicion, and further tests were done to confirm this. See Table 13.7

There was no doubt that the pathology had changed quite significantly, in terms of the reticulocyte count and the bone showing hyperactivity – clearly the picture is no longer that of aplastic anemia (despite the persistent pancytopenia).

The new condition was strongly suspected to be paroxysmal nocturnal hemoglobinuria (PNH). This disease has been mentioned before and its characteristics will be discussed in Chapter 23. A neutrophil alkaline phosphatase test was done and this was markedly decreased. There are only two conditions that cause a decreased NAP – chronic myelocytic leukemia (CML) and PNH. There is no evidence of CML in this patient. The suspected PNH was later confirmed by flow cytometry (CD58 and CD59).

8. The patient was placed on high doses of steroids, and he gradually improved. After 2 years, he had gone into complete remission apart from a constant slightly reduced platelet count. (Remission is very unusual in these cases but is nevertheless more common than in aplastic anemia.)

Comment

1. Most cases of aplastic anemia are idiopathic.
2. Conversion of aplastic anemia to PNH is uncommon. PNH is somewhat more responsive to therapy than aplasia, particularly to steroids.
3. Patients with aplastic anemia are very prone to infections, and when these have progressed to sepsis the diagnosis of complications can be very difficult.

CASE #42. (EXAMINE TABLE 13.8)

DISCUSSION:

There is clearly a pancytopenia. As far as the general pathology is concerned, there are several clues:

1. The leuko-erythroblastic reaction in the FBC suggests either bone marrow infiltration or severe marrow stress (e.g., acute hemorrhage or hemolysis, of which there are no suggestion here).
2. The previous mastectomy raises the question as to whether this could be an occult relapse of her carcinoma with spread to bone. This would be very unusual but is certainly possible.

Table 13.8

Patient	Age	Sex	Race	Altitude
Mrs J de L	59 yrs	Female	White	2,500 ft

This patient presented to her family doctor with a story of tiredness, shortness of breath and easy bruising. On examination he confirmed the bruising and thought the patient was anemic. General examination revealed no abnormalities except for an old mastectomy scar. On referral, these findings were confirmed; in addition there was some bony tenderness found. She also complained of severe headaches. The radical mastectomy had been done 12 years previously.

	Value	Units	Reference range Low	High	Permitted range Low	High
Red cell count	2.98	$\times 10^{12}$/l	3.91	4.94	2.89	3.07
Hemoglobin (Hb)	8.1	g/dl	12.4	15.5	7.8	8.4
Hematocrit (Hct)	0.24	l/l	0.37	0.47	0.23	0.25
Mean cell volume	81	fl	80	99	79.4	82.6
Mean cell Hb	27.2	pg	27	31.5	26.6	27.7
Mean cell Hb conc.	33.6	g/dl	31.5	34.5	32.9	34.2
Red cell dist. width	16.9	%	11.6	14	16.9	16.9
Retic count %	0.22	%	0.25	0.75	0.2	0.2
Retic absolute (abs.)	6.6	$\times 10^9$/l	30	100	6.4	6.8
White cell count	3.64	$\times 10^9$/l	4	10	3.37	3.91
Corrected WCC	3.53	$\times 10^9$/l				
Neutrophils abs.	0.94	$\times 10^9$/l	2	7	0.87	1.01
Band cells abs.	0.40		0	0	0.36	0.44
Lymphocytes abs.	1.27	$\times 10^9$/l	1	3	1.18	1.37
Monocytes abs.	0.26	$\times 10^9$/l	0.2	1	0.24	0.28
Eosinophils abs.	0.21	$\times 10^9$/l	0.02	0.5	0.20	0.23
Basophils abs.	0.04	$\times 10^9$/l	0.02	0.1	0.04	0.04
Blasts		%	0	0		
Promyelocytes	3	%	0	0		
Myelocytes	5	%	0	0		
Metamyelocytes	6	%	0	0		
Normoblasts	3	/100 WBC	0	0		
Platelet count	61.2	$\times 10^9$/l	150	400	55.1	67.3
Sedimentation	49	mm/h	0	20	47	51
Morphology	There is a pancytopenia as well as a leuko-erythroblastic reaction. The red cells are normochromic and show considerable anisocytosis with numerous elliptical and tear-drop poikilocytes.					

Accordingly, bone marrow aspiration and biopsy were done. The results confirmed adenocarcinomatous deposits throughout the marrow, consistent with origin in the breast.

CASE #42 (EXAMINE TABLE 13.9)

After red cell transfusion, bone marrow studies were embarked upon. Attempted aspiration had yielded no marrow. A biopsy, in summary, showed a markedly hypocellular marrow with normoblastic erythropoiesis;

Table 13.9

Patient	Age	Sex	Race	Altitude
Mr D J C	58 yrs	Male	White	5,000 ft

This patient has a long and involved history, over 4 years. He originally presented to his family doctor and later to an internist with symptoms of exhaustion, easy bruising, and prolonged bleeding from injuries. His original FBC follows.

	Value	Units	Reference range Low	High	Permitted range Low	High
Red cell count	2.04	$\times 10^{12}$/l	4.03	5.09	1.98	2.10
Hemoglobin (Hb)	7.5	g/dl	12.7	15.9	7.2	7.8
Hematocrit (Hct)	0.22	l/l	0.38	0.49	0.21	0.23
Mean cell volume	107.8	fl	80	99	105.6	110.0
Mean cell Hb	36.8	pg	27	31.5	36.0	37.5
Mean cell Hb conc.	34.1	g/dl	31.5	34.5	33.4	34.8
Red cell dist. width	18.8	%	11.6	14	18.8	18.8
Retic count %	1.85	0.1	0.3		1.8	1.9
Retic absolute (abs.)	37.7	$\times 10^9$/l	30	100	36.6	38.9
White cell count	0.8	$\times 10^9$/l	4	10	0.74	0.86
Neutrophils abs.	0.24	$\times 10^9$/l	2	7	0.22	0.25
Band cells abs.	0.00		0	0	0	0
Lymphocytes abs.	0.53	$\times 10^9$/l	1	3	0.49	0.57
Monocytes abs.	0.02	$\times 10^9$/l	0.2	1	0.02	0.02
Eosinophils abs.	0.01	$\times 10^9$/l	0.02	0.5	0.01	0.01
Basophils abs.	0.00	$\times 10^9$/l	0.02	0.1	0.00	0.00
Blasts		%	0	0		
Promyelocytes		%	0	0		
Myelocytes		%	0	0		
Metamyelocytes		%	0	0		
Normoblasts	0	/100 WBC	0	0		
Platelet count	58.0	$\times 10^9$/l	150	400	52.2	63.8
Sedimentation	52	mm/h	0	20	49	55
Morphology	Anisocytosis + Macrocytosis +					

scattered eosinophils and plasma cells were seen, but there was no evidence of malignancy.

The patient had at that time been diagnosed as an aplastic anemia. This diagnosis is suspect because of the very high RDW. Detailed morphology would have been very helpful. Supportive therapy only was offered, and the patient did reasonably well until a few months ago, when he had deteriorated clinically. His FBC was repeated (Table 13.10), whereupon he was referred.

DISCUSSION OF FBC IN TABLE 13.10

1. The blood picture has clearly deteriorated but in addition it now seems obvious that aplastic anemia was incorrect, for several reasons:

   a. The RDW in aplastic anemia is only mildly raised, if at all.
   b. Significant anisopoikilocytosis is most unusual in true aplastic anemia.
   c. Blasts are not found in aplastic anemia.

Table 13.10

	Value	Units	Reference range Low	High	Permitted range Low	High
Red cell count	2.09	× 10^{12}/l	4.03	5.09	2.03	2.15
Hemoglobin (Hb)	8	g/dl	12.7	15.9	7.7	8.3
Hematocrit (Hct)	0.22	l/l	0.38	0.49	0.21	0.23
Mean cell volume	105.8	fl	80	99	103.7	107.9
Mean cell Hb	38.3	pg	27	31.5	37.5	39.0
Mean cell Hb conc.	36.2	g/dl	31.5	34.5	35.5	36.9
Red cell dist. width	19.9	%	11.6	14	19.9	19.9
White cell count	0.4	× 10^9/l	4	10	0.37	0.43
Neutrophils abs.	0.06	× 10^9/l	2	7	0.06	0.06
Band cells abs.	0.00		0	0.00	0.00	0.00
Lymphocytes abs.	0.01	× 10^9/l	1	3	0.01	0.01
Monocytes abs.	0.02	× 10^9/l	0.2	1	0.02	0.02
Eosinophils abs.	0.01	× 10^9/l	0.02	0.5	0.01	0.01
Basophils abs.	0.00	× 10^9/l	0.02	0.1	0.00	0.00
Blasts	3	%	0	0		
Promyelocytes		%	0	0		
Myelocytes		%	0	0		
Metamyelocytes		%	0	0		
Normoblasts	0	/100 WBC	0	0		
Platelet Count	15.0	× 10^9/l	150	400	13.5	16.5
Morphology	Anisocytosis + poikilocytosis + macrocytosis + fragmentation + elliptocytes +					

2. Consequently it was felt that the patient had either a hypoplastic acute leukemia (rather unlikely in view of the length of history and assuming that the pathology has not changed in the interim) or hypoplastic myelodysplasia.
3. The bone marrow studies were repeated. In summary, the marrow remained hypocellular, but there was fairly convincing evidence of dysplasia.
4. The patient was treated supportively, with filgastrim and platelet transfusion. Unfortunately, he developed septicemia which was intractable.

!

Comment

1. Factors against the diagnosis of aplastic anemia are a high RDW, splenomegaly, absence of mild macrocytosis, the presence of blasts, or dysplastic changes (unless there is transformation to PNH).
2. Aplastic marrow is found in aplastic anemia, PNH, the hypoplastic variant of acute leukemia, and the hypoplastic variant of myelodysplasia.

CASE #43 (TABLE 13.11)

Table 13.11

Patient	Age	Sex	Race	Altitude
Miss J D	26 yrs	Female	Black	5,000 ft

This patient had presented to hospital complaining of marked weakness and tiredness, as well as a feeling of fullness in her upper abdomen. On examination, she was found to be very pale. Her eyes showed pronounced pingueculae, and the spleen was massively enlarged.

	Value	Units	Reference range Low	High	Permitted range Low	High
Red cell count	3.44	× 10^{12}/l	4.03	5.09	3.34	3.54
Hemoglobin (Hb)	9.8	g/dl	12.7	15.9	9.5	10.1
Hematocrit (Hct)	0.30	l/l	0.38	0.49	0.29	0.31
Mean cell volume	88	fl	80	99	86.2	89.8
Mean cell Hb	28.5	pg	27	31.5	27.9	29.1
Mean cell Hb conc.	32.4	g/dl	31.5	34.5	31.7	33.0
Red cell dist. width	12.7	%	11.6	14	12.7	12.7
Retic count %	0.2	0.1	0.3		0.2	0.2
Retic absolute (abs.)	6.9	× 10^9/l	30	100	6.7	7.1
White cell count	2.97	× 10^9/l	3.5	10	2.75	3.19
Corrected WCC	2.83	× 10^9/l				
Neutrophils abs.	0.98	× 10^9/l	1.5	7	0.91	1.06
Band cells abs.	0.00		0	0	0.00	0.00
Lymphocytes abs.	1.69	× 10^9/l	1	3	1.56	1.81
Monocytes abs.	0.26	× 10^9/l	0.2	1	0.24	0.28
Eosinophils abs.	0.03	× 10^9/l	0.02	0.5	0.03	0.04
Basophils abs.	0.01	× 10^9/l	0.02	0.1	0.01	0.01
Blasts		%	0	0		
Promyelocytes		%	0	0		
Myelocytes		%	0	0		
Metamyelocytes		%	0	0		
Normoblasts	5	/100 WBC	0	0		
Platelet count	111.0	× 10^9/l	150	400	99.9	122.1
Sedimentation	33	mm/h	0	20	31	35
Morphology	There is a mild pancytopenia. The red cells are normochromic and normocytic.					

DISCUSSION:

1. **THE ANATOMICAL DIAGNOSIS** on the FBC is clearly a pancytopenia. This is mild. The normal MCV and morphology would tend to exclude megaloblastosis, as does the splenomegaly. Myelodysplasia (in this case the chronic myelomonocytic type) also can be excluded, since the monocyte count is low, there is no evidence of dysplasia morphologically, and the RDW is normal. The likeliest possibilities here are

   a. **INFILTRATION OR OTHER PATHOLOGY OF BOTH THE SPLEEN AND MARROW.** Some conditions would be more likely than others:

i. Leukemic infiltration would be unlikely in view of the completely normal morphology.

ii. Lymphomatous infiltration is possible.

iii. Secondary malignancy of both the marrow and spleen is most uncommon.

iv. Infections, usually chronic, affecting the reticulo-endothelial system and particularly the spleen and marrow, such as kala-azar. The latter would have to be considered in endemic areas.

v. Storage diseases. These are rare.

b. **A PRIMARY PATHOLOGY OF THE SPLEEN WITH HYPERSPLENISM.**

2. One clinical feature provided **A VERY STRONG CLUE TO THE SPECIFIC DIAGNOSIS** – the **PINGUECULAE**, suggesting Gaucher disease. A bone marrow aspirate confirmed this, as did the specific enzyme assay. She also on X-ray had the typical Erlenmeyer flask appearance of the lower femora, and the acid phosphatase level was high. What is extremely unusual is the appearance of this disease in a black.

Exercise Cases

CASE #44 (EXAMINE TABLE 13.12)

Questions

1. What do you think is the anatomical diagnosis? Try to state this as precisely as possible.

_____

2. What are the general possibilities?

_____

3 What would be your first step in investigating these possibilities?

_____

Answers:

1. "Pancytopenia" would be acceptable. Better would be "pancytopenia with moderate macrocytosis of the red cells."

2. If one takes into account the high RDW, the low retic count and the absence of splenomegaly, there are really only two practical possibilities: megaloblastosis and myelodysplasia.

Table 13.12

Patient	Age	Sex	Race	Altitude
Mr C J	81	Male	White	5,000 ft

The patient is a retired Appeal Court justice. He complained only of marked tiredness and a sore tongue. Examination revealed only pallor and some glossitis. There was no splenomegaly.

	Value	Units	Reference range Low	Reference range High	Permitted range Low	Permitted range High
Red cell count	**2.61**	$\times 10^{12}$/l	4.77	5.83	2.53	2.69
Hemoglobin (Hb)	**9.7**	g/dl	13.8	18.0	9.4	10.0
Hematocrit (Hct)	**0.31**	l/l	0.42	0.53	0.30	0.32
Mean cell volume	**118**	fl	80	99	109.7	126.3
Mean cell Hb	37.2	pg	27	31.5	36.4	37.9
Mean cell Hb conc.	31.5	g/dl	31.5	34.5	30.9	32.1
Red cell dist. width	**18.7**	%	11.6	14	18.7	18.7
Retic count %	**0.11**	%	0.27	1.00	0.1	0.1
Retic absolute (abs.)	**2.9**	$\times 10^9$/l	30	100	2.8	3.0
White cell count	**3.11**	$\times 10^9$/l	4	10	2.88	3.34
Corrected WCC	**2.99**	$\times 10^9$/l				
Neutrophils abs.	**1.22**	$\times 10^9$/l	2	7	1.12	1.31
Stab cells abs.	0.00		0	0.00	0.00	0.00
Lymphocytes abs.	1.47	$\times 10^9$/l	1	3	1.36	1.58
Monocytes abs.	0.22	$\times 10^9$/l	0.2	1	0.20	0.24
Eosinophils abs.	0.16	$\times 10^9$/l	0.02	0.5	0.15	0.17
Basophils abs.	0.04	$\times 10^9$/l	0.02	0.1	0.04	0.04
Blasts		%	0	0		
Promyelocytes		%	0	0		
Myelocytes		%	0	0		
Metamyelocytes		%	0	0		
Normoblasts	4	/100 WBC	0	0		
Platelet Count	**81.0**	$\times 10^9$/l	150	400	74.9	87.1
Sedimentation	**51**	mm/h	0	10	48	54

3. As a first step, get a morphological assessment of the blood smear. See Table 13.13

Table 13.13

Morphological assessment of FBC in case #44	
Morphology	There is a pancytopenia. The red cells are normochromic and show marked anisocytosis with oval macrocytes, tear-drop poikilocytes, and some fragmentation. Occasional Howell–Jolly bodies and punctate basophilia are observed. The neutrophils show a prominent right shift.

Further Questions

1. How has the morphology helped you?

_____

2. Do you think this conclusion is sufficient for the diagnosis and to institute treatment?

_____

3 If not, what would you do to complete your diagnosis?

_____

4 What are the commonest causes of a right shift of the neutrophils?

_____

_____

Answers:

1. The features are now very strongly in favor of megaloblastic anemia.
2. No. First, myelodysplasia is by no means impossible as the diagnosis. Secondly, it is always better to identify the exact cause before any treatment.
3. Vitamin B_{12} and folate levels. In view of the patient's age, it might be acceptable to institute a combined therapy without further ado were these results to reveal a clear diagnosis.
4. Iron deficiency, megaloblastic anemia, renal insufficiency.

Further tests were done (Table 13.14)

Table 13.14

	Value	Units	Reference range Low	High
S-Urea	5.1	mmol/l	2.1	7.1
S-Creatinine	81	mmol/l	62	115
S-Sodium	138	mmol/l	136	145
S-Potassium	5.3	mmol/l	3.5	5.1
S-Bilirubin (total)	39.8	μmol/l	6.8	34.2
S-Bilirubin (direct)	7.9	μmol/l	1.7	8.6
S-Bilirubin (indirect)	31.9	μmol/l	5.1	25.6
S-LDH	1980	IU/l	90	180
S-Vitamin B_{12}	94.2	pg/ml	193	982
S-Folate	8.2	ng/ml	3.0	17.0
RBC-Folate	201.3	ng/ml	93.0	641.0
S-Gastrin 61yrs	331.2	ng/ml	10.0	100.0

Further Questions

1. How have the results in Table 13.14 helped you?
2. Why was the serum potassium estimated? What do you think of the raised level?
3. Do you think you have enough data to institute treatment?

Answers

1. The raised LDH and indirect bilirubin strongly favor megaloblastosis. This is strengthened by the low vitamin B_{12} level, suggesting possibly a pernicious anemia. This possibility in turn is strengthened by the very high gastrin levels.
2. Serum potassium is frequently slightly raised in megaloblastic anemia. It is important to measure this, and to monitor the level once treatment is instituted since this drives the potassium from the extracellular fluid into the intracellular compartment, which potentially can cause significant hypokalemia.
3. Strictly speaking one should confirm megaloblastosis with a bone marrow aspirate, and in all younger patients, this should be done. Because of the age of the patient, treatment with vitamin B_{12} injections was started immediately and his condition monitored. He responded dramatically and completely, and remained well 2 years later.

CASE #45 (TABLES 13.15 AND 13.16)

Table 13.15

Patient	Age	Sex	Race	Altitude
Mr J D	55 yrs	Male	Black	2,500 ft

The patient is a railway worker. He consulted his GP with symptoms of tiredness, malaise, and anorexia. He was found to be mildly jaundiced with an enlarged irregular hepatomegaly and considerable ascites. Some blood tests were performed and then the patient was referred. The local laboratory was evidently a level 1 lab.

	Value	Units	Reference range Low	High
Red cell count	3.11	$\times 10^{12}$/l	4.64	5.67
Hemoglobin (Hb)	9.8	g/dl	13.4	17.5
Hematocrit (Hct)	0.33	l/l	0.41	0.52
Mean cell volume	107	fl	80	99
Mean cell Hb conc.	29.4	g/dl	31.5	34.5
White cell count	3.2	$\times 10^9$/l	4	10
Neutrophils	39.0	%		
Lymphocytes	44.0	%		
Monocytes	7.0	%		
Eosinophils	8.0	%		
Basophils	2.0	%		
Neutrophils abs.	1.25	$\times 10^9$/l	2	7
Lymphocytes abs.	1.41	$\times 10^9$/l	1	3
Monocytes abs.	0.22	$\times 10^9$/l	0.2	1
Eosinophils abs.	0.26	$\times 10^9$/l	0.02	0.5
Basophils abs.	0.06	$\times 10^9$/l	0.02	0.1
Platelet count	102.0	$\times 10^9$/l	150	400
Sedimentation	35	mm/h	0	10
Morphology	Pancytopenia. Anisocytosis + Macrocytosis +			

Table 13.16

	Value	Units	Reference range Low	High
S-Protein (total)	77	g/l	64	83
S-Albumin	28	g/l	34	48
S-Globulin	49.0	g/l	30	35
S-Bilirubin (total)	56.7	µmol/l	6.8	34.2
S-Bilirubin (direct)	17.2	µmol/l	1.7	8.6
S-Bilirubin (indirect)	39.5	µmol/l	5.1	25.6
S-ALP	187	IU/l	53	128
S-gGT	88	IU/l	8	37
S-ALT	59	IU/l	19	40
S-AST	49	IU/l	13	32
S-LDH	270	IU/l	90	180

Questions

1. From the hematological point of view, what is the first-stage diagnosis?

2. What are the general pathology possibilities in terms of the given facts?

3 What further data would you like to have to be more certain?

Answers

1. Pancytopenia.
2. The hepatomegaly, ascites, and liver functions suggest chronic liver disease. No mention is made of the spleen size but one possible cause is hypersplenism. Alternatively, the pancytopenia could be the result of several semi-independent factors:

   a. The anemia could be due to liver disease per se.
   b. The thrombocytopenia could be due to platelet adhesion to the endothelium in the cirrhotic nodules.
   c. The neutropenia could be because the patient is black, at least in part.

3. One would like to know:

   a. The size of the spleen. If the ascites makes accurate palpation difficult, it could be done by sonography.

Table 13.17

Case #45 cont. Further examination.

In consultation, the patient denied ever having abused alcohol. He does remember an episode about 10 years before of quite severe illness with anorexia, nausea, vomiting, jaundice, painful abdomen and joints, and dark urine. This he said cleared up eventually.

On examination, he was mildly cachectic and wasted. He was jaundiced and pale. There was no purpura but he had hemangiomata across the front of his chest, several spider nevi and palmar erythema. His ascites was severe enough to make palpation very difficult. Sonography revealed an enlarged non-homogenous liver, a 14 cm spleen, and, with Doppler technology, clear evidence of portal hypertension.

The ascitic fluid was shown to be a transudate. Examination of a blood film showed the macrocytes to be round with numerous target cells and some stomatocytes. Iron studies showed no evidence of iron deficiency, and folate levels were normal.

Gastroscopy revealed moderate esophageal varices.

Hepatitis virus studies revealed: HbsAg positive; HbeAg positive; anti-Hbe positive; anti-HBc positive; anti-HBs negative. This is the picture of chronic HB infection without immunity.

At the same time, Doppler studies could be done to estimate portal flow rates.
   b. Whether he has varices.
   c. Whether the ascites is due to a transudate.
   d. What the shape of the macrocytes is.
   e. Whether there is evidence of iron or folate deficiency.
   f. The patient's alcoholic history and whether there has been hepatitis in the past. Viral studies would be essential.

See Table 13.17

Further Question

1. On the basis of this data, do you think you have enough to make a diagnosis of hypersplenism?

Answer

Although the evidence was very convincing, to be on the safe side, a marrow aspirate was advisable. This revealed a normocellular marrow with normal hematopoiesis.

!

Comment The value of splenomegaly in the diagnosis of pancytopenia should be clear from the above cases. An enlarged spleen effectively rules out aplastic anemia, Fanconi anemia, pernicious anemia, most cases of myelodysplasia (the only exception being chronic myelomonocytic leukemia), and most cases of folate deficiency (the exceptions being chronic liver disease and infiltrative conditions affecting both marrow and spleen).

Further Reading

Andreoli TE, Bennett JC, Carpenter CCJ, Plum F (eds) (1997). Cecil Essentials of Medicine. 4th edn. Philadelphia, PA: WB Saunders Company.

Epstein RJ (1996). Medicine for Examinations. 3rd edn. London: Churchill Livingstone.

Hoffbrand AV, Pettit JE (2001). Essential Haematology. 4th edn. Oxford: Blackwell Science.

Lewis SM, Bain B, Bates I (2006) Dacie and Lewis Practical Haematology. 10th edn. London: Churchill Livingstone.

As a preliminary diagnosis, "thrombocytosis" means an increase in the platelet count. It is preliminary because, until the diagnosis is confirmed, one usually has no certainty as to whether the case is one of thrombocytosis or thrombocythemia.

Defining Thrombocytosis and Thrombocythemia

Essentially, there are two groups of conditions characterized by a raised platelet count: "thrombocytosis" used for non-malignant increases and "thrombocythemia" used for malignant increase. Thrombocytosis is almost always a **REACTIVE** condition. Thrombocythemia may occur in any of the chronic myeloproliferative disorders. Essential thrombocythemia per se is essentially a diagnosis of exclusion; it follows that the reactive causes and the approach to them, as well as the exclusion of other chronic myeloproliferative disorders, must properly be understood.

The Anatomical Diagnosis

Clearly, this is a platelet count (PC) raised above the reference range. Care must be exercised in excluding artefactual causes, the only important one being marked fragmentation of the red cells (see below).

The General Pathology Causes

These are straightforward:

1. **SPURIOUS.** Due to red cell fragmentation – see below.

2. **REACTIVE.**
3. **PRIMARY.**

Reactive Thrombocytosis

This can occur as a result of the following:

1. **ACUTE HEMORRHAGE** (regularly). In the earliest stages after an **ACUTE HEMORRHAGE**, thrombocytosis may be the only abnormality – see Chapter 3. Later it can be accompanied by other changes.
2. **ACUTE HEMOLYSIS** (often). However, thrombocytosis **AS THE PRESENTING FEATURE** is very rare indeed. The FBC, other laboratory results, and clinical features are described in Chapter 10. As can be expected, they are very variable.
3. **SPLENECTOMY AND HYPOSPLENISM** (usually). While red cell changes will be prominent after **SPLENECTOMY** or with **HYPOSPLENISM**, occasionally thrombocytosis will be the most obvious feature. The main features are discussed in Chapter 4.
4. **CHRONIC INFLAMMATORY DISORDERS** (sometimes). Thrombocytosis is fairly frequently seen in active collagen vascular disease, tuberculosis, other **CHRONIC** granulomatous **INFECTIONS, AND INFLAMMATORY BOWEL DISEASE.** Usually, the other changes in the tests will be more obvious, but occasionally, thrombocytosis can alert one to the presence of an inflammatory condition.
5. **SOME ACUTE INFLAMMATORY DISORDERS.** Two acute infections that are said to be fairly commonly associated with thrombocytosis are osteomyelitis (presumably due to stimulation of the marrow in the infected bone) and gonococcal arthritis.

O.N. Beck, *Diagnostic Hematology*, DOI 10.1007/978-1-84800-295-1_14,
© Springer-Verlag London Limited 2009

6. **CERTAIN MALIGNANCIES** are rather frequently associated with thrombocytosis: carcinoma of the breast and lung, mesothelioma, and lymphomas.

7. **OTHER BONE MARROW IRRITANTS** (sometimes). This includes certain **STORAGE DISEASES AND MALIGNANCIES** affecting the marrow (but of course excluding the classical myeloproliferative diseases). Thrombocytosis occurs fairly commonly in multiple myelomatosis, although thrombocytopenia is the more frequent finding.

8. **SOME DRUGS**. The reason for thrombocytosis after epinephrine and corticosteroids is easily understood – release from the spleen. Vincristine also can cause thrombocytosis.

9. There is a subgroup called the **REBOUND** thrombocytoses. This can occur after any thrombocytopenia that has successfully been treated. It is commonly found:

   a. After splenectomy as mentioned, when done for non-hematological conditions, such as trauma.
   b. After alcohol withdrawal in patients with alcoholism (see Chapter 11).

Proliferative Thrombocytosis (Thrombocythemia)

Thrombocythemia may be found in any of the chronic myeloproliferative diseases. The pathogenesis is also malignant and thus the increase in platelets in these conditions can also be referred to as "thrombocythemia."

The platelets in any thrombocythemia vary considerably in their functionality. They may be very functional, leading to thrombotic episodes of various kinds. Alternatively, they may be dysfunctional and instead of thrombosis, they predispose to purpuric-type bleeding, often a slow oozing into the gut, etc., and presenting with an iron-deficiency anemia. The author has seen cases where both the above situations occur; presumably, this reflects different populations of platelets with their own functionality.

Specific Causes of Thrombocytosis

Acute Hemorrhage

(Briefly summarizing the changes described in Chapter 4):

1. **FBC CHANGES**. The platelet count can vary considerably, from very mildly raised to figures over $1,000 \times$ $10^9/l$. Morphologically, the platelets can show large forms, generally accepted as young platelets, and assumed to be functionally very active.

2. **FEATURES IN OTHER LABORATORY TESTS**. These largely depend on the underlying cause of the hemorrhage.

3. **COMMON CLINICAL ACCOMPANIMENTS**. These too largely depend on the underlying cause of the hemorrhage.

Acute Hemolysis

1. **FBC FEATURES**
   The platelet count is seldom very high. A mild neutrophilia with toxic granulation and a left shift is also commonly associated.

2. **FEATURES IN OTHER LABORATORY TESTS**
   These have been discussed in Chapters 6 and 10.

3. **COMMON CLINICAL ACCOMPANIMENTS**
   These are also discussed as described above.

Splenectomy

It was indicated in Chapter 2 that 25% or more of the circulating platelets produced in the marrow normally become sequestered in the spleen, with a constant turnover, being exchanged with the circulating platelets. It is to be expected therefore that splenectomy will produce a thrombocytosis. The platelet count will start rising in a day or so, generally peaking at around 7.0– 8.0 $\times$ $10^{12}/l$ in a week or so after the operation. Occasionally, however, the platelet count can reach 1.5–2.0 million on occasion.

It will remain at that level for at least a week or so. However, what happens thereafter is variable. One of three things can happen to the platelet count:

1. It gradually returns to normal over the next months (even up to 2 years).
2. It gradually comes down but always remain somewhat above normal.
3. It stays at very high levels permanently. This is a puzzling phenomenon. One obvious cause would be spleniculi that were not seen at the time of operation; spleniculi can be in very odd places, for example along the splenic artery behind the pancreas. Also, it has been suggested that it is the result of continuing anemia causing a hyperplastic marrow.

On the other hand, many other causes of a hyperplastic marrow are not necessarily accompanied by thrombocytosis.

Hyposplenism

There are a number of conditions where splenic function is lost or impaired, as discussed in Chapter 2. The blood picture of splenectomy and hyposplenism have been discussed in Chapter 4.

Spurious Thrombocytosis

This is due to technical factors. The only important cause here is in the hyperfragmentation (of red cell) syndromes; the fragments are frequently so small and so many that they fall within the range of the expected platelet size and are counted as such. This error would be spotted very soon by a hematologist or experienced technologist were the film to be examined. Note also that this error should not occur in level 1 laboratories, or in any laboratory where the platelet count must be done, for whatever reason, in a counting chamber; in the counting chamber, the refractility of the platelet should make the distinction from a red cell fragment easy.

One very important point must be made: the platelets in the above conditions are all functional, and this type of thrombocytosis could be seen as a hypercoagulable state – it may well play a role in post-operative pulmonary embolism.

PROLIFERATIVE THROMBOCYTOSIS (THROMBOCYTHEMIA). The specific condition known as essential thrombocythemia (ET) is one of the chronic myeloproliferative diseases. The platelets vary considerably in their functionality, as mentioned above.

FBC FEATURES OF ESSENTIAL THROMBOCYTHEMIA

1. **THE PLATELET COUNT IS RAISED**, but this can be anything from mildly raised to extremely high. Platelets are also frequently reported as being variable in size, and giant forms can be found.
2. Sometimes **THE WCC IS MILDLY RAISED**. However, a basophil leukocytosis is extremely common (as with all chronic myeloproliferative disorders).

3. **THE HB, RCC, AND HCT ARE VERY VARIABLE**. They can be normal, but anemia can be found: in this case, it is commonly microcytic due to iron deficiency, but occasionally can be macrocytic due to increased folate utilization.

FEATURES IN OTHER LABORATORY TESTS

1. As with other chronic myeloproliferative disorders, **RAISED LDH AND URATE** are common.
2. **BONE MARROW BIOPSY** will show markedly increased megakaryocytes, but of course this is found in reactive thrombocytosis as well. However, in ET, there is typically an increase in reticulin and collagen fibers, and this may be in a highly suggestive pattern.

COMMON CLINICAL ACCOMPANIMENTS. These are very variable:

1. **THERE MAY BE NO SYMPTOMS**, and the raised platelet count is discovered accidentally or for the investigation of a mild splenomegaly.
2. **EFFECTS OF MICRO-VASCULAR OBSTRUCTION OR SLUDGING**. These can vary considerably: common are transient ischemic episodes and amaurosis fugax; occasionally one has seen migraine, petit mal epileptiform-like attacks, etc., which have disappeared once the platelets have been brought under control. Major thrombotic episodes are rare, but can be catastrophic.

Making the Diagnosis

As has already been indicated, the diagnosis of essential thrombocythemia, at the moment anyway, is one of exclusion – i.e., one must first thoroughly eliminate all the known causes of thrombocytosis before the diagnosis can be entertained. And the distinction is important, since the treatment of ET is very different, and very successful (and very expensive). The exclusion of reactive thrombocytosis is frequently a difficult and time-consuming process.

As usual, the approach to these questions depends to a large extent on how the patient presents:

Clinical Presentation

1. **OBVIOUS FEATURES COMPATIBLE WITH REACTIVE THROMBOCYTOSIS:**

a. **SPLENECTOMY**
b. **DERMATITIS HERPETIFORMIS** (hyposplenism associated with gluten enteropathy)
c. **SICKLE DISEASE AND GLUTEN ENTEROPATHY** are often clinically obvious (hyposplenism)
d. Clinically obvious **ACUTE HEMORRHAGE**
e. **ACUTE HEMOLYSIS** and **CHRONIC INFLAMMATORY DISORDERS** are usually clinically obvious

2. **CLINICALLY DIFFICULT DISORDERS (OCCULT OR AMBIGUOUS FEATURES)**:

a. **OCCULT ACUTE HEMORRHAGE**
b. Possible **ACUTE HEMOLYSIS** with atypical presentation
c. **MANY CHRONIC INFLAMMATORY DISORDERS AND MALIGNANCIES** are very difficult to exclude confidently

3. **FEATURES OF MICRO-VASCULAR OBSTRUCTION OR SLUDGING** are suggestive but not diagnostic of ET. Purpuric manifestations (due to ineffectiveness of the platelets) is far more significant as a pointer to ET. The most important features are neurological symptoms, such as amaurosis fugax, "absences," migraine and the like, all of which are strongly in favor of the diagnosis of ET.
4. **FEATURES STRONGLY SUGGESTIVE OF ET:** Purpura in the face of a high PC is very suggestive of ET. TIAs of various kinds are strongly suggestive of ET. Unfortunately, splenomegaly has little differentiating value.

The Clinical Examination

Figure 14.1 offers suggestions on **SPECIFIC ASPECTS** of the examination of a patient in whom thrombocytosis is known or suspected; clearly, it is part of the overall examination as depicted in Fig. 5.4.

Comments of Fig. 14.1

It can be seen that thrombocytosis and thrombocythemia tend to have few or no distinctive clinical signs. There is no doubt that ET is a difficult diagnosis to make, since it is essentially by exclusion, and the number of conditions to exclude is high.

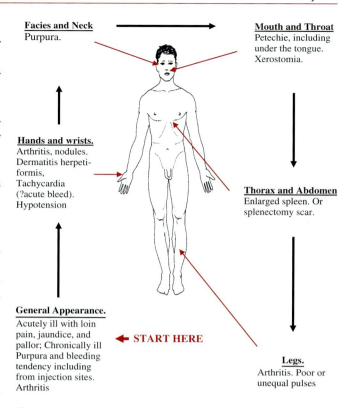

Facies and Neck
Purpura.

Mouth and Throat
Petechie, including under the tongue. Xerostomia.

Hands and wrists.
Arthritis, nodules. Dermatitis herpetiformis, Tachycardia (?acute bleed). Hypotension

Thorax and Abdomen
Enlarged spleen. Or splenectomy scar.

General Appearance.
Acutely ill with loin pain, jaundice, and pallor; Chronically ill Purpura and bleeding tendency including from injection sites. Arthritis

← **START HERE**

Legs.
Arthritis. Poor or unequal pulses

Fig. 14.1 Thrombocytosis: Clinical Examination

THE FBC FEATURES ARE SELDOM OF ASSISTANCE, EXCEPT:

1. The higher the platelet count the more likely is the diagnosis of ET. Anything over $1,000 \times 10^{12}/l$ is presumed to be ET unless very strong evidence of a secondary cause is found. Even then, it can be very difficult.
2. **A RAISED BASOPHIL LEUKOCYTE COUNT.** It is unfortunately not always present.
3. **FEATURES OF IRON DEFICIENCY** may be present due to chronic oozing (ineffective platelets).

Otherwise, presentation with a raised platelet count without any or only with vague symptoms is fairly common. The height of the platelet count is not really of much help, as mentioned. However, abnormal platelet shapes with giant forms are more in keeping with ET.

Other Investigations

The only test of value here is the bone marrow examination, but at best is only confirmatory of other findings. Raised LDH levels are also helpful.

Optional Advanced Reading

There are very few "advanced" causes of thrombocytosis. One very interesting condition is the so-called 5q-deletion myelodysplasia: this is characterized by dysplastic features in the marrow but with a raised platelet count, occurring typically in elderly women and with a relatively good prognosis.

Teaching Cases

We shall begin with summaries of two cases that have already been presented elsewhere.

CASE #46

It will be recalled from Chapter 2 that a case was presented that illustrated the effect of acute hemorrhage on the platelet count. The patient had suffered a large silent bleed from a duodenal ulcer, and the FBC 1 h afterward showed a marked thrombocytosis. Since there was no clinical evidence at that time of a bleed, a FBC taken at the time would be very alarming. It is essential that the possibility of large occult bleeds always be kept in mind; follow-up FBCs are essential.

Table 14.1

Case #47, originally case #35			Reference range		Permitted range	
	Value	Units	Low	High	Low	High
Red cell count	4.21	$\times 10^{12}$/l	4.03	5.09	4.08	4.34
Hemoglobin (Hb)	**11.2**	g/dl	12.7	15.9	10.8	11.6
Hematocrit (Hct)	**0.36**	l/l	0.38	0.49	0.35	0.37
Mean cell volume	85.1	fl	80	99	83.4	86.8
Mean cell Hb	26.6	pg	27	31.5	26.1	27.1
Mean cell Hb conc.	31.3	g/dl	31.5	34.5	30.6	31.9
Red cell dist. Width	15.9	%	11.6	14	15.9	15.9
Retic count	**2.4**	%			2.3	2.5
Retic absolute (abs.)	**101**	$\times 10^9$/l	30	100	98	104.1
White cell count	**13.88**	$\times 10^9$/l	4	10	12.84	14.92
Neutrophils abs.	**10.72**	$\times 10^9$/l	2	7	9.91	11.52
Band cells abs.	**0.50**		0	0.00	0.45	0.55
Lymphocytes abs.	1.46	$\times 10^9$/l	1	3	1.35	1.57
Monocytes abs.	0.79	$\times 10^9$/l	0.2	1	0.73	0.85
Eosinophils abs.	0.31	$\times 10^9$/l	0.02	0.5	0.28	0.33
Basophils abs.	0.11	$\times 10^9$/l	0.02	0.1	0.10	0.12
Normoblasts	0	/100 WBC	0	0		
Platelet count	**224.4**	$\times 10^9$/l	150	400	202.0	246.8
Sedimentation	**44**	mm/h	0	20	42	46
Morphology	The red cells are normochromic and normocytic. Rouleaux formation persists. The neutrophils show a moderate right shift. There is a mild neutrophilia. The platelet count is now normal.					

CASE #47

This patient with thrombocytopenia had been intensively investigated for SLE. She was eventually submitted to endoscopic splenectomy. Eighteen hours after the surgery, this FBC was obtained.

DISCUSSION

1. The normal platelet count is noted. However, from the following day, the count rose steadily, reaching a count of 756×10^{12}/l. Over a period of weeks, it settled down at 171.
2. The Hb has normalized because the patient had been transfused prior to surgery.
3. The neutrophilia now reflects, at least in part, the effect of surgery and mild bleeding, as does the reticulocyte count.

CASE #48 (EXAMINE TABLE 14.2)

NOTE THAT NO MORPHOLOGICAL COMMENT WAS SUPPLIED.
DISCUSSION

1. On the face of it, the diagnosis of ankylosing spondylitis (AS) seems reasonable. However, the gastrointestinal findings are possibly very relevant, in view of the thrombocytosis – i.e., it may represent a recent colonic bleed. Accordingly a colonoscopy was carried out, and features very suggestive of Crohn disease in the proximal colon and cecum were seen. This was confirmed histologically.
2. The relationship of Crohn disease to a form of ankylosing spondylitis is well known.

Table 14.2

Patient	Age	Sex	Race	Altitude
Mrs R J	37 yrs	Female	White	500 ft

This patient presented with moderately severe chronic pain in her lower back and hips with stiffness as well as swelling and pain in both knees; all these symptoms had been slowly worsening. A diagnosis had been made of ankylosing spondylitis, reinforced by the finding of HLA-DR4 positivity, and positive X-ray studies of the sacro-iliac joints. A FBC revealed thrombocytosis, and further opinion was sought. Further enquiry revealed vague generalized colicky abdominal pain with exacerbations. There was no clear history of bleeding but this was a concern. Examination revealed a moderately obese woman; the only positive feature was a tender fullness in the right iliac fossa, which was originally thought to be impacted feces, since she had complained of chronic constipation with episodes of painful diarrhea. There was no evidence of psoriasis. The FBC shown was one that accompanied her from the country laboratory.

	Value	Units	Reference range Low	High
Red cell count	3.91	$\times 10^{12}$/l	3.8	4.8
Hemoglobin (Hb)	12.3	g/dl	12	15
Hematocrit (Hct)	0.38	l/l	0.36	0.46
Mean cell volume	**98**	fl	80	99
Mean cell Hb	31.5	pg	27	31.5
Mean cell Hb conc.	32.1	g/dl	31.5	34.5
Retic count	0.25	%	0.25	0.75
White cell count	9.87	$\times 10^9$/l	4	10
Neutrophils abs.	6.91	$\times 10^9$/l	2	7
Lymphocytes abs.	1.58	$\times 10^9$/l	1	3
Monocytes abs.	0.79	$\times 10^9$/l	0.2	1
Eosinophils abs.	0.49	$\times 10^9$/l	0.02	0.5
Basophils abs.	0.10	$\times 10^9$/l	0.02	0.1
Platelet count	**629.0**	$\times 10^9$/l	150	400
Sedimentation	**51**	mm/h	0	20

3. Note the high normal MCV. A serum vitamin B$_{12}$ level was done, and this was just below normal, suggesting very strongly that a megaloblastic anemia was in the process of developing.

4. Thrombocytosis as a feature of inflammatory bowel disease is also well known. However, it may (rarely) occur in AS. Thus, while thrombocytosis seldom points to a specific diagnosis, it is very valuable in pointing one to a general one.

CASE #49 (EXAMINE TABLE 14.3)

DISCUSSION

1. There are some definite pointers to this being a case of thrombocythemia:

   a. The absence of any known secondary causes.
   b. The neurological symptoms.
   c. The fact that the platelet count had increased considerably in a short period of time without there being any clear cause for this.

Table 14.3

Patient	Age	Sex	Race	Altitude
Mrs D T	42 yrs	Female	White	2,500 ft

The patient is a housewife. She presented to her family doctor with blurring of vision and severe headaches. A FBC was done, and it was noted that the platelet count was 752×10^{12}/l. She was then referred. She was seen 1 month later. She described the visual disturbance as occurring suddenly and out of the blue; there was no true double vision. The headaches were of two types: one appeared to be typical of migraine with characteristic fortification spectra and nausea, and the other occurred either on coughing or when, after doing aerobics, she would lie down, then on sitting up get a sudden severe frontal headache. Otherwise, the history and examination were non-contributory. There was no splenomegaly.

	Value	Units	Reference range Low	High	Permitted range Low	High
Red cell count	**4.99**	$\times 10^{12}$/l	3.91	4.94	4.84	5.14
Hemoglobin (Hb)	13.9	g/dl	12.4	15.5	13.4	14.4
Hematocrit (Hct)	0.42	l/l	0.37	0.47	0.41	0.43
Mean cell volume	84	fl	80	99	82.3	85.7
Mean cell Hb	27.9	pg	27	31.5	27.3	28.4
Mean cell Hb conc.	33.2	g/dl	31.5	34.5	32.5	33.8
Red cell dist. width	14.9	%	11.6	14	14.9	14.9
White cell count	**10.5**	$\times 10^9$/l	4	10	9.71	11.29
Neutrophils abs.	**8.43**	$\times 10^9$/l	2	7	7.80	9.06
Lymphocytes abs.	1.42	$\times 10^9$/l	1	3	1.31	1.52
Monocytes abs.	0.20	$\times 10^9$/l	0.2	1	0.18	0.21
Eosinophils abs.	0.22	$\times 10^9$/l	0.02	0.5	0.20	0.24
Basophils abs.	0.23	$\times 10^9$/l	0.02	0.1	0.21	0.25
Normoblasts	0	/100 WBC	0	0		
Platelet count	**907.0**	$\times 10^9$/l	150	400	704.7	861.3
Morphology	The red cells are normochromic and normocytic. There is a marked thrombocytosis as well as a very mild neutrophilia.					

   d. The red and white cell counts are slightly raised, with a mild basophil leukocytosis.
   e. Note that the height of the count is **NOT** of particular assistance – many secondary causes can produce a count higher than found in this patient.

2. Very many different neurological symptoms can be found in ET, ranging from classical TIAs to migraine-type headaches to absences resembling petit mal epilepsy to serious depression.

3. The patient was prescribed β–interferon, 5,000,000 units subcutaneously three times a week for 6 months; it was arranged with her family doctor to supervise the injections. The patient entered complete remission within 5 months. Three years later, her platelet count rose mildly again, never exceeding 500×10^{12}/l; she was asymptomatic and was treated with small doses of hydroxyurea.

Exercise Case

CASE #50 (TABLE 14.4)

Table 14.4 Note that the abnormal results have deliberately not been highlighted

Patient	Age	Sex	Race	Altitude		
Mr J F	41 yrs	Male	White	2,500 ft		
About 6 months after the patient discussed as case #49 above, the same family doctor telephoned for a consultation after faxing a FBC. The doctor said he had an identical patient to Mrs D T, and wanted to know if he could commence β–interferon therapy. The faxed FBC follows.						
				Reference range	Permitted range	
	Value	Units	Low	High	Low	High
Red cell count	4.65	× 10¹²/l	4.64	5.67	4.51	4.79
Hemoglobin (Hb)	14.6	g/dl	13.4	17.5	14.1	15.1
Hematocrit (Hct)	0.45	l/l	0.41	0.52	0.44	0.46
Mean cell volume	96.5	fl	80	99	94.6	98.4
Mean cell Hb	31.4	pg	27	31.5	30.8	32.0
Mean cell Hb conc.	32.5	g/dl	31.5	34.5	31.9	33.2
Red cell dist. width	14.7	%	11.6	14	13.6	15.8
White cell count	17.6	× 10⁹/l	4	10	16.28	18.92
Corrected WCC	17.25	× 10⁹/l				
Neutrophils abs.	10.07	× 10⁹/l	2	7	9.31	10.82
Band cells abs.	0.76		0	0	0.68	0.83
Lymphocytes abs.	3.83	× 10⁹/l	1	3	3.47	4.29
Monocytes abs.	0.81	× 10⁹/l	0.2	1	0.75	0.87
Eosinophils abs.	0.86	× 10⁹/l	0.02	0.5	0.80	0.93
Basophils abs.	0.51	× 10⁹/l	0.02	0.1	0.47	0.55
Blasts		%	0	0		
Promyelocytes	1	%	0	0		
Myelocytes	2	%	0	0		
Metamyelocytes	2	%	0	0		
Normoblasts	2	/100 WBC	0	0		
Platelet count	1,012.1	× 10⁹/l	150	400	910.9	1,113.3
Morphology	The red cells are normochromic and normocytic. There is a leukocytosis with a left shift and basophil increase. There is a marked thrombocytosis.					

Questions

1. Do you think the family doctor was correct in considering this patient's disease the same as that in case #49? If so, give your reasons. If not, what do you think is the diagnosis, and why?

   _____

   _____

   _____

2. How would you go about confirming your suspicion? Mention both clinical and laboratory examinations.

   _____

   _____

Answers:

1. Although at first glance the two cases appear similar, particularly since it is the thrombocytosis that is the prominent abnormal feature, a careful examination reveals some possible contradictory features. While Mrs T's WCC was also raised, in this case the increase is more substantial. In addition, there is a mild left shift; while this is not unheard of in ET, it is very unusual. The same goes for the normoblasts. The basophil leukocytosis is also far more prominent. It was felt that chronic myelocytic leukemia should be excluded.

2. Clinically, search must be made for an enlarged spleen. From the laboratory point of view, a neutrophil alkaline phosphatase (NAP) test must be requested; if this turns out to be low, the Philadelphia chromosome must be looked for. In addition, the LDH and uric acid levels should be measured.

Table 14.5

Follow-up of Case #50 (Table 14.5).
The doctor was told to refer the patient. In brief, the spleen was found to be enlarged 4 cm below the costal margin. The LDH and urate levels were found to be considerably raised. The NAP was 2 units (normal 15–100). The Philadelphia chromosome was positive.

Comments

1. Once again the logical progression in the diagnostic process is shown to be very important. In this case, the correct anatomical diagnosis is critical. In particular, the danger of focusing only on one abnormal feature is highlighted.

2. Again, the value of finding an enlarged spleen is valuable. Splenomegaly is virtually a sine qua non in CML, whereas in very many cases ET does not show an enlarged spleen, even on sonography.

3. The classic presentation of CML, with a markedly raised WCC and massive spleen, is not always present – the early case may show a mild granulocytosis and splenomegaly, gradually worsening with time.

!

Further Readings

Andreoli TE, Bennett JC, Carpenter CCJ, Plum F (eds). (1997). Cecil Essentials of Medicine. 4th edn. Philadelphia: WB Saunders Company.

Epstein RJ. (1996). Medicine for Examinations. 3rd edn. Churchill Livingstone.

Hoffbrand AV, Pettit JE (2001). Essential Haematology. 4th edn. Oxford: Blackwell Science.

Lewis SM, Bain B, Bates I (2006). Dacie and Lewis Practical Haematology. 10th edn. Churchill Livingstone.

Leukocytosis (a generic term indicating an increase in the count of one or more of the white cells series) is one of the commonest findings in the FBC; it can also be among the most helpful findings in general clinical work. Consequently, this topic is explored at length. The chapter is long since it covers increases of a great many types of "white" cell.

Defining Leukocytosis

There are several problems with the term.

1. **LEUKOCYTES COMPRISE A NUMBER OF DIF-FERENT TYPES OF CELL,** which are not necessarily related to each other biologically, and increases in their numbers generally have different causes.
2. **MODERN COUNTERS,** including those capable of doing differential counts, will all, **IN THE FIRST INSTANCE,** count all nucleated cells in the peripheral blood as leukocytes. Cells that are thus counted can be

a. **NEUTROPHILS, MONOCYTES, LYMPHO-CYTES, EOSINOPHILS, AND BASOPHILS.**
b. **PRECURSORS** of the above.
c. **NORMOBLASTS** (i.e., red cell precursors).
d. Leukemic **BLASTS.**
e. Atypical and immature lymphocytes.
f. **PLASMA CELLS, PLASMABLASTS** (essentially leukemic blasts with features suggesting plasma cell origin).
g. "**LYMPHOMABLASTS**" (this is where certain lymphomas, notably lymphoblastic lymphomas) enter a leukemic phase, with these blasts appearing in the peripheral blood.
h. Very rarely indeed, **NON-HEMOPOIETIC CELLS.** These may be benign, as in endothelial cells (occurring with endothelial damage during venepuncture); or malignant, such as carcinoma

O.N. Beck, *Diagnostic Hematology*, DOI 10.1007/978-1-84800-295-1_15,
© Springer-Verlag London Limited 2009

cells, presumably in the process of metastasizing. They are always too few to interfere with the significance of the total white cell count, but are included here for completeness.

It can be seen from the above that "leukocytosis" as a first-stage diagnosis is generally unsatisfactory. For example, in a patient recovering from say an acute hemolytic episode, 50% or more of the so-called white cells may be normoblasts (red cell precursors and counted initially as white cells because they are nucleated). These added to a normal white cell count would make the total very high. It would be seriously misleading to refer to this as a leukocytosis. Similarly, the term "leukocytosis" used to describe an infiltration of the blood by blasts would be very misleading. Thus, "leukocytosis" should not be used as an anatomical diagnosis except in specific circumstances, for example, when all the cell types normally comprising the leukocytes are increased more or less in their normal proportions to each other, with or without a left shift; this can be difficult to interpret.

> Thus, the term "leukocytosis" should only be used as a preliminary to making the first-stage diagnosis.

It follows that identification of the exact nature of a leukocytosis is mandatory. The technology of blood counters is advancing all the time, and some of the instruments are getting quite reliable in "diagnosing" whether there are "white" cells present that are not of the five basic types normally found, and even whether they are abnormal or not. However, as things stand at the moment, they cannot fully be relied upon. Consequently, one must make sure that manual differential counts are done in all cases where there is the slightest doubt as to the nature of a leukocytosis (or indeed a leukopenia). How is the end-user to judge whether in fact a manual differential was done by the lab, by looking at a FBC report?

a. **AUTOMATIC DIFFERENTIAL COUNTERS COUNT TENS OF THOUSANDS OF CELLS,** and their differential is virtually always expressed as a decimal, e.g., neutrophils of 55.1%. When a count is done manually, only 100 cells are counted, and thus the percentage will be in round figures.

b. Clearly, if **A DETAILED MORPHOLOGICAL COMMENT** about the leukocytes is provided, one can be sure that the results are reliable.

The modern practice is to discuss increases or decreases in any of the white cells in terms of their

absolute numbers (per mm³). There is one exception to this – the so-called neutrophil:lymphocyte ratio, normally about 3:2 in persons 6 years of age and over. This ratio has a restricted importance, but within those restrictions is extremely valuable; reversal of this ratio suggests a viral infection, but can have a more serious implication. It should be used only if:

1. **THE ABSOLUTE NEUTROPHIL AND LYMPHOCYTE COUNTS ARE WITHIN THEIR REFERENCE RANGES.** If the "reversal" is due to an absolute **LYMPHOCYTOSIS,** then **THAT** is the point of departure (see later in this chapter), not the reversal; if it is due to an absolute **NEUTROPENIA, THAT** then is the point of departure (Chapter 12).
2. The patient is 6 years of age or more.

Before discussing the approach to a raised white cell count, some practical examples will be given to demonstrate some of the points raised above, since misinterpretation at this level can throw one off the track seriously. The following results (Tables 15.1, 15.2, 15.3, and, 15.4) are all from an adult Caucasian female (the WCC and Neutrophil Count in Blacks (and Yemenite Jews) are normally lower).

EXAMPLE #1 (TABLE 15.1)

Table 15.1

Example #1	Value	Units	Reference range Low	High	Permitted range Low	High
White cell count	4.29	× 10⁹/l	4	10	3.97	4.61
Neutrophils	48.7	%				
Band cells		%				
Lymphocytes	27.8	%				
Monocytes	10.1	%				
Eosinophils	**11.3**	%				
Basophils	2.1	%				
Neutrophils abs.	2.09	× 10⁹/l	2	7	1.93	2.25
Band cells abs.	0.00		0	0	0.00	0.00
Lymphocytes abs.	1.19	× 10⁹/l	1	3	1.10	1.28
Monocytes abs.	0.43	× 10⁹/l	0.2	1	0.40	0.47
Eosinophils abs.	**0.48**	× 10⁹/l	0.02	0.5	0.45	0.52
Basophils abs.	0.09	× 10⁹/l	0.02	0.1	0.08	0.10
Normoblasts	0	/100 WBC	0	0		

1. The total white cell count is on the low side, but is still within the reference range.
2. The **EOSINOPHIL PERCENTAGE** is far higher than is generally encountered, and one would be tempted to think of the causes of an eosinophilia. However, the

ABSOLUTE COUNT is normal, and this is overriding. If the absolute count were not looked at, further investigations for eosinophilia might have been undertaken (unnecessarily).

3. The same considerations apply to the monocyte and basophil percentages.
4. All the results are decimals, indicating that this is an instrument count (this does not mean that it has not been checked).
5. If one were to add up the percent figure, they would total 100. Therefore, no other cells (e.g., precursors) were detected. This statement **DOES NOT** apply to normoblasts, since they are reported separately, as per 100 WBC.

EXAMPLE #2 (TABLE 15.2)

Table 15.2

Example #2	Value	Units	Reference range Low	Reference range High	Permitted range Low	Permitted range High
White cell count	4.97	$\times 10^9/l$	4	10	4.60	5.34
Neutrophils	**41.1**	%				
Band cells		%				
Lymphocytes	**45.1**	%				
Monocytes	8.6	%				
Eosinophils	4.1	%				
Basophils	1.1	%				
Neutrophils abs.	**2.04**	$\times 10^9/l$	2	7	1.89	2.20
Band cells abs.	0.00		0	0	0.00	0.00
Lymphocytes abs.	**2.24**	$\times 10^9/l$	1	3	2.07	2.41
Monocytes abs.	0.43	$\times 10^9/l$	0.2	1	0.40	0.46
Eosinophils abs.	0.20	$\times 10^9/l$	0.02	0.5	0.19	0.22
Basophils abs.	0.05	$\times 10^9/l$	0.02	0.1	0.05	0.06
Normoblasts	0	/100 WBC	0	0		

1. The neutrophil:lymphocyte ratio is reversed, but the absolute levels are within their reference ranges.
2. The results are again reported in decimals, indicating an instrument count. There is also no morphological comment. This is somewhat disturbing: the lymphocyte morphology should have been looked at; while it is unlikely that this represents anything more than a viral infection, it could be something else. And even in the case of a probable viral infection, the morphology of the lymphocytes may throw considerable light on the actual cause (e.g., infectious mononucleosis). One should ask the laboratory to review the smear, particularly if the findings persist after a week or two. Had the following comment been appended (Table 15.3), all would have been well:

Table 15.3

Morphological comment on example #2
Morphology   There is a reversal of the neutrophil:lymphocyte ratio. Many of the lymphocytes are atypical with increased light-blue cytoplasm, and a somewhat immature nucleus; their appearance suggests a viral infection. Should the picture persist after 2 weeks, please contact the laboratory.

EXAMPLE #3 (TABLE 15.4)

Table 15.4

Example #3	Value	Units	Reference range Low	Reference range High	Permitted range Low	Permitted range High
White cell count	9.81	$\times 10^9/l$	4	10	9.07	10.55
Neutrophils	43.5	%				
Band cells.		%				
Lymphocytes	**51.4**	%				
Monocytes	2.9	%				
Eosinophils	1.3	%				
Basophils	0.9	%				
Neutrophils abs.	4.27	$\times 10^9/l$	2	7	3.95	4.59
Band cells abs.	0.00		0	0	0.00	0.00
Lymphocytes abs.	**5.04**	$\times 10^9/l$	1	3	4.66	5.42
Monocytes abs.	0.28	$\times 10^9/l$	0.2	1	0.26	0.31
Eosinophils abs.	0.13	$\times 10^9/l$	0.02	0.5	0.12	0.14
Basophils abs.	0.09	$\times 10^9/l$	0.02	0.1	0.08	0.09
Normoblasts	0	/100 WBC	0	0		

1. At first sight this report may be interpreted as representing a reversal of the N:L ratio. This would be incorrect: the true abnormality is a mild absolute lymphocytosis. While the causes of a reversal are very similar to those of a mild lymphocytosis, they can be consistent with something more ominous.
2. A morphological comment is **MANDATORY** in all cases of absolute lymphocytosis.

EXAMPLE #4 (EXAMINE TABLE 15.5)

1. This patient was recovering from an acute hemolytic episode, hence the normoblastemia.
2. The normoblasts are not part of the differential count, but are reported separately; thus the total white cell count must be corrected.
3. If correction had not been done, a false impression of a leukocytosis would have been created.

Table 15.5

Example #4	Value	Units	Reference range Low	Reference range High	Permitted range Low	Permitted range High
White cell count	**13.3**	× 10⁹/l	4	10	12.30	14.30
Corrected WCC	9.71	× 10⁹/l				
Neutrophils	62.0	%				
Band cells		%				
Lymphocytes	30.0	%				
Monocytes	5.0	%				
Eosinophils	2.0	%				
Basophils	1.0	%				
Neutrophils abs.	6.02	× 10⁹/l	2	7	5.57	6.47
Band cells abs.	0.00				0.00	0.00
Lymphocytes abs.	2.91	× 10⁹/l	1	3	2.69	3.13
Monocytes abs.	0.49	× 10⁹/l	0.2	1	0.45	0.52
Eosinophils abs.	0.19	× 10⁹/l	0.02	0.5	0.18	0.21
Basophils abs.	0.10	× 10⁹/l	0.02	0.1	0.09	0.10
Normoblasts	**37**	/100 WBC	0	0		

Morphology: The total white cell count has been corrected for the raised normoblast count.

The Approach to a Raised White Cell Count

STEP 1: "What is the abnormality and what form does it take?" **THE ABNORMALITY IS AN INCREASE IN ONE OR MORE OF THE USUAL COMPONENTS OF THE WHITE CELL SERIES.** The specific cell type involved is identified, i.e., neutrophils, eosinophils, reversal of the N:L ratio, etc.

STEP 2: "How severe is the increase?" An indication of severity is supplied in the sections dealing with the individual changes. The significance and sometimes the likely general diagnosis can be much influenced by the degree or intensity of the particular leukocytosis. Note that the decision with respect to severity based on the counts alone is sometimes rather arbitrary.

STEP 3: "What white cell morphological features frequently associated with increased cell counts are present?" These features can sometimes be of great assistance in considering the general pathology causes.

Only now can one state **THE ANATOMICAL DIAGNOSIS** as say "reversal of the N:L ratio," or "severe neutrophilia," "mild eosinophilia," etc.

The next step is to try to **DEFINE THE GENERAL PATHOLOGY.** The importance of proceeding methodically from "anatomical" to "general" to "specific" is especially important in the leukocytoses, for the following reason.

The ultimate aim is to identify the actual cause of the particular type of leukocytosis one is dealing with. If one

looks at "leukocytosis" (or any of the component cell increases) in any hematology text, one will find that it provides **LONG** lists of causes, which one is expected to consult and thereby somehow finding the cause appropriate to the particular case. How this is to be done is not properly explained. In other words, the proper sequential process as recommended in this book, i.e., going from anatomical to general to specific causes, is bypassed, taking one straight from anatomical to specific causes.

Also, consulting these lists is a thankless task, because they often do not give an idea of the frequency with which different ones are responsible for the change. The compilers of these lists often make them as complete as possible, with the result that very rare causes, sometimes only one or two reported cases, make it on to the list – which to the author's mind is silly. If the **GENERAL** causes are remembered and processed properly, it will be found that lists seldom need to be consulted.

IN CONSIDERING THE GENERAL CAUSES, TWO SETS OF PRINCIPLES ARE VERY USEFUL:

1. **AN INCREASE IN NUMBERS** of one or more of the white cells may be

   a. **ACUTE** (essentially a **CLINICAL** decision). The causes here are relatively short lived, since the normal marrow cannot, in general, sustain a prolonged severe **REACTIVE** increase in the relevant white cell count for more than a week or two. While the marrow reserves of the white cells are large, and in the case of neutrophils, enormous, the utilization of these cells in combating whatever the cause of the increase was is similarly very large. Eventually the marrow becomes exhausted if the cause persists, and leukopenia will supervene.

   b. **CHRONIC** (essentially a **FBC** decision). Chronic rises in one or other of the white cells are either malignant conditions, or the marrow has reached a steady state of high production in relation to the utilization. This and related issues are discussed in the Optional Advanced Reading section at the end of the chapter.

      Thus, previous counts and follow-up counts can make an extremely valuable contribution to the diagnostic process.

2. **AN INCREASE IN THE NUMBERS OF ANY OF THE WHITE CELLS CAN BE BROADLY DIVIDED** into three groups of causes, in the broadest terms:

   a. **PHYSIOLOGICAL**.

   b. **REACTIVE.** The leukocytes are reactive to a large number of stimuli, but the reactions are biologically relatively specific to the cell type. Thus, for example, the reaction to parasites is essentially by the eosinophil; of bacterial infection by the neutrophil.

c. **PRIMARY PROLIFERATIVE**.

There is a strong but not exact overlap between two sets of criteria; that is to say,

a. Acute rises are always reactive, but reactive rises may be acute or chronic.
b. Malignant rises are usually more or less chronic, but can be **FAIRLY** acute.

The major task is to identify which of these is responsible, and this can sometimes be very difficult, often requiring extensive further investigations, as well as thorough clinical evaluation.

General Investigations in the Leukocytoses

While the FBC and the morphological appearances of the cells often give a good indication of what the pathological process is, one very frequently is required to do further investigations, for different reasons:

1. To identify the nature of the proliferation: whether it is benign or malignant, what the origin of the cells is, and so on.
2. What the specific increases mean in clinical terms.

The various investigations can be grouped into various classes. Which tests are used and in what order are largely determined by both the clinical features and the FBC results:

1. **CLINICAL.** The general clinical features very often provide sufficient information for the increases to be explained, in part or completely. Nevertheless, further investigations are often required.
2. **BIOCHEMICAL INVESTIGATIONS.** Inflammatory markers (e.g., pro-calcitonin and neutrophil elastase) and acute phase reactants (e.g., CRP and SAA) fall into this category. Their utility is frequently excellent.
3. **MICROBIOLOGICAL INVESTIGATIONS.** These are often mandatory.
4. **RADIOLOGICAL AND RADIONUCLIDE INVESTIGATIONS.** The X-ray appearances of various affected regions are often highly suggestive or even diagnostic; radionuclide identification (such as gallium scans) can identify where deep infective lesions lie.
5. **IMMUNOLOGICAL.** Traditional serological tests are very often decisive. In addition, however, developments in the field of cell surface and cytoplasmic structures (i.e., **IMMUNOPHENOTYPING**) have now become commonplace, and their utility is often decisive. So important have these become that something should be known about them. The physiological basis of immunophenotyping is that almost all cells exhibit, normally, sets of specific antigens on their surface, and to an extent in the cytoplasm. These are referred to as clusters of differentiation ("CD"), and individual antigens are (usually) identified by a CD number. Thus, CD19 on the surface of a lymphocyte identifies the cell as a B-cell. These are all identified with monoclonal antibodies, usually by flow cytometry.

In any normal population of cells, there is a known range of antigens present in any group of cells. Of singular importance is when the percentage of a specific CD is far higher in a population of cells than it should be; this is interpreted as representing a clone of cells, in most cases malignant.

From the hematological point of view, our main interest in the results of immunophenotyping lies in some specific areas (this section is simplified for the general reader):

a. Whether an increase in a number of cells represents a clone or not – **PARTICULARLY WHETHER A LYMPHOCYTOSIS IS PROBABLY MALIGNANT OR NOT.** This technique is very useful where there is a lymphocytosis for which no cause can be found and there are no clinical features to suggest malignancy.
b. If the cells indeed represent a clone, what specifically is the nature, e.g., B-cell, T-cell, etc. From the patterns that emerge, one can also get a good idea as to the actual pathology, such as "large cell undifferentiated lymphoma," and so on. This distinction is important since it has prognostic and therapeutic implications.
c. The identification of blasts and other primitive cells that are morphologically either undifferentiated or susceptible of differing explanations.
d. A number of other less common conditions can also be identified with this method, such as paroxysmal nocturnal hemoglobinuria.

6. **CYTOGENETIC STUDIES.** These too are assuming greater and greater importance, especially in the hematological malignancies. They have diagnostic, prognostic, and therapeutic implications.
7. **BONE MARROW EXAMINATION.** Generally speaking, these are only required (and then are of enormous importance) in the malignant conditions. At the time of bone marrow aspiration, marrow is also drawn for cytogenetic and immunophenotyping studies, and occasionally for microbiology.

We can now return to our methodical evaluation, having made the anatomical diagnosis. The different white cell types are to a large extent biologically unrelated, and thus each has to be discussed separately, except that occasionally one is faced with a generalized increase in all the white cell elements – i.e., a general leukocytosis.

General Leukocytosis

There is sometimes no option but to use this term, even if temporarily. It is used to describe an increase in all (or most of) the different species of white cell, especially when there is no clear preponderance of any one of the cell types.

In terms of general pathology, the causes are **CHRONIC MYELOPROLIFERATIVE DISORDER, INFECTION,** and **SYSTEMIC MALIGNANCY.** In practice, this type of picture can represent one of the following:

1. **CHRONIC MYELOCYTIC LEUKEMIA.** The presence of an enlarged spleen would be of great significance.
2. **MYELOFIBROSIS.** One would have to look at the red cell picture for evidence of typical changes with this condition. The presence of an enlarged spleen would be of great significance.
3. **LEUKEMOID REACTION.** It sometimes occurs in a non-malignant cause of neutrophilia that many or even all of the other white cell species are increased as well, in a non-specific kind of way. The clinical features are extremely important and a thorough clinical examination is of the essence.
4. **LEUKOERYTHROBLASTIC REACTION.** See Example #5, Table 15.6.

Making the Diagnosis in a Case of General Leukocytosis

There are a number of factors that influence the decision: **THE HEIGHT OF THE TOTAL WHITE CELL COUNT; THE PREDOMINANT CELL/S COMPRISING THE INCREASE; THE CLINICAL FEATURES** particularly the presence of a severe infection or a

Table 15.6 Observe that the WCC has been corrected for the presence of normoblasts

Example #5			Reference range		Permitted range	
	Value	Units	Low	High	Low	High
White cell count	**31.94**	$\times 10^9/l$	4	10	29.54	34.34
Corrected WCC	**29.85**	$\times 10^9/l$				
Neutrophils	52.0	%				
Band cells	11.0	%				
Lymphocytes	19.0	%				
Monocytes	4.0	%				
Eosinophils	3.0	%				
Basophils	3.0	%				
Neutrophils abs.	**16.61**	$\times 10^9/l$	2	7	15.36	17.85
Band cells abs.	**3.51**		0	0.00	3.16	3.86
Lymphocytes abs.	**6.07**	$\times 10^9/l$	1	3	5.61	6.52
Monocytes abs.	**1.28**	$\times 10^9/l$	0.2	1	1.18	1.37
Eosinophils abs.	**0.96**	$\times 10^9/l$	0.02	0.5	0.89	1.03
Basophils abs.	**0.96**	$\times 10^9/l$	0.02	0.1	0.89	1.03
Blasts		%	0	0		
Promyelocytes	**2**	%	0	0		
Myelocytes	**3**	%	0	0		
Metamyelocytes	3	%	0	0		
Normoblasts	7	/100 WBC	0	0		

malignancy; **THE SIZE OF THE SPLEEN;** and **THE HISTORY. SPECIAL LABORATORY TESTS** also play a very significant role in the final decision.

1. **THE PRESENCE OF A SEVERE INFECTION.** This can very often be diagnosed clinically, but can if necessary be identified with a very high CRP, gallium scanning, CAT scanning. But these are not necessarily enough: **THERE SHOULD BE NO CONTRADICTORY EVIDENCE** from other aspects of the examination, e.g., the spleen should not be massively enlarged; the history of the leukocytosis should be short, or at least in consonance with the length of the present disease, and there should not be evidence in previous FBCs of an unexplained leukocytosis.
2. **THE PRESENCE OF CERTAIN RAPIDLY GROWING NEOPLASMS WITH A LOT OF NECROSIS.** These usually are intra-abdominal and should be detectable with special radiology. Certain laboratory tests can also help, such as chromogranin A, urine for metanephrines. The CRP is usually much lower than in an infection, although fever may be as prominent.
3. **THE SIZE OF THE SPLEEN.** A spleen that is massively enlarged, and particularly a truly enormous spleen, tends to rule out a leukemoid reaction and favor either CML or MF. This is not to say that patients with either of these diseases cannot at the same time develop a severe infection. This can be a very difficult diagnosis and is important to make. Therefore, all ancillary data should be considered

even if the diagnosis seems clear. On the other hand, there is a stage in the development of both MF and CML when the spleen is sub-massive in size, and great care must once again be exercised in the interpretation of the other features not to miss these.

4. **THE HISTORY.** Previous FBCs can be an invaluable guide. A similar picture (even vaguely similar) present for a significant time before the current episode should strengthen the possibility of a myeloproliferative condition as opposed to a leukemoid reaction.

5. **FBC APPEARANCES.** A number of features should be looked for: teardrop poikilocytes, elliptocytes, normoblasts, blast count, and basophil count. With respect to the latter, if the basophil count is disproportionately high the chances are strongly in favor of CML or MF (it is unusual for ulcerative colitis (UC), myxedema, or pox-virus infections to present with a leukemoid reaction – if it does, one should then suspect a paracolic abscess or pustular pseudodiverticulae, in the case of UC). With respect to the blast count, if it is greater than 5%, the condition is most unlikely to be a leukemoid reaction; if it is greater than 10% it is most likely to be a CML, in which case consideration must be given as to whether it has entered the accelerated phase or even progressed to acute leukemia.

6. **BONE MARROW APPEARANCES.** Again the presence and number of blasts and basophils are of great importance. Increase in reticulin is against a leukemoid reaction. The presence of frank fibrosis is in favor of a MF.

7. **SPECIAL LABORATORY INVESTIGATIONS.** The following are of particular value in this context:

a. CRP, SAA, pro-calcitonin, neutrophil elastase
b. Levels of vitamin B_{12} and its binders
c. Blood, urine, pus swab, catheter, and intravenous line and sputum cultures
d. Cytogenetic studies, for the Philadelphia chromosome

Features in Favor of Myelofibrosis

1. Previous FBCs showing a suggestive pattern.
2. In the current FBC: large number of teardrop poikilocytes, elliptocytes, and normoblasts; disproportionate basophil leukocytosis.
3. Raised vitamin B_{12} and B_{12} binders.
4. An enormous spleen. Again, these other features in the presence of a sub-massive spleen should make one suspicious of a MF.
5. Features of clinical cachexia (as opposed to CML) but no evidence of severe infection.

6. Laboratory markers of acute infection either negative or mildly raised.
7. Philadelphia chromosome negative.

Features in Favor of Chronic Myelocytic Leukemia

1. Previous FBCs showing a suggestive pattern.
2. In the current FBC: blasts greater than 5%; basophil leukocytosis.
3. Raised vitamin B_{12} and B_{12} binders.
4. An enormous spleen. Again, these other features in the presence of a sub-massive spleen should make one suspicious of a CML.
5. Features of clinical cachexia can only be found when the disease has transformed (characterized especially by a very high blast count).
6. No evidence of severe infection. Laboratory markers of acute infection either negative or mildly raised.
7. Philadelphia chromosome positive.

Features in Favor of a Leukemoid Reaction

1. Previous FBCs would be normal or at least show no evidence of proliferative disease.
2. The current FBC: blasts less than 5% (usually absent); no prominent basophil leukocytosis; prominent toxic granulation, and Döhle bodies.
3. Vitamin B_{12} and B_{12} binders are normal.
4. A sub-massive spleen at the most.
5. Clinical features of severe infection or sepsis.
6. Laboratory markers of acute infection markedly raised
7. Philadelphia chromosome negative.

Neutrophilia

It is assumed that the anatomical diagnosis has been made of an **ISOLATED ABSOLUTE NEUTROPHILIA.** However, in the latter type of case, it is very helpful to be more explicit (if possible), e.g., "severe neutrophilia with a moderate left shift, toxic granulation, and Döhle bodies" (see below).

Neutrophilia can vary in intensity. The division into mild, moderate, and so on is somewhat arbitrary, but clinical experience suggests that the different degrees of neutrophilia have at least a general range of causes associated with them; and the following ranges are reasonable (referring here to **ABSOLUTE NEUTROPHIL COUNTS** $\times 10^9$/l):

1. **MILD:** 7.1–12.0
2. **MODERATE:** 12.0–20.0
3. **SEVERE:** 20.0–30.0
4. **LEUKEMOID REACTION:** 30.0–50.0 (or more). This means a marked neutrophilia plus an intense left shift (but excluding anything more than isolated blasts), and the major diagnostic problem is the differentiation from a chronic myeloproliferative disorder.

Associated Features in the FBC That May Occur with Neutrophilia

Several common morphological findings are often associated. Their presence or absence may point one in different general directions. These findings are as follows:

1. **A LEFT SHIFT.** This means the appearance in the peripheral blood of precursors of the mature neutrophil, normally only found in the marrow. Note that a left shift can occur in the absence of neutrophilia; this phenomenon has to do with the marrow reserves of neutrophils, and is discussed in the Optional Advanced Reading section below. The degree of the left shift, i.e., which precursor forms are the earliest seen, also has some diagnostic value. A left shift can occur in

   a. **A NORMAL PREGNANCY.** Here it is accompanied by a mild neutrophilia; the left shift is mild (only band forms); toxic granulation and Döhle bodies are absent.
   b. **A BACTERIAL INFECTION,** and occasionally other types of infection – in the latter this is a difficult problem, since it is not certain to what extent a sub-clinical bacterial superinfection is responsible for the left shift. The left shift may be severe enough to involve very early forms. However, blasts will hardly ever be seen – if they are, one must think of something in addition. A leukemoid reaction can be found.
   c. **TOXEMIAS,** including keto-acidosis, acute porphyria, pre-eclampsia.
   d. **MYELOPROLIFERATIVE DISEASE** – see under b.

2. **TOXIC GRANULATION.** The neutrophil granules are normally barely visible, staining neutrally with routine stains (hence the name). With bacterial infections, and sometimes with other types of infection, some of the primary granules stain prominently, and this is called "toxic granulation." Note however that there are other causes of dark-staining granules; normally these would not be confused by the laboratory, but it may be that you are working with a laboratory staffed only by more junior technologists, who could in this way miss the granules or apparent granules of the Alder-Reilly phenomenon and the Chediak–Higashi syndrome, which are rare inherited disorders. As indicated before, it is up to the user of a laboratory to assure herself of its expertise. An important tip is that in these two conditions, the "granules" appear in other leukocyte series as well, which never happens with pure toxic granulation.
3. **DÖHLE BODIES.** These almost always mean a bacterial infection; again, however, there is a rare inherited condition, known as the May–Hegglin anomaly, where similar-looking structures occur.

The General Causes of Neutrophilia

This is a rather restricted list, comprising:

1. Infection.
2. Inflammation.
3. Malignancy.
4. Reactive and physiological. This is not a traditional general pathology category but in the case of the blood should perhaps be created.

The Reactive and Physiological Causes of Neutrophilia

Neutrophilia can occur in response to a number of physiological stimuli. It is usually short lived and is only of clinical importance from two aspects:

1. One cannot automatically assume that neutrophilia implies, say, an infection or other pathology.
2. The presence of neutrophilia in the absence of an evident pathological cause may alert one to the possibility of an underlying process to which the neutrophilia could be a physiological reaction, e.g., occult hemorrhage.

The causes are as follows:

1. **PREGNANCY.** A mild neutrophilia is fairly common in pregnancy, usually becoming obvious around the middle of pregnancy.
2. **ACUTE HEMORRHAGE.** This has been discussed in Chapter 4.
3. **ACUTE HEMOLYSIS.**
4. **PHYSICAL EXERCISE.**
5. **TOXEMIA.** A large number of toxins may be responsible for a mild neutrophilia, such as keto-acidosis, organophosphate poisoning. This includes a non-pathological reaction to some drugs, e.g., lithium.

Infective Causes of Neutrophilia

Bacterial infections are by far the most important infective cause for a neutrophilia. It can sometimes occur with fungal and even viral infections, but there is always the suspicion that in these cases the neutrophilia is due to bacterial superinfection.

Bacterial Infection

This can be a primary infection, such as lobar pneumonia, osteomyelitis, abscess, etc., or secondary bacterial infection such as bronchopneumonia secondary to a viral bronchitis – in which case the picture can be more complex, often showing features of a viral infection as well (this will be discussed later). The features are strongly influenced by the course the infection follows, and this in turn depends on the interplay between the virulence of the organism, the site of infection, and the effectiveness of the host response. If an infection does not resolve within about 2 weeks, either due to lack of treatment or a disturbance of the balance between virulence and resistance, the character of the disorder changes, as will the clinical and laboratory features.

The neutrophil count has one particular and specific other virtue: when it appears in the course of a chronic disease, it tends to suggest either superadded infection, extension of the disease, or necrosis (e.g., malignant transformation); however, it is particularly in disorders of hollow muscular organs such as the bowel that sudden neutrophilia is valuable, since it suggests development of a peritonitis or abscess (or, in the case of a hernia, the development of strangulation), especially when evaluated in conjunction with the activity tests. This type of complication may be difficult to suspect otherwise.

The Acute Phase

1. **FBC FEATURES.**

   a. The severity varies extremely: the highest neutrophil counts can be found with pus under pressure, e.g., osteomyelitis, and with septicemia. Very broadly, the intensity of the changes to be described tends to parallel the severity of infection. Apart from this, no definite guidelines can be given – there is too much individual variation.

   b. Bacterial infections are frequently accompanied by

      i. **A LEFT SHIFT,** which can sometimes be very severe. Band cells are the stage immediately preceding the mature neutrophil, and sometimes, when following up cases of acute infection, etc., a band cell count is useful to monitor progress. Some laboratories routinely report this; if not, you can ask for it. Reporting band cell counts should be mandatory for patients in the ICU.

      ii. **TOXIC GRANULATION AND/OR DÖHLE BODIES**. Note that in very early infection, and sometimes late in a severe acute infection, these changes can occur without neutrophilia. There may even sometimes be neutropenia. In these cases, they have the same basic clinical implications as neutrophilia per se. The dynamics of these changes are discussed in the Optional Advanced Reading section.

   c. The platelet count varies, from mildly raised to decreased to normal. A decreased platelet count can have many causes in this context – see Chapter 11. An increased platelet count is probably due to direct stimulation of the marrow.

   d. The red cells typically show minimal if any changes, except when severe complications of the infection result.

2. **FEATURES IN OTHER LABORATORY TESTS.**

   a. The acute phase proteins are raised, notably the CRP and the SAA. These respond faster than the ESR (and come down sooner with resolution of the infection). It takes up to a day for the ESR to respond, and thus if the infection is very acute, the ESR can be normal while the CRP is raised.

   b. A variety of more esoteric tests are available, such as pro-calcitonin and neutrophil elastase; these are generally only used in complex cases, where there is uncertainty about the role of infection when there are more than one possible causes of a neutrophilia present.

3. CLINICAL ACCOMPANIMENTS.

There are both general and specific features. General features of acute infection are well known. The specific features depend on the site of infection, whether it is enclosed or not, whether there is organ dysfunction as a result, and the nature of the response. Occasionally, a neutrophilia can present without an obvious clinical disorder; this then becomes a diagnostic conundrum.

The Subacute and Chronic Phases

1. FBC FEATURES.

 a. Several things can happen with the neutrophil count, largely depending on the severity of the underlying infection. The commonest finding is that the neutrophil count decreases, even to normal, but that other changes, such as a left shift, persist; this may be accompanied by a monocytosis. If the infection is severe enough, the marrow may become depleted and a neutropenia can supervene. True chronicity if reasonably stable may well show a more or less normal white cell count and picture.
 b. The ESR will tend to be quite significantly increased.
 c. Red cell changes will supervene (see Anemia of Chronic Disorders in Chapter 8).

2. FEATURES IN OTHER LABORATORY TESTS.

Some of the acute phase proteins will show fairly prominent changes: these are therefore sometimes referred to as chronic phase proteins (see Chapter 2). One can also expect the development of typical patterns on serum protein electrophoresis.

3. CLINICAL FEATURES.

These again will have general features, in this case malaise, perhaps weight loss and so on; and features specific to the site and cause of the infection.

Other Infection

Mild neutrophilia may be found irregularly with infections due to a number of other organisms, e.g., fungal. It is likely that bacterial superinfection plays a role here.

Inflammatory Causes of Neutrophilia

A variety of inflammatory conditions where no obvious known infective cause is responsible, and with diverse etiologies, can have an associated neutrophilia:

1. **TISSUE NECROSIS,** as seen (sometimes) with myocardial infarction, trauma including post-operative, and burns.
2. **AUTOIMMUNE DISORDERS** if acute can show a fairly significant neutrophilia.
3. **ACUTE GOUT** can show quite a prominent neutrophilia.
4. **CHRONIC CONDITIONS WITH SUPERIMPOSED ACUTE EPISODES** can also show neutrophilia.

The features of the white cell count, differential and morphology, are largely similar to those of infections; left shift, toxic granulation, and Döhle bodies occur quite frequently, but are typically less prominent than with infections – this however does not help in the differential diagnosis. However, other features of the FBC may well be abnormal as well, particularly with extensive burns.

Malignancies as Causes of Neutrophilia

Certain malignancies are quite regularly associated with neutrophilia, such as neural crest tumors, and probably reflecting necrosis in the tumor.

Having described the various causes, we can now look at the likely causes of different degrees of severity of neutrophilia. One important point must be made: a marked neutrophilia **AS AN ISOLATED FINDING** is very rarely **IN ITSELF** a malignant condition (**UNLIKE THE SITUATION WITH LYMPHOCYTOSIS, WHERE THE HIGHER THE LYMPHOCYTE COUNT THE MORE LIKELY IT IS THAT IT IS IN ITSELF A MALIGNANCY**). The malignant condition presenting as an isolated neutrophilia is chronic neutrophilic leukemia – a rare condition and difficult to diagnose.

Making the Diagnosis in a Case of Neutrophilia

CLINICAL EVALUATION is all-important. The specific direction one takes depends to an extent on the severity of the neutrophilia as well as the clinical severity. In brief

1. **WITH A SEVERE NEUTROPHILIA OR LEUKEMOID REACTION,** there can be no doubt that one is dealing with something serious, such as a septicemia. Sometimes, however, the cause is occult, and deep abscesses (e.g., sub-phrenic) and certain malignancies,

usually intra-abdominal, should be looked for. Typical tests here would be blood, urine and sputum cultures, pro-calcitonin levels, CRP levels, then if necessary specialized radiology and gallium scans.

2. **MODERATE NEUTROPHILIA** also generally indicates organic disease, including those mentioned above. The possible range of conditions is large – any bacterial infection, severe toxemia, non-infective disorders in the acute phase, such as rheumatoid arthritis and gout, and malignancies with tissue necrosis. Again, a thorough clinical examination may provide valuable clues. However, failing a clear indication by the clinical features, a great many special investigations are likely to be necessary.

3. **MILD NEUTROPHILIA.** It is here that most practical problems arise. The first order of business is to exclude a physiological or purely reactive cause, such as

   a. **PREGNANCY.** However, even if she is pregnant, one cannot automatically assume that there is no underlying organic cause, such as a urinary tract infection or acute appendicitis (which can present very atypically in pregnancy).

   b. **HEMORRHAGE AND HEMOLYSIS,** especially of occult.

   c. **A SILENT MYOCARDIAL INFARCTION** or other tissue necrosis.

   d. **POISONS.**

These having been excluded, the approach is essentially as described above.

A NUMBER OF FAIRLY TYPICAL CLINICAL PRESENTATIONS ARE PRESENTED A LITTLE LATER.

To Summarize the Laboratory Investigations

THE FBC FEATURES: A left shift, toxic granulation, and Döhle bodies can be of some assistance in neutrophilia but generally their presence is rather indicative of severity than the cause, and they must be correlated with and consonant with the clinical features. Note that, unlike with many other FBC appearances, there is nothing the FBC can say as to where the cause is, or what its nature is. Even the specific diagnosis is a clinical one, in this case.

OTHER LABORATORY FEATURES are generally of great importance in the conditions suggested by the findings. There are three groups:

1. **ACUTE PHASE RESPONSE TESTS.** These range from the ESR, to the CRP and SAA, to typical patterns seen on serum protein electrophoresis.

2. **SPECIFIC TESTS TO IDENTIFY THE CAUSATIVE ORGANISMS,** where these are responsible. The choice of tests largely depends on the nature of the FBC findings plus clinical input. The decision is a **CLINICAL** one.

3. **TESTS TO IDENTIFY THE SITE** of occult infections or infiltrations. These are generally radiological or radionuclide investigations.

Representative Clinical Presentations

By and large there are three very common ways in which a neutrophilia can present clinically, and the evaluation should usually start with these in mind.

1. **A MILD TO PERHAPS MODERATE NEUTROPHILIA** in an ill patient, frequently pyrexial with a tachycardia, and perhaps confused and showing features of the primary cause – tonsillitis, otitis, cystitis, appendicitis, etc. The neutrophilia is commonly accompanied by a left shift and toxic granulation, but in milder cases need not be, especially in the early stages. In general practice, this would be by far the commonest presentation (and indeed is one of the commonest of all presentations in practice), and would be found after hemorrhage or hemolysis, or in any of a myriad of bacterial infections, like otitis media, tonsillitis, appendicitis, cystitis, but sometimes also in toxemias, such as keto-acidosis. Points of interest are as follows:

   a. If the patient had had a previous chronic but stable condition, and especially if previous (normal) leukocyte counts are available, the appearance of a neutrophilia strongly suggests the development of a complication. For example, a vasculitis may show increased neutrophilia where flare-ups or decreased response to therapy have occurred. Because it is often very difficult to know what is going on in the abdomen in chronic disease, the appearance of neutrophilia is also of particular value here, such as in ulcerative colitis (normally not associated with significant neutrophilia) having developed pustular pseudodiverticulae.

The sudden appearance of a neutrophilia in a patient with an existing general medical or surgical condition should never be ignored.

!

b) Diabetes should always be excluded; if it is present, the patient may be in a keto-acidotic state, which in itself can cause the neutrophilia, etc. This sort of case requires great care – one cannot ascribe the neutrophilia only to the keto-acidosis without considerable further investigation and exclusion of an infection (and acute infection is a classic cause of destabilizing diabetes and precipitating diabetic ketosis).

c) When in doubt as to the diagnosis, it is useful to remember that the worse the blood changes, the more likely it is that there is an infection.

2. **THE SEVERELY ILL PATIENT,** shocked, prostrated, and usually pyrexial. A source for septicemia can usually be found, such as a urinary tract infection and pelvic inflammatory disease. Here the neutrophilia can be marked, but if the process has persisted for a week or so, the marrow might have become exhausted, producing a neutropenia but with the left shift and toxic changes persisting.

3. **THE RAISED NEUTROPHIL COUNT IN AN OTHERWISE APPARENTLY MORE OR LESS WELL PATIENT.** This is **GENERALLY A CHRONIC NEUTROPHILIA** and the conditions to consider are pregnancy, exposure to toxins, a stable chronic bacterial infection (e.g., an intracellular infection such as due to brucella), chronic myelocytic leukemia, myelofibrosis, Cushing syndrome, subacute to chronic cholecystitis, etc. **IF, HOWEVER, IT OCCURS ACUTELY,** one must consider an acute infective or necrotic complication of the underlying condition. It may require considerable investigation to identify the cause, from extensive serological and microbiological testing to gallium scans, etc.

4. **RECURRENT EPISODES OF MILD TO MODERATE NEUTROPHILIA, OFTEN WITH EPISODIC SYMPTOMS.** These are quite a common presentation and can be exasperatingly difficult to get to the bottom of. Generally, no specific symptoms pointing to an organ can easily be elicited, although direct questioning may sometimes be of assistance. Conditions to consider are as follows:

a) **CHRONIC INFECTIONS** especially involving the marrow, such as tuberculosis, cryptococcosis, brucellosis, ehrlichiosis, toxoplasmosis, Q fever, EB virus and CMV infections, occasionally hepatitis. In these cases, there may be intermittent abnormalities of the other cell lines, such as mild anemia for no obvious cause, thrombocytosis, or thrombocytopenia. Bone marrow biopsy will often show granulomata.

b) **SUBACUTE TO CHRONIC INFECTIONS** in certain organs, often with acute flare-ups. Notable here is cholecystitis, where presenting symptoms are in any case often very vague or even absent.

The latter three groups of cases are complex and at the general practice level should be referred.

Particular note must be taken of the case where the neutrophil count apparently stabilizes or even drops, and the CRP continues to increase; this is potentially a very dangerous situation, since it may mean that the marrow is becoming exhausted; sudden deterioration and even death can supervene. Note that for this type of change to be picked up, cumulative reports are extremely useful, else they may be missed.

These issues are discussed in the Optional Advanced Reading section.

Monocytosis

Monocytosis as an isolated phenomenon is unusual. It may be found in the recovery phase of an acute infection and with certain fungal infections and in tuberculosis and malaria. **IN TUBERCULOSIS,** monocytosis is a very significant feature, strongly suggesting activity; in certain centers it is taken to be a sufficient reason to institute therapy. Advanced aspects are discussed in the Optional Advanced Reading section.

Making the Diagnosis in Monocytosis

Once again this is an entirely clinical enterprise. Search should be made for a resolving acute infection, certain chronic infections, and malaria. An unusual cause is chronic myelomonocytic leukemia (a myelodysplastic syndrome) – this should always be referred. Otherwise, if no cause can be found and the monocytosis persists, it is advisable also to refer the patient.

Lymphocytosis

It is assumed that the anatomical diagnosis has been made of an **ISOLATED ABSOLUTE LYMPHOCYTOSIS.** Again, morphological features may be very helpful, and thus a more explicit (if possible) anatomical diagnosis can be made, e.g., "Severe lymphocytosis with atypical lymphocytes."

The division of lymphocytosis into mild, moderate, and so on is again somewhat arbitrary, but clinical experience suggests that the different degrees of lymphocytosis have at least a general range of causes associated with them; and the following ranges are reasonable (referring here to **ABSOLUTE LYMPHO-CYTE COUNTS** $\times 10^9$/l):

1. **MILD:** 4.1–8.0
2. **MODERATE:** 8.1–20.0
3. **SEVERE:** 20.1 and upward

Associated Features in the FBC That May Occur with Lymphocytosis

Unlike with neutrophilia, specific morphological features are much less complex. The most important of these is "atypical lymphocytes."

> **"Atypical" Lymphocytes** This comment is very common in FBC reports. All viral infections have a tendency to produce atypical lymphocytes – those of infectious mononucleosis (IM) are often morphologically different and thus recognizable as such. Atypical lymphocytes generally are simply lymphocytes that are being stimulated to undergo blast transformation as part of the immune response to the infection.
>
> There are, however, two points of note:
>
> 1. Sometimes the so-called atypical lymphocytes are in fact N(atural) K(iller) cells, whose significance is often obscure.
> 2. The "atypical" lymphocytes are sometimes in fact abnormal lymphocytes, as found in lymphomas, etc. It is thus critically important that the FBC of any patient with reported "atypical lymphocytes," particularly where the clinical evidence of a viral infection is weak be repeated in 10 days or so.

Morphologically the lymphocytes may appear obviously malignant, in which case the count is often, but not always, very high.

The presence of generalized lymphadenopathy and splenomegaly do not necessarily indicate a malignant process.

The General Causes of Lymphocytosis

This again is a rather restricted list, comprising

1. Infection
2. Inflammation
3. Malignancy

Infective Causes of Lymphocytosis

1. **VIRAL INFECTIONS** are by far the most common. There are two groups:

   a. **THOSE WHERE THE VIRUS CAUSES LYMPHOCYTOSIS DIRECTLY.** The most important of these is the group known as the mononucleosis syndromes. The reference condition is of course infectious mononucleosis.

> **Infectious Mononucleosis and the Mononucleosis Syndromes** *IM is a common disease, due to EB virus infection. The hematological features include absolute lymphocytosis with characteristic atypical lymphocytes and positive heterophile antibodies. Associated features can be thrombocytopenia and autoimmune hemolytic anemia. Many other conditions mimic IM in many respects, such as CMV infection, toxoplasmosis, cat-scratch disease; the notable feature is that they are all negative for heterophile antibodies, and the classic atypical lymphocytes are seldom found.*

   b. **POST-VIRAL INFECTIONS.** Here the virus first causes a lymphopenia followed in a few days by a lymphocytosis. Important causes here are mumps, chickenpox, infective hepatitis, and certain respiratory viruses. Of interest is that the atypical lymphocytes can resemble those found in infectious mononucleosis.

   Note that the above types of picture are sometimes referred to as a "reactive" lymphocytosis.

2. **OTHER ORGANISMS.**

   a) In childhood, **BORDETELLA PERTUSSIS** infection is the classic cause of **INFECTIOUS LYMPHOCYTOSIS.**
   b) **TOXOPLASMOSIS** can also occur in the adult. The lymphocytosis is usually only relative, and atypical lymphocytes are absent.

c) **ACUTE INFECTIOUS LYMPHOCYTOSIS** occurs mainly in children, but cases in teenagers are described. No etiological agent has yet been identified. The lymphocytosis is typically quite marked, and atypical lymphocytes are largely absent.

Inflammatory Causes of Lymphocytosis

Lymphocytosis can be found in association with a number of inflammatory conditions, such as **HEALING TUBERCULOSIS, BRUCELLOSIS, SYPHILIS, INFLAMMATORY BOWEL DISEASE, VASCULITIS,** and **DRUG HYPERSENSITIVITY**; occasionally in **THYROTOXICOSIS** and **ADDISON DISEASE** (in the latter two presumably reflecting the autoimmune status of these conditions). Also some peculiar, apparently benign, conditions associated with chronic lymphadenopathy and **SOMETIMES** producing lymphocytosis have been described. Their status is still uncertain.

Malignant Lymphocytosis

To reiterate, malignancy associated with lymphocytosis entails that the lymphocytosis itself may be a malignant proliferation, unlike the situation with neutrophilia.

1. This occurs **REGULARLY** in chronic lymphocytic leukemia (CLL).
2. Lymphocytosis **SOMETIMES** occurs in the so-called non-Hodgkin lymphomas (NHL). The lymphocytosis in these conditions is of two general types:

   a. **"OVERFLOW"** – when lymphoma cells spill into the peripheral blood from the tumor mass, perhaps due to intercurrent stress. This form can apply to any of the lymphomas, from mature (i.e., resembling normal lymphocytes) to immature lymphoma cells (perhaps even resembling blasts).
   b. If and when the lymphoma enters the so-called **LEUKEMIC PHASE.** This is usually a late event, and is permanent (i.e., not (obviously) related to stress).

Occasionally, the lymphoma cells in the peripheral blood have specific, identifiable, morphological features, such as in some of the cutaneous T-cell lymphomas.

Note from the above:

1. One must be careful in assessing the significance of blast-like forms in the peripheral blood in the case of high-grade lymphomas.

2. The FBC plays a distinctly secondary role in the diagnosis of the lymphomas (but not in CLL). The above section is important at the general level only because of their relevance in the differential diagnosis of lymphocytosis.
3. The differing significance of malignancy as causes of neutrophilia and lymphocytosis is again emphasized: neutrophilia can occur as a **REACTION TO MALIGNANCY,** while **LYMPHOCYTOSIS CAN BE MALIGNANT.**

Distinguishing between the different causes of malignant lymphocytosis is a specialist activity, and can be exceptionally involved.

Making the Diagnosis in a Case of Lymphocytosis

THE FIRST AND OVERRIDING CONCERN IS WHETHER THE LYMPHOCYTOSIS IS MALIGNANT OR NOT (AND THE LYMPHOCYTOSIS NEED NOT BE SEVERE FOR IT TO BE MALIGNANT). There are a number of clinical and routine laboratory features that **MAY** help in this decision. For example,

1. In a patient with generalized lymphadenopathy, involvement of the epitrochlear nodes suggests a non-Hodgkin lymphoma (NHL).
2. In a patient with generalized lymphadenopathy, involvement of the infraclavicular nodes is more in keeping with a Hodgkin lymphoma (HL) or chronic lymphocytic leukemia (CLL) than a NHL.
3. In an elderly patient presenting for the first time in years with a chronic sore throat and enlarged tonsils, the possibility is strong that he has CLL, even before there is significant lymphocytosis or other lymphadenopathy.
4. NHL can infiltrate tissues anywhere, with many possible presentations, including hydronephrosis, pleural effusion.
5. HL characteristically presents with a history of significant weight loss, malaise, night sweats, and sometimes pruritus and pain occurring in one or other of the enlarged lymph node groups within minutes of taking alcohol. By contrast, systemic features are late in NHL.
6. Any of the above can **PRESENT** with an acute hemolytic anemia, with anemia, jaundice, an enlarged and perhaps tender spleen, and with characteristic changes in the blood.

7. On the other hand, there are some benign conditions that sometimes have typical presentations, such as the young, socially and sexually active person presenting with severe malaise, severe pharyngitis, generalized lymphadenopathy, and tender hepatosplenomegaly; these features may be very suspicious of infectious mononucleosis, particularly where other cases have occurred at the time.

Note that there is no place for an exclusively clinical diagnosis in any of these cases, whether presenting with any of the clinical features mentioned or with lymphocytosis alone. However, what tests to ask for is often a matter of considerable judgment, depending on the presentation.

1. In an adult, a **SEVERE LYMPHOCYTOSIS** must always be regarded as malignant, until proven otherwise (and this can be very difficult – there are a number of strange conditions associated with generalized lymphadenopathy and lymphocytosis whose malignant status is not clear). The relevant further investigations here are very complex and need referral. In brief, they would encompass bone marrow aspiration, biopsy, and cytogenetic and immunophenotyping studies (see below), as well as lymph node biopsy. Other tests of value are β-2-microglobulin, protein electrophoresis, and immunoglobulins.

2. Often, **MODERATE AND MILD LYMPHOCYTOSES** also turn out eventually to be malignant, but it must be emphasized that usually a benign cause is responsible, even if the clinical presentations can be very similar. In view of the very large number of possible causes of a benign lymphocytosis, extensive clinical assessment is necessary to exclude viral infections (in particular EB virus and cytomegalovirus) and various chronic states such as healing tuberculosis, brucellosis, syphilis, inflammatory bowel disease, vasculitis, and some miscellaneous conditions like drug hypersensitivity, thyrotoxicosis, and Addison disease. The relevant blood tests would follow from the clinical assessment.

Failing an answer, the suspicion of an early malignancy will come to mind. The first order of business will be to see that this is not a transient condition. Should it persist (say over 3 weeks), thorough clinical examination (often involving expensive radiology) may disclose enlargement of deep nodes, tissue infiltration, skin lesions. Thereafter, the problem should be approached as described under "severe lymphocytosis." Under no circumstances can the condition be ignored.

Representative Clinical Presentations

Broadly speaking, one can identify three general modes of presentation:

1. **THE ACUTELY ILL PATIENT,** probably with evidence of an infection, sometimes with a tender lymphadenopathy and sub-massive splenomegaly. The absolute lymphocyte count can be as high as $20.0 \times 10^9/l$, but more usually around $10.0–13.0 \times 10^9/l$. The finding of atypical lymphocytes will clearly support the diagnosis. Identification of the specific virus responsible is of course beyond the scope of this book. The acute infectious causes are always self-limiting and seldom cause more than a mild absolute lymphocytosis. Other investigations may be needed, notably virological and serological tests, including Epstein–Barr virus antibodies. If such a lymphocytosis does not resolve in a few weeks, it needs also to be referred.

2. **THE PATIENT IN WHOM LYMPHOCYTOSIS HAS BEEN DISCOVERED ACCIDENTALLY OR AFTER COMPLAINING OF VAGUE GENERALIZED SYMPTOMS.** There are a large number of possible causes. These may be

   a. **BENIGN,** as listed on page 329. The absolute lymphocyte count is seldom higher than $12.0 \times 10^9/l$; the presence of atypical lymphocytes would favor a viral cause, but this is by no means an absolute. The presence of a **TENDER** lymphadenopathy also supports the diagnosis; a non-tender adenopathy, particularly with glands greater than 2 cm in diameter, must raise suspicion of another pathology. The onus is thus on the clinician to search for and confirm these diseases.

   b. **MALIGNANT.**

      i. Clinical features can sometimes help, particularly in relation to the blood findings. Generally, however, clinical features are unreliable.
      ii. The FBC may be very convincing:

         - The height of the lymphocyte count. Anything above say $20.0 \times 10^9/l$ (in an adult) is virtually certain to be malignant.
         - Obviously malignant-appearing cells.

The approach in the cases where the clinical and FBC features are not convincing is

a. Serological and biochemical tests as discussed above
b. Symptomatic treatment and repeat of the FBC in 14 days
c. Referral if you are in any way concerned

3. **THE CHRONICALLY ILL PATIENT WITH FEATURES SUGGESTIVE OF A PROGRESSIVE DISEASE.** There are a number of conditions in this group, showing an associated lymphocytosis **THAT IS NOT NECESSARILY MALIGNANT.** The approach is essentially clinical, and details cannot be entered into. These are further discussed in the Optional Advanced section.

In general terms, the higher the lymphocyte count, the more likely it is that it is a malignancy.

Eosinophilia

Eosinophilia is an abnormal accumulation of eosinophils in the blood **OR ANY TISSUE.** It is one of the more specifically informative of the cytoses, and yet its significance is often overlooked. When it is considered that

1. A quarter of the world's population suffers from parasitic disease,
2. In a great many of these the clinical features are not specific to the type of organism and demonstrate fairly similar clinical features, and in any case can be compatible with other disease,
3. Eosinophilia is an extremely valuable marker of the presence of very many parasitoses,
4. With world travel having increased to unprecedented levels such that large number of travelers and expatriates from the first world are exposed to these,
5. With significant immigration from undeveloped countries, medical personnel in developed countries should be aware of the possibilities of parasitosis,

then it should be realized that eosinophilia cannot be ignored. One problem is that it is found in a number of non-parasitic conditions.

While the severity of neutrophilia is only in general terms suggestive of the etiology, with **EOSINOPHILIA THE SEVERITY POINTS DIRECTLY AT THE RANGE OF POSSIBLE CAUSES.**

Note that biologically eosinophilia is a two-edged sword. Its granules contain a number of highly potent molecules that are very toxic to tissues – as well as to parasites, presumably their original "intended" target and which then would be seen as a beneficial effect. Thus eosinophilia occuring for reasons other than parasitoses can have many side effects, due to tissue damage. The existence of eosinophilia should prompt a wide range of clinical investigations.

The criteria for severity (i.e., mild, moderate, or severe) have changed in recent years. Eosinophilia is one of the very few situations in hematology where the standard groups of general pathologies are not very appropriate, since the causes are frequently not easily categorized in this way. Thus, a combination of traditional causes and regional descriptions is used.

Mild Eosinophilia

The absolute eosinophil count is between 0.45 and 1.50 × 10^9/l. There is a distinct diurnal variation, peaking in the early evening, and with an inverse relationship to cortisol levels. The commonest general causes are

1. **ALLERGIES**
2. **CERTAIN DRUGS**

    a. Para-aminosalicylic acid and chlorpromazine
    b. Some antibiotics, notably penicillins, streptomycins, sulphonamides, and nitrofurantoin
    c. Gold (often also causes neutropenia)
    d. Tryptophan: the eosinophilia-myalgia syndrome (this is most likely due to an impurity in the tryptophan)

3. **PARASITOSES.** Some parasitoses cause only a mild eosinophilia; these are those with minimal if any tissue invasion, such as with many gut parasites. The eosinophilia-causing parasitoses will be discussed separately.
4. **OTHER INFECTIONS.** It is very uncommon for other organisms to cause an eosinophilia. One of the very few non-parasitic infections that regularly cause eosinophilia is **COCCIDIOIDOMYCOSIS,** a fungal infection. This starts out as a flu-like illness, later with polyarthralgia and erythema nodosum and erythema multiforme, pulmonary infiltrates, pleural effusion, and eosinophilia.
5. **MANY SKIN DISEASES** (including some that are not obviously allergic), such as eczema, exfoliative dermatitis, mycosis fungoides, psoriasis, can sometimes be accompanied by a mild eosinophilia.

    Less common causes include
6. **MALIGNANT DISEASE** such as Hodgkin lymphoma (± 20% of these have a mild to moderate eosinophilia). It may also be found in melanoma and brain tumors. It can also occur as part of the leukocytosis in the myeloproliferative disorders.
7. **SOME COLLAGEN DISEASES,** such as polyarteritis nodosa and the Churg–Strauss syndrome, and systemic lupus erythematosis.
8. **CERTAIN IMMUNE DEFICIENCIES,** and occasionally some endocrine deficiency states (classically Addison disease).
9. A mild eosinophilia is sometimes seen in resolving bacterial infections, as the neutrophilia starts to wane.

Moderate Eosinophilia

The absolute eosinophil count is between 1.50 and 5.00 × 10^9/l. The causes here are more severe forms of the above, but allergic causes, endocrine causes, malignancies, and immune deficiencies are distinctly less common. **PARASITIC INFESTATIONS ARE GENERALLY ONES FIRST CONSIDERATION.** Thereafter, causes mentioned under severe eosinophilia should be considered.

Severe Eosinophilia

The absolute eosinophil count is above 5.00 × 10^9/l. The important groups of causes are as follows:

1. **CERTAIN SKIN DISEASES** like **DERMATITIS HERPETIFORMIS** (see "The Malabsorption Syndromes" in Chapter 4), and **PEMPHIGUS.**
2. **INFILTRATION OF VARIOUS SOFT TISSUES, WITH EOSINOPHILIA.** This occurs

   a. In the life cycle of many parasites, such as visceral larva migrans (due to larvae of the cat and dog tapeworm – Toxocara cati and Toxocara canis, respectively – migrating through the tissues).
   b. Some parasites take up permanent residence in the tissues; some of these can cause marked eosinophilia.
   c. In a number of idiopathic conditions, such as eosinophilic myositis and fasciitis.
   d. In the gut and lungs, these often take specific forms – see next.

3. **GASTROINTESTINAL CAUSES. EOSINOPHILIC GASTROENTEROPATHY** can present in different ways, varying with the histological appearances. These are obstructive (mainly antral involvement), classical malabsorption (mainly small bowel mucosa), and ascites (serosal involvement). The significant diagnostic factor is pronounced peripheral eosinophilia. In the malabsorption form, there is evidence of iron deficiency, hypoproteinemia (with edema), hypocalcemia, increased fat in the stools, and an abnormal D-xylose test. The condition responds dramatically to steroids, but it is strongly recommended that a course of albendazole (at least) be given before steroids.

4. **RESPIRATORY CAUSES.** There are six fairly well-defined syndromes of pulmonary infiltrates with peripheral eosinophilia.

   a. **LÖFFLER SYNDROME.** This term is typically applied to patients with transient pulmonary infiltrates, sometimes with asthma, and with peripheral eosinophilia for which no cause can be found. It must be distinguished from eosinophilic pneumonia and other conditions with pulmonary infiltrates. It appears that a prominent cause of this syndrome is passage through the lungs of parasitic larvae as part of their life cycle, and the infiltrates and sometimes the eosinophilia then disappear. It is most common with Ascaris, Schistosoma, Filaria, Hookworm, and Strongyloides.
   b. **CHRONIC EOSINOPHILIC PNEUMONIA.**
   c. **ACUTE IDIOPATHIC EOSINOPHILIC PNEUMONIA,** often with pleural effusion.
   d. **ALLERGIC BRONCHOPULMONARY ASPERGILLOSIS (ABPA),** occurring primarily in the asthmatic patient.
   e. **TROPICAL EOSINOPHILIA.** This was discussed in Chapter 4.
   f. **SOME COLLAGEN DISEASES** affecting the lung, such as polyarteritis nodosa and the Churg–Strauss syndrome.

5. **EOSINOPHILIC LEUKEMIA** and **THE HYPEREOSINOPHILIC SYNDROME.** The diagnosis can be very difficult, and indeed the line between the two is often very vague indeed.

   a. **THE HYPEREOSINOPHILIC SYNDROME.** While it frequently has some very suggestive features, it remains a diagnosis of exclusion. It is a serious disease with high mortality unless treated. It has a tendency to considerable tissue involvement, such as endomyocardial fibrosis with a high risk of thrombotic complications; pulmonary infiltrates; skin lesions (angio-edema, urticaria, vasculitis); and most significantly, neurological complications such as psychoses, ataxia, coma, mononeuritis multiplex and peripheral neuropathy. The criteria for diagnosis are

      i. An absolute eosinophil count of 1.5 × 10^9/l, for longer than 6 months.
      ii. Organ dysfunction as described above.
      iii. No other known cause can be found.

   b. **EOSINOPHILIC LEUKEMIA** is a very difficult diagnosis. One needs the presence of unmistakable eosinophilic blasts in the context of a myelocytic leukemia to even entertain the diagnosis.

Parasitoses and Eosinophilia

Not all parasitoses result in eosinophilia:

1. **THE PARASITES MOST LIABLE BY FAR TO CAUSE EOSINOPHILIA** are the **HELMINTHS**

(worms). **ISOSPORA BELLI** and **DIENTAMEBA FRAGILIS** (whose pathogenicity is disputed) are the only non-helminths that regularly cause eosinophilia. Again, **NOT ALL HELMINTHS CAUSE EOSINO-PHILIA.** Those that do not are the ones that inhabit the lumen of the gut without attachment to the wall or invasion, such as:

a **ENTEROBIUS VERMICULARIS**
b **TRICHURIS TRICHURA**
c **TAENIA SAGINATA**
d **TAENIA SOLIUM,** except when eggs hatch in the bowel and the larvae invade the tissues
e **DIPHYLLOBOTHRIUM LATUM**
f **METAGONIMUS YOKOGAWAI**
g **ECHINOSTOMA** spp.

2. **THE DEGREE OF EOSINOPHILIA CAUSED BY DIFFERENT HELMINTHS VARIES** partly with which type of helminth it is and to what extent it invades the tissues.

　　a. **PRIMARILY INTESTINAL HELMINTHS** that cause eosinophilia. The eosinophilia is mild, and is because of attachment or other involvement of the gut wall. Occasionally, however, the larvae can enter the tissues when the eosinophilia will increase as described under 2b) below.

　　　　Of the nematodes (round worms), the typical example is **HYMENOLEPIS NANA;** this shares with Strongyloides a unique characteristic – auto-infection; this is described later.

　　　　Many of the intestinal trematodes (flukes) will cause a mild to moderate eosinophilia. These include **FASCIOLOPSIS BUSKI** (Southeast Asia, China, India) and **HETEROPHYES HETERO-PHYES** (Orient, Africa, Middle East. The latter is ingested in raw or undercooked fish, and only will cause eosinophilia if and when it invades the tissues).

　　b. **HELMINTHS WITH A TISSUE MIGRATORY PHASE.** With these the temporary eosinophilia can be marked. In the non-invasive phase the eosino-philia is typically mild. Typical causes here are hookworm (**NECATOR AMERICANUS** in the New World and **ANCYLOSTOMA DUODE-NALE** in the Old World) that will cause severe eosinophilia when they pass through the lungs. Visceral larva migrans (due to migrating larvae of the cat and dog tapeworms, **T. CATI** and **CANIS,** respectively) migrate generally with a profound eosinophilia.

　　c. **HELMINTHS WHICH BECOME TISSUE RESI-DENTS.** The nematodes all cause eosinophilia, namely the filariae (important ones are Wuchereria bancrofti, Abegia, and Oncocerca). The trematodes however do not except when they pass through the lungs, e.g., schistosoma.

3. Note that markedly severe parasitic eosinophilia only occurs when there is a hypersensitivity or immune complex-type reaction in lymph or blood.

　　NOTES:

1. The eating of raw or undercooked fish, typically found in people of Scandinavian, Eskimo, Japanese, and Jewish extraction, as well as some African tribes), can have a number of pathological consequences. As far as worms are concerned, the two most important ones are **D. LATUM** and **H. HETEROPHYES.**

2. Auto-infection is an interesting phenomenon and is found in two helminths: Strongyloides and Hymenole-pis. With these parasites eggs released by the adult may hatch in the small bowel and again enter the tissues. Patients can thus be infected for life.

3. Strongyloides has other interesting and important features. It may cause malabsorption, along with diarrhea and abdominal pain and associated with a marked eosinophilia, although most cases are asymptomatic. This infection is common in South-east Asia and is found also in expatriates living in the area and soldiers who had served there. It must be differentiated from eosinophilic gastroen-teropathy, and this can be very difficult, since stool examination for ova is not very sensitive. Note that in the immune-compromised, the eosino-philia tends to disappear, making the diagnosis even more difficult.

4. There are a number of drugs that are associated with eosinophilia; they mostly also are hepatotoxic, such as halothane.

Table 15.7 summarizes **THE DEGREE OF EOSINO-PHILIA** at the different stages of the life cycles of most common parasitoses.

Making the Diagnosis in a Case of Eosinophilia

In practice, there are two typical scenarios:

1. One is faced with a patient who, for various reasons, is suspected of having a parasitosis. The reasons may be episodes of diarrhea and abdominal pain, or simply malaise, but all occurring in a patient who is a recent immigrant or traveler from a developing country.

Table 15.7 Expected Degree of Eosinophilia in Various Parasitoses

Parasite	Origin	Stage	Site	Remarks	Degree
Hookworm	Soil (larvae)	Infection	Skin	Allergic rx.	+ +
		10 days	Lungs	Löffler	+ +
				Ova swallowed	
			Bowel	Adult worm	± to + +
Schistosoma	Water (Cercariae)	Infection	Skin	Swimmer's itch	+ +
		2 weeks	Lymph, blood	Katayama syndrome	+ +
			Lungs	Löffler	+ +
			Liver	Granulomas	– to +
Ascaris	Fecal ingestion	Infection	Gut	Penetrate	+ +
			Blood, lymph		?
			Lungs	Löffler	+ +
			Bronchi	(swallowed)	
			Gut	Adult worm	– to +
Strongyloides	Wet soil	Infection	Skin		+ +
		and reinfection	Lungs	Löffler	+ +

2. On the other hand, it frequently happens that a patient has very non-specific symptoms, and one is forced to do a FBC, in which one finds eosinophilia.

Regardless of the clinical presentation, one is guided by the severity of the eosinophilia.

Mild and Moderate Eosinophilia

One is concerned first with **THE EXCLUSION OF THE COMMON CAUSES.** One must remember that causes of severe eosinophilia may fortuitously be picked up in the early stages, and thus cannot be excluded when considering a mild eosinophilia.

1. **THE HISTORY CAN BE VERY INFORMATIVE:**

   a. **ATOPY,** such as wheezing, rhinitis, eczema, asthma. In the case of asthma, it is important to ask whether there has been a sudden deterioration (see under **ALLERGIC BRONCHOPULMONARY ASPERGILLOSIS** (ABPA) below)
   b. **DRUG INGESTION** or a recent general anesthetic (Halothane)
   c. **ANY SKIN LESIONS,** especially if pruritic
   d. **RECENT TRAVEL** to or from a developing country
   e. **WEIGHT LOSS, NIGHT SWEATS,** and other features suggesting a malignancy
   f. **RECURRENT DIARRHEA,** steatorrhea, weight loss
   g. **MENTAL CONFUSION,** neuropathies, etc.
   h. **JOINT AND MUSCLE DISEASE**

2. **ON EXAMINATION THERE MAY BE LITTLE TO FIND.** Conversely, there may be features of

   a. **SKIN DISEASE,** such as mycosis fungoides, melanoma, eczema, and psoriasis

   b. **GENERAL MALIGNANCY,** especially Hodgkin disease
   c. **MALABSORPTION**
   d. **CONNECTIVE TISSUE DISORDERS**
   e. **ASTHMA AND RHINITIS**

ALLERGIC BRONCHOPULMONARY ASPERGILLOSIS (ABPA). In essence, the patient presents with an exacerbation of atopic asthma, with the production of rubbery brown sputum plugs with large numbers of aspergilli on culture. X-ray of the chest shows upper lobe infiltrates and peripheral linear shadows. The eosinophil count is almost always greater than $1.0 \times 10^9/l$, and the IgE level is greater than 2,000 ng/ml, and specific IgE to **ASPERGILLUS FUMIGATUS** is strongly positive (NB: this is negative in an aspergilloma).

Severe Eosinophilia

A diagnosis here is very important, considering the serious nature of many of the causes, and can be very difficult.

1. Again, **THE HISTORY CAN BE VERY INFORMATIVE** or at least suggestive. Symptoms may point to a number of clinical regions:

   a. **THE TRAVEL HISTORY** is again very important.
   b. The presence of domestic **CATS AND DOGS.**
   c. **CHEST,** e.g., recent onset of "asthma" and cough, or even pulmonary embolism.
   d. **HEART,** e.g., cardiac failure, palpitations, missed beats.
   e. **GIT,** e.g., malabsorption, diarrhea, abdominal pain.

f. **MUSCLES AND JOINTS,** e.g., arthritis, muscle stiffness.
g. **CNS,** e.g., confusion, movement disorders, etc.

2. **ON EXAMINATION, THERE MAY BE FEATURES OF**

a. **SKIN DISEASE,** such as pemphigus and dermatitis herpetiformis.
b. **TISSUE INFILTRATION** including pulmonary crackles and rhonchi. Tissue involvement may be a thickening of the skin in places: of the many causes (acromegaly, scleroderma, leprosy), eosinophilic fasciitis can be considered. This is characterized by swelling and tightness of the skin of the trunk and proximal limbs with induration. The skin is shiny with an orange peel appearance, and eosinophilia is prominent.
c. **CARDIAC INVOLVEMENT** with cardiac failure and dysrhythmias.
d. **NEUROLOGICAL DAMAGE,** as described above in the hypersosinophilic syndrome.
e. **ACUTE SEVERE AUTOIMMUNE DISEASES,** particularly with generalized involvement.

THE RESULTS OF OTHER TESTS ARE SOMETIMES VERY SUGGESTIVE.

FBC FEATURES: AN ASSOCIATED MICROCYTIC ANEMIA is suggestive of iron deficiency, which can be confirmed by iron studies. If it is proven, this may indicate chronic bleeding. Bleeding may be associated with a number of parasitic infestations, such as from varices due to portal hypertension as a result of schistosomiasis; however, the classic association is with hookworm infestation. Each worm ingests 0.2 ml of blood from the mucosa per day, and since infestation can involve thousands of worms, it is easy to see that iron deficiency can develop very readily.

Note, however, that a microcytic anemia in these cases can also indicate chronic disease.

OTHER TESTS. Apart from iron studies as indicated above, the IgE levels are sometimes of assistance. IgE levels will generally parallel the eosinophilia in allergic conditions and parasitoses; their level is very much more variable in other causes, particularly infiltrative conditions.

In addition, serial stool and urine samples for parasites and ova are essential; allergen testing, lung functions, and chest X-rays, etc., all may be indicated (the clinical evaluation is essential to decide where to look). Bone marrow examination is hardly ever called for – only in cases where eosinophilic leukemia is suspected.

It happens quite frequently that no cause can be found for an eosinophilia. If it is mild it can conveniently be treated expectantly. However, if it is severe, it potentially represents a dangerous disease. Here an empirical approach is called for.

1. Parasitoses must be excluded as far as possible. This implies the following:

a. Three stools are submitted for analysis.
b. Day and night blood samples are submitted for filariae.
c. Skin snips are taken for filariae, where geographical factors are compatible.
d. A selection of serological tests are requested, depending on the local prevalences.

2. There are no positive diagnostic clinical features.
3. In 40% of cases, these tests will all be negative.

The patient is now treated empirically, with a series of drugs, giving time for a response to be noted before proceeding:

a. Metronidazole (high dose for 10 days).
b. A standard course of albendazole.
c. A standard course of praziquantel.
d. If necessary, a course of diethylcarbamazine. This is very toxic however, and ivermectine (if available) is now recommended.
e. Failing all this, one then must consider the diagnosis of hypereosinophilic syndrome (HES), even in the absence of typical clinical features and complications. Note that on no account should antihistamines be administered to these patients – rapid degranulation of eosinophils can lead to profound CNS damage in HES.

ALL SEVERE EOSINOPHILIAS SHOULD IDEALLY BE REFERRED.

Basophil Leukocytosis

This is characteristically found in the chronic myeloproliferative disorders (see later in this chapter). Otherwise, it can be found in hypersensitivity reactions, myxedema, ulcerative colitis, and pox-virus infections.

Unusual Causes of Leukocytosis

These will be mentioned and described but briefly, since their diagnosis and management are highly specialized. However, the fact that these are unusual does not lessen their great importance – they comprise "diagnoses that one cannot afford to miss." Aspects of the malignant lymphocytoses have already been discussed. Modern classification has become very complex. The FAB (French–American–British) classification is still useful, but the modern trend is to correlate the predominant type of cell with the clinical features, the cytogenetic and immunophenotypic abnormalities, and the prognosis. For our purposes we will begin with a traditional approach.

The Acute Leukemias

Acute leukemia is by definition an infiltration of the **BONE MARROW** by blasts; **THERE ARE NOT NECESSARILY BLASTS IN THE PERIPHERAL BLOOD.** The diagnosis is then part of the differential of the particular presentation, and leukemic infiltration of the marrow can present in the blood in different ways. The "classical" **BLASTIC INFILTRATION** of the blood is not likely to be missed, but atypical appearances are fairly common.

Uncommonly, acute leukemia may be discovered by accident on a FBC. Typically, the patient presents with progressive malaise, pallor, easy bleeding, and bruising and sometimes an acute infection. These are all very nonspecific, and it is obvious that without a FBC, the diagnosis could not be made. Occasionally the features are more specific: tissue infiltration, especially gum hypertrophy, is found in monocytic or monoblastic types of leukemia.

Lymphoblastic Leukemias

These are most common in children, but by no means uncommon in adults. The prognosis with treatment is excellent in children, but progressively deteriorates with increasing age. Common presenting features are those of anemia and low platelets. There is a subtype, the Burkitt type ALL, that is more serious, presenting typically with prominent tissue infiltration, especially in the jaws or abdomen.

Non-lymphoblastic Leukemias

There are several varieties, including myeloblastic, monoblastic, megakaryocytic, and erythroblastic leukemias. Generally speaking, the prognosis is poor, but is improving, particularly with advances in transplantation.

High-Grade Lymphomas in a Leukemic Phase

These can mimic the acute leukemias very closely, but there are a number of clinical and other features which frequently put one on the right road.

THE FBC FEATURES OF THE ACUTE LEUKEMIAS can be very variable and non-specific. There are several possible pictures:

1. The general diagnosis may be obvious, with a normocytic anemia, thrombocytopenia, and a very high WCC with numerous blasts to be seen. If blasts are seen, their morphology may be very suggestive, but in no circumstances can the specific diagnosis be made on the blood – a marrow aspiration is mandatory.
2. The FBC may not show much abnormality apart from the high WCC with blasts.
3. Occasionally, the picture may be that of a pancytopenia or bicytopenia. A thorough examination may reveal some blasts. There may be evidence of dysplastic changes.
4. The leukoerythroblastic blood picture. Blasts can occur in this picture even when it is not caused by leukemia. However, in this case they generally are few and far between. A leukoerythroblastic picture with prominent blasts should always prompt an exclusion of acute leukemia.
5. Not much to see at all.

The diagnosis can only be made with certainty on the bone marrow. In the marrow of the acute leukemias, the traditional FAB classification plus the results of cytochemical stains are essentially only a starting point. A summary of the FAB classification and the cytochemical reactions of the cells is given in the Optional Advanced Reading section. The final diagnosis increasingly demands chromosomal analysis and, in many cases, immunophenotyping.

In the typical (or "classic") case of acute leukemia, there is a very high leukocyte count, with at least 30% of cells being identified as blasts (30% being the diagnostic level required for diagnosis in the peripheral blood – with rare exceptions). High-grade lymphomas in the leukemic phase can present identically. The identity of the blasts is of course the next step, and this is usually not a trivial matter, requiring expert assessment.

Features in Other Tests

THE BONE MARROW APPEARANCES. These are usually characteristic. The marrow is markedly hypercellular with an obvious infiltration by blasts. The blasts may have a recognizable morphology, as myeloblasts, monoblasts, lymphoblasts, and the like. This cannot be relied upon, except occasionally there are distinctive morphological features:

1. AUER RODS. Their presence in the cytoplasm of the blasts proves them to be of myeloblastic origin.
2. LARGE BLASTS WITH A CHARACTERISTIC BLUE CYTOPLASM CONTAINING NUMEROUS VACUOLES indicate a lymphoblastic origin.

Rarely, the marrow may be hypoplastic, and the diagnosis can be very difficult.

Further tests on the marrow are

1. CYTOCHEMICAL STAINS, notable peroxidase, non-specific esterase, and PAS. Specific patterns are very informative, but their use is gradually being superseded by:
2. CYTOGENETIC STUDIES, which are becoming more and more relevant, having diagnostic, prognostic, and therapeutic implications.
3. IMMUNOPHENOTYPING is also generally performed and are generally regarded as the gold standard of diagnosis. The results, however, are sometimes not clear.

In the monoblastic leukemias, serum muramidase may be markedly raised.

The Chronic Leukemias

These can be divided broadly into myelocytic and lymphocytic.

Chronic Lymphocytic Leukemia (CLL)

This is typically a disease of older people, with an insidious onset, generalized lymphadenopathy, and a usually slow gradual progression to anemia and thrombocytopenia, and very occasionally to blast transformation (Richter syndrome).

CLL presents typically with generalized lymphadenopathy, and enlarged spleen, often with pallor, and sometimes with some unusual features:

1. Autoimmune hemolytic anemia
2. Skin lesions such as herpes zoster
3. Occasionally with purpura

Once again the features are by no means obviously classically those of CLL. Without a FBC (to start with) one would have no way of knowing what is going on.

It used always to be said that CLL is a very benign form of leukemia and almost never needs specific treatment, and that the patients usually die of old age before the leukemia can progress significantly. This is a serious misapprehension. Modern studies involving advanced diagnostic techniques, sophisticated epidemiological studies, and advances in therapeutic modalities and the response to them, have shown that the above conclusion applies to less than half of all patients with CLL. About one third of patients have very aggressive disease.

The Laboratory Features of Chronic Lymphocytic Leukemia

The features vary quite a lot with various stages of the disease and with the presence of complications.

THE EARLY PHASE. The patient may present only with a mild chronic lymphocytosis. Atypical lymphocytes may be present but not primitive ones. In this stage, the patient may not have any lymphocytosis or splenomegaly – in fact there may well be no positive features.

THE ESTABLISHED PHASE. This is the typical appearance, with high absolute lymphocyte count, sometimes showing atypical features. However, the more progressive and aggressive variants may show cells of increasing primitiveness, anemia, and thrombocytopenia. These features are often accompanied by clinical features of weight loss, malaise, and weakness. These findings have significant implications for prognosis and therapy.

COMPLICATIONS. The most important of these is the Richter syndrome, which is a form of acute transformation.

THE LEUKEMIC PHASE OF A LOW-GRADE LYMPHOMA IS MUCH LESS COMMON, but otherwise has much the same features. However, there are rare other lymphoproliferative disorders causing a lymphocytosis and their distinction can be very difficult – and the distinction is important, since the malignant status of some of these is open to question.

In all these cases, bone marrow aspiration, biopsy, cytogenetics, and immunophenotyping are essential investigations.

Chronic Myelocytic Leukemia (CML)

This again is a disease of older people; however, the diagnosis is being made in younger people. CML presents typically with a large, often very large, spleen, and perhaps some pallor and malaise – basically rather non-specific.

There is a juvenile form that is very aggressive, but generally CML is a disease that slowly progresses to worsening anemia and eventual transformation to acute leukemia. It is one of the chronic myeloproliferative disorders (i.e., CML, PV, ET and Myelofibrosis (MF)). Again, diagnosis is impossible without special tests.

The Laboratory Features of Chronic Myelocytic Leukemia

FBC Features

1. **THE RED CELLS.** There is usually a mild normocytic anemia. Sometimes the MCV is raised; this is usually due to a combination of two factors:

   a. The high WCC causing a spurious rise. It will be remembered from Chapter 6 that the larger white cells are also sized by the counter, but normally their number is so low relative to the red cells (~99:1) that they have no practical effect on the MCV. In any very high WCC, however, this effect may become noticeable.

   b. In any highly active marrow, the utilization of folate for DNA synthesis may cause relative deficiency of folate, causing a (true) macrocytosis.

   The morphology of the red cells is generally unremarkable unless folate deficiency is significant.

2. **THE LEUKOCYTES.** The WCC is raised, usually markedly, although in early cases the increase can be mild. There is characteristically a basophil leukocytosis. There is a significant left shift including many myelocytes. Until the disease enters the progressive phase, blasts usually account for less than 10% of cells. Occasional normoblasts can be seen.

3. **THE PLATELETS.** These are often somewhat increased, sometimes quite markedly, although in the progressive phase a thrombocytopenia may develop.

Bone Marrow Appearances

In the stable phase, the marrow is typically markedly hyperactive with a M:E ratio usually greater than 10:1.

Blasts account for 10% of cells or less. Megaloblastic change might be observed.

In the progressive phase, the blast count rises progressively. Note that these are not always myeloblasts – in 20% of cases they are lymphoblasts. The basophil leukocytosis may decrease.

Features in Other Tests

1. The LDH and urate are very often raised.
2. PCR for Philadelphia chromosome is positive.
3. The neutrophil alkaline phosphatase test shows a marked decrease.
4. Vitamin B_{12} and its binders are raised.
5. Culture of cells in the marrow, or FISH analysis, will reveal the Philadelphia chromosome.

A Brief Note About the Chronic Myeloproliferative Disorders (MPD)

Chronic myelocytic leukemia (CML), polycythemia vera (PV), essential thrombocythemia (ET), and myelofibrosis (MF) are the best known of these. Others include chronic neutrophilic leukemia (CNL) and possibly the myelodysplastic syndromes (MDS), as well as a group of conditions where the specific diagnosis is unclear and that are referred to as undifferentiated MPD. For our purposes, we concentrate on the four classical disorders and their diagnosis.

One major problem with these is that they tend to present with features that can also be found in a number of benign conditions:

1. In the case of CML: the leukemoid reaction
2. In the case of PV: reactive erythrocytosis
3. In the case of ET: reactive thrombocytosis
4. In the case of MF: various combinations of the above

Another problem is that these conditions sometimes transform into one of the others.

It is clear therefore that specific diagnosis is very important; it is often, however, very difficult. The easiest to diagnose is CML, where practically all are Philadelphia chromosome positive. The biggest problem has always lain with the others. Cytogenetic and immunophenotyping studies have always had poor sensitivity and specificity.

The latest development is the JAK2 PCR.[1] This mutation has been found to be positive in

1. ± 75% of cases of PV
2. ± 50% of cases of ET
3. ± 50% of cases of MF
4. ± 20% of cases of CNL and UMPD

The test thus has poor sensitivity and reasonable specificity for PV – i.e., you use this test to (try to) ***exclude*** the clinical/laboratory diagnosis of PV.

Making the Diagnosis

It should be clear that, since the leukemias generally have the tendency to present in non-specific ways, laboratory investigations should be requested whenever the suspicion of a serious pathology exists. It should not be concluded, however, that the clinical features are not important. Clinical evidence of complications influences choice of therapy. Nevertheless, the first step in all cases is the FBC. This generally provides at least a provisional diagnosis, with confirmation being provided mainly by bone marrow studies, including cytochemistry, cytogenetics, and immunophenotyping. The laboratory's role is of overriding importance and there is very little that the clinician can (or should) do without the laboratory. These cases should be referred.

Of much greater importance for the generalist is **THE PREVENTION OF THE TUMOR LYSIS SYNDROME** (i.e., while the patient is being sent to the specialist). This syndrome can occur in any malignancy, whether or not on treatment. In the leukemias it is especially likely in the lymphoblastic leukemias, especially when corticosteroid treatment is given. It is due to a massive breakdown in cells with the release of uric acid and with other biochemical abnormalities. Characteristically it presents as an acute renal failure, and laboratory tests will reveal

1. Hyperuricemia. This is the major cause of renal damage.
2. Hypocalcemia.
3. Hyperkalemia.
4. Hyperphosphatemia.
5. Raised LDH.
6. Raised creatinine and urea.

Preventive strategies include leukopheresis before commencing treatment, allopurinol, and vigorous hydration and alkalinization of the urine.

Teaching Cases

A few short cases (mostly excerpts) will first be shown to illustrate some pitfalls.

CASE #51

This case has already briefly been alluded to. The patient was a 19-year-old girl with an acute abdomen, and the important issue was to exclude an atypical urinary tract infection or mesenteric adenitis as causes. A urinalysis revealed a few inflammatory cells; the FBC revealed a mild neutrophilia, compatible with appendicitis and not with a urinary tract infection or mesenteric adenitis (where one might have expected a lymphocytosis).

CASE #52 (TABLE 15.8)

Table 15.8

Patient	Age	Sex	Race	Altitude
Miss E v L	24	Female	White	2,500 ft

The patient presented to her family doctor at the 20th week of pregnancy. Her complaint was burning and frequency of micturition. The BP and pulse rate was normal, and she was apyrexial. There was mild suprapubic tenderness. The fetal size and heart rate were normal.

			Reference range		Permitted range	
	Value	Units	Low	High	Low	High
White cell count	**12.1**	$\times 10^9/l$	4	10	11.19	13.01
Neutrophils	69.0	%				
Band cells		%				
Lymphocytes	23.0	%				
Monocytes	5.0	%				
Eosinophils	3.0	%				
Basophils	0.0	%				
Neutrophils abs.	**8.35**	$\times 10^9/l$	2	7	7.72	8.98
Band cells abs.	0.00		0	0	0.00	0.00
Lymphocytes abs.	2.78	$\times 10^9/l$	1	3	2.57	2.99
Monocytes abs.	0.61	$\times 10^9/l$	0.2	1	0.56	0.65
Eosinophils abs.	0.36	$\times 10^9/l$	0.02	0.5	0.34	0.39
Basophils abs.	0.00	$\times 10^9/l$	0.02	0.1	0.00	0.00
Normoblasts	0	/100 WBC	0	0		
Platelet count	224.0	$\times 10^9/l$	150	400	201.6	246.4
Sedimentation	**33**	mm/h	0	20	31	35

DISCUSSION

Clearly the anatomical diagnosis is that of isolated mild neutrophilia. Of the general causes infection seems the most obvious, but one cannot exclude a purely physiological cause, in this case pregnancy.

Table 15.9

	Value	Units	Reference range Low	Reference range High	Permitted range Low	Permitted range High
White cell count	**11.7**	$\times 10^9/l$	4	10	10.82	12.58
Neutrophils	72.0	%				
Band cells	0	%				
Lymphocytes	22.0	%				
Monocytes	5.0	%				
Eosinophils	1.0	%				
Basophils	0.0	%				
Neutrophils abs.	**8.42**	$\times 10^9/l$	2	7	7.79	9.06
Band cells abs.	0.00		0	0	0.00	0.00
Lymphocytes abs.	2.57	$\times 10^9/l$	1	3	2.38	2.77
Monocytes abs.	0.59	$\times 10^9/l$	0.2	1	0.54	0.63
Eosinophils abs.	0.12	$\times 10^9/l$	0.02	0.5	0.11	0.13
Basophils abs.	0.00	$\times 10^9/l$	0.02	0.1	0.00	0.00
Normoblasts	0	/100 WBC	0	0		
Platelet count	231.0	$\times 10^9/l$	150	400	207.9	254.1
Sedimentation	**30**	mm/h	0	20	29	32

Isolating the specific cause could be easy (e.g., a positive bacterial culture and response to antibiotic therapy). In this case, the symptoms are somewhat suggestive of a lower urinary tract infection, and the neutrophilia and raised ESR were thought to support this.

However, proving a physiological cause could be difficult, especially in a case such as this. Her practice records showed the following excerpt from a FBC of 4 weeks before, when she had been entirely asymptomatic (see Table 15.9).

The conclusion was reached that the neutrophilia was physiological, and did not in itself necessarily point to a bacterial infection. Urine cellularity and culture were negative, and antibiotics were not used. The patient settled down on conservative management. There are a few points to note:

1. There was evidently no left shift. A mild left shift too can be physiological, so long as it does not go further than band cells.
2. There was effectively no change in the two analyses – if one looks at the range of permitted values, it can be seen that the repeat results fall well within the first result's permitted ranges.
3. The raised ESR is normal for this stage of pregnancy.
4. The importance of referring to (and keeping) previous records is emphasized.

Note, however, that the picture in suspected appendicitis can be more difficult.

1. Up to 20% of acute appendicitis cases present atypically.
2. Mesenteric adenitis can also present with a mild neutrophilia – the reason is unknown, but possibly has to

do with erosion of the bowel epithelium due to the swollen Peyer's patches, with secondary infection.

CASE #53 (TABLE 15.10)

Table 15.10

Mrs M B	29 yrs	Female	White	5,000

The patient had been referred by a pulmonologist. He had been treating her for 4 years for refractory, adult-onset asthma. Clinically she was severely Cushingoid.

	Value	Units	Reference range Low	Reference range High	Permitted range Low	Permitted range High
Red cell count	4.13	$\times 10^{12}/l$	4.03	5.09	4.01	4.25
Hemoglobin (Hb)	13	g/dl	12.7	15.9	12.5	13.5
Hematocrit (Hct)	0.38	l/l	0.38	0.49	0.37	0.40
Mean cell volume	93.2	fl	80	99	91.3	95.1
Mean cell Hb	31.5	pg	27	31.5	30.8	32.1
Mean cell Hb conc.	33.8	g/dl	31.5	34.5	33.1	34.4
Red cell dist. width	13.8	%	11.6	14	13.8	13.8
Retic count	0.8	%	0.1	0.9	0.8	0.8
Retic absolute	33.0	$\times 10^9/l$	30	100	32.0	34.0
White cell count	**16.5**	$\times 10^9/l$	4	10	15.26	17.74
Neutrophils abs.	**8.42**	$\times 10^9/l$	2	7	7.78	9.05
Band cells abs.	**0.50**		0	0	0.45	0.54
Lymphocytes abs.	**5.94**	$\times 10^9/l$	1	3	5.49	6.39
Monocytes abs.	**1.16**	$\times 10^9/l$	0.2	1	1.07	1.24
Eosinophils abs.	0.00	$\times 10^9/l$	0.02	0.5	0.00	0.00
Basophils abs.	0.00	$\times 10^9/l$	0.02	0.1	0.00	0.00
Normoblasts	0	/100 WBC	0	0		
Platelet count	357.0	$\times 10^9/l$	150	400	321.3	392.7
Sedimentation	22	mm/h	0	20	21	23

DISCUSSION

The anatomical diagnosis is not quite straightforward: there is clearly a mild neutrophilia with a mild left shift; however, there is also a mild lymphocytosis and monocytosis. In view of the clinical features it was decided to use neutrophilia as a starting point.

In Chapter 16, a similar patient will be presented, except that she shows a polycythemia. The "cytoses" that can be found with Cushing pictures are most commonly a neutrophilia (often, as in this case, with a mild left shift), then polycythemia, then, unusually, erythrocytosis and thrombocytosis.

Note the absence of eosinophils. In a level 4 laboratory, where thousands of cells are counted, absence of eosinophils is abnormal.

However, the mild monocytosis and lymphocytosis are a source for concern. With great difficulty and with the assistance of her pulmonologist and a psychologist the patient was weaned off the oral steroids (these patients tend to show great psychological dependence on oral steroids. Note that inhaled steroids are not associated with Cushingoid features, being destroyed in the first pass through the liver). Gradually the counts all returned to normal. There is no clear explanation for the lymphocytosis and monocytosis.

CASE #54 (TABLE 15.11)

This table shows the FBC that was seen by his doctor.

Table 15.11

Patient	Age	Sex		Race	Altitude	
Mr S L	39 yrs	Male		Black	5,000 ft	

The patient presented to his doctor feeling tired, with a cough. The doctor thought the patient looked underweight, and ordered a FBC. He diagnosed a neutropenia and referred him for a marrow aspirate and then to a specialist.

	Value	Units	Reference range Low	High	Permitted range Low	High
Red cell count	4.57	$\times 10^{12}$/l	4.77	5.83	4.43	4.71
Hemoglobin (Hb)	13.9	g/dl	13.8	18.0	13.4	14.4
Hematocrit (Hct)	0.44	l/l	0.42	0.53	0.43	0.45
Mean cell volume	96.4	fl	80	99	94.5	98.3
Mean cell Hb	30.4	pg	27	31.5	29.8	31.0
Mean cell Hb conc.	31.6	g/dl	31.5	34.5	30.9	32.2
Red cell dist. width	14.5	%	11.6	14	13.4	15.6
White cell count	4.06	$\times 10^9$/l	3.5	10	3.76	4.36
Neutrophils	39.6	%				
Band cells		%	0			
Lymphocytes	49.1	%				
Monocytes	4.5	%				
Eosinophils	5.9	%				
Basophils	0.9	%				
Neutrophils abs.	1.61	$\times 10^9$/l	1.5	7	1.49	1.73
Band cells abs.	0.00		0	0.00	0.00	0.00
Lymphocytes abs.	1.99	$\times 10^9$/l	1	3	1.84	2.14
Monocytes abs.	0.18	$\times 10^9$/l	0.2	1	0.17	0.20
Eosinophils abs.	0.24	$\times 10^9$/l	0.02	0.5	0.22	0.26
Basophils abs.	0.04	$\times 10^9$/l	0.02	0.1	0.03	0.04
Blasts		%	0	0		
Promyelocytes		%	0	0		
Myelocytes		%	0	0		
Metamyelocytes		%	0	0		
Normoblasts	0	/100 WBC	0	0		
Platelet count	271	$\times 10^9$/l	150	400	240	300
Sedimentation	9	mm/h	0	10	0	0

DISCUSSION

On the face of it, there appeared to be a **NEUTROPENIA.** However, the family doctor was evidently unaware that, in Blacks, the lower limit of normal for the neutrophil count is 1.5×10^9/l, and not 2.0 as is it for Caucasians. This was unfortunate for the patient since it lead to a marrow aspiration for which there was insufficient indication at that time. (The marrow was reported as "reactive.") There is indeed **A REVERSAL OF THE NEUTROPHIL:LYMPHOCYTE RATIO,** in keeping with a viral infection. The picture settled down in a few weeks.

CASE #55 (TABLE 15.12)

Table 15.12

Patient	Age	Sex	Race	Altitude
Mrs M S	56 yrs	Female	White	5,000 ft

This patient had had numerous problems. Schistosomiasis had been successfully treated 10 years prior, but since then has had persistent "bladder problems." She also had a cholecystectomy and experienced considerable bloating. She was undergoing treatment for a spastic colon. Her doctor reported that two recent FBCs had shown rises in some of the white cell series, in an "irregular fashion." The red cells and platelets were always within their reference ranges.

Date of test ⟶	14–05	27–06	13–11	11–12
White cell count	16.0	18.4	15.5	12.6
Neutrophils %	81.1	59.8	57.3	53
Band cells %				
Lymphocytes %	17.2	32.2	33.3	38
Monocytes %	0.4	5.5	5.0	4
Eosinophils %	1.0	1.3	3.0	4
Basophils %	0.3	1.2	1.4	1
Neutrophils abs.	12.98	11.00	8.88	6.7
Band cells abs.	0.00			
Lymphocytes abs.	2.75	5.9	5.16	4.8
Monocytes abs.	0.06	1.01	0.78	0.5
Eosinophils abs.	0.16	0.24	0.47	0.5
Basophils abs.	0.05	0.22	0.22	0.12

This type of case is very troubling. It will be seen that, taking all the results into consideration, not even an anatomical diagnosis can be made, making it extremely difficult to know how to proceed.

Extensive investigation of the patient revealed no known source of leukocytosis. In particular there was no clinical change that the patient could report in the course of the months during which the tests were done. A single FBC taken at any time during the course could have prompted very different thinking, from allergy to early CLL to a chronic infection, and so on.

Clinical judgment is imperative particularly in borderline cases. Note that this type of problem, especially with the white cell series, is not uncommon. The major lesson to learn is, in the case of a mild alteration in any of the counts and there is no obvious clinical cause, repeating the count (and demanding a morphological assessment) is probably the safest route to follow.

On the other hand, this type of presentation cannot be ignored. At least regular follow-up is required, in the absence of a diagnosis.

As a matter of interest, because of the spastic colon and cholecystectomy, a search was made for hiatal hernia, and this was proven (Saint's triad).

CASE #56 (TABLE 15.13)

Table 15.13

Patient	Age	Sex	Race	Altitude
Mr E M	63 yrs	Male	Black	5,000 ft

The patient was referred to a surgeon for investigation of nausea, vomiting, heartburn, and weight loss. Gastroscopy revealed a chronic penetrating intrapyloric ulcer. He was also noticed to be pale. An urgent FBC was requested and a preliminary report was phoned through, as follows: Hb 7.2, WCC 10.2, Platelets 210. The surgeon assumed that this reflected chronic bleeding and started a transfusion. When the complete FBC report reached him (again telephoned urgently), he referred the patient.

	Value	Units	Reference range Low	High	Permitted range Low	High
Red cell count	2.45	$\times 10^{12}/l$	4.77	5.83	2.38	2.52
Hemoglobin (Hb)	7.2	g/dl	13.8	18.0	6.9	7.5
Hematocrit (Hct)	0.22	l/l	0.42	0.53	0.21	0.23
Mean cell volume	90	fl	80	99	88.2	91.8
Mean cell Hb	29.4	pg	27	31.5	28.8	30.0
Mean cell Hb conc.	32.7	g/dl	31.5	34.5	32.0	33.3
Red cell dist. width	18.1	%	11.6	14	16.7	19.5
White cell count	10.2	$\times 10^9/l$	3.5	10	9.44	10.97
Neutrophils abs.	2.14	$\times 10^9/l$	1.5	7	1.98	2.30
Band cells abs.	0.00		0	0	0.00	0.00
Lymphocytes abs.	3.06	$\times 10^9/l$	1	3	2.83	3.29
Monocytes abs.	0.10	$\times 10^9/l$	0.2	1	0.09	0.11
Eosinophils abs.	0.10	$\times 10^9/l$	0.02	0.5	0.09	0.11
Basophils abs.	0.31	$\times 10^9/l$	0.02	0.1	0.28	0.33
Blasts	44	%	0	0		
Normoblasts	1	/100 WBC	0	0		
Platelet count	210.0	$\times 10^9/l$	150	400	189.0	231.0

DISCUSSION

The anatomical diagnosis in this case, as far as the white cells are concerned, is in fact a big problem: there is not a leukocytosis in the traditional sense at all. The presence of blasts is highly significant, and one is justified in saying that the first stage diagnosis, provisionally at any rate, is "Leukocytosis: probable acute leukemia." The matter cannot, however, be left there: the diagnosis must be confirmed and then the type and severity of the leukemia must be established.

1. The importance of doing a full FBC with morphology is again emphasized. The traditional usage of requesting only a Hb and WCC (particularly by surgeons) is to be deprecated.
2. A leukemia can, and often does, present atypically, both clinically and in the FBC, as this case clearly indicates.
3. Further developments in this case were

a. Bone marrow aspiration revealed prominent infiltration by extremely primitive blasts. Cytochemical stains were all negative.
b. Immunophenotyping (in summary) revealed the presence of blasts which were strongly suggestive of myeloid origin (CD117+, CD34++, CD45+, CD33+, and CD13+), although there were in addition some features (dim CD11b and bright HLA-Dr) which were suggestive of a monoblastic component.

CASE #57 (TABLE 15.14)

X-ray of this patient's chest in Emergency had revealed right upper lobe and lingular consolidation. Further specific investigations revealed the diagnosis (Tables 15.14 and 15.15).

Table 15.14

Patient	Age	Sex	Race	Altitude
Mr X M	37 yrs	Male	Black	5,000 ft

The patient presented at the Emergency Department with pneumonia and atypical grand mal seizures. He had lost weight and was weak. His sputum was yellowish with tinges of blood. When the results of a FBC, routine biochemical profile and CRP were received he was admitted.

	Value	Units	Reference range Low	High	Permitted range Low	High
Red cell count	3.59	$\times 10^{12}/l$	4.77	5.83	3.48	3.70
Hemoglobin (Hb)	12.2	g/dl	13.8	18.0	11.8	12.6
Hematocrit (Hct)	0.36	l/l	0.42	0.53	0.35	0.37
Mean cell volume	99.1	fl	80	99	97.1	101.1
Mean cell Hb	34.0	pg	27	31.5	33.3	34.7
Mean cell Hb conc.	34.3	g/dl	31.5	34.5	33.6	35.0
Red cell dist. width	18.5	%	11.6	14	17.1	19.9
White cell count	16.33	$\times 10^9/l$	3.5	10	15.11	17.55
Neutrophils	88.8	%				
Band cells		%				
Lymphocytes	7.2	%				
Monocytes	2.2	%				
Eosinophils	0.1	%				
Basophils	0.0	%				
Neutrophils abs.	14.50	$\times 10^9/l$	1.5	7	13.41	15.59
Band cells abs.	0.00		0	0.00	0.00	0.00
Lymphocytes abs.	1.18	$\times 10^9/l$	1	3	1.09	1.26
Monocytes abs.	0.36	$\times 10^9/l$	0.2	1	0.33	0.39
Eosinophils abs.	0.02	$\times 10^9/l$	0.02	0.5	0.02	0.02
Basophils abs.	0.01	$\times 10^9/l$	0.02	0.1	0.01	0.01
Blasts		%	0	0		
Promyelocytes		%	0	0		
Myelocytes	1.7	%	0	0		
Metamyelocytes		%	0	0		
Normoblasts	0	/100 WBC	0	0		
Platelet count	243.0	$\times 10^9/l$	150	400	218.7	267.3
Morphology	The red cells show moderate anisocytosis with numerous round macrocytes and target cells. There is a neutrophilia with a significant left shift, as well as considerable dysplasia.					

Table 15.15

	Value	Units	Reference range Low	High
S-Urea	**27.2**	mmol/l	2.1	7.1
S-Creatinine	**172**	mmol/l	62	115
S-Urea:creatinine	**158.1**			
S-Sodium	**126**	mmol/l	136	145
S-Potassium	**5.2**	mmol/l	3.5	5.1
S-Chloride	101.00	mmol/l	98	108
S-Total CO$_2$	**16**	mmol/l	22	28
S-Anion gap	14.2	mmol/l	5	14
S-Glucose	5.6	mmol/l	3.9	5.8
S-Osmolarity	276	mmol/l	275	295
S-Osmolality	276.2	mmol/kg	275	295
S-Osmolar gap	0.0		–6	6
S-Uric acid	**0.63**	mmol/l	0.21	0.42
S-Calcium (total)	2.23	mmol/l	2.2	2.55
S-Calcium (corrected)	**2.65**	mmol/l	2.2	2.55
S-Magnesium	1.07	mmol/l	0.66	1.07
S-Phosphate	**2.45**	mmol/l	0.87	1.45
S-Protein (total)	**119**	g/l	64	83
S-Albumin	**19**	g/l	34	48
S-Globulin	**100.0**	g/l	30	35
S-Bilirubin (total)	11.9	μmol/l	6.8	34.2
S-Bilirubin (direct)	3.1	μmol/l	1.7	8.6
S-Bilirubin (indirect)	8.8	μmol/l	5.1	25.6
S-ALP	64	IU/l	53	128
S-gGT	**40**	IU/l	8	37
S-ALT	24	IU/l	19	40
S-AST	**84**	IU/l	13	32
S-LDH	**462**	IU/l	90	180
C-Reactive protein	**268.3**	mg/l	0.0	10.0

DISCUSSION

1. There is a mild anemia, marginally macrocytic. This type of anemia has been discussed in Chapter 9. Very briefly, the round macrocytes and target cells are suggestive of liver disease or hypothyroidism.
2. There is a moderate neutrophilia. It may seem strange that a left shift could be reported without the presence of band cells; however, the presence of even a few myelocytes or metamyelocytes indicates a significant left shift. With promyelocytes present it would be even more significant. Dysplastic changes are common in this condition.
3. The lymphocyte percentage seems low, but in absolute terms the count is normal.

The routine biochemistry (see Table 15.15) revealed renal failure as well as some liver disease, profound hypoalbuminemia, and a gammopathy. The markedly raised CRP almost certainly indicated a bacterial infection. Hyponatremia seems characteristic of this patient's disease.

SPECIFIC INVESTIGATIONS

1. HIV antibodies were positive on three occasions.
2. CD4/CD8 count revealed the following (reference ranges are given in brackets):

Lymphocytes absolute:	1,900 × 10^6/l	
CD4 + cell count:	70.3	(560–2,700)
CD4 + cell %:	3.7	(27–76)
CD8 + cell count:	1,328.1	(236–895)
CD8 + cell %:	69.9	(16–43)
CD4 +:CD8 + ratio:	0.05	(1.00–3.50)

The patient thus has AIDS, explaining most of the clinical features.

The nature of the pneumonia needed to be established. Sputum examination with Auramine staining revealed 1+ acid- and alcohol-fast bacilli per 100 oil-immersion fields. PCR examination confirmed tuberculosis.

CASE #58 (TABLE 15.16)

This case is another manifestation of proven AIDS.

Table 15.16

Patient	Age	Sex	Race	Altitude
Mr B M	35 yrs	Male	Black	5,000 ft

The patient presented with weakness and weight loss and was found to have a generalized lymphadenopathy. The chest was clear.

	Value	Units	Reference range Low	High	Permitted range Low	High
Red cell count	**3.53**	× 10^{12}/l	4.77	5.83	3.42	3.64
Hemoglobin (Hb)	**11.2**	g/dl	13.8	18.0	10.8	11.6
Hematocrit (Hct)	**0.32**	l/l	0.42	0.53	0.32	0.33
Mean cell volume	92	fl	80	99	90.2	93.8
Mean cell Hb	31.7	pg	27	31.5	31.1	32.4
Mean cell Hb conc.	34.5	g/dl	31.5	34.5	33.8	35.2
Red cell dist. width	**16.3**	%	11.6	14	15.1	17.5
White cell count	5.5	× 10^9/l	3.5	10	5.09	5.91
Neutrophils	40.8	%				
Band cells		%				
Lymphocytes	32.3	%				
Monocytes	**20.8**	%				
Eosinophils	0.2	%				
Basophils	0.1	%				
Neutrophils abs.	2.24	× 10^9/l	1.5	7	2.08	2.41
Band cells abs.	0.00		0	0.00	0.00	0.00
Lymphocytes abs.	1.78	× 10^9/l	1	3	1.64	1.91
Monocytes abs.	**1.14**	× 10^9/l	0.2	1	1.06	1.23
Eosinophils abs.	0.01	× 10^9/l	0.02	0.5	0.01	0.01
Basophils abs.	0.01	× 10^9/l	0.02	0.1	0.01	0.01
Blasts		%	0	0		
Promyelocytes		%	0	0		
Myelocytes		%	0	0		
Metamyelocytes		%	0	0		
Normoblasts	0	/100 WBC	0	0		
Platelet count	227.0	× 10^9/l	150	400	204.3	249.7
Morphology	There is a mild normocytic anemia. There is a significant monocytosis; many of the monocytes are atypical. There are also a small number of granular cells with blue cytoplasm resembling NK cells.					

DISCUSSION

1. The white cell reaction to the HIV infection is very different from that in Case #57.
2. Note that in AIDS almost any abnormal blood picture can be found.

CASE #59 (TABLE 15.17)

Table 15.17

Patient	Age	Sex	Race	Altitude		
Mrs M T	67 yrs	Female	White	5,000 ft		

The patient has a long history of the complications of severe hypertension. This is now under control, and the patient feels reasonably well. Some weeks ago the patient developed a sore throat, and her doctor saw mildly enlarged tonsils. He ordered a FBC (presented here). Throat swabs taken at the time yielded normal flora.

	Value	Units	Reference range Low	Reference range High	Permitted range Low	Permitted range High
Red cell count	4.55	$\times 10^{12}$/l	4.03	5.09	4.41	4.69
Hemoglobin (Hb)	15.2	g/dl	12.7	15.9	14.7	15.7
Hematocrit (Hct)	0.46	l/l	0.38	0.49	0.45	0.47
Mean cell volume	101	fl	80	99	99.0	103.0
Mean cell Hb	33.4	pg	27	31.5	32.7	34.1
Mean cell Hb conc.	33.1	g/dl	31.5	34.5	32.4	33.7
Red cell dist. width	14.6	%	11.6	14	14.6	14.6
Retic count		%			0.0	0.0
Retic absolute (abs)	0.0	$\times 10^9$/l	50	100	0.0	0.0
White cell count	11.7	$\times 10^9$/l	4	10	10.82	12.58
Neutrophils	41.0	%			41.0	41.0
Band cells		%	0	0		
Lymphocytes	52.0	%			52.0	52.0
Monocytes	5.0	%			5.0	5.0
Eosinophils	1.0	%			1.0	1.0
Basophils	1.0	%			1.0	1.0
Neutrophils abs.	4.80	$\times 10^9$/l	2	7	4.44	5.16
Band cells abs.	0.00		0	0.00	0.00	0.00
Lymphocytes abs.	6.08	$\times 10^9$/l	1	3	5.63	6.54
Monocytes abs.	0.59	$\times 10^9$/l	0.2	1	0.54	0.63
Eosinophils abs.	0.12	$\times 10^9$/l	0.02	0.5	0.11	0.13
Basophils abs.	0.12	$\times 10^9$/l	0.02	0.1	0.11	0.13
Blasts		%	0	0		
Promyelocytes		%	0	0		
Myelocytes		%	0	0		
Metamyelocytes		%	0	0		
Normoblasts	0	/100	0	0		
		WBC				
Platelet count	260.0	$\times 10^9$/l	150	400	234.0	286.0
Sedimentation	5	mm/h	0	20	5	5
Morphology	There is a mild absolute lymphocytosis. The lymphocytes are small and mature, with only a few atypical forms.					

DISCUSSION

The anatomical diagnosis clearly is mild lymphocytosis. Of the general causes, the most important to keep in mind, in this age-group, is lymphoid malignancy, and the fact that the lymphocytosis is mild by no means is against malignancy. Small mature lymphocytes could fit in with malignancy, but are less likely with infective causes, at least in an adult.

The general pathology diagnosis came from clinical considerations, as it so often does. As mentioned before, a sore throat developing in an elderly patient should never be passed off as trivial. Fortunately, the doctor was aware of the problem and referred the patient. Nevertheless, it could be a completely benign manifestation, and possibly a repeat of the FBC in a month or so to see if the pattern persisted may have been optimal. Thorough examination, clinical and radiological, revealed no evidence of lymphadenopathy or splenomegaly.

The sore throat had in the meantime settled down. A repeat FBC showed that in fact there was no significant change in the lymphocytosis. Blood was submitted for immunophenotyping and this showed a population of small cells with the following phenotype: CD19, CD5, CD20, CD23, CD45, with lambda light chain restriction. This picture is compatible with a low-grade B-cell lymphoproliferative disease, most likely CLL. (Note that CD5 is normally a T-cell marker, but becomes atypically positive in CLL, a B-cell disease.)

The diagnosis of CLL stage 0 was made (stage 0 refers to the presence only of a malignant lymphocytosis).

In view of the diagnosis, the patient's condition, and the fact that no treatment was in any case contemplated, a bone marrow aspirate and biopsy, also for cytogenetics, was postponed and the patient treated expectantly. The important things to watch for on follow-up are features of progression and the development of symptoms:

1. The doubling time of the lymphocytosis
2. The development of lymphadenopathy and splenomegaly
3. The development of anemia and/or thrombocytopenia
4. The development of "B" symptoms – weight loss, fever, night sweats, malaise

Staging is fairly complex, but in principle if the lymphocyte count doubles in 6 months or less, or any of the other features develop, specific therapy must be considered. (It should be mentioned that modern developments in the epidemiology of the disease especially the cytogenetics and phenotype and of new therapeutic modalities will probably result in the near future in a reappraisal of this policy).

CASE # 60 (EXAMINE TABLE 15.18)

DISCUSSION

The first-stage diagnosis is clear: mild lymphocytosis. Of the general causes, the most important to keep in mind is

Table 15.18

Patient	Age	Sex	Race	Altitude		
Miss J T	21 yrs	Female	White	5,000 ft		

The patient is a fifth year medical student and enjoys an active and liberated social life. She presented with severe malaise, sore throat, and she palpated her own enlarged neck glands and spleen. She was mildly pyrexial and had generalized purpura. She had severe pharyngitis with a tonsillar membrane, a tender liver, and jaundice.

	Value	Units	Reference range Low	Reference range High	Permitted range Low	Permitted range High
Red cell count	4.11	$\times 10^{12}/l$	4.03	5.09	3.99	4.23
Hemoglobin (Hb)	12.9	g/dl	12.7	15.9	12.4	13.4
Hematocrit (Hct)	0.36	l/l	0.38	0.49	0.35	0.37
Mean cell volume	87	fl	80	99	85.3	88.7
Mean cell Hb	31.4	pg	27	31.5	30.8	32.0
Mean cell Hb conc.	36.1	g/dl	31.5	34.5	35.4	36.8
Red cell dist. width	13.5	%	11.6	14	13.5	13.5
Retic count %						
Retic absolute (abs.)		$\times 10^9/l$	50	100		
White cell count	**14.21**	$\times 10^9/l$	4	10	13.14	15.28
Neutrophils	**36.5**	%				
Band cells		%				
Lymphocytes	**55.3**	%			55.3	55.3
Monocytes	4.1	%			4.1	4.1
Eosinophils	3.1	%			3.1	3.1
Basophils	1.0	%			1.0	1.0
Neutrophils abs.	5.19	$\times 10^9/l$	2	7	4.80	5.58
Band cells abs.	0.00		0	0.00	0.00	0.00
Lymphocytes abs.	**7.86**	$\times 10^9/l$	1	3	7.27	8.45
Monocytes abs.	0.58	$\times 10^9/l$	0.2	1	0.54	0.63
Eosinophils abs.	0.44	$\times 10^9/l$	0.02	0.5	0.41	0.47
Basophils abs.	0.14	$\times 10^9/l$	0.02	0.1	0.13	0.15
Blasts		%	0	0		
Promyelocytes		%	0	0		
Myelocytes		%	0	0		
Metamyelocytes		%	0	0		
Normoblasts	0	/100 WBC	0	0		
Platelet count	**9.8**	$\times 10^9/l$	150	400	8.8	10.8
Sedimentation	**24**	mm/h	0	20	35	39
Morphology	There is a mild absolute lymphocytosis, and there are numerous atypical lymphocytes morphologically resembling those found in infectious mononucleosis. There is also marked thrombocytopenia.					

lymphoid malignancy. If it were a malignancy, it would most likely be a lymphoma, since CLL is extremely rare in young people (note though that the youngest recorded case was in a patient in his twenties).

Because of the solid lead provided by the morphology, the diagnosis of infectious mononucleosis (IM) was immediately considered. Without this comment a more elaborate investigative strategy would have needed to be followed.

1. It was considered that, with one exception, all the clinical and FBC features were entirely consistent with IM.
2. The exception was held to be the thrombocytopenia. First, one could be sure that this was a true thrombocytopenia since

   a. The patient had purpura.
   b. The morphologist made no comment about any causes of spurious thrombocytopenia visible on the smear, i.e., platelet satellitism or excessive clumping.

3. In addition, the very tender liver and jaundice were thought to be atypical. Liver functions were requested. See Table 15.19.

   Table 15.19 shows clear evidence of hepatitis. Hepatitis virus studies for hepatitis A and C were done and were all negative. Hepatitis B antibodies were positive and showed an immune pattern (the patient had been routinely immunized).

4. It was decided to confirm the diagnosis of IM. The following tests were done:

   a. Throat swab for culture: this revealed normal flora.
   b. Monospot test for heterophile antibodies: this was strongly positive.
   c. Epstein–Barr viral antibodies: the IgM was strongly positive indicating a recent infection; the IgG was negative.

COMMENT

1. While ITP is very uncommon as a presenting feature of IM, it can occur. Slightly more common is an autoimmune hemolytic anemia.
2. True IM hepatitis occurs in less than 10% of cases. It normally resolves without treatment.
3. Because of the purpura this patient was put on steroids, with a very successful result. Normally steroids are not necessary or indicated in this disease.

Table 15.19

	Value	Units	Reference range Low	Reference range High
S-Protein (total)	79.0	g/l	64	83
S-Albumin	45.0	g/l	34	48
S-Globulin	34.0	g/l	30	35
S-Bilirubin (total)	**51.1**	µmol/l	6.8	34.2
S-Bilirubin (direct)	**22.4**	µmol/l	1.7	8.6
S-Bilirubin (indirect)	**28.7**	µmol/l	5.1	25.6
S-ALP	**196**	IU/l	53	128
S-gGT	**69**	IU/l	8	37
S-ALT	**74**	IU/l	19	40
S-AST	**68**	IU/l	13	32
S-LDH	**301**	IU/l	90	180
U-Bilirubin	**+ +**	" + "		
U-Urobilin	**+ + +**	" + "		

4. Other causes of the IM syndrome exist. Most are due to other viruses. The monospot test is usually negative in them.

5. IM has a tendency to relapse often. Of interest is that the atypical lymphocytes are usually not nearly as prominent in relapses; also the monospot test is usually negative. The history and previous records in such a patient are thus very important.

6. Observe the close parallels between this case and the one immediately preceding.

CASE # 61 (TABLE 15.20)

Table 15.20

Patient	Age	Sex	Race	Altitude
Mr F C	25 yrs	Male	White	5,000 ft

The patient complained to his family doctor of easy bleeding after injuries and of epistaxis. A hemostatic screen and FBC were requested. The screen was entirely normal but the FBC showed a marked eosinophilia. Several stool samples for ova were negative. The doctor telephoned for advice. It was suggested that the patient be given a course of metronidazole 800 mg daily for 10 days, and then to repeat the FBC; if the eosinophilia persisted he was to be referred (the doctor was also warned about prescribing any antihistamines). When the patient was seen on referral, on further questioning he revealed that he was a diamond miner. He was convinced that there were dangers in his work place, particularly the water being suspect. He had no neurological, respiratory, or indeed any other symptoms. He was an ardent dog lover, indeed owning several. On examination he was quite normal and apparently healthy. There was no clinical evidence of neurological, respiratory, skin, or ocular involvement.

	Value	Units	Reference range Low	Reference range High	Permitted range Low	Permitted range High
Red cell count	5.31	$\times 10^{12}$/l	4.77	5.83	4.65	5.97
Hemoglobin (Hb)	15.7	g/dl	13.8	18.0	15.2	16.2
Hematocrit (Hct)	0.46	l/l	0.42	0.53	0.45	0.48
Mean cell volume	87	fl	80	99	77.9	96.1
Mean cell Hb	29.6	pg	27	31.5	26.5	32.7
Mean cell Hb conc.	34.0	g/dl	31.5	34.5	33.3	34.7
Red cell dist. width	13.8	%	11.6	14	12.8	14.8
White cell count	13.2	$\times 10^9$/l	4	10	11.88	14.52
Neutrophils abs.	5.41	$\times 10^9$/l	2	7	4.87	5.95
Band cells abs.	0.00		0	0.00	0.00	0.00
Lymphocytes abs.	3.43	$\times 10^9$/l	1	3	3.09	3.78
Monocytes abs.	0.13	$\times 10^9$/l	0.2	1	0.12	0.15
Eosinophils abs.	**4.09**	$\times 10^9$/l	0.02	0.5	3.68	4.50
Basophils abs.	0.13	$\times 10^9$/l	0.02	0.1	0.12	0.15
Blasts		%	0	0		
Promyelocytes		%	0	0		
Myelocytes		%	0	0		
Metamyelocytes		%	0	0		
Normoblasts	0	/100 WBC	0	0		
Platelet count	229.0	$\times 10^9$/l	150	400	200.4	257.6
Sedimentation	**21**	mm/h	0	10	21	21

Table 15.21

	Value	Units	Reference range Low	Reference range High
S-Uric acid	0.39	mmol/l	0.21	0.42
S-Immunoglobulin G	8.94	g/l	2.5	12
S-Immunoglobulin M	1.55	g/l	0.19	1.93
S-Immunoglobulin A	0.87	g/l	0.07	0.94
S-Immunoglobulin E	**171**	IU/ml	10	150
C-Reactive protein	**15.6**	mg/l	0.0	10.0

DISCUSSION

1. The repeat FBC confirmed the marked eosinophilia. The anatomical diagnosis was thus clear.

2. A number of possibly relevant further tests were requested. See Table 15.21.

   The results were not of much assistance.

3. The clinical features also were of no help. The history, however, was somewhat suggestive, first of a water-borne parasite or allergen, and second his exposure to dogs.

4. Consequently, the following possibilities were considered:

   a. Systemic parasitoses, notable Toxocara
   b. Tropical eosinophilia
   c. Löffler eosinophilia
   d. Pulmonary infiltrates and polyarteritis nodosa
   e. Hypereosinophilic syndrome

   Each of these was considered in turn.

5. Several stool samples had already been shown as negative for ova. Blood samples taken morning and midnight for filaria were negative, and a few skin snips were submitted for filaria, which were negative. It must be emphasized that these tests are not enough to exclude filariasis – properly the patient should be given a loading dose of diethylcarbamazine (DEC) or ivermectine to mobilize the filaria and then repeat the test. These drugs were not, however, available. X-ray of the chest revealed no abnormality, particularly no pulmonary infiltrates. Lung function tests revealed no evidence of airways obstruction, which was very much against the Churg–Strauss syndrome. While the history of exposure to dogs was suggestive, the following facts were relevant:

   a. The patient gave the assurance that his dogs were regularly dewormed.
   b. The clinical features were against this being a visceral larva migrans, and the degree of eosinophilia in this disease is usually very much higher.

No diagnosis could be reached at that stage. It had previously been suggested to the doctor that the local water supply and work place conditions be investigated – no significant departures from acceptable standards were found.

The patient was given a three-day course of albendazole and the FBC was repeated after a week. The eosinophilia had markedly improved and continued to do so.

CASE #62 (TABLES 15.22 AND 15.23)

Table 15.22

Patient	Age	Sex	Race	Altitude
Mrs M L	35 yrs	Female	White	5,000 ft

The history was of recurrent attacks of loin pain, burning, and frequency of micturition during the pregnancy and birth of a child 3 months before, with recent deterioration and eventual prostration. Due to financial restrictions, she had had treatment only intermittently, and had had no treatment at all for 3 months. She suddenly collapsed and was admitted to a private hospital. On examination she was shocked, with rigors, full bounding pulses, and a blood pressure of 90/60. Urine output appeared still to be reasonable. The chest was clinically clear, and there was marked tenderness over both loins. The temperature was 40.9°C. The diagnosis was made of early septic shock.

	Value	Units	Reference range Low	Reference range High	Permitted range Low	Permitted range High
Red cell count	**3.78**	$\times 10^{12}$/l	4.03	5.09	3.67	3.89
Hemoglobin (Hb)	**11.5**	g/dl	12.7	15.9	11.1	11.9
Hematocrit (Hct)	**0.33**	l/l	0.38	0.49	0.32	0.34
Mean cell volume	86.6	fl	80	99	84.9	88.3
Mean cell Hb	30.4	pg	27	31.5	29.8	31.0
Mean cell Hb conc.	35.1	g/dl	31.5	34.5	34.4	35.8
Red cell dist. width	13.7	%	11.6	14	13.7	13.7
Retic count %	0.5	0.1	0.3		0.5	0.5
Retic absolute (abs.)	**18.9**	$\times 10^9$/l	30	100	18.3	19.5
White cell count	6.06	$\times 10^9$/l	4	10	5.61	6.51
Neutrophils	**70.0**	%				
Band cells	**4.0**	%	0	0		
Lymphocytes	7.0	%				
Monocytes	3.0	%				
Eosinophils	5.0	%				
Basophils	1.0	%				
Neutrophils abs.	4.24	$\times 10^9$/l	2	7	3.92	4.50
Band cells abs.	**0.25**		0	0.00	0.76	0.93
Lymphocytes abs.	**0.42**	$\times 10^9$/l	1	3	0.39	0.46
Monocytes abs.	**0.18**	$\times 10^9$/l	0.2	1	0.17	0.20
Eosinophils abs.	0.30	$\times 10^9$/l	0.02	0.5	0.28	0.33
Basophils abs.	0.06	$\times 10^9$/l	0.02	0.1	0.06	0.07
Blasts	0	%	0	0		
Promyelocytes	**1**	%	0	0		
Myelocytes	**4**	%	0	0		
Metamyelocytes	**5**	%	0	0		
Normoblasts	0	/100 WBC	0	0		
Platelet count	144.0	$\times 10^9$/l	150	400	129.6	158.4
Sedimentation	**115**	mm/h	0	20	109	121
Morphology	The red cells are normochromic and normocytic. The neutrophils show a significant left shift. Examination of thick and thin smears for malaria was negative.					

Table 15.23

	Value	Units	Reference range Low	Reference range High
S-Urea	**7.9**	mmol/l	2.1	7.1
S-Creatinine	**154**	mmol/l	62	115
S-Urea:creatinine	51.3			
S-Sodium	138	mmol/l	136	145
S-Potassium	3.6	mmol/l	3.5	5.1
S-Chloride	106	mmol/l	98	108
S-Total CO$_2$	24.5	mmol/l	22	28
S-Anion gap	11.1	mmol/l	5	14
S-Glucose	5.8	mmol/l	3.9	5.8
S-Osmolarity	279	mmol/l	275	295
S-Bilirubin total	12	mmol/l	0	17
S-Bilirubin conj.	2	mmol/l	0	6
S-LDH	481	U/l	266	500
C-Reactive protein	**257.7**	mg/l	0.0	10.0

For further results, see Table 15.23

An urgent X-ray of the chest revealed no pathology and that of the abdomen revealed only non-specific changes.

Because of the danger of DIC, various tests were done to exclude this. This topic will be covered extensively later in the book. Suffice it to say that there was no evidence of DIC in this patient.

DISCUSSION

From the hematological point of view the anatomical diagnosis is only that of a normocytic anemia and a significant left shift of the neutrophils.

The phenomenon of the left shift without a neutrophilia is very important, suggesting exhaustion of marrow neutrophil reserves (see the Optional Advanced Reading section for a discussion of this phenomenon), and thus is a potentially very dangerous finding, requiring urgent intervention, particularly in the clinical context like that of our patient. The danger is reinforced by the markedly raised CRP and ESR.

These findings and the clinical features strongly suggested a general pathology diagnosis of severe overwhelming infection.

Urine and blood samples were collected for culture. In the meantime, broad-spectrum antibiotics were prescribed while awaiting the results, together with intensive support of hydration and blood pressure. **KLEBSIELLA PNEUMONIAE** was cultured on numerous occasions from both fluids. The patient responded very well, and within 5 days the FBC had almost normalized. The CRP also normalized very rapidly, but the ESR took 10 days to normalize.

The major lesson to learn from this case is that a normal WCC can be found in very severe infection.

Exercise Cases

CASE #63 (TABLES 15.24 AND 15.25)

Table 15.24

Patient	Age	Sex	Race	Altitude
Mr C T	34 yrs	Male	White	2,500 ft

The patient is a foreman on a large farm, mostly agricultural. He was discovered by some farm laborers in a state of collapse and very confused. He was transported to the city. On admission he was found to be stuporose, hypotensive, hyper-salivating, and with constricted pupils. Initially he was thought to have had a stroke. An MRI and some blood tests were arranged.

	Value	Units	Reference range Low	Reference range High	Permitted range Low	Permitted range High
Red cell count	4.51	$\times 10^{12}$/l	4.64	5.67	4.37	4.65
Hemoglobin (Hb)	13.1	g/dl	13.4	17.5	12.6	13.6
Hematocrit (Hct)	0.40	l/l	0.41	0.52	0.38	0.41
Mean cell volume	87.9	fl	80	99	86.1	89.7
Mean cell Hb	29.0	pg	27	31.5	28.5	29.6
Mean cell Hb conc.	33.0	g/dl	31.5	34.5	32.4	33.7
Red cell dist. width	13.8	%	11.6	14	13.4	14.2
White cell count	21.7	$\times 10^9$/l	4	10	20.07	23.33
Neutrophils	78.1	%				
Band cells		%	0	0		
Lymphocytes	11.7	%				
Monocytes	0.2	%				
Eosinophils	9.9	%				
Basophils	0.1	%				
Neutrophils abs.	16.95	$\times 10^9$/l	2	7	15.68	18.22
Band cells abs.	0.00		0	0.00	0.00	0.00
Lymphocytes abs.	2.54	$\times 10^9$/l	1	3	2.35	2.73
Monocytes abs.	0.04	$\times 10^9$/l	0.2	1	0.04	0.05
Eosinophils abs.	2.15	$\times 10^9$/l	0.02	0.5	1.99	2.31
Basophils abs.	0.02	$\times 10^9$/l	0.02	0.1	0.02	0.02
Normoblasts	0	/100 WBC	0	0		
Platelet count	363.0	$\times 10^9$/l	150	400	335.8	390.2

Table 15.25

Case #63 cont.	Value	Units	Reference range Low	Reference range High
S-Urea	5.0	mmol/l	2.1	7.1
S-Creatinine	86	mmol/l	62	115
S-Urea:creatinine	58.1			
S-Sodium	137	mmol/l	136	145
S-Potassium	2.9	mmol/l	3.5	5.1
S-Chloride	106.00	mmol/l	98	108
S-Total CO_2	14	mmol/l	22	28
S-Anion gap	19.9	mmol/l	5	14
S-Glucose	11	mmol/l	3.9	5.8
S-Osmolarity	280	mmol/l	275	295
S-Calcium (total)	2.47	mmol/l	2.2	2.55
S-Phosphate	1.71	mmol/l	0.87	1.45

We shall work through the problem in stages.

Questions

1. From the hematological point of view, what is the "anatomical" diagnosis?

_____

2. Given these possibilities, how do you think the FBC altered the clinical suspicion?

_____

_____

Answers

1. A moderate neutrophilia without any evidence of a left shift.
2. The possibility of this being an inflammatory/infective condition, such as a cerebral abscess, now became prominent. Members of the family who had come along could shed no light on what had happened, but confirmed that the patient had been very well up to the time he left for the fields. A lumbar puncture was performed but the CSF was normal apart from a mild increase in protein. The MRI revealed no abnormality in the brain.

Further Developments

Clearly there was a diagnostic problem. A large number of other tests were requested, including a drug profile. In the mean time, however, a colleague who had been raised on a farm happened to be present and thought he recognized the problem, partly from the clinical appearance and from a residual smell. He suggested a further urgent test – see Table 15.26. An urgent phone call to the farm elicited the following history from a worker: he had been supervising spraying crops when a defect in the machinery occurred, and the foreman had been busy trying to fix it.

Table 15.26

	Value	Units	Reference ranges Low	Reference ranges High
S-Cholinesterase	397	IU/l	4,300	11,200

Questions

1. What is the diagnosis?

_____

2. What methodological error did the first attending clinician commit?

_____

3. What then are the general pathology possibilities of this presentation?

_____

_____

_____

4. What other laboratory results are in conformity with the diagnosis?

_____

5. What do you think of the eosinophilia?

_____

_____

6. Do you think morphology of the films could have been of assistance?

_____

Answers

1. Organophosphate poisoning.
2. He went straight from the anatomical diagnosis (neutrophilia) to a consideration of specific causes, concentrating exclusively on infection.
3. Infection, inflammation, malignancy, reactive, and physiological. In this case, the importance of the clinical features in reaching the general diagnosis (the history and the appearance) is made clear. It is also clear that a huge amount of money and time could possibly have been saved by a strict methodological approach.
4. The mild acidosis and raised phosphate levels.
5. The eosinophilia is not regarded as a classic response to this form of poisoning. However, this example does show that eosinophilia can be a fairly non-specific reaction in many cases. The case would need to be followed up to ensure that there is not an independent cause for the eosinophilia (farmers appear particularly prone to parasitic infestation).
6. The presence of toxic granulation and Döhle bodies would at least have been consistent with a diagnosis of toxic exposure. (In fact, the morphology revealed marked toxic granulation.)

CASE #64 (EXAMINE TABLE 15.27)

Questions

1. With reference only to the FBC, what can you make of the "anatomical" diagnosis?

_____

_____

Table 15.27

Patient	Age	Sex	Race	Altitude
Mr G vd M	61 yrs	Male	White	5,000 ft

The patient presented to his GP with fever, rigors, chest pain, and general body pains. He had had prostatic carcinoma diagnosed 5 years previously and was receiving chemotherapy. His hypertension was basically well controlled. On examination, his abdomen was very obese and distended with a palpable spleen, and no obvious ascites. An X-ray of the chest revealed consolidation of the right lower lobe. A FBC done at that time is shown. He was referred and admitted.

	Value	Units	Reference range Low	High	Permitted range Low	High
Red cell count	4.11	$\times 10^{12}$/l	3.91	4.94	3.99	4.23
Hemoglobin (Hb)	**11.9**	g/dl	12.4	15.5	11.5	12.3
Hematocrit (Hct)	**0.35**	l/l	0.37	0.47	0.34	0.36
Mean cell volume	84.4	fl	80	99	82.7	86.1
Mean cell Hb	29.0	pg	27	31.5	28.4	29.5
Mean cell Hb conc.	34.3	g/dl	31.5	34.5	33.6	35.0
Red cell dist. width	21.1	%	11.6	14	21.1	21.1
White cell count	**55.7**	$\times 10^9$/l	4	10	51.52	59.88
Corrected WCC	**52.06**	$\times 10^9$/l				
Neutrophils	**57.0**	%			57.0	57.0
Band cells	**5.0**	%	0	0		
Lymphocytes	5.0	%				
Monocytes	8.0	%				
Eosinophils	2.0	%				
Basophils	4.0	%				
Neutrophils abs.	**31.75**	$\times 10^9$/l	2	7	29.37	34.13
Band cells abs.	**2.79**		0	0.00	2.51	3.06
Lymphocytes abs.	2.79	$\times 10^9$/l	1	3	2.58	2.99
Monocytes abs.	**4.46**	$\times 10^9$/l	0.2	1	4.12	4.79
Eosinophils abs.	**1.11**	$\times 10^9$/l	0.02	0.5	1.03	1.20
Basophils abs.	**2.23**	$\times 10^9$/l	0.02	0.1	2.06	2.40
Blasts		%	0	0		
Promyelocytes	**3**	%	0	0		
Myelocytes	**7**	%	0	0		
Metamyelocytes	**4**	%	0	0		
Normoblasts	**7**	/100 WBC	0	0		
Platelet count	**754.0**	$\times 10^9$/l	150	400	678.6	829.4
Sedimentation	**47**	mm/h	0	20	45	49
Morphology	The following flags were on the report: Anisocytosis +. Poikilocytosis +.					

2. What are the general pathology diagnoses applicable?

_____

3. What are the features so far available that are for and against each possibility?

_____

_____

_____

_____

_____

4. What is lacking in the FBC from the laboratory that could help with the diagnosis as well as with the assessment of the general condition?

_____

_____

_____

5. All in all, we are not much closer to the diagnosis. What would you do next?

_____

_____

Answers

1. This is complex. From the red cell point of view we have a mild normocytic anemia. We are primarily concerned with the white cells. There is a generalized leukocytosis with a marked left shift, as well as normoblasts – i.e., this is a leukoerythroblastic reaction.
2. Chronic myelocytic leukemia, myelofibrosis, and a leukemoid reaction.
3. **CML. FOR:** The enlarged spleen, the basophil leukocytosis, possibly the thrombocytosis.
   AGAINST: nothing.
   MF. FOR: The enlarged spleen, the basophil leukocytosis, possibly the thrombocytosis.
   AGAINST: nothing.
   LEUKEMOID REACTION. FOR: The lobar consolidation and systemic features strongly suggest a pneumonia, particularly since the patient's immune system may be depressed because of chemotherapy.
   AGAINST: The enlarged spleen would only be against the diagnosis if it were massive. The ESR could be expected to be much higher. The basophil leukocytosis is rather high, somewhat against the diagnosis, but it is possible. The level of thrombocytosis is unusual for an infection but not against it.
4. It is clear that the smear was looked at, since there is a count of all the precursors (which cannot as yet be done by an instrument). It also seems clear that this was done by a technologist, since only the white cells received attention. The two flags given under "Morphology" are in fact machine generated, and the morphology of the red cells can have much to offer here, as will be shown in a minute. It will also be shown that these flags were inaccurate. The other test that would have been helpful is the reticulocyte count, since the patient probably has pneumonia and is thus in danger of hypoxia, which would probably be shown up in the retic count.
5. The following were done: a repeat FBC with full morphology and retic count; blood and sputum cultures; LDH and urate levels; vitamin B_{12} and binders (as well

Table 15.28

	Value	Units	Reference range Low	Reference range High	Permitted range Low	Permitted range High
Red cell count	**3.97**	$\times 10^{12}$/l	4.77	5.83	3.47	4.47
Hemoglobin (Hb)	**11.5**	g/dl	13.8	18.0	11.1	11.9
Hematocrit (Hct)	**0.35**	l/l	0.42	0.53	0.34	0.36
Mean cell volume	87	fl	80	99	77.9	96.1
Mean cell Hb	29.0	pg	27	31.5	25.9	32.0
Mean cell Hb conc.	33.3	g/dl	31.5	34.5	32.6	34.0
Red cell dist. width	**19.9**	%	11.6	14	18.4	21.4
Retic count	1.9	%	0.27	0.80	1.8	2.0
Retic absolute (abs.)	75.4	$\times 10^9$/l	30	100	67.9	83.0
White cell count	**56.2**	$\times 10^9$/l	4	10	50.58	61.82
Corrected WCC	**51.09**	$\times 10^9$/l				
Neutrophils	53.0	%				
Band cells	8.0	%	0	0		
Lymphocytes	9.0	%				
Monocytes	2.0	%				
Eosinophils	3.0	%				
Basophils	3.0	%				
Neutrophils abs.	**29.79**	$\times 10^9$/l	2	7	26.81	32.76
Band cells abs.	**4.50**		0	0.00	4.05	4.95
Lymphocytes abs.	5.06	$\times 10^9$/l	1	3	4.55	5.56
Monocytes abs.	1.12	$\times 10^9$/l	0.2	1	1.01	1.24
Eosinophils abs.	**1.69**	$\times 10^9$/l	0.02	0.5	1.52	1.85
Basophils abs.	**1.69**	$\times 10^9$/l	0.02	0.1	1.52	1.85
Blasts		%	0	0		
Promyelocytes	**3**	%	0	0		
Myelocytes	**8**	%	0	0		
Metamyelocytes	**9**	%	0	0		
Normoblasts	**10**	/100 WBC	0	0		
Platelet count	**698.0**	$\times 10^9$/l	150	400	610.8	785.3
Sedimentation	**44**	mm/h	0	10	44	44
Morphology		There is a leukoerythroblastic reaction. The red cells show moderate anisocytosis with a number of elliptocytes and teardrop poikilocytes. The neutrophils show a left shift with prominent toxic granulation and some Döhle bodies.				

as tests to assess the general condition). The results are shown in Tables 15.28 and 15.29. Also an ultrasound examination of the abdomen to assess the size of the spleen was performed.

Blood and sputum cultures were consistently negative. Ultrasound examination of the abdomen revealed a massive spleen (21 cm).

Questions

1. How have these various results affected the probabilities of the general pathology causes?

_____

_____

_____

Table 15.29

	Value	Units	Reference range Low	Reference range High
S-Urea	4.8	mol/l	2.1	7.1
S-Creatinine	87	mmol/l	62	115
S-Urea:creatinine	55.2			
S-Sodium	137	mmol/l	136	145
S-Potassium	3.6	mmol/l	3.5	5.1
S-Chloride	103.00	mmol/l	98	108
S-Total CO$_2$	25.2	mmol/l	22	28
S-Anion gap	12.4	mmol/l	5	14
S-Glucose	4.9	mmol/l	3.9	5.8
S-Osmolarity	**269**	mmol/l	275	295
S-Uric acid	**0.45**	mmol/l	0.21	0.42
S-Protein (total)	64	g/l	64	83
S-Albumin	36	g/l	34	48
S-Globulin	28.0	g/l	30	35
S-a1-globulin	1.2	g/l		1.9
S-a2-globulin	**8.1**	g/l	5	7
S-B-globulin	6.5	g/l	5	8
S-g-globulin	**12.2**	g/l	6	10
S-Bilirubin (total)	21	µmol/l	6.8	34.2
S-Bilirubin (direct)	3	µmol/l	1.7	8.6
S-Bilirubin (indirect)	18.0	µmol/l	5.1	25.6
S-ALP	**207**	IU/l	53	128
S-gGT	**209**	IU/l	8	37
S-ALT	**39**	IU/l	19	40
S-AST	**43**	IU/l	13	32
S-LDH	**1,755**	IU/l	90	180
C-Reactive protein	**182.6**	mg/l	0.0	10.0
S-Vitamin B$_{12}$	**1,068**	pg/ml	193	982

2. What would you do to confirm the diagnosis?

_____

_____

Answers

1. The leukemoid reaction is much less likely, because of the massive spleen, the raised LDH, urate, and of course the basophil leukocytosis. The possibility of a chronic myeloproliferative condition is correspondingly stronger.
2. In our view, the most important **DIAGNOSTIC** test in these circumstances is doing a neutrophil alkaline phosphatase (NAP) test and looking for the Philadelphia chromosome. These days it is possible to look for the chromosome in peripheral blood with a PCR technique. If this is positive it will confirm the diagnosis of CML. A bone marrow aspirate and biopsy may then not be necessary. In this case, the NAP was 1 unit

(normal range 15–100), and the PCR was unequivocally positive.

Optional Advanced Reading

Neutrophilia

In complex cases, particularly in the ICU, the interpretation of neutrophilia can be very difficult, and knowledge of some of the dynamics of neutrophil production and disposal will be of assistance.

The marrow reserves of neutrophils are enormous – at least 10 times the size of the circulating pool. In addition, the rate of production of neutrophils is rapid, and can be made more rapid by the effect of certain inflammatory cytokines. Finally, the natural disposal of neutrophils – apoptosis – can be inhibited by other inflammatory cytokines (and that may indeed be the case with some cytogenetic disorders, as in CML).

Thus in an on-going infection say, the resultant neutrophilia can reach very high values, for an appreciable length of time, and can even be sustained for a time, depending on the balance of forces.

However, these reserves are not limitless, and should the infection be severe enough and persist long enough, the neutrophilia cannot be sustained, and indeed some very interesting things can happen. These changes are summarized in Table 15.30. The stages described (by the author) are fairly arbitrary but appear clinically valid.

Table 15.30

Stage	Degree of stimulus	Neutrophil count	Left shift
I	Very small (e.g., a boil)	Probably normal	None
II	Mild to moderate (such as a septic laceration)	Mild to moderate increase	None
III	Increasingly severe (such as a pulp space abscess)	Moderate increase	Yes
IVa	Severe (such as osteomyelitis)	Marked increase	Marked
IVb	Severe (such as severe peritonitis)	Above + normoblasts	Marked
V	Severe but stable with a healthy marrow (such as a subacute abscess under pressure)	Moderate to marked increase	Decreased or none
VIa	Severe, deteriorating (such as worsening septicemia)	Tend to decrease	Yes
VIb	Marrow failing (such as fulminant septicemia)	Further decrease	Yes
VII	Marrow exhaustion	Neutropenia	Yes

A Note on the Interpretation of Activity Tests in Infection

In acute infection, the ESR is too slow in response to be as useful as the CRP. However, the problem with the CRP (and the other activity tests) is that they can rise with other infections, such as viral, and with tissue necrosis. This is usually only a problem when the etiological factor is uncertain, and where the CRP is below about 100; anything over this level is almost certainly bacterial.

Chronic Neutrophilia

A particularly knotty problem is the case of a chronically raised neutrophil count in an otherwise apparently more or less well patient. The conditions to consider are as follows:

1. **A STABLE CHRONIC BACTERIAL INFECTION** (e.g., an intracellular infection such as due to brucella, chlamydia, or rickettsia.
2. **CONTINUING INFECTION** from a chronic abscess.
3. **CUSHING SYNDROME.** The increased bone marrow stimulus due to the increased cortisol (or analogue producing a "Cushingoid appearance") most commonly results in a neutrophilia; erythrocytosis accompanies this less frequently, and true polycythemia and essential thrombocythemia are the least common.
4. **CHRONIC NEUTROPHILIC LEUKEMIA** is a rare condition, characterized by splenomegaly, mature circulating neutrophils, and normal NAP and absent Philadelphia chromosome (in most cases, it would seem).
5. **CHRONIC LITHIUM THERAPY** (the neutrophilia is benign and needs no specific attention, so long as the dosage of lithium is controlled).

Monocytosis

Unusual causes of (usually chronic) monocytosis can alert you to what is going on in what is otherwise an obscure case. The problem in is that usually the monocytosis in these cases occurs in association with other, more obvious changes in the FBC.

It should be remembered that the monocyte is the source of all the macrophages in the body: Kuppfer cells, glial cells, pulmonary alveolar macrophages, Langerhans cells in the skin, and pleural and peritoneal macrophages. In addition, the dendritic cells of lymph tissue also derive from macrophages, and this serves to remind us of the close relationship the macrophages (and therefore monocytes) have with the immune system. Also, macrophages are particularly prominent lining the sinusoids of the spleen, serving to remind us of the role the macrophages play in red cell breakdown and extravascular hemolysis – indeed, monocytosis is often found in hemolytic states. Finally, they can form giant cells, physiologically as in osteoclasts, and pathologically, in the various granulomas, reminding us of the role macrophages play in granulomatous inflammation.

To summarize **THE FURTHER CAUSES OF MONOCYTOSIS:**

1. **REACTIVE**
   a. Intracellular infections
   b. Tuberculosis, brucellosis, leprosy
   c. Histoplasmosis, cryptococcosis
   d. Toxoplasmosis, leishmaniasis
   e. Foreign material, such as beryllium, moulds
   f. Miscellaneous, such as hemolysis, pulmonary hemosiderosis

2. **NEOPLASTIC**
   a. Acute monoblastic leukemia (FAB M5)
   b. Acute myelomonocytic leukemia (FAB M4)
   c. Chronic myelomonocytic leukemia (a form of myelodysplasia)
   d. Histiocytic lymphomas and related conditions

3. **IDIOPATHIC**
   a. Wegener's granulomatosis
   b. Sarcoidosis
   c. Langerhans cell proliferation syndromes

The FAB Classification of the Acute Leukemias

1. **THE ACUTE LYMPHOBLASTIC LEUKEMIAS.**
   FAB L1: Lymphoblasts without any pleomorphism.
   FAB L2: Lymphoblasts showing pleomorphism.
   FAB L3: Lymphoblasts with large blue cytoplasm containing many vacuoles. This is characteristic of the Burkitt type of leukemia.

2. **THE ACUTE NON-LYMPHOBLASTIC LEUKEMIAS.**
   FAB M1: Recognizable myeloblasts without any differentiation.

FAB M2: Recognizable myeloblasts showing some features of differentiation. Auer rods may be present.

FAB M3: The primitive cells are abnormal promyelocytes. They too may show Auer rods and they particularly are frequently related to a DIC-type bleeding tendency.

FAB M4: Recognizable myeloblasts plus monoblasts.

FAB M5: The primitive cells are monoblasts.

FAB M6: Among the primitive cells are a significant number of erythroblasts (i.e., erythroleukemia), and the rest are morphologically myeloblasts.

FAB M7: The primitive cells have some megakaryocytic features.

There is also a class known as the FAB M0: this is an acute leukemia where the morphological features cannot allow distinction between lympho- and non-lymphoblastic characteristics.

A (SIMPLIFIED) SUMMARY OF THE CYTO-CHEMICAL REACTIONS IN THE ACUTE LEUKE-MIAS. See Table 15.31.

Note that exceptions occur regularly in the patterns.

Table 15.31

	Peroxidase	PAS	Non-specific esterase
Lymphoblastic	Negative	Positive	Negative
Myeloblastic	Positive + +	Negative	Negative
Monoblastic	Positive +−	Negative	Positive
Erythroblastic	Positive +−	Positive	Negative

Reference

1. Tefferi A, Lasho TL, Gilliland A, Kralovics R, Cazzola M, Skoda RC (2005). N Eng J Med 353: 1416–1417.

Further Reading

Andreoli TE, Bennett JC, Carpenter CCJ, Plum F (eds) (1997). Cecil Essentials of Medicine. 4th edn. Philadelphia: WB Saunders Company.

Epstein RJ (1996). Medicine for Examinations. 3rd edn. Churchill Livingstone.

Hoffbrand AV, Pettit JE (2001). Essential Haematology. 4th edn. Oxford: Blackwell Science.

Lewis SM, Bain B, Bates I (2006). Dacie and Lewis Practical Haematology. 10th edn. Churchill Livingstone.

Polycythemia

16

Defining Polycythemia

To repeat, to facilitate diagnosis, in this book we use this term to indicate **AN INCREASE IN ALL THREE CELL LINES.** It is very important to understand that any of the causes presented here can present only with erythrocytosis – but the approach to this is different and more involved; where all three lines are raised, the approach is simpler and time-saving.

The anatomical diagnosis (i.e., "polycythemia") has been reached as follows:

STEP 1: "Where is the primary abnormality? It is in **ALL THREE CELL LINES OF THE FBC**.

STEP 2: "What form does it take?" The abnormality is **AN INCREASE IN ALL THREE CELL LINES**.

STEP 3: "Are the increases reasonably in proportion to one another or not?" (in many cases of chronic myeloid leukemia, for example, the WCC is markedly raised and the RCC and PC mildly raised – this sort of case should be approached as CML rather than polycythemia). If "yes," then only now can one state the anatomical diagnosis as "polycythemia."

> **!** AN IMPORTANT JUDGMENT CALL: WHERE TWO OR MORE CELL LINES ARE INCREASED, THE *RELATIVE* INCREASES SHOULD BE EVALUATED. IF AN INCREASE IS DISPROPORTIONATE THEN THE INITIAL POINT OF DEPARTURE IS OF THE INCREASE IN *THAT* CELL COUNT.

General Causes of Polycythemia

At the general level there are only three general causes of significance:

1. Chronic myeloproliferative disease
2. Increased circulating cortisol or cortisol-like substances
3. Decreased plasma volume, causing hemoconcentration

Chronic Myeloproliferative Disease

Although all the chronic myeloproliferative diseases (chronic myelocytic leukemia (CML), essential thrombocythemia (ET), primary myelofibrosis (PM), and polycythemia vera (PV)) are associated with increased production of one or other or all of the blood cells, the classical one associated with increase in all cell lines more or less in proportion is **POLYCYTHEMIA VERA**. The chronic myeloproliferative disorders **ARE LOW-GRADE MALIGNANCIES OF THE HEMOPOIETIC TISSUES AND TEND TO HAVE FEATURES IN COMMON.**

FBC Features

1. Increases in one or more of the three cell lines that are not reactive, and the increases can frequently reach very high levels.
2. Basophil leukocytosis.
3. Transformation to acute leukemia in all, but far more commonly in some than in others.
4. The red cells can show features of iron deficiency in some of them, due to chronic oozing (or in the case of polycythemia vera, repeated venesection).

Features in Other Laboratory Tests

1. Raised LDH
2. Raised urate
3. Raised serum vitamin B_{12} levels

O.N. Beck, *Diagnostic Hematology*, DOI 10.1007/978-1-84800-295-1_16,
© Springer-Verlag London Limited 2009

Common Clinical Features

Splenomegaly is very common indeed. Otherwise they vary considerably with the different forms of chronic myeloproliferative disease. Without blood tests it would be impossible to reach a diagnosis.

> **Summary of Features in Favor of a Chronic Myeloproliferative Disorder** A patient with splenomegaly and showing a *chronic* increase (by reference to previous or repeat FBCs) in one or more of the three cell lines, with no evidence of a stimulus relevant to the cell line/s in question; basophil leukocytosis, and raised LDH and often urate levels.

> **Summary of Features Against the Diagnosis of a Chronic Myeloproliferative Disorder**
>
> 1. A patient showing an acute increase in one, or perhaps two, of the three cell lines
> 2. An increase in a cell line that is clearly reactive (e.g., to hypoxia, acute infection, bleeding)
> 3. Absence of basophil leukocytosis, raised LDH and/or splenomegaly

THE SPECIFIC CAUSE OF MYELOPROLIFERATIVE POLYCYTHEMIA WITH ALL CELL LINES BEING INCREASED MORE OR LESS EQUALLY IS POLYCYTHEMIA VERA. Nevertheless, one must bear the other chronic myeloproliferative disorders in mind.

Specific Causes of Polycythemia

Classical Polycythemia Vera (i.e., with All Three Cell Lines Increased)

Characteristic Features of PV

1. **FEATURES IN THE FBC**.

   a. **INCREASED HCT AND HB, AND USUALLY INCREASED RCC**, unless the patient is iron deficient as a result of repeated venesection or chronic GIT oozing. Indeed, the red cell morphology is normal unless iron deficiency exists. When all three cell lines are increased, they are increased more or less in proportion (PV can initially sometimes present as erythrocytosis only, in which case the approach is that described in Chapter 17).

   b. **INCREASED PC AND WCC**, and especially **BASOPHIL LEUKOCYTOSIS**.

   c. In uncomplicated PV, the **ESR IS CHARACTERISTICALLY LOW NORMAL** and the RDW is normal (i.e., if these are abnormal you must consider another diagnosis or a complication).

2. **FEATURES IN OTHER LABORATORY TESTS**.

   a. **DECREASED OR LOW-NORMAL EPO**.
   b. **OXYGEN SATURATION** > 92%.
   c. Raised **NEUTROPHIL ALKALINE PHOSPHATASE** score.
   d. There is an **INCREASE IN RED CELL MASS AND TOTAL BLOOD VOLUME**, which can be measured with radionuclide dilution techniques.

3. **COMMON CLINICAL ACCOMPANIMENTS**.

   a. **THROMBOSES**. These are very common. They may be arterial or venous, superficial or deep, trivial or catastrophic.
   b. Paradoxically, patients may also show a tendency to **EASY BLEEDING AND BRUISING**, due mainly to platelet dysfunction.
   c. **NEUROLOGICAL FEATURES** (due to hyperviscosity, platelet thrombi, or both) ranging from mild subjective symptoms to serious damage.
   d. **AQUAGENIC PRURITUS** (itch when in contact with water, typically experienced when getting out of the bath).
   e. **PLETHORA**.
   f. **SPLENOMEGALY**.
   g. **HYPERTENSION**

There is no specific confirmatory test. The histological picture of PV on a bone marrow biopsy can be typical and very suggestive. It tends to show fairly characteristic findings:

1. Variable increase in fibrous tissue. This is apart from the development of overt myelofibrosis, which occurs in ± 25% of cases.
2. Paratrabecular clustering of hemopoietic cells.

A fairly new technical development in diagnosis is the assay of erythropoietin-dependent colonies (the blast-forming units – or BFUs) on cell culture. (This technique was developed from the clustered appearance of the hemopoietic cells on biopsy in this condition.) It appears to hold considerable promise. Unfortunately it is only available in research and some tertiary centers. It is likely to be of the greatest value in cases with atypical presentation. Generally, in the typical case as we have described above, it is difficult to see what other diagnosis could be arrived at. As a general rule, the stronger the circumstantial evidence, the more likely is the diagnosis.

Polycythemia vera can present in other ways. From the clinical point of view, not all patients have pruritus; not all patients have splenomegaly; not all patients are hypertensive. From the FBC point of view there similarly are many variants. These presentations are summarized later.

Increased Circulating Cortisol or Cortisol-Like Hormones

The commonest of these is **CUSHING SYNDROME** (a specific cause), but iatrogenic hypercortisolism is very common. The clinical features are essentially identical.

Characteristic Features of Cushing syndrome

FEATURES IN THE FBC

While true polycythemia does occur, it is more commonly a leukocytosis (mainly a neutrophilia); however, **BASOPHIL LEUKOCYTOSIS IS NOT A FEATURE.** The reticulocyte count is normal.

FEATURES IN OTHER LABORATORY TESTS

1. The LDH is usually normal.
2. The urate level is mostly normal.
3. The EPO level is normal.
4. The plasma cortisol level is raised in classical Cushing syndrome and the ACTH levels would be low (unless we are dealing with a **CUSHING DISEASE** (i.e., of pituitary origin)). Strictly speaking, in iatrogenic Cushing the cortisol level should be low; however, some of the proprietary cortisone preparations cross-react with the test reagent, giving a spurious high result.

CLINICAL FEATURES

The most clinically valuable are

1. Obesity of a specific distribution (central obesity, moon face, buffalo hump).
2. Hirsutism (a difficult diagnosis in a male).
3. Purple striae especially in the axillae.
4. Plethora
   (but there are very many exceptions).

The confirmatory tests in the first instance are measurements of ACTH and cortisol levels.

Dehydration

The features of dehydration have been discussed in Chapter 4. Note again that usually dehydration causes only a rise in the Hct.

Making the Diagnosis

As in most hematological disorders, the approach depends on how the patient presents: clinical presentation is often decisive or bears a significant role in the diagnosis.

THE FIRST AND MOST CRUCIAL DECISION TO BE MADE IS WHETHER THE INCREASE IN CELL COUNTS IS A TRUE INCREASE OR THE RESULT OF DEHYDRATION. This is largely a clinical decision but is reinforced by the results of biochemical tests, such as osmolality, etc.

Note that for dehydration to present with polycythemia it needs to be very acute, extensive, and recent. Diagnosing this is not always as easy as it sounds – see Case #66. That is to say, if dehydration is not obvious, it should nevertheless be kept in the back of one mind while other possibilities are explored. A very important cause here is third-space losses which are not always clinically apparent.

The Clinical Examination

Figure 16.1 offers suggestions on **SPECIFIC ASPECTS** of the examination of a patient in whom it is known that all three cell lines are increased; clearly it is part of the overall examination as is depicted in Fig. 5.4. Figure 16.1 also offers a more general clinical approach to the **PLETHORIC** patient.

The clinical features of **CUSHING SYNDROME** are often obvious, but one is often caught out by very atypical presentations, e.g., with generalized obesity only, and the diagnosis may be missed, particularly in males where hirsutism can be very difficult to establish.

Differentiating the Possible Causes

THE DIFFERENTIATION OF DEHYDRATION generally should not pose a problem, using clinical features and results of urea, creatinine, and osmolality

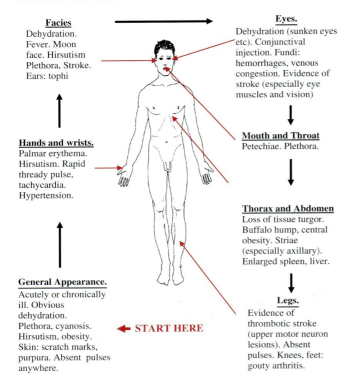

Facies
Dehydration.
Fever. Moon
face. Hirsutism
Plethora, Stroke.
Ears: tophi

Hands and wrists.
Palmar erythema.
Hirsutism. Rapid
thready pulse,
tachycardia.
Hypertension.

General Appearance.
Acutely or chronically
ill. Obvious
dehydration.
Plethora, cyanosis.
Hirsutism, obesity.
Skin: scratch marks,
purpura. Absent pulses
anywhere.

Eyes.
Dehydration (sunken eyes
etc). Conjunctival
injection. Fundi:
hemorrhages, venous
congestion. Evidence of
stroke (especially eye
muscles and vision)

Mouth and Throat
Petechiae. Plethora.

Thorax and Abdomen
Loss of tissue turgor.
Buffalo hump, central
obesity. Striae
(especially axillary).
Enlarged spleen, liver.

Legs.
Evidence of
thrombotic stroke
(upper motor neuron
lesions). Absent
pulses. Knees, feet:
gouty arthritis.

◄ **START HERE**

Fig. 16.1 Polycythemia: examination

estimations. The features in the FBC are not very help-ful, with one exception: if the Hct is 60 l/l or more, for all practical purposes this would be virtually diagnostic of a true increase in cell mass and **NOT** dehydration. The reasons are complicated and not fully understood; it is really just a trick of the trade. The absence of common features of the other two disorders is also helpful.

The correct approach then would be to correct the fluid and electrolyte status and repeat the count in a week; if the count remains high further attention should be given to the other causes. It is only when no firm diagnosis can be reached that blood volume studies **MAY** be indicated.

DIFFERENTIATING BETWEEN POLYCYTHE-MIA VERA AND CUSHING SYNDROME if the clin-ical features are indeterminate:

THE FBC. Generally, the FBC is not a great deal of help, apart from

1. Basophil leukocytosis is strongly in favor of PV.
2. The presence of microcytic red cells is in favor of PV. However, if the dominant picture is that of microcyto-sis, then the guidelines in Chapter 8 should be followed.
3. Cushing syndrome is generally accompanied by an eosinopenia (not an easy diagnosis to make, especially in a level 1 lab).

OTHER TESTS are often necessary. The following may be decisive:

1. **CORTISOL AND ACTH LEVELS** – abnormal in Cushing syndrome. Note that early Cushing may have cortisol levels still within the normal range; how-ever, of enormous value to the diagnosis is that the normal diurnal variation is lost. Thus blood for corti-sol levels should be taken at 8.00 AM and 12 midnight.
2. **UREA, CREATININE AND ELECTROLYTES** – usually unaffected in PV.
3. **URIC ACID** – tendency to be raised in PV.
4. **LDH** – classically moderately raised in PV.
5. **ERYTHROPOIETIN** (EPO) – of little help.
6. **BONE MARROW EXAMINATION**. This can be typical and almost diagnostic of PV. One important point – stainable iron is seldom found in the marrow even in the absence of regular venesections or chronic oozing; this does not imply iron deficiency (ferritin levels are usually normal in this type of case) – it is most likely due to the very rapid turnover of red cells in the marrow, and hence of iron. This point is particu-larly relevant since you may be tempted to prescribe iron therapy – the effect of this may be an **INCREASE** in Hct. This applies particularly to patients who are being venesected – the therapeutic effect of venesection is by making the patient iron deficient.
7. **THE PRESENCE OF KARYOTYPE ABNORMAL-ITIES** (although only 15–20% of PV cases show these) in the marrow are very strongly suggestive of poly-cythemia vera.
8. **SPLENOMEGALY** – strongly suggestive of PV rather than Cushing syndrome.
9. **BLOOD VOLUME STUDIES**. These are very rarely indicated.

A Word About Blood Volume Studies

1. It is sometimes stated that the definitive diagno-sis of PV requires measurement of the red cell mass. Many years ago, the Polycythemia Vera Study Group (PVSG) established entry criteria for cases to be studied as a research project. The *major* criteria were total red cell volume (TRCV) of $\geq$ 36 ml/kg ($\female$) or $\geq$ 32 ml/kg ($\male$); arterial oxygen saturation (Sao_2) $\geq$ 92%; and splenome-galy. It was clearly important to objectively docu-ment patients with PV; these tests will be much less helpful in distinguishing Cushing syndrome.
2. They will not clearly distinguish PV from aty-pical presentations of the other chronic myelo-proliferative conditions.

3. It is difficult to see what other diagnosis could be made in a patient with an increase in all three cell lines, in the absence of features suggestive of Cushing syndrome or dehydration, especially when other clinical and laboratory features as described are present.

4. In any case, there has recently been a major diagnostic breakthrough – the PCR for the JAK2 gene, although it is usually not necessary.

The above arguments do not apply to erythrocytosis (i.e., where only the Hct is raised). However, even in that case, resorting to TRCV studies is only occasionally required, as you will see in the next chapter.

It is easy to see that the root of the problem was one of nomenclature – confusing polycythemia with erythrocytosis. See Chapter 1.

Using the JAK2 PCR Since the diagnosis of PV can sometimes be very difficult, it may be tempting to turn to the JAK2 PCR for the diagnosis. However, as has been indicated in Chapter 15, its sensitivity and specificity are not adequate for this purpose – it is not, for example, nearly as useful as the Philadelphia chromosome in the diagnosis of CML.

The point should once again be made: it is only when the two approaches – clinical and laboratory – are combined that clarity is reached. Often it is the FBC that directs clinical attention appropriately.

Clinical Features in Favor of P. Vera

SPLENOMEGALY
EVIDENCE OF ARTERIAL THROMBOTIC DISEASE
PRURITUS ESPECIALLY ASSOCIATED WITH WATER
NO EVIDENCE SUGGESTIVE OF CUSHING SYNDROME OR DEHYDRATION

Clinical Features in Favor of Cushing Syndrome

CENTRAL OBESITY PATTERN, BUFFALO HUMP, MOON FACE.

HIRSUTISM, SINGLE CROP ACNE, PURPLE STRIAE, PLETHORA.
NO EVIDENCE OF PV – E.G., PRURITUS, SPLENOMEGALY.
NO EVIDENCE SUGGESTIVE OF DEHYDRATION.

Diagnostic difficulties with PV relate to the fact that the raised Hct may be the only feature. One third of patients with PV do not have a raised WCC; half the patients do not have a raised platelet count. These cases are discussed in later chapters. Sometimes PV can present with one of its complications, the diagnosis then requiring considerable clinical skill and thoroughness. The most important complications are

1. Arterial or venous thrombosis
2. Gout or hyperuricemia
3. Myelofibrosis
4. Hyperviscosity syndrome. This is discussed in Chapter 22.

A Practical Summary of the Diagnostic Approach

If the clinical features suggest dehydration: Confirm or exclude with biochemical tests, i.e., Na^{1+} and osmolality in blood and urine; blood urea and creatinine; blood volume studies only as a last resort.

If the clinical features suggest hypercortisolism: Confirm or exclude with biochemical tests – plasma cortisol and ACTH levels as a first step.

If the clinical and FBC features are compatible with PV (i.e., clinical features or complications as above, basophil leukocytosis, raised LDH): No specific confirmatory features exist. Diagnosis strengthened by low-normal EPO, typical features on bone marrow biopsy and cytogenetics.

If the clinical and FBC features are completely non-contributory: The whole gamut of investigations as discussed above will be necessary. In addition, the small possibility exists that you are dealing with multiple pathologies, particularly pure erythrocytosis plus other causes of leukocytosis and thrombocytosis, such as infection, bleeding, infiltration, etc. Thus the investigations discussed in the next chapter may also be necessary. Thus:

1. Blood and urine osmolality and Na^{1+}, urea, and creatinine
2. Erythropoietin, cortisol, and ACTH
3. Lung function tests and blood gas studies – Pao_2, Sao_2, Pco_2, etc.
4. Bone marrow biopsy and cytogenetics
5. Blood volume studies
6. Sonographic and radiological studies for tumors, etc.
7. Only if still seriously uncertain should the JAK2 PCR be done (it is very expensive).

2. Erythrocytosis with or without basophil leukocytosis and normal morphology
3. Microcythemia with hypochromic red cells and a right shift of the neutrophils
4. Increase in all cell lines with basophil leukocytosis as well as features suggesting transformation to myelofibrosis – left shift, tear-drop poikilocytes, and fragments.

FBC Features *Strongly* in Favor of a New Case of Polycythemia Vera (i.e., There Is a Proportionate Increase in White Cells, Platelets, and Hematocrit)

1. NO OR MINIMAL LEFT SHIFT OF NEUTROPHILS
2. HEMATOCRIT $\geq$ 60 L/L
3. BASOPHIL LEUKOCYTOSIS

Atypical Presentations

POLYCYTHEMIA VERA presents with typical clinical features fairly commonly, but frequently not. It is with these cases only that advanced investigations are warranted. Thus, frequently the clinical features are negative or vague and reliance is placed on the FBC and subsequent laboratory tests.

By and large, if the clinical or the FBC features of polycythemia are obvious, no problems should be experienced. However, when they are not, it is generally advisable to refer the patient (and since the confirmation and management of polycythemia vera and Cushing syndrome are complex, they will need to be referred anyway, but only after at least a provisional diagnosis).

A Summary of the Ways P. Vera Can Present on FBC

1. Proportionate increase in all three cell lines, with basophil leukocytosis and normal morphology

Teaching Cases

CASE #65 (TABLE 16.1)

Table 16.1

Patient	Age	Sex	Race	Altitude
Mr S F	24 yrs	Male	White	2,500 ft

He had been feeling "heavy in the head" for some time, with tinnitus. Friends had noticed that his eyes were "bloodshot." He itches after a bath and especially when in contact with cold water. He is hypertensive and the spleen is just palpable. He is lean and athletic.

	Value	Units	Reference range Low	Reference range High	Permitted range Low	Permitted range High
Red cell count	**6.89**	$\times 10^{12}$/l	4.64	5.67	6.68	7.10
Hemoglobin (Hb)	**20.1**	g/dl	13.4	17.5	19.4	20.8
Hematocrit (Hct)	**0.60**	l/l	0.41	0.52	0.58	0.62
Mean cell volume	87	fl	80	99	85.3	88.7
Mean cell Hb	29.2	pg	27	31.5	28.6	29.8
Mean cell Hb conc.	33.5	g/dl	31.5	34.5	32.9	34.2
Red cell dist. width	**14.1**	%	11.6	14	13.7	14.5
Retic. count %	0.27	%	0.26	0.77	0.3	0.3
Retic. absolute (abs.)	18.6	$\times 10^9$/l	30	100	17.2	20.0
White cell count	**12.9**	$\times 10^9$/l	4	10	11.93	13.87
Neutrophils abs.	**7.35**	$\times 10^9$/l	2	7	6.80	7.90
Band cells abs.	0		0	0	0	0
Lymphocytes abs.	3.74	$\times 10^9$/l	1	3	3.46	4.02
Monocytes abs.	0.77	$\times 10^9$/l	0.2	1	0.72	0.83
Eosinophils abs.	0.52	$\times 10^9$/l	0.02	0.5	0.48	0.55
Basophils abs.	**0.52**	$\times 10^9$/l	0.02	0.1	0.48	0.55
Normoblasts	0	/100 WBC	0	0		
Platelet count	**504.0**	$\times 10^9$/l	150	400	466.2	541.8
Sedimentation	**0**	mm/h	0	10	0	1

DISCUSSION

THE CLINICAL FEATURES are, in this case, highly suggestive, if all of them are taken into account – the water-related ("aquagenic") pruritus, the hypertension, and the splenomegaly. Even before the FBC was done, the possibility of PV could have very strongly been raised. But it should be made perfectly clear that by no means could the diagnosis be made without the FBC (and what follows therefrom). The latter is therefore the essence of this chapter.

WITH RESPECT TO THE FBC: There is no doubt about the anatomical diagnosis, i.e., polycythemia. Looking at all three cell lines (i.e., the Hct, the WCC, and the PC), we see that:

1. All three cell lines are increased.
2. They are increased more or less in proportion. The fact they are increased in proportion does not exclude the possibility of another myeloproliferative disease, i.e., chronic myeloid leukemia (CML) or myelofibrosis. However, this would not be one's first thought in the above case. One may have to return to this possibility if further investigation proves fruitless or contradictory.

THE POSSIBLE GENERAL CAUSES ARE

1. **MYELOPROLIFERATIVE DISEASE.** For further evidence of this, we need to have the LDH and urate levels (see Table 16.2), and certain clinical features. Points in favor of a myeloproliferative cause in this patient are basophil leukocytosis, raised LDH and urate levels, and splenomegaly; as well as the absence of dehydration and Cushingoid features. There are no points against the diagnosis.
2. **CUSHING SYNDROME.** There are no clinical features to suggest this. There is no evident obesity (hirsutism can be very difficult to establish in a male). The overwhelming evidence in favor of PV would suggest that Cushing syndrome only be reconsidered if other evidence were to turn up.
3. **DEHYDRATION**. Again, nothing to suggest this. Dehydration leading to polycythemia would almost always be a dramatic picture.

Table 16.2 displays the results of various biochemical investigations.

NOTES

1. With any cythemia, a basophil leucocytosis very strongly suggests a chronic myeloproliferative disorder.
2. The raised **URIC ACID** and **LDH** are characteristic of all the chronic myeloproliferative disorders.
3. The results in **RED** (in Table 16.2) are all normal and argue strongly against dehydration. Also there is no suggestion of a hypokalemic alkalosis with increased anion gap, which would be in keeping with a Cushing syndrome.

Table 16.2

	Value	Units	Reference range Low	High
S-Urea	**4.9**	mmol/l	2.1	7.1
S-Creatinine	81	mmol/l	62	115
S-Sodium	**138**	mmol/l	136	145
S-Potassium	4.5	mmol/l	3.5	5.1
S-Chloride	105.00	mmol/l	98	108
S-Total CO_2	25	mmol/l	22	28
S-Anion gap	12.5	mmol/l	5	14
S-Glucose	5.1	mmol/l	3.9	5.8
S-Osmolarity	**276**	mmol/l	275	295
S-Uric acid	**0.51**	mmol/l	0.21	0.42
S-Calcium (total)	2.36	mmol/l	2.2	2.55
S-Magnesium	0.91	mmol/l	0.66	1.07
S-Phosphate	0.96	mmol/l	0.87	1.45
S-Bilirubin (total)	21.1	mmol/l	6.8	34.2
S-Bilirubin (direct)	5.1	mmol/l	1.7	8.6
S-Bilirubin (indirect)	16.0	mmol/l	5.1	25.6
S-ALP	98	IU/l	53	128
S-gGT	31	IU/l	8	37
S-ALT	32	IU/l	19	40
S-AST	22	IU/l	13	32
S-LDH	**473**	IU/l	90	180

CONFIRMING THE DIAGNOSIS, I.E., THE SPECIfic Diagnosis

One can almost certainly exclude dehydration in this case, and there is no positive evidence for Cushing. Clearly the most obvious condition to consider is PV; the aquagenic pruritus in particular is a very important pointer. It is true that the age of presentation is unusual – the median age is about 55 years; only 5% of PV cases are under 40 years. But cases may, and do, present at virtually any adult age.

The normal RDW is characteristic of uncomplicated PV, as is the low-normal ESR.

There are no specific or "gold-standard" tests that can be used to confirm PV. Bone marrow and cytogenetic studies if positive are very suggestive indeed, but not specific (yet). Ultimately **IT IS A DIAGNOSIS OF EXCLUSION**; in this case the positive features are so strong that one would be hard put NOT to make the diagnosis of polycythemia vera. In the typical case, if all or most of the characteristic features mentioned above are present, the diagnosis can be made confidently. The following points should be made, however,

1. The overlap between the different chronic myeloproliferative disorders (i.e., PV, CML, essential thrombocythemia, and myelofibrosis) has already been mentioned.
2. A high index of suspicion is required in the differential diagnosis.

If there is any doubt at all, it is advisable to refer the patient.

> **Comment** This patient also demonstrates the effect of a certain form of therapy. To see this in perspective, we present a brief overview of possible therapeutic approaches and their sometimes confusing effects on the FBC.

Treatment of Polycythemia Vera and Its Effects

There are various modes of treating polycythemia vera, and the effects on the FBC are variable:

1. ^{32}**P. RADIO-ACTIVE PHOSPHORUS** causes a low-grade irradiation of the marrow, producing a reduction in all three lines. Generally speaking it results in a more or less normal FBC (for roughly 2 years, but this is very variable).
2. **VARIOUS CYTOSTATICS.** Hydroxyurea is very effective at reducing the Hct and the WCC, but less so with the platelet count. Since the platelet count can be significantly raised and is partly responsible for one of the most serious complications of PV, viz., arterial (and other) thrombosis, it is sometimes necessary to use another agent. Note that one almost inevitable side effect of using hydroxyurea is macrocytosis, often very marked; in these cases the vitamin B_{12} and folate levels are normal, and the macrocytosis is a result of the pharmacological effect of hydroxyurea – interference with DNA synthesis. High-dosage folate helps but seldom reduces the MCV to normal (and the MCV is a useful test for patient compliance, unless the dosage required is very low).
3. **VENESECTION.** This was for years the mainstay of treatment for the condition. It is important to realize that the treatment works by making the patient iron deficient (each unit of venesected blood will contain 250 mg iron). Remember also that iron-deficient cells are very rigid (i.e., poorly deformable); in ordinary iron deficiency the red cell count is lower and the effect of this on the micro-circulation tends to be less pronounced; but in PV there are very large numbers of these cells, with an effect, as yet unquantified, on the micro-circulation.

The effect of venesection on the FBC is interesting, and can be very confusing if not understood. The above patient was venesected, at first three times a week, then

Table 16.3

	Value	Units	Reference range Low	Reference range High	Permitted range Low	Permitted range High
Red cell count	**6.21**	$\times 10^{12}$/l	4.64	5.67	6.02	6.40
Hemoglobin (Hb)	14.1	g/dl	13.4	17.5	13.6	14.6
Hematocrit (Hct)	0.45	l/l	0.41	0.52	0.44	0.46
Mean cell volume	**71**	fl	80	99	69.6	72.4
Mean cell Hb	**22.7**	pg	27	31.5	22.3	23.2
Mean cell Hb conc.	**31.3**	g/dl	31.5	34.5	30.7	32.0
Red cell dist. width	**16.6**	%	11.6	14	16.1	17.1
Retic. count %	**0.51**	%	0.26	0.77	0.5	0.5
Retic. absolute	**31.7**	$\times 10^9$/l	30	100	29.3	34.0
White cell count	**12.1**	$\times 10^9$/l	4	10	11.19	13.01
Neutrophils abs.	6.66	$\times 10^9$/l	2	7	6.16	7.15
Lymphocytes abs.	3.87	$\times 10^9$/l	1	3	3.58	4.16
Monocytes abs.	0.48	$\times 10^9$/l	0.2	1	0.45	0.52
Eosinophils abs.	**0.61**	$\times 10^9$/l	0.02	0.5	0.56	0.65
Basophils abs.	**0.48**	$\times 10^9$/l	0.02	0.1	0.45	0.52
Platelet count	**613.0**	$\times 10^9$/l	150	400	567.0	659.0
Sedimentation	1	mm/h	0	10	1	1

as the Hct fell, less frequently, and ultimately kept at a Hct of about 0.45 l/l. Table 16.3 shows the FBC after 4 months of regular venesection.

There are a number of very instructive points arising out of this count:

1. The **RED CELL INDICES** are peculiar. The RCC remains very high, but the MCV is low (this phenomenon is known as microcythemia, as explained in Chapter 8). It was stated that the aim of venesection is to make the patient iron deficient, and it was seen in Chapter 8 that iron deficiency is characteristically microcytic (and hypochromic – see the MCH). What is odd here is the raised RCC, which is NOT a feature of iron deficiency. The pattern **IS**, however, characteristic of thalassemia (see Chapter 8). The raised RDW is characteristic of iron deficiency, as was seen in Chapter 8.
2. The **RETICULOCYTE COUNT** is on the low side, which is a characteristic feature of **CHRONIC** iron deficiency without a recent acute bleed.
3. Iron studies will usually be of great assistance.
4. The point has already been made that an increased RCC by itself can be misleading in the clinical sense, which this case serves to illustrate.
5. The high **PLATELET COUNT** and **WCC** are not improved by venesection, and indeed could even be worsened temporarily immediately after a venesection (see Chapter 4). The potential for thrombosis is still significant.
6. One could have trouble in a level 1 laboratory, particularly in the case where the patient has been venesected, since the RCC will not be done (and therefore a

MCV could not be reported) and would in any case be unreliable. Clinical judgment would be even more important.

7. The case originally presented is perhaps the characteristic one. However, a fairly common complication of PV (in a new case – i.e., one that has not yet been venesected) is chronic bleeding, usually from the gut, for various reasons such as stasis, platelet dysfunction, and so on, and they may thus **PRESENT** with the second picture. One would expect that the raised RCC, WCC, and PC would give one the clue but:

a. Early PV often presents **ONLY** with erythrocytosis (see Chapter 17), and despite a normal platelet count the platelets can be dysfunctional and thus the patient can still bleed.

b. The basophil leukocytosis is often very mild at first and can be overlooked.

In consequence, the picture can easily be confused with that of thalassemia, particularly thalassemia minor (see Chapter 8, where the distinction was discussed).

CASE #66 (TABLES 16.4, 16.5, AND 16.6)

Examine Table 16.4. This case occurred at a mission hospital in Bangladesh, with a level 2 laboratory.

DISCUSSION

The clinical features were the primary consideration; indeed the patient was considered very seriously ill, if not critical. The diagnosis of dehydration was made almost immediately. Considerations of etiology were delayed, and after blood was drawn he was actively rehydrated. Dehydration dominated the clinical picture, and the results in Table 16.5 were considered before those of the FBC.

These results show hyponatremic dehydration with hyperchloremic acidosis. Were it not for the experience

Table 16.4

Patient	Age	Sex	Race	Altitude
Mr K G	34 yrs	Male	Indian	1,000 ft
The patient is a very poor man, without a family, and living in a shack on the banks of a polluted river in Bangladesh. He was taken ill very suddenly, with thirst, muscle cramps, dry skin, sunken eyes, prostration, and rapid pulse rate. There was no evidence of trauma, no pyrexia, no cough, no chest pain, no abdominal pain, or vomiting, but there was a mild watery diarrhea with considerable abdominal distention. He was admitted urgently to a rural clinic. He was found to be very thin and malnourished.				

Table 16.5

	Value	Units	Reference range Low	Reference range High
S-Urea	10.9	mmol/l	2.1	7.1
S-Creatinine	141	mmol/l	62	115
S-Urea:creatinine	77.3			
S-Sodium	129	mmol/l	136	145
S-Potassium	2.4	mmol/l	3.5	5.1
S-Chloride	114.00	mmol/l	98	108
S-Total CO$_2$	18	mmol/l	22	28
S-Anion gap	−0.6	mmol/l	5	14
S-Glucose	3.9	mmol/l	3.9	5.8
S-Osmolarity	264	mmol/l	275	295
S-Uric acid	0.51	mmol/l	0.21	0.42
U-Sodium	11	mmol/l		

Table 16.6

	Value	Units	Reference range Low	Reference range High	Permitted range Low	Permitted range High
Red cell count	6.39	× 10^{12}/l	4.64	5.67	6.20	6.58
Hemoglobin (Hb)	19.1	g/dl	13.4	17.5	18.4	19.8
Hematocrit (Hct)	0.56	l/l	0.41	0.52	0.54	0.57
Mean cell volume	87	fl	80	99	85.3	88.7
Mean cell Hb	29.9	pg	27	31.5	29.3	30.5
Mean cell Hb conc.	34.4	g/dl	31.5	34.5	33.7	35.0
White cell count	12.1	× 10^9/l	4	10	11.19	13.01
Neutrophils abs.	7.14	× 10^9/l	2	7	6.60	7.67
Band cells abs.	1.09		0	0.00	0.98	1.20
Lymphocytes abs.	3.27	× 10^9/l	1	3	3.02	3.51
Monocytes abs.	0.61	× 10^9/l	0.2	1	0.56	0.65
Eosinophils abs.	0.00	× 10^9/l	0.02	0.5	0.00	0.00
Basophils abs.	0.00	× 10^9/l	0.02	0.1	0.00	0.00
Normoblasts	0	/100 WBC	0	0		
Platelet count	419.0	× 10^9/l	150	400	377.1	460.9

of the personnel, this case would have been a problem – there was no reason to be found for dehydration.

About an hour after admission he commenced explosive diarrhea. Dark-ground examination of the stool revealed comma-shaped bacilli of Vibrio species, and the diagnosis of cholera was made. Note that the features of dehydration were the result of massive fluid loss into the gut, **BEFORE** diarrhea was obvious – indeed, the patient could have died from shock before diarrhea started. The patient could of course have presented with erythrocytosis alone.

We shall concentrate for teaching purposes on the FBC. See Table 16.6

DISCUSSION

Again, the **ANATOMICAL DIAGNOSIS, POLYCYTHEMIA**, is obvious. Reaching the general cause has required further data (Table 16.5).

In a case like this, the usual methodical approach is bypassed. However, for the sake of completeness, of the possible general causes, there is nothing to support PV or Cushing syndrome, although there is no reason why this patient could not otherwise have either of these conditions.

The following two cases are examples of complex and potentially misleading presentations, and which perhaps should always be referred.

CASE #67 (EXAMINE TABLE 16.7)

DISCUSSION

The clinical features are really of very little assistance, except for the massively enlarged spleen – which,

Table 16.7

Patient	Age	Sex	Race	Altitude		
Mrs K S	61 yrs	Female	White	5,000 ft		
She presents with progressive lassitude slowly deteriorating over the last 6 months. There is no pruritus. She is mildly hypertensive and the spleen is 20 cm enlarged. There is no obesity or hirsutism.						
				Reference range		Permitted range
	Value	Units	Low	High	Low	High
Red cell count	**5.73**	× 10¹²/l	4.03	5.09	5.56	5.90
Hemoglobin (Hb)	**16.5**	g/dl	12.7	15.9	15.9	17.1
Hematocrit (Hct)	**50.00**	l/l	0.38	0.49	48.50	51.50
Mean cell volume	85	fl	80	99	83.3	86.7
Mean cell Hb	28.8	pg	27	31.5	28.2	29.4
Mean cell Hb conc.	31.0	g/dl	31.5	34.5	30.4	31.6
Red cell dist. width	15.1	%	11.6	14	15.1	15.1
Retic. count %	1.1	%	0.3	0.8	1.1	1.1
Retic. absolute (abs.)	63.0	× 10⁹/l	30	100	61.1	64.9
White cell count	**17.1**	× 10⁹/l	4	10	15.82	18.38
Neutrophils abs.	**10.09**	× 10⁹/l	2	7	9.33	10.85
Lymphocytes abs.	**4.10**	× 10⁹/l	1	3	3.80	4.41
Monocytes abs.	0.51	× 10⁹/l	0.2	1	0.47	0.55
Eosinophils abs.	0.34	× 10⁹/l	0.02	0.5	0.32	0.37
Basophils abs.	**0.86**	× 10⁹/l	0.02	0.1	0.79	0.92
Blasts %		%	0	0		
Promyelocytes %		%	0	0		
Myelocytes %	**1**	%	0	0		
Metamyelocytes %	**2**	%	0	0		
Band cells %	**4**	%	0	0		
Normoblasts	**2**	/100 WBC	0	0		
Platelet count	**541.0**	× 10⁹/l	150	400	486.9	595.1
Sedimentation	7	mm/h	0	20	7	7
Morphology	The red cells are normochromic and normocytic and show mild anisocytosis. The neutrophil series shows a marked left shift.					

however, has a large range of possible causes. There is inherently very little indication to do a FBC, yet without it, the investigation of a large spleen would be more or less fruitless.

This case illustrates the difficulties that can arise where all three cell lines are increased. Different patterns can occur, particularly when the rise in counts is not close to being in proportion. Depending on which line is worst affected, or indeed, as the author has seen, when the increase in one cell line is noticed and concentrated upon without noticing the rest of the picture, diagnoses such as chronic myelogenous leukemia or essential thrombocythemia can be made. In this case, it will be seen that reaching the correct diagnosis requires

1. A full understanding of what the "anatomical" diagnosis – polycythemia – **CAN** mean.
2. The importance of the clinical features in the process.
3. The importance of proceeding methodically. Specifically, when one considers the general causes, one must proceed from the anatomical diagnosis of "polycythemia" to the general possibility of "myeloproliferative disease" rather than leaping immediately to the diagnosis of PV.

Observe that

1. Again, **ALL THREE CELL LINES** are increased.
2. They are again more or less in proportion, but the WCC is suspiciously high.
3. The spleen is far too large for a typical case of PV.

WHAT CLUES CAN BE FOUND IN THE REST OF THE FBC?

1. **THE BASOPHIL COUNT** is again considerably increased. With any cythemia, a basophil leukocytosis very strongly suggests a chronic myeloproliferative disorder.
2. Of great concern is the presence of **LEUKOCYTE PRECURSORS**. This certainly can occur in PV if it is beginning to transform to myelofibrosis (and which in fact is a possibility in this case); however, the red cell morphology shows no features suggestive of myelofibrosis, and thus the left shift suggests that there is something odd.

WHAT CLUES CAN BE FOUND IN THE ROUTINE BIOCHEMICAL/SEROLOGICAL TESTS? See Table 16.8.

The uric acid and LDH are again raised, thus in favor of a chronic myeloproliferative disorder. However, the renal function is impaired, which might have relevance to the hypertension and the raised urate.

Table 16.8

	Value	Units	Reference range Low	High
S-Sodium	**134**	mmol/l	136	145
S-Chloride	108	mmol/l	98	108
S-Urea	**9.2**	mmol/l	2.1	7.1
S-Creatinine	**136**	mmol/l	62	115
S-Uric acid	**0.51**	mmol/l	0.21	0.42
S-Bilirubin (total)	21.1	μmol/l	6.8	34.2
S-ALP	98	IU/l	53	128
S-Ggt	31	IU/l	8	37
S-ALT	32	IU/l	19	40
S-AST	22	IU/l	13	32
S-LDH	**358**	IU/l	90	180
S-Osmolality	286	mmol/kg	275	295

Thus of the three general causes, dehydration can almost certainly be excluded, Cushing's is most unlikely, and so far the evidence points to a myeloproliferative condition.

WHAT CLUES CAN BE FOUND IN THE CLINICAL FEATURES?

The absence of pruritus, while fairly unusual, is by no means against the diagnosis of PV. The size of the spleen, however, is cause for concern, and two other conditions must therefore be considered in this presentation – chronic myelogenous leukemia and myelofibrosis. The hypertension probably has little or nothing to do with the blood disease.

ASSESSMENT AND FURTHER INVESTIGATION

There are a number of atypical features, mainly the size of the spleen and the abnormal WCC and differential, sufficient to reconsider one's first diagnosis. In this case a neutrophil alkaline phosphatase (NAP) test was requested, and showed a result of 0 units (normal: 15–100). Some doubt was raised by the consultant hematologist as to the accuracy of this result, since the test was done on anticoagulated blood. It was repeated on slides made from fresh blood at the bedside, and the result was 2 units. There are only two conditions that cause a decreased NAP: chronic myelogenous leukemia (CML) and paroxysmal nocturnal hemoglobinuria (PNH). PNH would not enter into the differential diagnosis of this case, and CML would have to be excluded. A bone marrow specimen for the Philadelphia chromosome was submitted, and the result was positive, and early CML was diagnosed.

It is clear that the diagnosis of the chronic myeloproliferative disorders can be difficult. They can overlap both hematologically and clinically – indeed, occasionally one must be satisfied with a diagnosis of "chronic myeloproliferative disorder – unclassified," and wait and see what develops. But it is clear that one needs to be conscious of alternative explanations for this type of case, and it is here that discrepancies in laboratory and clinical findings require careful consideration.

CASE #68 (EXAMINE TABLE 16.9)

This case illustrates another set of problems

DISCUSSION

The clinical features were strongly suggestive of Cushing syndrome. Polycythemia has traditionally been recognized as a characteristic feature. However, true polycythemia is less common than leukocytosis, which is largely neutrophilia (but remember that eosinopenia is also characteristic).

The results of adrenocortical function are shown in Table 16.10.

The features would be strongly indicative of classic Cushing syndrome, were the history not available. Chronic

Table 16.9

Patient	Age	Sex	Race	Altitude
Mrs A	49 yrs	Female	White	2,300 ft

The patient was referred by a pulmonologist for the investigation of a moderate neutrophilia. She had been in his care for 4 years for severe adult-onset asthma. She showed marked central obesity, hirsutism, violaceous striae right up to the axillae, mild hypertension, and persistent glycosuria.

	Value	Units	Reference range Low	High	Permitted range Low	High
Red cell count	**5.11**	× 10¹²/l	3.91	4.94	4.96	5.26
Hemoglobin (Hb)	**16.1**	g/dl	12.4	15.5	15.5	16.7
Hematocrit (Hct)	0.47	l/l	0.37	0.47	0.46	0.48
Mean cell volume	92	fl	80	99	90.2	93.8
Mean cell Hb	31.5	pg	27	31.5	30.9	32.1
Mean cell Hb conc.	34.2	g/dl	31.5	34.5	33.6	34.9
Red cell dist. width	13.1	%	11.6	14	13.1	13.1
Retic. count %	0.59	%	0.25	0.75	0.6	0.6
Retic. absolute (abs.)	30.1	× 10⁹/l	30	100	29.2	31.1
White cell count	**14.56**	× 10⁹/l	4	10	13.47	15.65
Neutrophils abs.	**10.48**	× 10⁹/l	2	7	9.70	11.27
Band cells abs.	0		0	0	0	0
Lymphocytes abs.	2.91	× 10⁹/l	1	3	2.69	3.13
Monocytes abs.	0.91	× 10⁹/l	0.2	1	0.81	0.94
Eosinophils abs.	**0.0**	× 10⁹/l	0.02	0.5	0.13	0.16
Basophils abs.	0.15	× 10⁹/l	0.02	0.1	0.13	0.16
Normoblasts	0	/100 WBC	0	0		
Platelet count	**449.0**	× 10⁹/l	150	400	395.1	482.9
Sedimentation	1	mm/h	0	20	1	1

Table 16.10

			Low	High
S-ACTH	0.2	ng/l	0.9	46.0
S-Cortisol	891	nmol/l	38	690

severe asthma is often treated with oral corticosteroids (as was confirmed in this patient). However, were this case one of iatrogenic Cushing's, one would expect the patient's true cortisol level to be almost undetectable (suppression by prednisone). But, depending on the method of assay, the prednisone molecule cross-reacts with cortisol in the assay, and is thus measured as cortisol. The point that is made is that iatrogenic Cushing's is also a cause of hematological cythemias.

Diagnostic Conundrums – When to Refer

1. Occasionally you will come across cases that appear not to fit into any of the categories.
2. Some cases presenting with the clinical features of PV can have very different causes.
3. Any patient who does not respond appropriately to therapy.

The larger the spleen at the time of first diagnosis, the sooner you consider CML and MF as possible causes.

Optional Advanced Reading

The Formal Definition of Polycythemia Vera

Currently, the formal criteria for the diagnosis of polycythemia vera are

1. A red cell mass more than 25% above the predicted mean normal value for the patient based on body surface area.
2. No evidence of secondary causes and oxygen saturation of over 92%.

PLUS ONE OF
3. Palpable splenomegaly.
4. Abnormal karyotype.

OR TWO OF
5. Platelet count $>400 \times 10^9/l$.
6. Absolute neutrophil count $>10 \times 10^9/l$.
7. Confirmed splenomegaly in the absence of liver disease.
8. Characteristic cell culture patterns **OR** a decreased EPO.

Further Causes of Polycythemia

There is only one other significant further cause of polycythemia (although erythrocytosis appears to be much more common) to be discussed: that due to chronically increased androgens (either iatrogenic or self-administered, or from androgen-secreting tumors).

Polycythemia vera will sometimes present with a (fairly common) complication already present, i.e., myelofibrosis. The larger the spleen, the more one should suspect myelofibrosis. Indeed, it has been said that the larger the spleen at time of presentation, the greater the chance that the disease will progress to myelofibrosis.

There is an increased tendency for arterial thrombosis in any cause of polycythemia (or erythrocytosis). One problem is that most patients present at an age when underlying arterial disease is common, and polycythemia may not be thought of. Polycythemia (and the increased viscosity that it causes) may be seen as a precipitating or contributory factor in many cases of arterial thrombosis; this is especially so when the platelet count is very high.

Arterial involvement can vary from complete occlusions of large arteries to transient episodes to non-specific cerebral symptoms (such as headaches, loss of memory, dizziness, visual disturbances, and so on), although these mild symptoms may be due to poor perfusion rather than actual obstruction. It is probable that many of the lesions are related to the raised platelet count. Micro-vascular lesions especially in the toes are suspicious of obstruction by platelet aggregates (as in essential thrombocythemia).

Venous occlusion varies from superficial to deep vein thrombosis, including splanchnic involvement.

In polycythemia vera the oxygen-carrying **CAPACITY** of the blood is basically increased (since there is more circulating hemoglobin); this causes a decrease in blood flow in the capillary beds. As a result of the raised Hct, the viscosity increases, aggravated by the decreased flow (blood being a non-Newtonian fluid). If the Hct is not too high, the two processes will cancel, and the oxygen **DELIVERY** to the tissues is probably slightly improved – unless the platelet count is very high, with the production of platelet aggregates, a known cause of micro-vascular obstruction. At very high Hcts, however, the viscosity rises so much that blood flow, and therefore tissue oxygenation, may be compromised.

The Natural History of PV (in the Absence of Thrombosis)

Generally speaking, it is estimated that by the time the diagnosis is made, the patient has had the disease for about 7 years. Once diagnosed, three phases have been recognized:

1. The proliferative phase. In this phase, phlebotomy and/or myelo-suppression is necessary. It lasts for 2–8 years. The only complications likely to be seen are thrombotic, usually in poorly managed cases.
2. The stable phase is characterized by little need for treatment, and lasts for 2–5 years. It should be seen as a transitional stage.
3. The terminal phase is characterized by the development of complications, notably myelofibrosis or a myelodysplastic syndrome.

Management Issues, Complications, and Their Effect on the FBC

Obviously the patient must be monitored frequently to keep the Hct at an acceptable level. Non-compliance can be a significant problem in these cases. Apart from this, however, there is an important aspect that needs discussion, and these are the important complications.

1. It has been indicated that the diagnosis in the classical case can be made by reference to the clinical features and those in the various blood tests. It is only when the presentation is atypical that further investigations may be needed (e.g., Philadelphia chromosome, bone marrow aspiration, biopsy, and cytogenetics).
2. Four complications must be watched for and treated; also, certain forms of treatment of the basic condition seem to be associated with certain complications, and this can influence one's choice of treatment:

   a. **TRANSFORMATION**. PV can transform into any of the chronic myeloproliferative conditions, but by far the commonest is to myelofibrosis. The latter can be a very difficult decision, and this is why various other baseline studies are necessary, particularly if the patient sees another doctor at that time. Thus, if you are going to treat the patient yourself, it is advisable to do a bone marrow aspirate, biopsy, and cytogenetic studies first – not so much to confirm the diagnosis, but to facilitate evaluation in the future if and when the patient's condition deteriorates.

   b. **TRANSFORMATION TO ACUTE LEUKEMIA** is probably no more common than found in the general population.

   c. **TENDENCY TO THROMBOSIS**, particularly arterial thrombosis. Indeed this is the largest single cause of death in these patients. They should all be on prophylactic low-dose aspirin.

   d. **HYPOXIA.** Venesection as a long-term therapy is still commonly used. One problem is that a significant number of hypochromic and microcytic cells **DECREASE** the deformability of red cells; this may interfere with proper diffusion of O_2 and thus tissue oxygenation, but the effect is probably offset by the fact that the cells are small. But a very high Hct can cause sufficient sludging to interfere with flow through the capillary beds. For this and numerous other reasons, other modalities of treatment are sometimes preferred. A further discussion of this topic is to be found below. Please do not venesect your patients without having studied this section.

Choice of Therapy

Careful interpretation of the FBC, integrated with the clinical features, is very important in assessing the choice of therapy. About 15% of patients have an abnormal karyotype at the time of diagnosis, and this too may have relevance to the choice of therapy. Any form of therapy, including venesection, appears to be associated with an increase in karyotype abnormalities, but this is particularly so with ^{32}P and cytostatic agents. The significance of these changes, however, is not clear – there is no definite evidence that these changes are associated with a greater tendency to transformation.

VENESECTION. Venesection is very effective in controlling the Hct but not the WCC or the platelet count. A raised WCC in this context is of little concern, but the platelets are significant. Venesection is always indicated:

1. In the "acute" phase, covering the patient with aspirin daily
2. With significant obstructive vascular lesions, accompanied by cytostatic therapy and aspirin
3. When urgent surgery is indicated

However, venesection is somewhat dangerous in three groups of patients:

1. The elderly. Much less blood (about half) should be removed per venesection, and then only about once every 2 weeks.
2. Any patient who weighs less than 50 kg. Again, only about half a unit should be removed, also once every 2 weeks at the most.
3. Patients who have associated severe chronic respiratory disease.

There is no clear evidence that the incidence of transformation to leukemia is increased with venesection alone as therapy.

PV is a well-known cause of the hyperviscosity syndrome. It is important that the Hct be kept below ± 50 l/l. A high Hct is in itself a well-known predisposing factor to thrombosis.

THE EFFECT ON THE FBC OF REPEATED VENESECTION. The typical effect of repeated venesection has already been shown.

CYTOSTATICS. Apart from their use as indicated above, there is a particular concern with the raised platelet count, particularly if moderately or markedly high, as an independent cause of vascular obstruction. It has already been noted that venesection does not affect the platelet count, and therapy with **HYDROXYUREA** (a commonly used agent) is not always successful in controlling the platelets. The platelet count can be successfully treated with:

1. **BUSULPHAN** (myeleran). **IN GENERAL THE USE OF BUSULPHAN IS DISCOURAGED** (complications include pulmonary fibrosis and an increased incidence of acute leukemia), but it is very effective in controlling the platelet count, and most importantly, once the count is well within the reference range, the dosage required drops dramatically and is generally then only required intermittently. At this dosage, leukemic transformation is only slightly higher than is found with venesection.

2. α-**INTERFERON**. There is no increased incidence of leukemic transformation.

3. **ANAGRELIDE**. The mechanism of its thrombocytopenic effect is not known.

4. High-dosage **CHLORAMBUCIL**.

The above drugs have no significant effect on the cell morphology.

HYDROXYUREA. This has become a mainstay of therapy. There is only a minimal increase in leukemic transformation. It has a significant and potentially confusing effect on the FBC:

The action of hydroxyurea is to inhibit DNA synthesis. Regular use therefore causes the red cells to become macrocytic, relatively unresponsive to folate. This is not a contra-indication to its use. (Increases in the transaminase levels to over twice normal are by contrast an indication to decrease or stop therapy.)

^{32}**PHOSPHORUS.** This is very effective but the incidence of leukemic transformation is about 10% higher than with venesection alone (although this has recently been disputed as being exaggerated). Its use is generally therefore limited to the older patients. It has no significant effect on cell morphology.

ASPIRIN. In low doses (100 mg/day), this is of great value in the early stages of therapy, whilst waiting for specific treatment to reduce the counts. It is claimed that the incidence of gastro-intestinal bleeding is 1.3 times the normal. Higher dosage, however, particularly combined with dipyrimadole, has a significant incidence of hemorrhage.

Exercise Cases

CASE #69 (TABLE 16.11)

Table 16.11

Patient	Age	Sex	Race	Altitude
Mr Q R	52 yrs	Male	Black	2,500 ft

The patient is a wealthy owner of a fleet of taxis. He presented acutely with severe pain in the left leg to a rural family doctor. The leg was found to be cold. The femoral pulse was present but the popliteal and posterior tibial pulses were absent. The provisional diagnosis was made of arterial thromboembolic disease. The other pulses were present and regular, but he noted that the left radial pulse was slightly delayed behind the right; there was very severe arcus senilis. The doctor decided provisionally that this was thrombotic rather than embolic. He also noted that the patient appeared plethoric. The blood pressure was normal and there was no splenomegaly. He gave the patient morphine, put up a heparin drip, and arranged urgently for transport. He drew blood for an urgent FBC and sent the patient to a surgeon in the city, 3 h away.

	Value	Units	Reference range Low	Reference range High	Permitted range Low	Permitted range High
Red cell count	**6.74**	$\times 10^{12}/l$	4.64	5.67	6.54	6.94
Hemoglobin (Hb)	**20.3**	g/dl	13.4	17.5	19.6	21.0
Hematocrit (Hct)	**0.59**	l/l	0.41	0.52	0.58	0.61
Mean cell volume	88	fl	80	99	86.2	89.8
Mean cell Hb	30.1	pg	27	31.5	29.5	30.7
Mean cell Hb conc.	34.2	g/dl	31.5	34.5	33.5	34.9
White cell count	**12.6**	$\times 10^9/l$	3.5	10	11.66	13.55
Neutrophils abs.	**9.95**	$\times 10^9/l$	1.5	7	9.21	10.70
Lymphocytes abs.	1.39	$\times 10^9/l$	1	3	1.28	1.49
Monocytes abs.	0.38	$\times 10^9/l$	0.2	1	0.35	0.41
Eosinophils abs.	0.25	$\times 10^9/l$	0.02	0.5	0.23	0.27
Basophils abs.	**0.63**	$\times 10^9/l$	0.02	0.1	0.58	0.68
Normoblasts	0	/100 WBC	0	0		
Platelet count	**479.0**	$\times 10^9/l$	150	400	431.1	526.9
Sedimentation	0	mm/h	0	10	0	0

Questions

1. From the hematological point of view, what is the "anatomical" diagnosis?

2. What is the probable general pathology diagnosis?

3. Why do you say this?

4. What is the special pathology (specific) diagnosis?

5. What other laboratory test result would you expect to be positive or abnormal?

6. What do you expect the erythropoietin result to be?

7. With which complication did the patient present?

8. Is this an unusual way of presentation?

9. Are the absence of splenomegaly and hypertension against the diagnosis of PV?

10. The patient had to be transported several hundred kilometers to a city. How would this affect subsequent management and what could the doctor do to minimize these problems?

Answers

1. Polycythemia. All three cell lines are clearly raised, and more or less in proportion.
2. Chronic myeloproliferative disease.
3. First, the prominent basophil leukocytosis; second, he presented with arterial thromboembolism; third, basophilic leukocytosis.
4. Polycythemia vera.
5. LDH and urate are typically raised.
6. Normal or below normal.
7. Arterial thrombosis.
8. No – indeed it is the largest single cause of death in PV.
9. Hypertension and splenomegaly have traditionally been regarded as characteristic of PV. Detailed investigations have shown that, while these are fairly common, they are by no means typical.
10. The important issue with respect to the FBC is in terms of prevention of further episodes. It frequently happens that patients in otherwise good health when requiring urgent surgery do not have a FBC done, or if so, only anemias are taken note of.

Subsequent Course

An urgent arterial bypass was performed and the leg saved. Arteriography revealed extensive calcific atheromatous lesions throughout the lower half of the body. The PV was treated successfully with hydroxyurea and low-dose busulphan (for the platelets) and the usual therapy for widespread atheromatosis was instituted.

Comments

Plethora can be difficult to assess in the Black skin. One needs a high index of suspicion. The clinical expertise of the family doctor in noticing the plethora is to be commended, since otherwise the PV would possibly not have been treated, exposing the patient to further episodes.

The role of thrombocytosis as part of polycythemia vera in the pathogenesis of arterial thrombosis is not clear. The incidence of thrombosis appears to be as high in those cases that do not have thrombocythemia.

Arterial thrombosis can occur without significant atheroma, but clearly the presence of atheromatosis will predispose to a much greater incidence.

CASE #70 (EXAMINE TABLE 16.12)

SUMMARY OF BONE MARROW ASPIRATE REPORT (requested by the referring physician; the aspiration and report were done by a laboratory):

Satisfactory aspirate.
Normo- to slightly hypercellular.
Megakaryocytes and platelets normal. ME ratio = 1.5:1
Erythropoiesis normoblastic.
Granulopoiesis and other cells normal.
Iron stain: no stainable iron present.

Questions

1. The RCC, Hct, WCC and differential, and platelet count are all completely normal. Do you think the original diagnosis could have been wrong?

2. If not, what features support the diagnosis?

3. What is your opinion of the marked macrocytosis?

4. The RDW is moderately raised, unusual in a polycythemia vera. What can this possibly mean?

5. There is no stainable iron in the marrow, yet the ferritin levels are raised. What could this mean?

Table 16.12

Patient	Age	Sex	Race	Altitude
Mrs B G	62 yrs	Female	White	5,000 ft

She had been diagnosed with PV 9 years previously. Her treatment for 4 years had been regular venesection. Her presenting symptoms had been regular transient ischemic episodes, and these had persisted despite this treatment. No FBCs from that period are available, and thus no idea of the control of the PV achieved is possible. She was then referred to another center where she was given ^{32}P. She was also found to be hypothyroid and thyroxine was prescribed. The ^{32}P controlled her counts well for a year and then she relapsed and was placed on hydroxyurea. She then moved to this city. She was found to be obese and clinically euthyroid; the BP was 142/94. The TIA's were as prominent as before. Neurological opinion in summary follows: the attacks occurred once to three times a day, characterized by occurring only in the erect position; bilateral blurring of vision and diplopia; dizziness. They last for 1–3 min.

	Value	Units	Reference range Low	Reference range High	Permitted range Low	Permitted range High
Red cell count	3.78	× 10^{12}/l	4.03	5.09	3.67	3.89
Hemoglobin (Hb)	14.1	g/dl	12.7	15.9	13.6	14.6
Hematocrit (Hct)	0.46	l/l	0.38	0.49	0.44	0.47
Mean cell volume	**121**	fl	80	99	118.6	123.4
Mean cell Hb	**37.3**	pg	27	31.5	36.6	38.0
Mean cell Hb conc.	30.8	g/dl	31.5	34.5	30.2	31.4
Red cell dist. width	**16.8**	%	11.6	14	16.7	16.9
White cell count	6.67	× 10^9/l	4	10	6.17	7.17
Neutrophils abs.	4.64	× 10^9/l	2	7	4.29	4.98
Lymphocytes abs.	1.52	× 10^9/l	1	3	1.41	1.63
Monocytes abs.	0.25	× 10^9/l	0.2	1	0.23	0.27
Eosinophils abs.	0.17	× 10^9/l	0.02	0.5	0.16	0.19
Basophils abs.	0.09	× 10^9/l	0.02	0.1	0.09	0.10
Normoblasts	0	/100 WBC	0	0		
Platelet count	241.0	× 10^9/l	150	400	216.9	265.1

	Value	Units	Reference range Low	Reference range High
S-Uric acid	0.39	mmol/l	0.21	0.42
S-LDH	**852**	IU/l	266	500
S-Total cholesterol	6	mmol/l		<5.2
S-Ferritin female	261.7	µg/l	14.0	233.1
S-Vitamin B$_{12}$	341	pg/ml	193	982
S-Folate	2.7	ng/ml	3.0	17.0
RBC-folate	154.6	ng/ml	93.0	641.0
S-T4	11.8	pmol/l	9.1	23.8
S-TSH	4.19	mIU/l	0.49	4.67
C-reactive protein	<5.0	mg/l	0.0	10.0

6. What would you think of the mildly raised ferritin levels?

_____

_____

7. The consultant neurologist was struck by the fact that all TIAs of this patient were clinically identical. What do you think this could mean?

_____

_____

_____

Answers

1. The only finding that gives one pause is the normal red cell count. An associated pathology is thus possible.

2. The following are very suggestive that the basic diagnosis was correct:

   a. The clinical history and response to therapy.
   b. The raised LDH.
   c. The TIA's.

3. It is well known that hydroxyurea causes a moderate rise in the MCV – indeed, it is used as a marker for compliance with therapy. However, the MCV in this case is higher than usually found. This may in part be due to the contribution made to the MCV by the hypothyroidism, except that she is euthyroid at present. The possibility exists that she has an associated folate deficiency; it would be wise to exclude this, since she would feel a great deal better if such existed and it were treated properly. A dietary history should be obtained.

4. As has been mentioned, a common complication of P. vera is transformation to myelofibrosis. If this were the case here, it would be very early indeed, and would require only observation. Somewhat more likely, however, is that the patient does indeed have a mild folate deficiency.

5. This is a very common finding in P. vera. Iron stores are in fact usually normal. It is thought that the very rapid turnover of red cells in the marrow is such that the iron in the sideroblasts is removed very quickly. This is probably not the whole story, however, since in this condition the cell turnover is probably not a great deal higher than normal.

6. The ferritin levels in this patient are not very elevated. They may reflect a number of phenomena:

   a. The residua of past transfusions (before the polycythemia developed).
   b. An early manifestation of hemochromatosis.
   c. A feature of chronic disease. In the presence of polycythemia, the typical picture of anemia of chronic disorders would of course not be obvious.
   d. Raised ferritin levels are discussed in greater detail in Chapter 20.

7. As was explained in Chapter 4, TIA's are the result in most cases of small emboli arising from the heart or great arteries above the heart, and lodging either in the vertebro-basilar or the internal carotid systems. While the attacks from vertebro-basilar embolization show considerable clinical variation in any one patient, those in the carotid system tend always to show the same pattern. This distinction is of value in various ways, but mainly to suggest where to look for the primary thrombosis. There are also some prognostic implications.

Further Reading

Andreoli TE, Bennett JC, Carpenter CCJ, Plum F (eds) (1997). Cecil Essentials of Medicine. 4th edn. Philadelphia: WB Saunders Company.

Epstein RJ (1996). Medicine for Examinations. 3rd edn. Churchill Livingstone.

Hoffbrand AV, Pettit JE (2001). Essential Haematology. 4th edn. Oxford: Blackwell Science.

Lewis SM, Bain B, Bates I (2006) Dacie and Lewis Practical Haematology. 10th edn. Churchill Livingstone.

Erythrocytosis

17

Defining Erythrocytosis

Strictly speaking, this term refers to an increase in the concentration of red cells, i.e., the RCC. Indeed, if asked in an examination to discuss causes of erythrocytosis, it is perfectly legitimate to discuss the erythrocytosis of thalassemia. However, the clinical content of this chapter is essentially to do with the **RAISED HEMATOCRIT,** which here is the focus and core problem we would identify in a FBC (i.e., the anatomical diagnosis). The pathophysiological mechanisms of the raised hematocrit have been discussed in Chapter 4.

- **STEP 1**: "Where is the abnormality and what form does it take?" The abnormality is an isolated increase, beyond the reference range for that sex and altitude, in the hematocrit.
- **STEP 2:** "Is the rest of the FBC more or less normal?" If the answer is "yes," one can state the anatomical diagnosis as "**ERYTHROCYTOSIS.**"

!

THERE ARE ONLY FOUR GENERAL CAUSES OF SIGNIFICANCE:

1. **DEHYDRATION.** This may be acute or chronic
2. **HYPOXIA**
3. **INAPPROPRIATE** (autonomous) **SECRETION OF ERYTHROPOIETIN** (EPO)
4. **CHRONIC MYELOPROLIFERATIVE DISEASE**

However, it must be stressed that a small percentage of cases remain very difficult to diagnose, even with sophisticated techniques, and one here adopts a wait-and-see attitude (plus, of course, symptomatic therapy). It is probably wise to refer these cases.

ALTHOUGH THE HCT, THE RCC, AND THE HB ARE OFTEN ALL RAISED, WE FOCUS ON AN INCREASE IN HCT, WHETHER OR NOT THERE IS A CONCOMITANT INCREASE IN RCC.

Dehydration

The pathophysiology of acute dehydration has been discussed in Chapter 4.

Gaisbock Syndrome, Often Known as Apparent Erythrocytosis (and Previously Called Stress Polycythemia)

!

This is a strange condition (and not at all uncommon). In most cases there appears to be a gradual reduction in plasma volume, causing hemo-concentration, until the viscosity reaches such a level that symptoms occur. Some workers have found, in addition, an expanded red cell volume in some cases. The condition is therefore probably not homogeneous. The mechanism in general is obscure.

Loss of plasma water presumably is mediated by blockage of the ADH secretion or its effect, but atrial natriuretic peptide or even the renin-angiotensin system could be involved. Interestingly, serum biochemical results are not very helpful in most cases. Logically, it would seem that the best way to definitively diagnose the condition is with blood volume studies; unfortunately these are often equivocal: the total red cell volume can become absolutely **INCREASED,** but not enough to offset the decrease in plasma volume. Very careful studies have shown that in ± 50% of cases, the red cell volume is at or near the upper limit of normal and the plasma

O.N. Beck, *Diagnostic Hematology*, DOI 10.1007/978-1-84800-295-1_17,
© Springer-Verlag London Limited 2009

volume is at or near the lower limit of normal; the two results in combination are sufficient to reflect **APPARENT (ACTUALLY A RELATIVE)** hemo-concentration.

For the sake of simplicity, however, at the general level, the pathogenesis is assumed to be a form of chronic dehydration. If the symptoms and signs of hyperviscosity are severe it is advisable to venesect the patient. However, this is only an emergency measure. The proper treatment, once the diagnosis is made (and this is often very difficult), is lifestyle management to control stress, stopping smoking, and avoiding diuretics of any kind, including alcohol. Practically speaking, if no other cause can be found, it is wise to institute lifestyle changes anyway and see the result. Gaisbock syndrome is characterized by the following:

FBC FEATURES (very similar to those of ordinary dehydration):

1. Increased Hct and Hb, and usually increased RCC. The reticulocyte count is normal. The ESR is normal unless there is an associated infective or infiltrative disorder.
2. The PC and WCC are normal.

FEATURES IN OTHER LABORATORY TESTS:

1. The LDH, urate, and EPO are normal.
2. Osmolality may be somewhat increased, but results of biochemicals like Na^{1+}, Cl^{1-}, urea, creatinine, plasma proteins are seldom helpful.

COMMON CLINICAL ACCOMPANIMENTS (very different from ordinary dehydration):

1. Plethoric, stressed facies
2. Often mild hypertension, probably as a result of stress

Sometimes blood volume studies are decisive; however, for various reasons these can be disappointing. Where the plasma volume is unquestionably decreased in the face of a normal red cell volume, the diagnosis should be clear – assuming that acute dehydration has been excluded.

Hypoxia

In contrast to polycythemia vera patients, those with **ERYTHROCYTOSIS CAUSED BY TISSUE HYPOXIA** usually benefit from a raised Hct (up to the point of clinical sludging or cyanosis, usually when the Hct goes above 55–60 l/l). We distinguish between **HYPOXEMIA AND HYPOXIA.**

HYPOXEMIA essentially means reduced arterial oxygen saturation (although strictly speaking it means reduced oxygen **CONTENT**); thus oxygen transport (i.e., the **AMOUNT** of oxygen carried per unit volume of blood per unit time) is lower for a given Hct than with a normal saturation. Thus **IT IS CHARACTERIZED BY DECREASED Pao_2.** It does **NOT** necessarily mean that tissue oxygenation is decreased (and that therefore EPO secretion would tend to increase in compensation). It is clear that the characteristics of the blood gas studies are very important in identifying the type of hypoxemia. The important causes of **HYPOXEMIA** (i.e., decreased Pao_2 at rest without inhaling pure oxygen) that may be **ASSOCIATED WITH ERYTHROCYTOSIS** are as follows:

1. **SHUNTING** of venous blood to the arterial system. The resulting admixture of blood with that of a low Pao_2 effectively dilutes the arterial oxygen content. The causes of such shunting in brief are:

   a. **CHRONIC LUNG DISEASES CAUSING VENTILATION/PERFUSION (V/Q) DEFECTS;** essentially some parts of the lungs are being perfused and not ventilated and others ventilated but not perfused. Thus a proportion of right ventricular blood effectively bypasses the lungs and goes directly to the left atrium. The **BLOOD GAS PICTURE** shows decreased Pao_2 that normalizes on 100% oxygen; low or normal $PaCo_2$ until it becomes severe. Note that **ACUTE SEVERE V/Q DEFECTS** (type 1 respiratory failure), e.g., ARDS, will **NOT** be associated with erythrocytosis, since it (erythrocytosis) takes time (months) to develop.

   b. **RIGHT-TO-LEFT INTRA-PULMONARY SHUNTS.** An example would be intra-pulmonary A-V fistulae; the commonest cause however is **SEVERE** V/Q mismatch, such that significant amounts of venous blood go directly into the arterial system. The blood gas picture shows decreased Pao_2 that does not normalize on 100% oxygen and normal $PaCo_2$.

   c. **RIGHT-TO-LEFT INTRA-CARDIAC SHUNTS,** such as Fallot's tetralogy, the Eisenmenger complex, etc. The blood gas picture is much as with b. above.

   d. Very occasionally, large **ARTERIOVENOUS FISTULAE,** again very much like b. above.

2. Predominantly **VENTILATORY DISORDERS,** such as chest wall deformities, high altitude, sedative overdose, morbid obesity. The blood gas picture shows decreased Pao_2 that normalizes on 100% oxygen as well as raised $PaCo_2$.

3. There is a subcategory called the sleep apnea syndromes, and which probably include what used to be known as the Pickwickian syndrome (i.e., the daytime sleepiness, erythrocytosis and cyanosis of gross obesity). This is discussed further in the Optional Advanced Reading section.

Note that pure diffusion defects do not ordinarily lead to erythrocytosis since the Pao_2 is normal or only slightly decreased. It decreases markedly however with exercise. Thus, where there is defective diffusion as an **ELEMENT** of any of the disease processes mentioned under 1 and 2, exercise will tend to decrease the Pao_2 even further.

HYPOXIA refers to the state of **EFFECTIVE** oxygenation of the tissues. It does not necessarily imply hypoxemia.

The important causes of **TISSUE HYPOXIA IN THE FACE OF A NORMAL Pao_2** can be grouped as follows:

1. **SEVERE POLYCYTHEMIA AND OTHER CAUSES OF IMPAIRED MICRO-CIRCULATION** or defective transport of oxygen from capillaries to tissues. This includes the hyperviscosity syndromes.
2. **SEVERE ANEMIA.**
3. **CAUSES OF INCREASED OXYGEN AFFINITY.**

   a. **TREATMENT OF KETO-ACIDOSIS** with insulin and large amounts of HCO_3^{2-}.
   b. **HIGH-AFFINITY HEMOGLOBINS.** These are rare and typically present in childhood, but occasionally one is surprised.
   c. **MASSIVE TRANSFUSION.**
   d. **MISCELLANEOUS.** Severe hypothermia, acidemia due to other causes, hypophosphatemia, myxedema.

These topics have been discussed at reasonable length, since the role of **HEMOGLOBIN** is critical in this regard. It may be worthwhile to reread the section on adaptation to hypoxia in Chapter 4. An essential point here is that EPO secretion and consequently reticulocytosis, in response to hypoxia, are intermittent reactions. **EPO LEVELS AND THE RETIC COUNT CAN BE NORMAL IN HYPOXIA.**

HYPOXIC ERYTHROCYTOSIS IS CHARACTERIZED BY

FBC FEATURES:

1. Increased Hct and Hb, and usually increased RCC.
2. The presence of "diffuse basophilia" in the morphological comment and a raised reticulocyte count will be very suggestive indeed. However, the retic count may be normal since EPO secretion is intermittent.
3. The RDW is usually normal.

4. The ESR is normal – indeed, may be very low, such as 0 mm/h.
5. The PC and WCC are normal.

FEATURES IN OTHER LABORATORY TESTS:

1. The LDH and urate are normal.
2. EPO is intermittently increased.
3. The effects of hemo-concentration will particularly affect results like urea, creatinine, osmolality, and plasma proteins.
4. Lung function tests will indicate disorders that may be responsible.

COMMON CLINICAL ACCOMPANIMENTS:

1. **A TENDENCY TO CENTRAL CYANOSIS.** Note however that central cyanosis does not necessarily mean hypoxia; from our point of view, the only important cause of central cyanosis is the one associated with erythrocytosis – see box.
2. **OTHERWISE** the clinical features very much depend on the underlying cause.

There is no routine specific confirmatory test, although serum and urine osmolality come close. The stronger the circumstantial evidence, the more likely is the diagnosis.

The Clinical Significance of Central Cyanosis
From our point of view, central cyanosis can be divided into those with and those without erythrocytosis.
Central cyanosis associated with erythrocytosis. These cases all have a decreased Pao_2:

1. Type I respiratory failure (severe V/Q mismatch)
2. Type II respiratory failure (alveolar hypoventilation)
3. Right-to-left shunts

Central cyanosis not associated with erythrocytosis. Here the Pao_2 is normal:

1. Mechanical obstruction, e.g., superior vena caval obstruction
2. Low-affinity hemoglobins, e.g., Hb Hammersmith
3. Pseudocyanosis, as found in methemoglobinemia

SMOKER'S ERYTHROCYTOSIS. Most smokers tend eventually to develop a degree of hypoxia. It is frequently assumed that this is due to the formation of carboxyhemoglobin; in fact this is at most only a small contributory cause. Other mechanisms are more complex, and are discussed in the Optional Advanced Reading section.

Inappropriate Secretion of Erythropoietin

There are a number of tumorous conditions where the level of circulating EPO is much increased, the best known being

1. Several kidney diseases – the commonest causes:

   a. Carcinoma
   b. Polycystic disease
   c. Obstructive nephropathy, including unilateral cases

2. Hepatic adenoma and carcinoma (uncommonly)
3. Uterine myomata (rarely)
4. Small cell carcinoma of the lung (extremely rarely)
5. Cerebellar hemangioblastoma (a very rare condition)

Early Polycythemia Vera

This can be a difficult clinical problem when presenting only as an erythrocytosis. The approach is essentially that as described in Chapter 16.

Making the Diagnosis

AGAIN, THE FIRST AND MOST CRUCIAL DECISION TO BE MADE IS WHETHER THE INCREASE IN CELL COUNTS IS A TRUE INCREASE OR THE RESULT OF DEHYDRATION. The correct diagnosis is critical since a great deal of time and money can be wasted in unnecessary investigations.

CLINICALLY, DEHYDRATION is generally (but need not be) obvious, among the first features that are noticed, and subsequent tests would merely confirm the dehydration and particularly its degree. Excluding dehydration must be one's first consideration, since otherwise unnecessary tests will be done, time will be wasted, and treatment is easy and definitive. This is not always as easy as it sounds. That is to say, if dehydration is not obvious, it should nevertheless be kept in the back of one's mind while other possibilities are explored. A very important cause here is third-space

losses which are not always clinically apparent. Note that there are undoubtedly cases where there is no clear history of a cause of dehydration, such as diarrhea and vomiting, and showing erythrocytosis and normal routine biochemical tests; the erythrocytosis resolves after increasing the fluid intake. Thus, one should always be cautious, and adopt a wait-and-see attitude where this is feasible.

In most cases, the diagnosis of HYPOXIA is not a problem. The presence of CYANOSIS is clearly suggestive, but not all cyanotic conditions are associated with erythrocytosis, such as in acute chest disease, asthma, methemoglobinemia, and nor are all cases of chronic chest disease causing erythrocytosis cyanotic at rest. Certain chronic lung disorders are common, and one cannot assume that they are causing hypoxia. Also, polycythemia vera itself can cause chest symptoms (due to increased work of the heart and sludging in pulmonary capillaries (pulmonary capillaries are wider than in the rest of the body, so the polycythemia must be severe to cause this; by the same token, one would expect to find some evidence of peripheral micro-vascular insufficiency). Otherwise the clinical features are usually obvious, i.e., chronic chest disease (primarily the "blue bloater"), and cyanotic congenital heart disease. However, if the chest is clinically clear, moves well, and the peak flow is normal, it is probably sufficient for the exclusion of hypoxia (of pulmonary origin). The sleep apnea/Pickwickian syndrome spectrum can be recognized fairly easily.

The clinical features of early POLYCYTHEMIA VERA are sometimes very suggestive; however, this is never enough to make the diagnosis, particularly in the present case where there is only an erythrocytosis.

The clinical features of GAISBOCK SYNDROME are too vague and open to other interpretations to allow the diagnosis without considerable further investigation. Stressful lifestyles are too common to be relied upon diagnostically.

It is only very occasionally that clinical features would point one directly to INAPPROPRIATE SECRETION OF EPO. Thus, IN A PLETHORIC PATIENT, the following should at least alert one to the possibility of the following:

1. A mass in the loin, perhaps with hematuria or even renal colic.
2. An enlarged nodular liver, with or without jaundice.
3. Clinically enlargement of one or both kidneys due to obstructive uropathy.
4. Prominent cerebellar signs.
5. Uterine myomata.
6. Very rarely indeed, the various features that can suggest carcinoma of the lung.

Figure 17.1 offers suggestions on **SPECIFIC ASPECTS** of the examination of a patient suspected or known to have a raised hematocrit. In the case where it is only suspected, this must include the possibility of PV; it is therefore included. Obvious triggers would include plethora, aquagenic pruritis. Clearly the schema presented is part of the overall examination is as is depicted in Fig. 5.4.

Note that there are algorithms that suggest that the first investigation to request in patients with erythrocytosis is blood and plasma volume studies. This cannot be endorsed: in most cases of acute dehydration their exclusion should not be difficult after a thorough clinical evaluation; in the case of suspected Gaisbock syndrome, these studies are too frequently ambiguous. If difficulty is experienced, or you suspect something other than these conditions, the patient should be referred.

Frequently the clinical features are basically unhelpful, and one relies heavily on the FBC (as a start). It is in these cases that blood volume studies may be indicated, although the results, as stated, may be ambiguous.

In practice, the problem resolves itself (i.e., in these circumstances, where the clinical features are inconclusive) into the **DIFFERENTIATION OF GAISBOCK SYNDROME, HYPOXIA, INAPPROPRIATE SECRETION OF EPO, AND EARLY POLYCYTHEMIA VERA.** The problems with each of these have been mentioned. The initial tests recommended in this type of situation are: the FBC, liver functions, urinalysis, blood gas analysis, EPO levels, and lung functions (and radiology).

FEATURES IN THE FBC THAT CAN ASSIST IN THE DIFFERENTIATION:

1. **DIFFUSE BASOPHILIA** (or reticulocytosis) would strongly favor hypoxia.
2. **BASOPHIL LEUKOCYTOSIS** would strongly favor early polycythemia vera.
3. A **HIGH RDW** could suggest a malignant circulation, especially if morphological comment indicated fragmented and burr cells.

FEATURES IN THE LIVER FUNCTIONS THAT CAN ASSIST IN THE DIFFERENTIATION:

1. These can be very deranged in cases of an EPO secreting carcinoma, or secondaries from the kidney.
2. Non-specific mild derangements are common in erythrocytosis.
3. Alcohol abuse in the case of Gaisbock syndrome may be evident.

FEATURES IN THE URINALYSIS THAT CAN ASSIST IN THE DIFFERENTIATION:

1. Hematuria or malignant cells may be found in the case of renal carcinoma.
2. Abnormal bile pigment patterns may be seen in liver disease.

FEATURES IN THE BLOOD GAS ANALYSIS THAT CAN ASSIST IN THE DIFFERENTIATION:

Hypoxemia will be in keeping with a hypoxic cause of the erythrocytosis.

FEATURES IN THE LUNG FUNCTIONS THAT CAN ASSIST IN THE DIFFERENTIATION:

The various patterns and their severity are beyond the scope of this book. They must be integrated with the blood gas analysis.

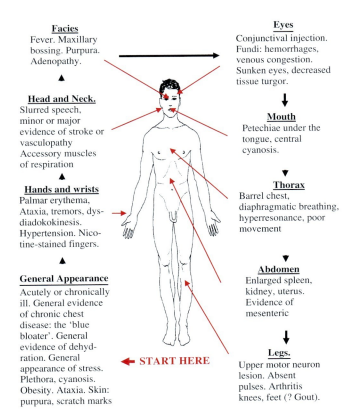

Facies
Fever. Maxillary bossing. Purpura. Adenopathy.

Head and Neck.
Slurred speech, minor or major evidence of stroke or vasculopathy Accessory muscles of respiration

Hands and wrists
Palmar erythema, Ataxia, tremors, dysdiadokokinesis. Hypertension. Nicotine-stained fingers.

General Appearance
Acutely or chronically ill. General evidence of chronic chest disease: the 'blue bloater'. General evidence of dehydration. General appearance of stress. Plethora, cyanosis. Obesity. Ataxia. Skin: purpura, scratch marks

← START HERE

Eyes
Conjunctival injection. Fundi: hemorrhages, venous congestion. Sunken eyes, decreased tissue turgor.

Mouth
Petechiae under the tongue, central cyanosis.

Thorax
Barrel chest, diaphragmatic breathing, hyperresonance, poor movement

Abdomen
Enlarged spleen, kidney, uterus. Evidence of mesenteric

Legs.
Upper motor neuron lesion. Absent pulses. Arthritis knees, feet (? Gout).

Fig. 17.1 The Patient with Plethora or Raised Hematocrit

EPO Levels

A clearly raised level is indicative of either hypoxia or inappropriate secretion, and will thus point one in those directions. A normal EPO does not exclude hypoxic causes.

The exclusion of cardio-pulmonary causes and inappropriate secretion of EPO are usually easy to exclude by the above process. **IN PRACTICE, THE MOST DIFFICULT CHOICE TO MAKE IS BETWEEN EARLY POLYCYTHEMIA AND GAISBOCK'S SYNDROME** (there is also an unusual and strange condition called idiopathic erythrocytosis. The nature of this condition is not understood; it may be a variant of PV. It is briefly discussed in the Optional Advanced Reading section). In these cases, one is forced to consider plasma volume studies; however, these may be very difficult to get done. It is quite acceptable in this case to treat the patient for Gaisbock and wait and see (with the obvious proviso that there is no evidence of arterial (or venous) thrombosis). Note that the Hct in Gaisbock syndrome can be quite markedly raised and may require venesection as an acute measure.

addition, the small possibility exists that you are dealing with multiple pathologies, particularly pure erythrocytosis plus other causes of leukocytosis and thrombocytosis, such as infection, bleeding, infiltration. Thus, the investigations discussed in the relevant chapters may also be necessary. Thus,

1. Blood and urine osmolality and Na^{1+}, urea, and creatinine
2. Erythropoietin, cortisol, and ACTH
3. Lung function tests and blood gas studies – Pa_{O_2}, Sa_{O_2}, Pc_{O_2}, etc.
4. Bone marrow biopsy and cytogenetics
5. Blood volume studies
6. P_{50} of the oxygen-dissociation curve
7. Sonographic and radiological studies for tumors, etc.

!

A Practical Summary of the Diagnostic Approach

If the clinical features suggest acute dehydration: Confirm or exclude with biochemical tests, i.e., Na^{1+} and osmolality in blood and urine; blood urea and creatinine; blood volume studies only as a last resort.

If the clinical features suggest hypoxia. Confirm or exclude with radiology of the chest, lung functions, blood gases.

If the clinical features suggest Gaisbock syndrome. Try to confirm or exclude with blood volume studies if seriously uncertain.

If the clinical features suggest inappropriate EPO production. Confirm or exclude with EPO levels, clinical and radiological evidence of neoplastic and related causes.

If the clinical features suggest high-affinity hemoglobin (commencing in childhood, family history). Confirm or exclude with Hb electrophoresis and P_{50} of the oxygen-dissociation curve.

If the clinical and FBC features are compatible with PV (i.e., clinical features or complications as above, basophil leukocytosis, raised LDH). No specific confirmatory features exist. Diagnosis strengthened by low-normal EPO, typical features on bone marrow biopsy, and cytogenetics.

If the clinical and FBC features are completely non-contributory. The whole gamut of investigations as discussed above will be necessary. In

Teaching Cases

CASE #71 (EXAMINE TABLE 17.1)

DISCUSSION

There should be no problem with the **ANATOMICAL DIAGNOSIS**, i.e., **ERYTHROCYTOSIS.** The **RCC**, the **HB,** and the **HCT** are all markedly raised. This case illustrates why the clinical features should always be integrated with the laboratory findings. Thus, while the general causes should all be considered, i.e., chronic hypoxia, Gaisbock syndrome, inappropriate secretion of EPO, or early polycythemia, the clinical features are so overwhelmingly those of dehydration that this must be the first consideration. Hemo-concentration occurs very rapidly in extensive second-degree burns and the Hct can reach 55 in an hour. (This is not the case with third-degree burns, where eschar formation tends to limit exudation.) The dehydration can also be seen in many of the biochemistry results (Table 5.2). Note that as a matter of interest, this patient could easily have presented with **POLYCYTHEMIA.**

These patients require huge amounts of crystalloid replacement. The patient was handled properly. She stabilized and the hematological and biochemical results rapidly returned to normal. On the third day, however, she deteriorated and developed toxic shock syndrome and was transferred to an ICU in the city. The subsequent course is discussed in Chapter 23.

Table 17.1

Patient	Age	Sex	Race	Altitude
Mrs DT	43 yrs	Female	White	2,200 ft

The patient suffered 40% second-degree burns after an accident on the farm. The following is her FBC 90 min later, upon admission to a rural facility (with a level 1 laboratory).

	Value	Units	Reference range Low	High	Permitted range Low	High
Red cell count	6.41	$\times 10^{12}/l$	3.91	4.94		
Hemoglobin (Hb)	18.9	g/dl	12.4	15.5		
Hematocrit (Hct)	0.54	l/l	0.37	0.47		
Mean cell volume	84	fl	80	99		
Mean cell Hb	29.5	pg	27	31.5		
Mean cell Hb conc.	35.1	g/dl	31.5	34.5		
Retic count	0.71	%	0.25	0.75		
Retic absolute (abs.)	45.5	$\times 10^9/l$	30	100		
White cell count	10.7	$\times 10^9/l$	4	11		
Neutrophils abs.	7.60	$\times 10^9/l$	2	7		
Band cells abs.	0.11	$\times 10^9/l$	0	0		
Lymphocytes abs.	2.14	$\times 10^9/l$	1	3		
Monocytes abs.	0.86	$\times 10^9/l$	0.2	1		
Eosinophils abs.	0.00	$\times 10^9/l$	0.02	0.5		
Basophils abs.	0.00	$\times 10^9/l$	0.02	0.1		
Normoblasts	0	/100 WBC	0	0		
Platelet count	401.0	$\times 10^9/l$	150	400		
Sedimentation	10	mm/h	0	20		

The biochemical results of the above patient on admission are shown in Table 17.2. They clearly confirm the dehydration.

Table 17.2

	Value	Units	Reference range Low	High
S-Urea	8.3	mmol/l	2.1	7.1
S-Creatinine	120	mmol/l	62	115
S-Sodium	151	mmol/l	136	145
S-Potassium	5.1	mmol/l	3.5	5.1
S-Chloride	111	mmol/l	98	108
S-Total CO$_2$	21	mmol/l	22	28
S-Anion gap	23.1	mmol/l	5	14
S-Glucose	6.2	mmol/l	3.9	5.8
S-Osmolarity	303	mmol/l	275	295
S-Uric acid	0.42	mmol/l	0.21	0.42
S-Calcium (total)	2.51	mmol/l	2.2	2.55
S-Magnesium	1.14	mmol/l	0.66	1.07
S-Protein (total)	71	g/l	64	83

CASE #72 (TABLE 17.3)

Table 17.3

Patient	Age	Sex	Race	Altitude
Mrs Y T	37 yrs	Female	White	2,600 ft

The patient is a businesswoman, very hyperactive both in business and socially. She smokes and drinks fairly heavily. She complains of recent fatigue, headache, buzzing in the head, and decreased effort tolerance, especially recently when she also developed a productive cough. She is visibly under stress, the BP is 130/88, the pulse rate is 88/min, and she has a fine tremor in the hands.

	Value	Units	Reference range Low	High	Permitted range Low	High
Red cell count	6.49	$\times 10^{12}/l$	3.91	4.94	5.61	7.21
Hemoglobin (Hb)	19.6	g/dl	12.4	15.5	18.2	19.6
Hematocrit (Hct)	0.57	l/l	0.37	0.47	0.52	0.55
Mean cell volume	84	fl	80	99	75.2	92.8
Mean cell Hb	29.4	pg	27	31.5	26.4	32.6
Mean cell Hb conc.	35.2	g/dl	31.5	34.5	34.4	35.8
Red cell dist. width	14.1	%	11.6	14	15.8	15.8
Retic count	0.51	%	0.25	0.75	0.7	0.8
Retic absolute (abs.)	35.3	$\times 10^9/l$	26	100	31.0	39.1
White cell count	10.7	$\times 10^9/l$	4	11	9.63	11.77
Neutrophils abs.	7.60	$\times 10^9/l$	2	7	6.84	8.36
Band cells abs.	0.11	$\times 10^9/l$	0	0	0.10	0.12
Lymphocytes abs.	2.14	$\times 10^9/l$	1	3	1.93	2.35
Monocytes abs.	0.86	$\times 10^9/l$	0.2	1	0.77	0.94
Eosinophils abs.	0.00	$\times 10^9/l$	0.02	0.5	0.00	0.00
Basophils abs.	0.00	$\times 10^9/l$	0.02	0.1	0.00	0.00
Normoblasts	0	/100 WBC	0	0		
Platelet count	400.0	$\times 10^9/l$	150	400	360.1	434.1
Sedimentation	18	mm/h	0	20	14	16

DISCUSSION

Again, the anatomical diagnosis is fairly straightforward as that of **ERYTHROCYTOSIS,** apart from the slight neutrophilia that is probably related to a chest infection, or even to her stressful lifestyle.

When one considers the possible general causes, it will be seen that there are considerable difficulties. The count is very similar indeed to the one shown in Table 17.1. Indeed, as a general rule, the FBC is of very little aid in distinguishing the causes of erythrocytosis, **EXCEPT WHEN THERE IS RETICULOCYTOSIS OR A BASOPHIL LEUKOCYTOSIS.** Its value is in assisting in identifying the **PATHOLOGICAL STATE.** In this case, even the clinical features are open to different interpretations.

The FBC does not exclude an early or variant polycythemia vera. One must necessarily look at routine biochemical tests and the clinical picture. The biochemical tests were non-contributory except that the urate and LDH were normal, again against the diagnosis of P. vera. Bone marrow studies also were of no assistance.

The clinical picture is somewhat suggestive of a stress situation, and thus of Gaisbock syndrome. However, it can be seen that this diagnosis is very difficult, and blood volume studies could be helpful However, these were not at the time available, which was unfortunate since a number of expensive tests had to be performed that could otherwise have been avoided. Extensive radiological and sonographic studies failed to show any evidence of a cause for inappropriate secretions of EPO; chest X-rays and lung functions were normal. The possibilities that remained were Gaisbock syndrome and idiopathic erythrocytosis (see the Optional Advanced Reading section). It was decided to treat the patient provisionally as a Gaisbock, then wait and see.

The patient was venesected of 1 unit, treated with sedatives, advised to take a long holiday, and advised about her lifestyle. Unusually, she complied with the

regimen prescribed, and within 6 months her count had returned to normal.

CASE #73 (EXAMINE TABLE 17.4)

DISCUSSION

The anatomical diagnosis – **ERYTHROCYTOSIS** – is clear. The general causes will all need to be considered, but the clinical features should point one first in the direction of hypoxia. If there had been a reticulocytosis, this diagnosis would be very much strengthened; the fact that there is no reticulocytosis is not against the diagnosis, but it does imply greater vigilance. As a consequence, an X-ray of the chest and blood gas studies were done as a first priority, and are shown in Table 17.5.

The **X-RAY OF THE CHEST** revealed (in summary) pulmonary fibrosis but no cavities. The appearance was that of old tuberculosis.

Blood gas studies are shown in Table 17.5.

The clinical impression of hypoxia is confirmed. **NOTE:** The erythrocytosis is severe. The degree of erythrocytosis has little diagnostic value.

Table 17.4

Patient	Age	Sex	Race	Altitude
Mr G M	36 yrs	Male	Black	5,000 ft

This patient presented to a family doctor with a 2-week history of a productive cough. The doctor ordered a FBC that showed erythrocytosis; he was referred. He had had TB 6 years before; he states that he adhered to the full course of treatment at the time, but the general impression cast some doubt on this. He has experienced increasing effort intolerance for the last 3 years. He smokes eight cigarettes per day. On examination, there was a tinge of cyanosis with obvious plethora. The chest displayed poor movement with respiration and was generally hyperresonant. Auscultation revealed widespread inspiratory and expiratory rhonchi. Peak expiratory flow was 255 l.

	Value	Units	Reference range Low	Reference range High	Permitted range Low	Permitted range High
Red cell count	**6.68**	$\times 10^{12}/l$	4.77	5.83	6.48	6.88
Hemoglobin (Hb)	**21.7**	g/dl	13.8	18.0	20.9	22.5
Hematocrit (Hct)	**0.64**	l/l	0.42	0.53	0.62	0.66
Mean cell volume	95.7	fl	80	99	93.8	97.6
Mean cell Hb	32.5	pg	27	31.5	31.8	33.1
Mean cell Hb conc.	33.9	g/dl	31.5	34.5	33.3	34.6
Red cell dist. width	14.2	%	11.6	14	13.1	15.3
Retic count	0.9	%	0.27	0.80	0.8	1.0
Retic absolute	60.1	$\times 10^9/l$	30	100	55.6	64.6
White cell count	6.5	$\times 10^9/l$	3.5	10	6.01	6.99
Neutrophils abs.	3.58	$\times 10^9/l$	1.5	7	3.31	3.84
Lymphocytes abs.	2.34	$\times 10^9/l$	1	3	2.16	2.52
Monocytes abs.	0.33	$\times 10^9/l$	0.2	1	0.30	0.35
Eosinophils abs.	0.26	$\times 10^9/l$	0.02	0.5	0.24	0.28
Basophils abs.	0.00	$\times 10^9/l$	0.02	0.1	0.00	0.00
Normoblasts	0	/100 WBC	0	0		
Platelet count	223.0	$\times 10^9/l$	150	400	200.7	245.3

Table 17.5

	Value	Units	Reference Range Low	Reference Range High
B-P_H	7.371	mmol/l	7.35	7.45
B-P_{O_2}	**57.6**	mmHg	77	90
O_2 saturation	**88.6**	%	90	99
B-P_{CO_2}	36.6	mmHg	28	41
B-Base excess	**−3.6**	mmol/l	−2	3
Actual HCO_3^{2+}	20.9	mmol/l	21	29
B-STD HCO_3^{2+}	**21.3**	mmol/l	22	26

CASE #74 (EXAMINE TABLE 17.6)

DISCUSSION

This case of **ERYTHROCYTOSIS** presents several difficulties. Certainly, all the general causes would have to be considered. The gross obesity certainly points one to the possibilities of the Pickwickian syndrome and Cushing syndrome, but should these not be the answer, it would be advisable to consider all the causes.

1. Hypoxia of ventilatory origin, and here specifically the Pickwickian syndrome; in support of this is the story of disturbed sleep. Somewhat against this is the lack of cyanosis.

Table 17.6

Patient	Age	Sex	Race	Altitude
Miss M S	15 yrs	Female	White	5,000 ft

Erythrocytosis was discovered on a routine visit to a family doctor. There was no history of chest or heart disease, although exercise capacity is markedly impaired. She is 150 cm tall and weighs 117 kg. She had always been plump, but had gained weight markedly in the past 5 years. Distribution of fat is generalized. Her sleep is seriously disturbed. She has a high color, her palms are red and sweaty, and the BP is 110/66. There are no pruritus or striae. Examination of the cardiovascular and neurological systems is normal. The urine is clear. The chest expands 2 cm and the peak expiratory flow is 280 l.

	Value	Units	Reference range Low	Reference range High	Permitted range Low	Permitted range High
Red cell count	**5.99**	$\times 10^{12}$/l	4.03	5.09	5.81	6.17
Hemoglobin (Hb)	**16.3**	g/dl	12.7	15.9	15.7	16.9
Hematocrit (Hct)	**0.54**	l/l	0.38	0.49	0.52	0.55
Mean cell volume	89.9	fl	80	99	88.1	91.7
Mean cell Hb	27.2	pg	27	31.5	26.7	27.8
Mean cell Hb conc.	30.3	g/dl	31.5	34.5	29.7	30.9
Red cell dist. width	13	%	11.6	14	13.0	13.0
Retic count	1.6	%	0.3	1.8	1.6	1.6
Retic absolute	95.8	$\times 10^9$/l	30	100	93.0	98.7
White cell count	7.7	$\times 10^9$/l	4	10	7.12	8.28
Neutrophils abs.	4.63	$\times 10^9$/l	2	7	4.28	4.97
Lymphocytes abs.	2.47	$\times 10^9$/l	1	3	2.29	2.66
Monocytes abs.	0.52	$\times 10^9$/l	0.2	1	0.48	0.56
Eosinophils abs.	0.02	$\times 10^9$/l	0.02	0.5	0.02	0.02
Basophils abs.	0.05	$\times 10^9$/l	0.02	0.1	0.05	0.06
Platelet count	272.0	$\times 10^9$/l	150	400	244.8	299.2

Table 17.7

	Value	Units	Reference range Low	Reference range High
S-Urea	4.3	mmol/l	2.1	7.1
S-Creatinine	69	mmol/l	62	115
S-Urea:creatinine	62.3			
S-Sodium	141	mmol/l	136	145
S-Potassium	4.6	mmol/l	3.5	5.1
S-Chloride	108	mmol/l	98	108
S-Total CO_2	25	mmol/l	22	28
S-Anion gap	12.6	mmol/l	5	14
S-Glucose	5.3	mmol/l	3.9	5.8
S-Osmolarity	281	mmol/l	275	295
S-Bilirubin (total)	23	μmol/l	6.8	34.2
S-Bilirubin (direct)	2	μmol/l	1.7	8.6
S-Bilirubin (indirect)	21.0	μmol/l	5.1	25.6
S-ALP	73	IU/l	53	128
S-gGT	11	IU/l	8	37
S-ALT	20	IU/l	19	40
S-AST	25	IU/l	13	32
S-LDH	121	IU/l	90	180
S-Ferritin	76	μg/l	14.0	233.1
S-Iron	13.9	μmol/l	11.6	31.3
S-Transferrin	2.98	g/l	2.12	3.60
S-Fe saturation	20	%	15.0	35.0
S-Erythropoietin	11.9	ng/ml	10	55
S-ACTH	11.8	ng/l	0.0	46.0
S-Cortisol	**699**	nmol/l	38	690
S-T4	15.7	pmol/l	9.1	23.8
S-TSH	3.1	mIU/l	0.49	4.67

2. Atypical **CUSHING SYNDROME.** Erythrocytosis as an isolated feature is most unusual with Cushing but it can occur.
3. Because of her age, the possibility of a hereditary **HIGH-AFFINITY HEMOGLOBINOPATHY** should be considered.
4. Inappropriate EPO secretion **SHOULD NOT BE FORGOTTEN. THERE IS NOTHING CLINICAL TO SUGGEST THIS, BUT HER OBESITY MAKES EXAMINATION DIFFICULT.**

Thus, a number of investigations were performed (Tables 17.7 and 17.8).

DISCUSSION

1. The routine biochemical investigations are all non-contributory (or "normal").
2. There is nothing to suggest renal, hepatic disease, or thyroid disease.
3. The mildly raised cortisol is almost certainly not significant, in view of the obesity.
4. Iron studies had been requested by the GP who had the mistaken impression (apparently not uncommon at all) that, just as iron deficiency causes anemia, so does increased absorption of iron lead to polycythemia!
5. The low-normal EPO is a cause for concern. Could this be early polycythemia vera?

Table 17.8

	Value	Units	Reference range Low	Reference range High
B-P$_H$	**7.340**	mmol/l	7.35	7.45
B-P$_{O_2}$	**71.0**	mmHg	77	90
O_2 saturation	**86.0**	%	90	99
B-P$_{CO_2}$	**45.0**	mmHg	28	41

Blood gas studies were clearly relevant here, and later polysomnography.

The features of the blood gas analysis are very suggestive of a ventilatory disorder, in this case the Pickwickian/sleep apnea spectrum, and against early polycythemia or inappropriate EPO secretion.

Polysomnography revealed (in summary) classic features of obstructive sleep apnea.

HEMOGLOBIN STUDIES

Hb Electrophoresis (P$_H$ 8.6): Normal
HbA2 chromatography: 2.3
HbH inclusions: Absent

These hemoglobin studies did not reveal a known high-affinity disorder. However, not all of these can be demonstrated by these studies. Family studies however lent no support to the possibility.

The final diagnosis was therefore the so-called Pickwickian syndrome. Expert dietetic and eventually surgical advice was sought, and a device to detect and control apnea during sleep was used. She gradually lost a great deal of weight, and the FBC appearances are gradually improving.

Optional Advanced Reading

Notes in Regard to Erythrocytosis

A number of topics need to be discussed:

1. Tissue hypoxia in the face of a normal Pao$_2$
2. Inappropriate secretion of erythropoietin
3. Gaisbock syndrome
4. Idiopathic Erythrocytosis
5. Smoker's erythrocytosis
6. Oxygen transport in erythrocytosis and polycythemia

1. **TISSUE HYPOXIA IN THE FACE OF A NORMAL Pao$_2$ (INCREASED OXYGEN AFFINITY OF HB).** From our point of view, only a few are associated with erythrocytosis, since many of the conditions discussed do not last long enough for this to develop.

   a. **CONDITIONS TYPICALLY ASSOCIATED WITH ERYTHROCYTOSIS.**

      i. **HIGH-AFFINITY HEMOGLOBINS**. These are rare and typically present in childhood. Note however that one very well-known high-affinity hemoglobin, HbF, is **NOT** associated with erythrocytosis.
      ii. **MYXEDEMA**. This is seldom significant.
      iii. **CHRONIC HYPOPHOSPHATEMIA.** A rare cause and rarely manifesting in clinical erythrocytosis. This may be found in chronic proximal tubular dysfunction, osteomalacia, chronic use of phosphate-binding antacids, and hemodialysis.

   b. **CONDITIONS NOT ASSOCIATED WITH ERYTHROCYTOSIS.**

      i. **MASSIVE TRANSFUSION.** The large amount of citrate infused leads to a decrease in 2,3-BPG, thus increasing affinity. This is short lived (a matter of hours), until the enzyme systems are reactivated. However, in the critically ill, this can be a serious problem for those hours.
      ii. **TREATMENT OF KETO-ACIDOSIS.** This causes tissue hypoxia via at least two mechanisms.

         – **LARGE AMOUNTS OF HCO$_3^{2-}$** cause a shift in the oxygen-dissociation curve.
         – **2,3-BPG** is reduced and is associated with hypophosphatemia.

      iii. **A MISCELLANEOUS GROUP OF CONDITIONS.** Severe hypothermia, acidemia due to other causes.

2. **INAPPROPRIATE SECRETION OF ERYTHROPOIETIN.**

   The clinical features have been outlined before. From the laboratory point of view **THE CONDITION IS CHARACTERIZED BY**

   FBC FEATURES:

   a. Increased Hct and Hb, and usually increased RCC. The reticulocyte count is normal.
   b. **THE ESR MAY BE RAISED** in the more aggressive causes.
   c. **THE RDW** may be raised – as a non-specific finding in cases of malignancy (this may be due to the presence of a malignant circulation, and thus is typically only found with a large tumor mass).
   d. The PC and WCC are typically normal.
      If there is an associated anemia of chronic disorders, the picture may be very complicated.

   FEATURES IN OTHER LABORATORY TESTS:

   a. Routine biochemical tests are normal unless malignancy has caused independent changes.
   b. Erythropoietin levels are raised in most cases. If there is strong clinical suspicion of the condition, the EPO may have to be repeated a few times to find the positive result.

   COMMON CLINICAL ACCOMPANIMENTS:

   These are usually the result of the underlying cause.

3. **GAISBOCK SYNDROME.** As mentioned before, the pathogenesis and indeed the very nature of this

condition are obscure. In the pathogenesis, many factors appear to be responsible:

a. Hypertension
b. Smoking
c. Diuretics, e.g., for hypertension, but including beverages with diuretic effect such as alcohol
d. Obesity
e. Alcohol
f. Underlying renal disease
g. Increased catecholamine levels

It is thought that the interaction of some of these factors produces both increased red cell mass and decreased plasma volume.

It is also likely that this condition in some cases represents an intermediate phase in the development of polycythemia vera **OR** hypoxic erythrocytosis **OR** inappropriate secretion of EPO.

THE RISK OF VASCULAR OCCLUSION IN GAISBOCK SYNDROME.

This is a controversial issue, mainly because the diagnosis is so difficult to establish with certainty. In addition, the underlying conditions with which it is associated are independently associated with increased incidence of atheroma.

4. **IDIOPATHIC ERYTHROCYTOSIS** is an uncommon and ill-defined condition (or more correctly, probably a group of conditions). It can be defined, loosely, as an absolute erythrocytosis without other features that would permit classification as either Polycythemia vera or one of the other causes of true erythrocytosis. It could be argued that "early polycythemia vera" as discussed earlier in this chapter would fall under this heading; however, the natural history and clinical spectrum of this condition is too diverse to permit this in all but a percentage of cases.

Clinically, it seems that very many of them **PRESENT** with arterial occlusive disease; others present with features like headache and dizziness; and in others the finding is incidental. The course is very variable.

About 10% of cases go on develop the typical features of polycythemia vera, within about a decade of the first diagnosis.

A small percentage will develop, in time, clear features of one of the secondary causes.

The rest remain more or less stable. The incidence of cerebro-vascular accidents in these patients, if poorly controlled, is particularly high. Treatment is by venesection alone – there is no place for ^{32}P or chemotherapy.

5. **SMOKER'S ERYTHROCYTOSIS.**

The pathogenesis of this is complex. Numerous factors play a role.

a. **EFFECT OF CARBON MONOXIDE IN SMOKE.**

i. The affinity of CO for Hb is 200 times greater than that of oxygen; thus, small quantities of CO can convert large amounts of Hb to carboxyhemoglobin – here the oxygen-binding site of Hb is bound by CO.
ii. The ODC is shifted (of Hb not bound to CO) to the left, causing increased affinity for oxygen (i.e., less is released to the tissues).
iii. Myoglobin binds CO avidly, thus intracellular transport of oxygen in skeletal and myocardial muscle is impaired.

b. **CHRONIC CHEST DISEASE.** The effects of chronic smoking on lung histology are well known, ultimately producing chronic bronchitis and/or emphysema.

c. **REDISTRIBUTION OF BLOOD VOLUMES WITH CONTINUAL SMOKING.** It seems clear that there is a serious redistribution of plasma water, especially in the lungs. This is presumably the explanation for the **RAPID** (within a week or two) improvement of the Hct after smoking ceases; this cannot be due to a sudden change in carboxyhemoglobin, since this will take months to resolve.

6. **OXYGEN TRANSPORT IN POLYCYTHEMIA.**

Blood flow decreases linearly with increasing viscosity. The rate of oxygen transport by arterial blood is the result of multiple factors. The total blood volume also plays a part; in polycythemia the associated hypervolemia and vasodilatation in the micro-circulation permits increased oxygen transport. Thus with tissue hypoxia, polycythemia is beneficial because of the increased oxygen transport. In causes of polycythemia not associated with tissue hypoxia, however, there is no benefit to the patient; should the Hct be very high, to the point of sludging, erythrocytosis potentially has an adverse effect on oxygen delivery. This is offset by vasodilatation, but the addition of other factors, such as widespread arterial disease, hyperlipidemia, platelet micro-thrombi, and decreased red cell deformability, may combine to impair oxygen carriage.

Patients with P. vera have no need for increased oxygen carriage. Where there is vessel disease, e.g., arteriosclerosis, the additional effect of increased viscosity may lead to ischemia in the relevant area/s. Clearly this becomes more relevant with advancing age. This is also a factor in other causes of raised Hct, and the total blood volume is relevant to understand the effects. The decrease in cerebral blood flow is least severe in P. vera, with its expanded total blood volume, and worst in cases due to decreased plasma volume.

The Effect on Oxygen Transport of Treatment of Polycythemia (and Erythrocytosis)

Venesection will cause significant clinical improvement, in part due to the increased tissue oxygenation. In P. vera, the issue of venesections for relief of symptoms is not a problem, as long as it is remembered that venesections should not be repeated too frequently, particularly in older patients with a greater probability of vessel disease, or in those with TIA's, etc. In such a patient and in an emergency, it may be advisable to maintain blood volume with a plasma expander.

In patients with erythrocytosis secondary to tissue hypoxia, venesection must be judged very carefully, and only used to reduce the work load of the heart and the micro-vascular sludging.

Erythrocytosis in Perspective

The formal diagnosis is frequently very difficult and quite often wrong. In one series, 57 patients diagnosed as "polycythemia" (in this case clearly including erythrocytosis) were referred for blood volume and other studies at an experienced center. Only 15 of these (26%) turned out to be true P. vera. Another 15 had hypoxia or renal disease. Two had no abnormality, and the remaining 25 (44%) had reduced plasma volumes, most with hypertension, and, to my mind, fulfilling the criteria for Gaisbock syndrome – a grossly underestimated and under-diagnosed (and eminently treatable) condition.

The greatest risk in persons with poorly controlled P. vera is arterial thrombosis. The key word here is "controlled." It seems well established that mortality associated with P. vera is not much higher than that in the general population PROVIDED that the condition is efficiently managed with the full cooperation of the patient.

Serious sequelae are otherwise uncommon. Transformation to acute leukemia is probably no higher than the incidence in the general population; transformation to myelofibrosis is fairly common; transformation to other chronic myeloproliferative disorders is very rare. The development of polycythemia vera is very slow – it is estimated that by the time the diagnosis of the typical case is made, the process has been in operation for about 7 years. The significance of the development of arterial disease in this "incubation" period has not been clarified.

We present here two difficult and very unusual cases for those who are interested.

Advanced Teaching Cases

CASE #75 (TABLE 17.9)

Table 17.9

Patient	Age	Sex	Race	Altitude
Mr J J M	65 yrs	Male	White	5,000 ft

He had consulted a family doctor for lassitude and erythrocytosis was discovered. He was referred to an internist, who after investigation decided that this was a myeloproliferative disorder and prescribed ^{32}P. The effect lasted for only about 9 months. During this time he felt worse, and he sought a second opinion, having stopped his treatment. His symptoms are very vague. He has never smoked; there is no history of chest or heart disease; and he uses minimal alcohol. He is obese, with a very high color, but no cyanosis. The BP is 156/96. All pulses are normal. He is clinically euthyroid. The heart sounds are closed and the chest is clear. Palpation of the obese abdomen is impossible. A bone marrow examination at the time of the first consultation had been normal.

	Value	Units	Reference range Low	Reference range High	Permitted range Low	Permitted range High
Red cell count	**6.29**	$\times 10^{12}$/l	4.77	5.83	6.10	6.48
Hemoglobin (Hb)	**19.1**	g/dl	13.8	18.0	18.4	19.8
Hematocrit (Hct)	**0.57**	l/l	0.42	0.53	0.56	0.59
Mean cell volume	91	fl	80	99	84.6	97.4
Mean cell Hb	30.4	pg	27	31.5	29.8	31.0
Mean cell Hb conc.	33.4	g/dl	31.5	34.5	32.7	34.0
Red cell dist. width	13.5	%	11.6	14	13.5	13.5
Retic count	0.61	%	0.27	0.80	0.6	0.6
Retic absolute	38.4	$\times 10^9$/l	30	100	37.2	39.5
White cell count	7.89	$\times 10^9$/l	4	10	7.30	8.48
Neutrophils abs.	4.50	$\times 10^9$/l	2	7	4.16	4.83
Lymphocytes abs.	2.68	$\times 10^9$/l	1	3	2.48	2.88
Monocytes abs.	0.47	$\times 10^9$/l	0.2	1	0.44	0.51
Eosinophils abs.	0.16	$\times 10^9$/l	0.02	0.5	0.15	0.17
Basophils abs.	0.08	$\times 10^9$/l	0.02	0.1	0.07	0.08
Normoblasts	0	/100 WBC	0	0		
Platelet count	321.0	$\times 10^9$/l	150	400	296.9	345.1

DISCUSSION

The anatomical diagnosis of **ERYTHROCYTOSIS** is clear. There was nothing in the FBC to suggest a general cause; the normal basophil count is strongly against a myeloproliferative disorder but does not exclude it, and of course this is to be expected in idiopathic erythrocytosis. Similarly, the normal reticulocyte count does not exclude hypoxia. The patient was retired and living comfortably. Further investigations were thus done. X-ray of his chest revealed mild left ventricular hypertrophy only. Peak flow was 525 l/min. See Tables 17.10 and 17.11.

It can be seen that there is no evidence of hypoxia. Abbreviated lung function test results can be seen in Table 17.11. They are completely satisfactory.

The results of selected biochemical investigations are shown in Table 17.12.

Table 17.10

	Value	Units	Reference range	
			Low	High
B-Ph	7.390	mmol/l	7.35	7.45
B-Po$_2$	86.0	mmHg	77	90
O$_2$ saturation	94.0	%	90	99
Oxygen content	19.2	vol%	19.1	19.9
B-Pco$_2$	36.0	mmHg	28	41
B-Base excess	1.0	mmol/l	−2	3
Actual HCO$_3^{2+}$	24.0	mmol/l	21	29
B-STD HCO$_3^{2+}$	25.0	mmol/l	22	26

Table 17.11

Result	Units	% of normal
FVC	l	104
FEV$_1$	%	103
FEV$_1$% of FVC	l/s	99
PEF	l/s	165
FEF$_{25}$	l/s	120
FEF$_{50}$	l/s	66
FEF$_{75}$	l/s	76
MVV	l/min	107

Table 17.12

	Value	Units	Reference range	
			Low	High
S-Urea	5.7	mmol/l	2.1	7.1
S-Creatinine	93	mmol/l	62	115
S-Glucose	5.4	mmol/l	3.9	5.8
S-Osmolality	281	mmol/kg	275	295
S-Uric acid	0.38	mmol/l	0.21	0.42
S-ALP	99	IU/l	53	128
S-gGT	31	IU/l	8	37
S-ALT	34	IU/l	19	40
S-AST	28	IU/l	13	32
S-LDH	161	IU/l	90	180
C-Reactive protein	5.1	mg/l	0.0	10.0
S-Erythropoietin	41	ng/ml	10	55
S-ACTH	31.9	ng/l	0.0	46.0
S-Cortisol	401	nmol/l	38	690
S-T4	15.5	pmol/l	9.1	23.8
S-TSH	2.11	mIU/l	0.49	4.67

These results suggested that there was no gross kidney, liver, or adrenal disease, or a chronic inflammatory or infiltrative disorder. The high normal EPO is very much against a myeloproliferative disorder. Gaisbock syndrome could not be excluded but was considered unlikely. Blood volume studies were normal. The patient was provisionally put on hydroxyurea, which controlled the red cell count very well. Once again the patient complained that he felt worse. He was also referred for dietetic advice, and proceeded to lose 25 kg over the next 6 months, at the end of which his blood pressure normalized.

All in all, this case was a conundrum. (Part of) the solution came about quite fortuitously: the patient had advised his son to seek consultation, also for vague but evidently fairly severe general symptoms.

CASE #76 (TABLE 17.13)

Table 17.13

Patient	Age	Sex	Race	Altitude
Mr A M (son of J J)	40 yrs	Male	White	5,000 ft

The patient is a senior IT manager and is under constant heavy stress. His symptoms are tiredness, palpitations, insomnia. His BP is 142/90, the heart sounds are closed, and the chest is clinically normal. He is a very big man and obese, weighing 108 kg and 1.79 m tall. Systemic history and examination were all otherwise non-contributory, apart from frequent epigastric discomfort.

	Value	Units	Reference range		Permitted range	
			Low	High	Low	High
Red cell count	**6.89**	× 10^{12}/l	4.77	5.83	6.68	7.10
Hemoglobin (Hb)	**18.7**	g/dl	13.8	18.0	18.0	19.4
Hematocrit (Hct)	**0.54**	l/l	0.42	0.53	0.53	0.56
Mean cell volume	**78.8**	fl	80	99	73.3	84.3
Mean cell Hb	27.1	pg	27	31.5	26.6	27.7
Mean cell Hb conc.	34.4	g/dl	31.5	34.5	33.8	35.1
Red cell dist. width	15.7	%	11.6	14	15.7	15.7
Retic count	0.78	%	0.27	0.80	0.8	0.8
Retic absolute	53.7	× 10^9/l	26	100	52.1	55.4
White cell count	8.86	× 10^9/l	4	10	8.20	9.52
Neutrophils abs.	5.40	× 10^9/l	2	7	5.00	5.81
Lymphocytes abs.	2.84	× 10^9/l	1	3	2.62	3.05
Monocytes abs.	0.35	× 10^9/l	0.2	1	0.33	0.38
Eosinophils abs.	0.18	× 10^9/l	0.02	0.5	0.16	0.19
Basophils abs.	0.09	× 10^9/l	0.02	0.1	0.08	0.10
Normoblasts	0	/100 WBC	0	0		
Platelet count	295.0	× 10^9/l	150	400	272.9	317.1

DISCUSSION

The anatomical diagnosis from the hematological point of view was clearly **ERYTHROCYTOSIS;** more specifically there was a microcythemia. Of the general causes, the following appeared possible:

1. **ATYPICAL EARLY POLYCYTHEMIA,** despite the absence of basophil leukocytosis: the microcytosis could be the result of mild constant oozing from the gut, which occurs sometimes with P. vera. But this is rather unlikely – this tends particularly to occur in cases with associated raised platelets and which are frequently functionally abnormal.

2. **STRESS POLYCYTHEMIA (GAISBOCK),** where the microcytosis could be due to associated gastric bleeding (also associated with stress).

3. **IDIOPATHIC ERYTHROCYTOSIS.**

Table 17.14

	Value	Units	Reference range Low	Reference range High
B-P$_H$	7.460	mmol/l	7.35	7.45
B-P$_{O_2}$	83.7	mmHg	77	90
O$_2$ saturation	96.5	%	90	99
Oxygen content	19.2	vol%	19.1	19.9
B-P$_{CO_2}$	32.6	mmHg	28	41
B-Base excess	−1.0	mmol/l	−2	3
Std HCO$_3^{2+}$	23.8	mmol/l	21	29

Table 17.15

	Value	Units	Low	High
Body mass	108	kg		
Total blood volume	6,267	ml	5,940	8,640
Total red cell volume	3,196	ml		
Comment	Normal			

Table 17.16

	Value	Units	Reference range Low	Reference range High
S-Urea	4.1	mmol/l	2.1	7.1
S-Creatinine	78	mmol/l	62	115
S-Urea:creatinine	52.6			
S-Sodium	141	mmol/l	136	145
S-Potassium	3.9	mmol/l	3.5	5.1
S-Chloride	104.00	mmol/l	98	108
S-Total CO$_2$	27	mmol/l	22	28
S-Anion gap	13.9	mmol/l	5	14
S-Glucose	4.4	mmol/l	3.9	5.8
S-Osmolarity	280	mmol/l	275	295
S-Osmolality	284	mmol/kg	275	295
S-Osmolar gap	−4		-6	6
S-Uric acid	0.39	mmol/l	0.21	0.42
S-Phosphate	0.89	mmol/l	0.87	1.45
S-Bilirubin (total)	21.1	µmol/l	6.8	34.2
S-Bilirubin (direct)	5.1	µmol/l	1.7	8.6
S-Bilirubin (indirect)	16.0	µmol/l	5.1	25.6
S-ALP	100	IU/l	53	128
S-gGT	25	IU/l	8	37
S-ALT	31	IU/l	19	40
S-AST	27	IU/l	13	32
S-LDH	114	IU/l	90	180
S-Total cholesterol	6.1	mmol/l		<5.2
S-LDL cholesterol	5.4	mmol/l		<2.6
S-HDL cholesterol	0.7	mmol/l		>1.0
S-Triglycerides	1.1	mmol/l	0.8	1.5
C-Reactive protein	4.2	mg/l	0.0	10.0
S-Erythropoietin	14.5	ng/ml	10	55
S-ACTH	33.1	ng/ll	0.0	46.0
S-Cortisol	291	nmol/l	38	690
S-T4	15.2	pmol/l	9.1	23.8
S-TSH	1.98	mIU/l	0.49	4.67
S-Ferritin	14.9	µg/l	20.0	250.0
S-Iron	9.9	µmol/l	11.6	31.3
S-Transferrin	3.51	g/l	2.12	3.60
S-Fe saturation	0.1	%	20.0	50.0

Table 17.17

Patient: Mr J J M		Reference range		
	Value	Units	Low	High
ODC P$_{50}$	**37.3**	mmHg	24	28

Table 17.18

Patient: Mr A M		Reference range		
	Value	Units	Low	High
ODC P$_{50}$	**38.1**	mmHg	24	28

4. **THALASSEMIA.** This is unlikely, since both sides of the parentage were of north European origin, but is always possible.

As far as the rest of his complaints were concerned, the ECG was normal and the X-ray of the chest revealed no abnormality. Gastroscopy revealed superficial generalized gastric erosions, some of them tending to bleed, but no obvious ulceration. Attention was now focused on the erythrocytosis. Tables 17.14, 17.15, 17.16, 17.17, and 17.18 show the results of various relevant investigations.

Blood volume studies were done.

The lung functions were very similar to those of his father.

All in all, the results were ambiguous. However, eventually and on reflection, the fact that both father and son had presented with erythrocytosis for which no clear cause could be found led to the suspicion that a hereditary factor could be involved, and the only established hereditary cause of erythrocytosis is a high-affinity hemoglobin. Further questioning of both patients revealed that it had been remarked from their childhood that both had a "high color"; of greater interest is that the father had **NEVER** in his life, until 18 months before, **EVER** had a FBC; the son had indeed had FBCs but no comment had been made about a raised Hct. A final, rather vague clue was that the elder patient's wife phoned to say that her husband's neuro-psychological state had subtly changed – he was forgetful, with outbursts of anger and irrationality. A neurologist's opinion was sought and he could find no objective evidence of brain dysfunction.

An oxygen-dissociation curve was done on both patients, and the results (see Tables 17.7 and 17.8) were as follows:

Both curves are clearly shifted to the right. Extrapolating the results and testing various P$_{O_2}$ results, and assuming that their "normal" red cell count would have been 5.55, the shift in the curve would, to provide the oxygen carriage that such a red count would have provided, mean that the red cell count would have to rise.

By using a graph, for the blood to maintain reasonably normal oxygen content, the rise in RCC should be roughly **IN THE CASE OF THE FATHER** 6.41, and **IN THE**

CASE OF THE SON, 6.45. Thus, this would explain the erythrocytosis in the father. In the case of the son, the associated microcytosis, presumably as a result of iron deficiency, could have led to a further adaptation, or associated stress might have caused some plasma water loss.

This was a very salutary experience and emphasizes the need for a strict methodological approach – i.e., proceeding from the anatomical diagnosis to all the general causes first and not jumping immediately to a set of specific causes. The correct diagnosis here has considerable practical implications, since the high Hct is necessary for adequate tissue oxygenation. The father's hydroxyurea was stopped, and he was monitored for excessive whole blood viscosity. His cerebral symptoms improved substantially over a period of 6 months.

Exercise Case

CASE #77 (TABLE 17.19)

Table 17.19

Patient	Age	Sex	Race	Altitude
Mr A du B	31	Male	White	5,000 ft

He presented to his family doctor with a moderate attack of gastroenteritis. His general condition was good, but a FBC showed some abnormalities. Examination for the chest, heart, and abdomen was normal. Effort tolerance was usually excellent. He is a graphic designer.

	Value	Units	Reference range Low	High	Permitted range Low	High
Red cell count	**6.14**	$\times 10^{12}$/l	4.77	5.83	5.96	6.32
Hemoglobin (Hb)	**18.7**	g/dl	13.8	18.0	17.5	18.7
Hematocrit (Hct)	**0.54**	l/l	0.42	0.53	0.52	0.55
Mean cell volume	87.5	fl	80	99	81.4	93.6
Mean cell Hb	29.5	pg	27	31.5	28.9	30.1
Mean cell Hb conc.	33.7	g/dl	31.5	34.5	33.0	34.4
Red cell dist. width	**14.4**	%	11.6	14	14.4	14.4
Retic count		%	0.27	1.00	0.0	0.0
Retic absolute (abs.)		$\times 10^9$/l	30	100	0.0	0.0
White cell count	6.6	$\times 10^9$/l	4	10	6.11	7.10
Neutrophils	71.3	%				
Band cells		%	0	0		
Lymphocytes	14.5	%				
Monocytes	**13.4**	%				
Eosinophils	0.3	%				
Basophils	0.5	%				
Neutrophils abs.	4.71	$\times 10^9$/l	2	7	4.35	5.06
Band cells abs.	0.00		0	0.00	0.00	0.00
Lymphocytes abs.	0.96	$\times 10^9$/l	1	3	0.89	1.03
Monocytes abs.	0.88	$\times 10^9$/l	0.2	1	0.82	0.95
Eosinophils abs.	0.02	$\times 10^9$/l	0.02	0.5	0.02	0.02
Basophils abs.	0.03	$\times 10^9$/l	0.02	0.1	0.03	0.04
Normoblasts	0	/100 WBC	0	0		
Platelet count	264.0	$\times 10^9$/l	150	400	244.2	283.8
Sedimentation	2	mm/h	0	10	2	2

Questions

1. From the hematological point of view, what is the "anatomical" diagnosis?

   _____

2. What are the possible general pathology diagnoses and what are the features for and against each? What important question did the doctor not ask?

   _____
   _____
   _____
   _____

3. What would be needed to establish the special pathology (specific) diagnosis? What would you do? (List the steps and what you would then do depending on the results.)

   _____
   _____
   _____
   _____
   _____
   _____

4. What would you decide if all the tests were negative or normal?

   _____
   _____

5. What do you think of the high monocyte percentage?

   _____

Answers

1. Erythrocytosis.
2. There are several possibilities:

   a. Dehydration. For: the recent gastroenteritis; against: nothing.
   b. Gaisbock syndrome. For: nothing specific; against: nothing.
   c. Chronic chest and other disease causing hypoxemia. For: nothing; against: the clinical history.
   d. Early polycythemia vera. For; nothing; against: no basophil leukocytosis.
   e. Idiopathic erythrocytosis. For and against: nothing.
   f. An important aspect of the history of any such patient is his smoking history. In fact the patient had never been a smoker.

3. Potentially, a very large number of tests would be necessary. In view of the history, it was decided to rehydrate the patient and repeat the FBC in a week. The repeat FBC showed **NO CHANGE.** The following tests were done:

   a. Hb electrophoresis: normal
   b. P_{50} of the oxygen-dissociation curve: 27.2 mmHg (normal)
   c. Family studies: normal
   d. Blood volume studies: normal
   e. Effect of sedation and lifestyle management: none

4. This type of problem is not particularly unusual. It is possible that this patient's results lie just beyond the

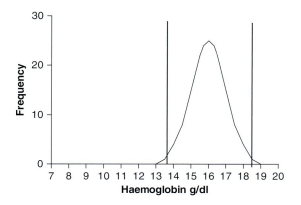

Fig. 17.2 The normal distribution of hemoglobin levels at 5,000 ft

2 SD limits of the normal range; this is depicted in Fig. 17.2.

A wait-and-see policy was adopted. The patient is followed up every year or two.

5. The high monocyte percentage is of little relevance, since the absolute monocyte count is normal.

Further Reading

Andreoli TE, Bennett JC, Carpenter CCJ, Plum F (eds) (1997). Cecil Essentials of Medicine. 4th edn. Philadelphia: WB Saunders Company.

Epstein RJ (1996). Medicine for Examinations. 3rd edn. Churchill Livingstone.

Hoffbrand AV, Pettit JE (2001). Essential Haematology, 4th edn. Oxford: Blackwell Science.

Lewis SM, Bain B, Bates I (2006). Dacie and Lewis Practical Haematology. 10th edn. Churchill Livingstone.

Defining "Bleeding Tendency"

The term "bleeding tendency" is necessarily a very general term for a large number of widely different presentations, with considerable overlap in many of their clinical, and indeed sometimes in their laboratory, presentations.

All that can be said at this stage is that a bleeding tendency is a presentation with bleeding in a patient in whom no anatomical cause for the bleeding (i.e., trauma to a vessel for one of many possible reasons) can be discovered. It is then inferred that the bleeding is due to a functional impairment of the normal hemostatic process. This impairment may be due to

1. A functional deficiency in the procoagulant mechanism. This may involve

   a. The platelets
   b. The procoagulant plasma components

2. A functional excess in anticoagulant mechanisms. This may be due to

   a. Anticoagulant drugs
   b. Natural anticoagulants

3. A functional excess in the fibrinolytic mechanism.

As was mentioned before, the first-stage diagnosis in the bleeding disorders is problematical. The reasons are threefold:

1. Unlike the disorders whose features are to do with changes in the blood cells, the first-stage diagnosis in the bleeding disorders is primarily clinical, for reasons that will appear.
2. Most cases of bleeding are not due to a bleeding disorder.

3. Separation of the bleeding disorders into diagnostic subgroups is difficult, with considerable overlap between groups, as well as overlap with non-pathological bleeding.

In Chapter 5 the identification of a so-called pathological bleed (i.e., not due to trauma to vessels but resulting from defects in the hemostatic mechanisms) was discussed extensively.

A very brief summary is presented under "Making the Diagnosis" below.

The Anatomical Diagnosis

It is clear that the first step is to identify the bleeding as pathological. In some cases, particularly those where the bleeding presentation mimics a more traditional picture, one is forced to use the hemostatic screen (HS) to confirm the possibility. This having been established, the **FIRST-STAGE DIAGNOSIS** is "Bleeding Tendency." Note that this is almost entirely clinical (very different from the situation with the FBC).

Reaching the general pathology diagnosis can be difficult. Once again we achieve this with a careful history and clinical examination.

The General Pathology Diagnosis

The following is a useful and practical division into various general pathology sub-categories. Broadly we can identify three: "**COAGULATION-DEFECT BLEEDS**," "**PURPURIC-TYPE BLEEDS**," and **MIXED** bleeds.

O.N. Beck, *Diagnostic Hematology*, DOI 10.1007/978-1-84800-295-1_18,
© Springer-Verlag London Limited 2009

"Coagulation Defect"

This term is used in quotes, since for convenience we include under this term bleeding tendencies due to disturbances of fibrinolysis.

The features depend very much on the severity of the defect – in effect the levels of circulating factor, in most cases. The laboratory and clinical features of each will be discussed under "**MAKING THE DIAGNOSIS.**"

1. **SEVERE HEREDITARY DEFICIENCIES OF FACTOR VIII OR IX** (hemophilias A and B).

    The factor level is so low (<1%) that any injury beyond a very superficial incision or abrasion is going to bleed persistently (after the initial hemostasis due to platelet activity (which is normal)). Minimal trauma to joints, usually unnoticed by the patient and affecting especially hinge joints such as the knee, ankle, and elbow, tends to lead to hemarthrosis. Internal injuries may lead to large hematomata that may cause compression and entrapment syndromes.

    A complicating factor with hemophilia A is the development, in about 10% of cases, of antibodies to infused factor VIII (this is less common with factor IX deficiency). This is a major problem and very difficult to manage.

2. **MODERATE DEFICIENCIES OF FACTORS VIII AND IX.**

    The factor level is between 1 and 5%, which is enough to cope with most small and medium injuries. Bleeding tends only to occur after severe trauma, or surgery. The characteristic clinical feature is the target joint. Its pathogenesis is as follows: as a child, usually around 6 years of age, a single joint (usually a knee) suffered a bleed after an injury (typically a sports injury as in rugby or soccer); the nature and cause of the bleed was not recognized and therefore not treated. As a result, the synovium became hyperplastic and hyperemic, making that joint vulnerable to further bleeds; this led eventually to a chronic arthropathy and destruction of the joint.

3. **MILD DEFICIENCIES OF FACTORS VIII AND IX.**

    The factor level is between 5 and 20%. Spontaneous bleeding will never occur; in fact bleeding will only occur after major trauma or surgery, if at all. Von Willebrand disease, discussed later, shows, as part of a rather complex pathogenesis, decreased factor VIII levels, usually around 20%.

4. **HEREDITARY DEFICIENCIES OF FACTORS V AND X.**

These patients tend only to bleed in unusual circumstances, and bleeding can be severe. Hemarthrosis or soft tissue hematomata are rare.

5. **ACQUIRED DEFICIENCIES**, most commonly of factors I, VIII, IX, and X.

    A variety of acquired, circulating inhibitors of non-activated, native factors can be responsible for severe bleeding tendencies. These can arise in three situations:

    a. **IN MULTIPLY-TRANSFUSED PATIENTS** usually suffering from a congenital deficiency of a clotting factor.

    b. As an **AUTOANTIBODY**. The most common of these is to factor VIII.

    c. **THE ANTICOAGULANTS** used therapeutically: heparin and the oral anti-coagulants (the latter also occasionally as a result of poisoning).

    d. Acquired deficiencies can also arise due to **ADSORPTION ON TO THE SURFACE OF PARAPROTEINS**, such as in myeloma. Factor X seems particularly prone to be adsorbed.

6. **DEFICIENCIES OF OTHER FACTORS.**

    Rarely, defects of **FACTORS I, II, VII, X, AND XI** occur. Most of these tend to experience epistaxis and menorrhagia, as well as bleeding from other sites. The incidence of hemarthosis varies a lot: with factors I, II, V, and X deficiencies, they occur in roughly two-thirds of cases; factor VII deficiency and the unusual combined deficiency of factors V and VII seldom experience hemarthrosis. **FACTOR XIII** deficiency can have very severe hemorrhagic phenomena of all types. However, the point must be stressed that these are rare and are usually suggested by the HS. The only ones of these that are relatively common are factor V, factor X, and the combined factor V and VII deficiencies. The clinically most severe of these rare deficiencies is factor X and XIII deficiencies.

7. **INCREASED FIBRINOLYSIS.**

    Abnormal activation of the plasminogen/plasmin system can be accompanied by severe bleeding. One important cause is activation of the fibrinolytic system (and the coagulation mechanism) by antigen–antibody complexes formed as a result of acute incompatibility of transfused red cells. Hemarthrosis is rare. Investigation of abnormal fibrinolysis – even suspecting its presence – is generally a highly specialized task.

8. **MULTIPLE DEFICIENCIES.**

    There are two quite common conditions where several factor deficiencies occur: chronic or acute liver disease, and DIC. Since, however, they are usually accompanied by platelet deficiencies or abnormalities, these are discussed later.

"Purpuric-Type" Defect

In all these cases, the coagulation tests are normal. The bleeding time is frequently prolonged. There are three general causes of this presentation:

1. **THROMBOCYTOPENIA.** This has been discussed in Chapter 11. Note that purpura and other bleeding phenomena only occur with a platelet count (PC) below 20×10^{12}/l **UNLESS:**

   a. The trauma is very severe.
   b. The platelets are also dysfunctional, as often occurs in myelodysplasia for example; in this type of case, severe bleeding has been observed with platelet counts of 60 or more.

      In thrombocytopenia it has been claimed that there is a linear relationship between the PC and the bleeding time, from about 70×10^{12}/l downward. In our unit we have not been convinced of this relationship.

2. **PLATELET FUNCTION DEFECTS.** These are briefly discussed later.
3. **VASCULAR DEFECTS** such as scurvy can sometimes present in this way.

The Danger of Serious Bleeding with Thrombocytopenia

Despite many attempts to prescribe the incidence of bleeding in thrombocytopenia in relation to the severity of the count, it is in fact largely unpredictable. If the platelets are functionally normal, it is frequently seen that patients running about in their daily activities with a PC of 5×10^9/l sometimes never bleed, except with significant injuries, and apart from mild purpura and perhaps some epistaxis or menorrhagia. This makes the decision to treat (and how to treat) sometimes very difficult. Practically speaking, if the count persists below 20 despite standard therapy, then it is incumbent always at least to try the various other options until they are exhausted.

Mixed Presentation

Many bleeding disorders affect both the platelets and the bleeding time, and the coagulation or fibrinolytic factors.

1. **VON WILLEBRAND DISEASE**
2. **LIVER DISEASE**
3. **DIC**
4. **DEFICIENCIES OF FACTORS II AND VII**

The Special Pathology Diagnosis

In the bleeding disorders, the specific diagnosis is always made by laboratory testing. The hemostatic screen (HS) unlike the FBC is not standard for all bleeding disorders; various parts are requested depending on the clinical features.

In principle, any features compatible with a purpuric-type lesion (see above) require a FBC with morphology.

1. If the platelet count is low and there are no contradictory features in the FBC or on clinical assessment, one can provisionally assume that the case can be approached as discussed in Chapter 11.
2. If the platelet count is normal and there are no contradictory features in the FBC or on clinical assessment, one must strongly suspect a platelet function defect.

> **Platelet Function Defects** Acquired platelet dysfunction is common, usually as a result of aspirin, NSAIDS and some antiplatelet medications. Uremia, significant acute alcohol ingestion and diabetes type II also cause significant dysfunction. In some of these cases, bleeding can be serious, even fatal. The numerous hereditary causes, however, are rare. The commonest and most important is von Willebrand disease. Others are Storage Pool Disease and the Bernard–Soulier syndrome. They typically present with purpuric-type bleeding, and in the case of von Willebrand disease, also with coagulation-defect bleeding as a result of factor VIII deficiency.
>
> For the general reader, it is sufficient to be able to suspect one of these conditions in a situation where a patient has purpuric-type bleeding with a normal platelet count. It is only von Willebrand disease that requires closer knowledge. It is described more fully later.
>
> Precise identification is only achieved in specialized laboratories.

In principle, any features compatible with a "coagulation-defect" lesion requires a version of the HS. What elements of the screen are requested depends on the clinical features, and usually the laboratory will be able to offer the correct advice. Generally speaking, however, it is most unwise to request a HS without a FBC.

1. Obvious prolonged secondary bleeding without evidence of critical illness or purpura will require platelet count (PC), PT, PTT, TT (thrombin time), and bleeding time (BT).

2. Unusual bleeding such as epistaxis without anatomical abnormalities or hypertension will require FBC, BT, PT, and PTT.
3. The ill patient, especially the shocked patient, requires BT, FBC, PT PTT, TT, and D-dimers.

Clearly, the specific diagnosis involves identifying precisely which factor/s is absent, decreased, or defective.

Making the Diagnosis

As indicated, the first step is to decide that the bleeding presentation is pathological. This is basically a clinical process. Sometimes, however, one is very unsure and primary recourse to the hemostatic screen (HS) is unavoidable.

Symptoms Suggesting Possible Pathological Bleeding

1. Proneness to easy bleeding, bruising, and bleeding into the skin
2. Recurrent painful swelling of the joints
3. Blue-black spots on the skin or mucosae. Blood-filled bullae on the mucosae
4. Bleeding, especially recurrent bleeding, from certain sites and where no obvious pathology exists, such as epistaxis, menorrhagia, hematuria
5. Bleeding presentation mimicking a well-known pattern but without many of or all of the expected associated features, such as hematemesis without any accompanying history of dyspepsia
6. Oozing during or after surgery or extraction
7. Bleeding from injection sites, or the gums or anus
8. Obvious spontaneous **PURPURA** especially if at least fairly generalized

Signs Suggesting Possible Pathological Bleeding

1. Acute hemarthrosis, muscle and/or soft tissue bleeds in the absence of trauma, or after inappropriately small trauma
2. Purpura
3. Perifollicular hemorrhages
4. Peutz-Jegher syndrome
5. Multiple telangiectases or angiomata

6. Periorbital bleeding
7. Periodontal infiltration and bleeding
8. Portal hypertension
9. Painful swollen joint/s
10. Chronic swollen or disorganized joints

The Clinical History

This may provide a very strong pointer to the nature of the bleeding disorder. The basic issues one makes enquiry about are

1. How wounds of different types stop bleeding or behave.
2. The pattern/s of spontaneous bleeding.
3. The family history.
4. The general medical and surgical history.

How Wounds of Different Types Stop Bleeding or Behave

There are a number of patterns:

1. **ABRASIONS, INCISIONS AND LACERATIONS** ooze but usually stop with local pressure: this picture is strongly suggestive of thrombocytopenia or platelet defect.
2. **ABRASIONS AND SUPERFICIAL INCISIONS** ooze but usually stop bleeding with local pressure; deep incisions and lacerations also stop but later recommence bleeding which is unresponsive to pressure: this picture is strongly suggestive of a coagulation defect.

The Pattern of Spontaneous Bleeding

1. **PURPURA, PETECHIAE, AND/OR ECCHYMOSES**. These features are strongly suggestive of thrombocytopenia or platelet defect.
2. **HEMARTHROSES OR SOFT TISSUE BLEEDS, OR RACCOON EYES,** suggest a coagulation-type bleed.
3. **BLEEDING FROM AN ORIFICE** without evidence of a local lesion may also suggest a coagulation-type bleed, but also disorders of platelets, usually secondary to a primary blood disease.
4. **PURPURA AND PERIFOLLICULAR HEMORRHAGES** with deep bone pain to percussion are very suggestive of scurvy.

The Family History

A positive family history is often a major clue in working out the general pathology. The patterns may be very revealing.

1. **A COAGULATION-TYPE BLEED WITH A SEX-LINKED INHERITANCE PATTERN** is very suggestive of hemophilia.

2. **A COAGULATION-TYPE BLEED WITH AN AUTOSOMAL (USUALLY DOMINANT) INHERITANCE** pattern is very suggestive of von Willebrand disease (and is usually associated with some purpuric-type features), or very rarely deficiencies of factors II, VII, or X.

3. **A COAGULATION-TYPE BLEED WITHOUT A POSITIVE FAMILY HISTORY** does not negate the possibility of a heritable defect. However, it does raise the possibility of

   a. **ACQUIRED COAGULATION DEFECTS**
   b. **UNDERLYING LIVER DISEASE OR BILIARY OBSTRUCTION**
   c. In a very ill patient, **HYPERFIBRINOLYSIS OR DIC**

4. **A PURPURIC-TYPE BLEED WITH AN AUTOSOMAL INHERITANCE PATTERN**, especially with a normal platelet count, suggests an inherited platelet function defect.

The General Medical and Surgical History

There are various possible scenarios.

1. **IN A PURPURIC-TYPE BLEED** there may be a history of a recent viral infection; alternatively there may be a history of the ingestion of various drugs, of the features of SLE, or of any of the cause of bone marrow failure. Any of these may reinforce the suggestion of thrombocytopenia.

2. **PATIENTS WITH HEART DISEASE OR PREVIOUS/EXISTING THROMBOTIC DISEASE** may be on anticoagulants; the dosage control may be poor resulting in a bleeding tendency.

3. **A HISTORY OF PROLONGED OOZING** during and after surgery. This may indicate moderate or even mild hemophilia, von Willebrand disease, liver disease, or Rendu-Osler-Weber disease (HHT).

4. The patient may have **FEATURES SUGGESTIVE OF LEUKEMIA, MYELOMA, MYELODYSPLASIA**. These are discussed elsewhere.

5. The patient may give a history of **ALCOHOLISM, PREVIOUS HEPATITIS OR BLOOD TRANSFUSION, OR BILIARY TRACT DISEASE.**

6. The patient may give a history of **RECURRENT EPISTAXIS OR MENORRHAGIA**.

7. There may be a history of **BLEEDING GUMS**. This is most commonly due to periodontal disease, but blood disorders that may be responsible are leukemic infiltration (especially AML M4 and M5), scurvy, DIC, thrombocytopenia.

Miscellaneous Causes of or Comments Related to Bleeding Disorders

1. **SENILE PURPURA**. This classically affects the dorsum of the forearms of patients who have been exposed to the sun for many years. It is due to solar damage to elastic tissue around the vessels. The vessels then become very susceptible to any shearing force experienced by the skin, such as scratching or rubbing (the forearms seem unduly prone to pruritus in the elderly).

2. **PSYCHOGENIC PURPURA**. This is a very strange condition. It undoubtedly is an entity. The patient is seriously neurotic or even psychotic, and presents with purpura occurring in crops, often in the same sites, and with a normal platelet count and coagulation profile. There are numerous theories as to the pathogenesis.

3. **COAGULATION-DEFECT TYPE BLEEDING IN A FEMALE**.

   a. **SEVERE, PURE, TYPICAL HEMOPHILIC-TYPE BLEEDING** in a female can only occur in:

      i. The very rare case of the female having a hemophilic father and carrier mother. Note that hemarthrosis is common.
      ii. Factor V or X deficiency. Hemarthrosis is very rare.
      iii. Acquired factor VIII deficiency. Hemarthrosis is common.

   b. **MILD, OCCASIONALLY EVEN MODERATE COAGULATION-TYPE BLEEDING** in a female may occur due to the hemophilic carrier state, especially with weighted lyonization. (Normally one of the X chromosomes is inactivated in a completely random manner. Sometimes by chance a majority of normal X chromosomes becomes inactivated.)

4. **BRUISING**, especially multiple bruising. While trauma, especially physical abuse, is the commonest cause, important conditions are

   a. **'SIMPLE EASY BRUISING'**. This is hardly a disease at all. It is found particularly in obese females in their thirties, and is probably due to subcutaneous fat interfering with the tissue support of the vessels.

b. **BRUISING CAN OCCUR OTHERWISE IN MOST OF THE DESCRIBED CONDITIONS.**

5. **LIVER DISEASE: HEMOSTATIC DEFECTS.** "Liver disease" is not a homogeneous concept. It embraces disorders from acute hepatitis to hepatic failure to alcoholism to obstructive liver disease to chronic hepatocellular liver disease. The features have been explored in Chapter 4. To summarize the hemostatic changes:

a. **ACUTE HEPATITIS.** The changes are usually mainly coagulation defects, affecting both the INR and the PTT. If there is a strong obstructive element, the changes discussed under point d. below will be obvious.

b. **IN HEPATIC FAILURE** the major changes too are coagulation defect in type, again affecting both the INR and the PTT, but typically with the additional effects on the fibrinolytic system and the D-Dimer test.

c. **IN ALCOHOLISM** the hemostatic changes are usually minimal unless chronic damage to the liver has occurred. See under point e. below.

d. **IN OBSTRUCTIVE LIVER DISEASE** the dominant abnormalities affect vitamin K metabolism and hence the INR.

e. **IN CHRONIC LIVER DISEASE** the changes will usually affect the PTT more than the INR.

6. **ALCOHOL ABUSE.** The hemostatic effects of chronic alcoholism and consequent liver disease are well known. However, before the stage of permanent liver damage, significant acute alcohol consumption, resulting in a blood alcohol level of > 0.2 g/dl, causes significant inhibition of platelet aggregation and prolongation of the bleeding time. In addition, flavonoids in red wine and red grape juice further inhibit normal platelet function.

The Clinical Examination of Suspected Bleeding Disorders

This has been discussed in Chapter 5. Figure 5.8 is reproduced here for convenience (See Fig. 18.1).

IN SUMMARY,

1. **A NUMBER OF CONDITIONS SHOULD BE RELATIVELY EASY TO IDENTIFY,** at least in general terms. Specific diagnosis always requires laboratory testing.

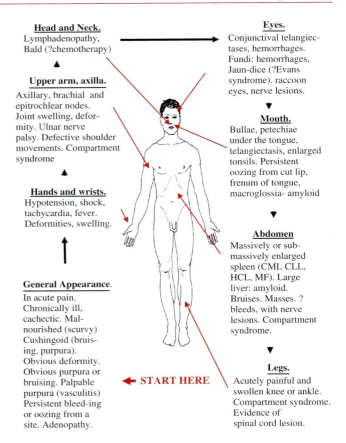

Head and Neck. Lymphadenopathy, Bald (?chemotherapy)

Upper arm, axilla. Axillary, brachial and epitrochlear nodes. Joint swelling, deformity. Ulnar nerve palsy. Defective shoulder movements. Compartment syndrome

Hands and wrists. Hypotension, shock, tachycardia, fever. Deformities, swelling.

General Appearance. In acute pain. Chronically ill, cachectic. Malnourished (scurvy) Cushingoid (bruising, purpura). Obvious deformity. Obvious purpura or bruising. Palpable purpura (vasculitis) Persistent bleed-ing or oozing from a site. Adenopathy.

← START HERE

Eyes. Conjunctival telangiectases, hemorrhages. Fundi: hemorrhages, Jaun-dice (?Evans syndrome). raccoon eyes, nerve lesions.

Mouth. Bullae, petechiae under the tongue, telangiectasis, enlarged tonsils. Persistent oozing from cut lip, frenum of tongue, macroglossia- amyloid

Abdomen Massively or sub-massively enlarged spleen (CML CLL, HCL, MF). Large liver: amyloid. Bruises. Masses. ? bleeds, with nerve lesions. Compartment syndrome.

Legs. Acutely painful and swollen knee or ankle. Compartment syndrome. Evidence of spinal cord lesion.

Fig. 18.1 Examination: bleeding tendency

a. **LIVER DISEASE** of various types including the cholestatic variety. The various patterns that may be found are shown in Tables 18.3, 18.4, 18.5. Frequently the clinical, biochemical, immunological and ultimately histological features will clinch the specific diagnosis. It will be seen that there are other conditions that can produce the same patterns, and it is clear that clinical input here is of the first importance.

b. **DIC** is usually strongly suggested or supported by the clinical conditions. It will be observed though that other conditions again can produce the same patterns, notably severe liver disease and massive transfusion. These however should be clinically recognizable. The pattern of the tests can be seen in Table 18.5

c. **THE BLEEDING TENDENCY OF RENAL FAILURE** also should be easily recognizable. It is shown in Table 18.6. The differentiation from other platelet dysfunctions would be by clinical and biochemical means.

d. **THE BLEEDING TENDENCIES THAT MAY BE FOUND** in myelodysplastic diseases, leukemias, aplastic anemias, and thrombocytopenia due to other causes should in most cases be identifiable from the clinical and FBC results.

e. Similarly, the differentiation of **BLEEDING TENDENCIES SECONDARY TO VASCULAR DISORDERS** is primarily clinical.

f. The patterns that may be found due to use of anticoagulants should be identifiable by the history.

2. **THE REST OF THE BLEEDING DISORDERS CONSTITUTE A DIAGNOSTIC PROBLEM**, and it is here that the HS, often supported by clinical features, is very important. Working from the patterns suggested in Tables 18.2, 18.3, 18.4, 18.5, 18.6, 18.7, 18.8 should enable a provisional diagnosis.

In the end, the final diagnosis will involve the laboratory.

The Characteristic Laboratory Features of the Most Important Coagulation-Type Bleeding Disorders

Note that only the most typical changes are described. The laboratory must be consulted. Complications in any of the conditions may show different results.

1. Moderate and severe hemophilia (A and B), deficiency of factors XI and XII, and circulating anticoagulants (Table 18.1)

Table 18.1

BT	PC	PT	PTT	D-Dimers
Normal	Normal	Normal	Prolonged	Normal

2. von Willebrand disease (Table 18.2)

Table 18.2

BT	PC	PT	PTT	D-Dimers
Prolonged	Normal	Normal	Prolonged	Normal

3. Chronic liver disease/cirrhosis (some cases) (Table 18.3)

Table 18.3

BT	PC	PT	PTT	D-Dimers
Normal	Decreased	Prolonged	Prolonged	Normal

4. Chronic liver disease, cholestatic liver disease, vitamin K deficiency, heparin therapy, deficiency of factors V, X, II, and I (Table 18.4)

Table 18.4

BT	PC	PT	PTT	D-Dimers
Normal	Normal	Prolonged	Prolonged	Normal

5. Liver failure, DIC, massive transfusion (Table 18.5)

Table 18.5

BT	PC	PT	PTT	D-Dimers
Prolonged	Decreased	Prolonged	Prolonged	Raised

6. Renal insufficiency, platelet function defects (Table 18.6)

Table 18.6

BT	PC	PT	PTT	D-Dimers
Prolonged	Normal	Normal	Normal	Normal

7. Early oral anticoagulation, factor VII deficiency (Table 18.7)

Table 18.7

BT	PC	PT	PTT	D-Dimers
Normal	Normal	Prolonged	Normal	Normal

8. Oral anticoagulants – chronic use (Table 18.8)

Table 18.8

BT	PC	PT	PTT	D-Dimers
Normal	Normal	Prolonged	Prolonged	Normal

Teaching Cases

CASE #78

This case, originally presented in Chapter 5 (as Case #8) is briefly reviewed. It will be remembered that this young girl developed a severe streptococcal tonsillitis, was placed on broad-spectrum antibiotics, ate virtually nothing for a week, then, feeling better, went for a ride on her bicycle. She fell off and suffered a minor closed injury to the right hip. The next morning she discovered a huge bruise down to her knee. The FBC was normal but the PT was markedly prolonged.

It was decided that this was probably a vitamin K deficiency due to the antibiotics, resulting in defective carboxylation of factors II, VII, IX, and X. She responded very well to vitamin K injections.

Vitamin K Deficiency It is not feasible to routinely measure vitamin K levels. Similarly, the levels of PIVKA's (see Chapter 2) are a research activity. Consequently, the diagnosis of vitamin K deficiency is essentially by derivation from clinical and laboratory features.

The most common causes of vitamin K deficiency are oral anticoagulants and antibiotic therapy. As long as one is aware of these, there should be no problem.

CASE #79 (TABLE 18.9)

This case was originally also presented in Chapter 5 (as Case #7). In brief, a man of 50 years presented with a history of having suddenly passed a lot of fresh blood per rectum. Clinically the patient was somewhat shocked. Further questioning revealed that he had been growing steadily weaker over the last few months, with severe lassitude and effort intolerance; he also had been troubled by numerous episodes of epistaxis and bleeding gums. His wounds stopped bleeding normally. Examination showed considerable pallor and scattered petechiae over the chest and thighs. There was no organomegaly. A FBC taken 30 min after admission and about 2 h after the bleeding appeared to have started is shown.

Table 18.9

	Value	Units	Reference range Low	Reference range High	Permitted range Low	Permitted range High
Red cell count	3.01	× 10¹²/l	4.64	5.67	2.92	3.10
Hemoglobin (Hb)	8.1	g/dl	13.4	17.5	7.8	8.4
Hematocrit (Hct)	0.25	l/l	0.41	0.52	0.24	0.26
Mean cell volume	83	fl	80	99	81.3	84.7
Mean cell Hb	26.9	pg	27	31.5	26.4	27.4
Mean cell Hb conc.	32.4	g/dl	31.5	34.5	31.8	33.1
Red cell dist. width	15.7	%	11.6	14	15.1	16.2
Retic count	1.71	%	0.26	0.77	1.7	1.8
Retic absolute	51.5	× 10⁹/l	30	100	47.6	55.3
White cell count	3.11	× 10⁹/l	4	10	2.88	3.34
Neutrophils	33.0	%				
Band cells		%				
Lymphocytes	57.5	%				
Monocytes	6.1	%				
Eosinophils	1.2	%				
Basophils	2.2	%				
Neutrophils abs.	1.03	× 10⁹/l	2	7	0.95	1.10
Lymphocytes abs.	1.79	× 10⁹/l	1	3	1.65	1.92
Monocytes abs.	0.19	× 10⁹/l	0.2	1	0.18	0.20
Eosinophils abs.	0.04	× 10⁹/l	0.02	0.5	0.03	0.04
Basophils abs.	0.07	× 10⁹/l	0.02	0.1	0.06	0.07
Blasts		%	0	0		
Promyelocytes		%	0	0		
Myelocytes		%	0	0		
Metamyelocytes		%	0	0		
Normoblasts	2	/100 WBC	0	0		
Platelet count	53.3	× 10⁹/l	150	400	78.1	88.3
Sedimentation	41	mm/h	0	10	39	43
Morphology	There is a pancytopenia with normocytic red cells. The red cells are normochromic and show mild anisocytosis. The neutrophils show prominent dysplastic changes.					

Notes on Table 18.9
1. There is a pancytopenia as well as evidence of dysplasia.
2. The FBC shows the effects of a recent bleed.
3. The significant point to note is that a platelet count of 53 is typically most unlikely to lead to gastro-intestinal bleeding, unless in addition they are functionally abnormal. The morphological comment about the dysplastic white cells is thus very significant.
4. A bone marrow examination revealed a myelodysplastic picture; it is known that the platelets in this disease can be markedly dysfunctional. Normal platelet morphology is the usual finding.

CASE #80 (TABLE 18.10)

Table 18.10

Patient	Age	Sex	Race	Altitude
Mr S de L	44 yrs	Male	White	5,000 ft

The patient complains of a recent onset of easy bleeding from any wounds, easy and sometimes apparently spontaneous bruising, episodes of hematemesis and rectal bleeding, and blood in the urine on occasion. He denies alcohol abuse, previous jaundice, or a positive family history. There is little to find on examination, apart from tenderness over the epigastrium; the abdomen is difficult to examine because of obesity, but the liver appears enlarged. He is not clinically anemic, but numerous bruises can be seen all over the body, and there are petechiae over the front of the chest and abdomen. When blood is drawn for examination, the puncture mark bleeds excessively.

	Value	Units	Reference range Low	Reference range High	Permitted range Low	Permitted range High
Red cell count	3.74	× 10¹²/l	4.77	5.83	3.63	3.85
Hemoglobin (Hb)	11.7	g/dl	13.8	18.0	11.3	12.1
Hematocrit (Hct)	0.38	l/l	0.42	0.53	0.37	0.39
Mean cell volume	101	fl	80	99	93.9	108.1
Mean cell Hb	31.3	pg	27	31.5	30.7	31.9
Mean cell Hb conc.	31.0	g/dl	31.5	34.5	30.4	31.6
Red cell dist. width	17.2	%	11.6	14	17.2	17.2
White cell count	4.77	× 10⁹/l				
Neutrophils abs.	2.91	× 10⁹/l	2	7	2.69	3.13
Band cells abs.	0.00	× 10⁹/l	0	0	0.00	0.00
Lymphocytes abs.	1.94	× 10⁹/l	1	3	1.79	2.08
Monocytes abs.	0.20	× 10⁹/l	0.2	1	0.19	0.22
Eosinophils abs.	0.05	× 10⁹/l	0.02	0.5	0.05	0.05
Basophils abs.	0.00	× 10⁹/l	0.02	0.1	0.00	0.00
Platelet count	21.3	× 10⁹/l	150	400	19.7	22.9
Morphology	There is a mild anemia. The red cells are normochromic and mildly macrocytic, and show numerous round macrocytes, target cells and some stomatocytes. There is a marked thrombocytopenia.					

DISCUSSION

1. There are clear indications of both purpuric and coagulation-defect bleeding. A strong possibility is liver disease, and the screen is constructed as follows: bleeding time, FBC, PT, PTT, FDPs, and D-dimers. See Table 18.11.
2. The features in the HS confirm that there are both purpuric-like and coagulation-defect types of problem.

Table 18.11

Test	Value	Units	Reference range	
Bleeding time	12	min	3	7
Platelet count	21.3	$\times 10^9$/l	140	440
PT	22	s	12	13
PTT	74	s	23	36
D-Dimers	0.29	mg/l	0	0.25

Table 18.12

	Value	Units	Reference range Low	High
S-Protein (total)	69	g/l	64	83
S-Albumin	30	g/l	34	48
S-Globulin	39.0	g/l	30	35
S-α1-globulin	1.3	g/l		1.9
S-α2-globulin	8.2	g/l	5	7
S-β-globulin	9.3	g/l	5	8
S-γ-globulin	11.3	g/l	6	10
S-Bilirubin (total)	38.9	μmol/l	6.8	34.2
S-Bilirubin (direct)	14.1	μmol/l	1.7	8.6
S-Bilirubin (indirect)	24.8	μmol/l	5.1	25.6
S-ALP	141	IU/l	53	128
S-gGT	61	IU/l	8	37
S-ALT	52	IU/l	19	40
S-AST	41	IU/l	13	32
S-LDH	231	IU/l	90	180
U-Bilirubin	+ +	"+"		
U-Urobilin	+ +	"+"		

3. There are several features that suggest the hepatic origin of the disorder – the clinical findings, the macrocytosis, and the morphology.

4. Accordingly, the liver function tests were performed. See Table 18.12.

5. The disturbed liver functions are obvious. Sonography of the abdomen revealed some ascites, and an enlarged non-homogeneous liver, and a slightly enlarged spleen. Doppler studies did not reveal portal hypertension.

6. The patient was given platelets, vitamin K, and fresh frozen plasma, and then a liver biopsy was done. This revealed cirrhosis, probably not related to alcohol.

7. Note that there are some other hemostatic complications of liver disease that were not demonstrated in this patient, such as DIC and hyperfibrinolysis.

CASE #81 (EXAMINE TABLES 18.13 AND 18.14)

DISCUSSION

The clinical diagnosis was questionable, particularly because of the marked synovial thickening: this is not a feature of osteoarthritis.

Table 18.13

Patient	Age	Sex	Race	Altitude
Master X J	11 yrs	Male	White	5,000 ft

This boy had presented 2 years before with a chronic swelling and pain in his left knee. No other joints were involved. He had stated that he had injured his knee many years before in a rugby practice, and it had never recovered. Investigations at the time had revealed a chronic osteoarthritis with a suggestion of synovial thickening. The diagnosis was made of post-traumatic osteoarthritis. Tests for immunological diseases proved negative. Otherwise he was well, completely asymptomatic. Eventually he was referred to a rheumatology unit for assessment.

A careful history, including from his mother, revealed that the original injury had indeed cleared up but slowly. However, subsequent rugby matches had resulted in repeated pain and swelling in that knee, often requiring bed rest. Further radiological examination confirmed the previous findings; the synovial thickening was marked. The general picture was very suggestive and certain tests were performed.

Table 18.14

Test	Value	Units	Reference range	
Bleeding time	4	min	3	7
Platelet count	213.6	$\times 10^9$/l	140	400
PT	12	s	12	13
PTT	47	s	23	36

The (mildly) prolonged PTT is extremely suggestive. Consequently, a factor VIII assay was performed, and this showed a factor level of 4% (reference range 70–150%). The diagnosis was made of a moderate factor VIII deficiency presenting as a target joint.

Endoscopic debridement was carried out and expert mobilization begun. The patient gradually recovered much of the use of his knee, although there had been quite significant destruction of cartilage at operation.

The problem was prevention of recurrence; most of the hyperplastic synovium was removed (it is virtually impossible to get to all of it). His sporting activities were reviewed and a supply of factor VIII was to be kept at home; in the event of an acute swelling the mother would administer the factor immediately as well as treat the swelling with ice packs.

It is likely that the patient may need a prosthesis when he reaches adulthood.

CASE #82 (EXAMINE TABLE 18.15)

It will be noted that the FBC is completely normal. Follow-up examination findings are seen in Tables 18.16 and 18.17.

Table 18.15

Patient	Age	Sex	Race	Altitude
Miss Y P	25 yrs	Female	Indian	5,000 ft

The patient is an admitted barrister but has not practiced due to severe psychological impairment. Her father, a family practitioner, referred her because he noticed purpura on the face and chest. He had requested a FBC, which follows.

			Reference range		Permitted range	
	Value	Units	Low	High	Low	High
Red cell count	4.29	$\times 10^{12}$/l	4.03	5.09	4.16	4.42
Hemoglobin (Hb)	13.4	g/dl	12.7	15.9	12.9	13.9
Hematocrit (Hct)	0.39	l/l	0.38	0.49	0.38	0.40
Mean cell volume	91	fl	80	99	89.2	92.8
Mean cell Hb	31.2	pg	27	31.5	30.6	31.9
Mean cell Hb conc.	34.3	g/dl	31.5	34.5	33.6	35.0
Red cell dist. width	12.2	%	11.6	14	12.2	12.2
White cell count	5.9	$\times 10^9$/l	4	10	5.46	6.34
Neutrophils abs.	3.61	$\times 10^9$/l	2	7	3.34	3.88
Lymphocytes abs.	1.50	$\times 10^9$/l	1	3	1.39	1.62
Monocytes abs.	0.43	$\times 10^9$/l	0.2	1	0.40	0.46
Eosinophils abs.	0.30	$\times 10^9$/l	0.02	0.5	0.28	0.32
Basophils abs.	0.05	$\times 10^9$/l	0.02	0.1	0.05	0.06
Platelet count	212.6	$\times 10^9$/l	150	400	191.3	233.9
Sedimentation	13	mm/h	0	20	12	14
Morphology	The film appearances are normal.					

Table 18.16

Further examination (case #82)

The patient was seen to be a thin, very disturbed-looking young woman. She spent the whole interview drawing elaborate patterns on the palms of her hands. She said that the "spots" mostly appeared on her face and arms; at present there were very few. The rest of the history was quite non-contributory. A number of tests were performed.

Table 18.17

Test	Value	Units	Reference range	
Bleeding time	4	min	3	7
PT	13	s	12	13
PTT	27	s	23	36

Note that the HS too was completely normal. Platelet aggregation tests also were quite normal, and it was concluded that the patient had psychogenic purpura.

CASE #83 (EXAMINE TABLES 18.18 AND 18.19)

DISCUSSION

1. Consulting Table 18.4 it will be seen that there is quite a large number of possible causes of this pattern: vitamin K deficiency, oral anticoagulants, heparin, liver

Table 18.18

Patient	Age	Sex	Race	Altitude
Mrs A de K	35 yrs	Female	White	5,000 ft

The patient had been traveling with her husband in his car when he had to brake very suddenly to avoid a collision. She was not wearing a seat belt, and banged her forehead on the padded dashboard of the car. She did not lose consciousness and indeed took no notice of the incident. The next morning she was astonished to see extensive bruising from the forehead down to her chin and neck. She denied any previous similar problem, or indeed any kind of bleeding disorder apart from mild menorrhagia all her life. Systematic history and examination were otherwise normal.

			Reference range		Permitted range	
	Value	Units	Low	High	Low	High
Red cell count	3.84	$\times 10^{12}$/l	4.03	5.09	3.72	3.96
Hemoglobin (Hb)	10.9	g/dl	12.7	15.9	10.5	11.3
Hematocrit (Hct)	0.31	l/l	0.38	0.49	0.31	0.32
Mean cell volume	82	fl	80	99	80.4	83.6
Mean cell Hb	28.4	pg	27	31.5	27.8	29.0
Mean cell Hb conc.	34.6	g/dl	31.5	34.5	33.9	35.3
Red cell dist. width	15.1	%	11.6	14	15.1	15.1
Retic absolute (abs.)	42.2	$\times 10^9$/l	30	100	41.0	43.5
White cell count	9.9	$\times 10^9$/l	4	10	9.16	10.64
Neutrophils abs.	7.53	$\times 10^9$/l	2	7	6.97	8.10
Lymphocytes abs.	1.49	$\times 10^9$/l	1	3	1.38	1.61
Monocytes abs.	0.55	$\times 10^9$/l	0.2	1	0.51	0.60
Eosinophils abs.	0.23	$\times 10^9$/l	0.02	0.5	0.21	0.24
Basophils abs.	0.09	$\times 10^9$/l	0.02	0.1	0.08	0.10
Platelet count	413.3	$\times 10^9$/l	150	400	372.0	454.6

Table 18.19

Test	Value	Units	Reference range	
Bleeding time	3.5	min	3	7
Platelet count	413.3	$\times 10^9$/l	140	440
PT	21	s	12	13
PTT	57	s	23	36

disease, deficiency of factors V, X, II, or fibrinogen, abnormal fibrinogens, and hyperfibrinolysis.

a. **ANTICOAGULANTS**. These were easy enough to exclude.

b. **LIVER DISEASE**. Clinically and by means of liver functions testing it was possible to exclude this fairly reliably.

c. **VITAMIN K DEFICIENCY**. The three important causes – diet, antibiotics and malabsorption – were fairly easy to exclude.

d. **HYPERFIBRINOLYSIS** practically only occurs with very ill people and with some malignancies, and there was nothing to suggest this possibility.

e. **DEFICIENCIES OF FACTORS I, II AND ABNORMAL FIBRINOGENS** are rare, and it was judged reasonable to proceed with the possibilities of factors V and X deficiency.

2. Specialized assay revealed normal factor X levels but a **FACTOR V LEVEL OF 8%**.

CASE #84 (EXAMINE TABLES 18.20 AND 18.21)

Table 18.20

Patient	Age	Sex	Race	Altitude
Miss J S	21 yrs	Female	White	5,000 ft

The patient was referred by a psychiatrist who was treating her for a major depressive condition, and had obtained from her a history of a bleeding tendency, and had noticed numerous bruises and purpura.

On systematic questioning, she said that she had experienced easy bruising and epistaxis from childhood. She had had cautery to Little's area. After the menarche she consistently had mild menorrhagia. She had never had joint or soft tissue bleeds. Her wounds stopped bleeding normally but always left marked keloids. The bleeding tendency had deteriorated in the last 9 months.

Table 18.21

Test	Value	Units	Reference Range	
Bleeding time	**8.5**	Min	3	7
Platelet count	230.1	$\times 10^9/l$	140	440
PT	12.6	S	12	13
PTT	29	S	23	36

The FBC was completely normal, with a platelet count of 230.1. The platelets were morphologically normal.

DISCUSSION

1. It would be jumping the gun to consider psychogenic purpura in this case – there is undoubtedly a bleeding tendency over and above purpura. How significant this is, however, is another question.
2. The prolonged bleeding time is of great significance. The possible causes of a prolonged bleeding time are

    a. Thrombocytopenia
    b. Vascular defect such as scurvy
    c. Platelet function defects

In this patient, there clearly was no thrombocytopenia or evidence of a vascular weakness. von Willebrand disease (most common forms) was excluded by the normal PTT. Thus, platelet function defects were considered. There was no evidence of renal failure or ingestion of aspirin or NSAIDS. Accordingly, platelet aggregation tests were arranged. These showed the following results (Table 18.22).

Table 18.22

Platelet aggregations	
Aggregant	Result
ADP	Normal
ADP 1/10 dilution	Normal
Epinephrine	**Decreased**
Collagen	**Decreased**
Ristocetin	Normal

This picture is classical of the so-called Storage Pool Disease – one of the classic hereditary platelet dysfunction diseases.

CASE #85 (TABLES 18.23 AND 18.24)

Table 18.23

Patient	Age	Sex	Race	Altitude
Mr J T	23 yrs	Male	Black	5,000 ft

This patient presented to his family practitioner with complaints of repeated severe epistaxis. The only tests he ordered were a FBC, a prothrombin time (PT) and a partial thromboplastin time. The FBC, PT, and PTT results are shown. The doctor packed the nose and referred the patient as a probable bleeding disorder.

	Value	Units	Reference range Low	Reference range High	Permitted range Low	Permitted range High
Red cell count	4.78	$\times 10^{12}/l$	4.77	5.83	4.64	4.92
Hemoglobin (Hb)	**12.9**	g/dl	13.8	18.0	12.4	13.4
Hematocrit (Hct)	**0.38**	l/l	0.42	0.53	0.37	0.39
Mean cell volume	**79.3**	fl	80	99	77.7	80.9
Mean cell Hb	27.0	pg	27	31.5	26.4	27.5
Mean cell Hb conc.	34.0	g/dl	31.5	34.5	33.4	34.7
Red cell dist. width	**16.1**	%	11.6	14	14.9	17.3
Retic count	**1.12**	%	0.27	0.80	1.0	1.2
Retic absolute (abs.)	53.5	$\times 10^9/l$	50	100	49.5	57.6
White cell count	5.98	$\times 10^9/l$	3.5	10	5.53	6.43
Neutrophils abs.	**2.13**	$\times 10^9/l$	1.5	7	1.97	2.29
Lymphocytes abs.	**2.92**	$\times 10^9/l$	1	3	2.70	3.14
Monocytes abs.	0.63	$\times x 10^9/l$	0.2	1	0.59	0.68
Eosinophils abs.	0.23	$\times 10^9/l$	0.02	0.5	0.22	0.25
Basophils abs.	0.06	$\times 10^9/l$	0.02	0.1	0.06	0.06
Normoblasts	0	/100 WBC	0	0		
Platelet count	301.3	$\times 10^9/l$	150	400	271.2	331.4
Sedimentation	9	mm/h	0	10	9	9
Morphology	There is a mild microcytic anemia. The red cells show anisocytosis and anisochromia. There is a reversal of the neutrophil: lymphocyte ratio.					

Table 18.24

Test	Value	Units	Reference Range	
PT	**17.0**	s	12	13
PTT	28	s	23	36

DISCUSSION

1. The FBC shows clear features of iron deficiency, most probably related to the repeated epistaxis. There are no features of a recent bleed, presumably because the nose was packed.
2. The prolonged PT requires explanation and if necessary further identification.
3. Further findings are presented in Table 18.25.

Table 18.25

Further examination (follow-up to case #85)
A detailed history revealed no other bleeding tendency and no positive family history of such a disorder. The epistaxis had only commenced about 2 years previously. The nose was carefully examined and dilated veins in Little's area were seen bilaterally.

4. The only disquieting feature with respect to a possible bleeding disorder was the prolonged PT. A clue was provided by the FBC – the reversal of the lymphocyte ratio. The patient revealed that he had recently had a severe influenza-like illness, for which his doctor had prescribed an antibiotic, the course of which he had completed 5 days ago. It was therefore suspected that the prolonged PT was due to vitamin K deficiency secondary to antibiotic therapy.
5. The patient was referred to an ENT surgeon who cauterized his Little's areas. The patient was given an injection of vitamin K. He recovered completely.
6. This case demonstrates the importance of a good history.

Exercise Case

CASE #86 (TABLES 18.26 AND 18.27)

Table 18.26

Patient	Age	Sex	Race	Altitude
Mr G B	30 yrs	Male	Black	Sea level

This patient is from Gabon and was referred with a diagnosis of "hemophilia A" by a dentist. He had consulted her because she had extracted two teeth from him 2 weeks previously, and the sockets were still oozing quite a lot, despite being packed. She had ordered a hemostatic screen.

On detailed questioning, he revealed that he had had mild bleeding tendencies since his childhood, mild enough for him not to have taken much notice of them. A superficial cut would stop bleeding rather slowly, then start again the next morning; a deep cut would only stop oozing 2 days later, and then could start up again. He does not bruise easily. He gets purpura with pressure – for example, after sleeping on his side, that side would show purpura in the morning. He had frequent epistaxis but has never had joint trouble. He had never had a transfusion. His maternal grandmother died of excessive bleeding after an operation; one of his brothers bled excessively after a circumcision. On examination he was somewhat pale but no other abnormal clinical features were found. His bleeding time was 10.5 min.

	Value	Units	Reference range Low	Reference range High	Permitted range Low	Permitted range High
Red cell count	4.64	$\times 10^{12}$/l	4.5	5.5	4.50	4.78
Hemoglobin (Hb)	13.0	g/dl	13	17	12.5	13.5
Hematocrit (Hct)	0.37	l/l	0.4	0.5	0.36	0.38
Mean cell volume	79.1	fl	80	99	77.5	80.7
Mean cell Hb	28.0	pg	27	31.5	27.5	28.6
Mean cell Hb conc.	35.4	g/dl	31.5	34.5	34.7	36.1
Red cell dist. width	16.1	%	11.6	14	16.1	16.1
Retic count	0.8	%	0.25	0.75	0.7	0.9
Retic absolute (abs.)	37.1	$\times 10^9$/l	50	100	33.4	40.8
White cell count	4.4	$\times 10^9$/l	3.5	10	4.07	4.73
Neutrophils abs.	1.81	$\times 10^9$/l	1.5	7	1.68	1.95
Lymphocytes abs.	2.13	$\times 10^9$/l	1	3	1.97	2.29
Monocytes abs.	0.27	$\times 10^9$/l	0.2	1	0.25	0.29
Eosinophils abs.	0.15	$\times 10^9$/l	0.02	0.5	0.13	0.16
Basophils abs.	0.04	$\times 10^9$/l	0.02	0.1	0.04	0.05
Platelet count	168.2	$\times 10^9$/l	150	400	151.4	185.0
Sedimentation	0	mm/h	0	10	0	0

Table 18.27

Test	Value	Units	Reference range	
Prothrombin time	12.4	s	11.5	13.5
PTT	51.3	s	23	35
Factor VIII	20	%	70	150
Factor IX	93	%	70	150

Questions

1. Do you think the dentist was correct in labeling this case as hemophilia A? Give reasons for your answer.

2. Purpura is classically a feature of thrombocytopenia. Do you think the laboratory could have made an error with the platelet count?

3. What do you think could be the explanation for this case?

4. How would you proceed to confirm your suspicion?

Answers

1. No. There are too many features that do not fit with hemophilia A. If this were hemophilia A it would have to be classified as a moderate case.

   a. Purpura is most unusual in hemophilia, especially moderate hemophilia.
   b. His family history is contradictory – a grand-**MOTHER** had died of bleeding.
   c. A prolonged bleeding time is not a feature of hemophilia.
   d. The factor VIII level is far too high for this type of bleeding.

2. No. Lab errors with the platelet count are usually underestimating the count rather than overestimating it.

3. The patient shows some features of both a coagulation-type disorder and a purpuric disorder. A strong possibility is von Willebrand disease. A factor VIII level of 20% in the face of both types of bleeding is extremely suggestive.

4. Some of the confirmatory tests for von Willebrand disease are extremely esoteric. However, it is possible to measure von Willebrand antigen directly as well as the ristocetin co-factor. The simplest way in many respects is to do platelet aggregation studies, although they are not always positive. See Table 18.28.

Note that these aggregation studies are characteristic of two diseases – von Willebrand disease and Bernard–Soulier disease. The latter is a rare functional platelet disorder that does not show coagulation-defect bleeding,

Table 18.28

Platelet aggregations	
Aggregant	Result
ADP	Normal
ADP 1/10 dilution	Normal
Epinephrine	Normal
Collagen	Normal
Ristocetin	**Absent**

and demonstrates giant platelets on the blood smear. Morphology was not provided on the FBC. A check on the morphology revealed normal-sized platelets. The ristocetin co-factor further confirmed the diagnosis.

The patient was given DDAVP whereupon his bleeding stopped dramatically.

Further Questions

1. What do you think about the red cell indices? What do you think they mean?

   _____

   _____

2. How would you confirm the diagnosis?

   _____

Answers

1. The hematocrit and MCV are decreased with a normal Hb and RCC. This probably indicates an early iron deficiency, in view of the constant bleeding. ACD and thalassemia cannot be excluded. However, the ESR of 0 mm is very much in favor of iron deficiency.
2. Iron studies, in the first instance. If they confirmed iron deficiency I would stop there. Otherwise I would look at markers of inflammatory or infiltrative disease, and do Hb electrophoresis.

Optional Advanced Reading

Only two topics will be discussed: hemophilia and disseminated intravascular coagulation (DIC).

Hemophilia

The reason this is discussed is that effective and prompt treatment of the manifestations of hemophilia will prevent crippling deformities as well as save lives. (Much of this material derives from general experience. However, valuable contributions came from the outstanding book by Duthie et al. (1994))

The bone and joint manifestations of hemophilia are as follows:

1. Hemarthrosis (75% of all hereditary coagulation-type bleeds)
2. Muscle hematomas
3. Cysts and pseudotumors

The Acute Hemarthrosis

Clinical Features

The most common joints involved are, in order of frequency,

1. Knee, elbow, ankle – accounting for the vast majority of clinical bleeds
2. Shoulder, wrist, hip

It is generally thought that the knee, ankle, and elbow are so commonly involved because they are hinge joints and tolerate sideways or rotary stresses with difficulty. This is probably not entirely true, since the hip, generally considered to be rarely involved, has been shown by advanced techniques to relatively commonly be affected by small bleeds, not detectable clinically.

There is a tendency to recurrent bleeds in any joint that has had a bleed before. This is unlike what happens with muscle bleeds.

Premonitory symptoms are common – abnormal sensations such as a "pricking" sensation or increased warmth, or slight stiffness, or weakness. This is very useful for both patient and doctor, permitting earlier specific therapy – indeed, the earlier the factor is given for a bleed the greater the chances are of avoiding permanent damage.

Once bleeding is established, the two most important symptoms are pain and swelling.

PAIN. This is the major complaint. It is partly due to a direct irritating effect of the blood itself, and partly due to the rapidity of distension. Both of these are important, as attested to by the following:

1. Pain on rapid distention occurs even when saline is injected.
2. In chronic joints there is a lot of fibrosis, and the amount of bleeding can be very little – a few milliliters only; aspiration of even this small amount leads to relief of pain.
3. Sometimes a patient can present with a painless chronic swelling.

Aspiration will yield blood plus synovial fluid, and is often followed by recurrence, which is also painless, but is now pure blood. Refilling with blood after aspiration of an acute bleed may also be painless. This is because the capsule is already stretched. Note that up to 220 ml blood have been aspirated from acute knees.

The pain subsides rapidly (within 4–6 h) after administration of factor (but takes 24 h without factor administration), since infused factor leads to clotting and further capsular swelling is stopped. However, the blood is not resorbed for several days.

SWELLING. It can be difficult to be sure what the cause of the swelling is, since apart from an acute bleed, it can also be a reactive sterile effusion, or of course a pyoarthrosis. Addicts know this and can claim to have had a bleed just to get the drug. The absence of swelling does not mean a minor bleed has not occurred. The size of the swelling depends on chronicity – i.e., the amount of fibrosis. The joint is held in flexion and is hard to palpate. There is usually one area where tenderness and joint swelling can be detected.

The acute swelling is also warm, and there can even be pyrexia, which can be a problem. The distinction from septic arthritis can be very difficult. There are a few pointers which may assist:

1. The pyrexia is never higher than 38.5°C in sterile hemarthrosis.
2. There is an increased incidence in immune-compromised patients, particularly those with AIDS.
3. Of importance is the rapidity of onset of pain and swelling. Hemarthrosis causes symptoms very much quicker than sepsis. Usually there is also tenderness – its absence suggests an effusion, particularly with underlying degenerative changes.

Ankle swelling distends anteriorly, below the malleoli; the elbow extends postero-laterally; and the shoulder anteriorly.

For those joints which are easily accessible clinically, the best way of measuring progress and the response to treatment is by daily measuring the circumference, after having marked one or more levels on the joint with an indelible ink.

There is of course loss of movement. The joint is held in flexion.

Nerve and vessel involvement by the swelling is uncommon but must always be looked for.

Management

For complications to be minimized, one must infuse factor within 4 h. If over 12 h have elapsed and the

hemarthrosis is severe and acute, it will often need aspiration and immobilization as well. If the bleed is days to weeks old and is still sore, hot, and painful, and feels doughy, then the blood has clotted. Check for antibodies and go on to arthroscopy if there is still some residual fluid, else go for long-term immobilization.

SPLINTING is rarely necessary in early minor bleeds. But if there is guarding, this is strongly recommended, otherwise one is likely to get very slow resorption or recurrence. Use compression bandages or padded POP as back splints ONLY, in the position of comfort. Relief of pain is the best indicator that bleeding has stopped. Ice packs should be used, 5 min on, 10 min off. After 24–48 h, re-position the POP, and change weekly.

ASPIRATION. This depends on

1. Size, severity of pain, and tension.
2. Loculation. A chronic joint often loculated, so aspiration generally is not very successful.
3. The time interval – aspiration is usually useless after 24 h.

Before aspiration, make sure there are no inhibitors otherwise a catastrophic hemarthrosis can ensue. Use a 20 bore needle. Try not to move the needle around once in the joint – rather milk the blood toward the needle. NEVER inject factor into a joint – there is a high risk of producing antibodies.

REHABILITATION. Mobilization should in most cases be started within 48 h.

Muscle Bleeds

There is no tendency to repeat bleeds in the same muscle (except in the iliacus) probably because of fibrosis obliterating vascular tissue later on (early on of course there is increased vascularity due to granuloma formation).

These bleeds are most commonly spontaneous, even occurring in sleep (and very commonly after intramuscular injections). Small bleeds are resorbed, but large volumes frequently form cysts. These may become complicated by progressive necrosis or atrophy of overlying tissues, and can thus present at the body surface, through the skin, with infection and abscess formation.

Clinical Features

Bleeding into muscle is much more insidious than into joints. Pain is the predominant symptom but may take days to reach the intensity of an acute hemarthrosis, and is determined by tension. There is a rapid reactive spasm of the muscle, typically in flexion. Nerve involvement occurs in about one third of cases, two thirds in ilio-psoas bleeds. Vascular involvement is not clinically significant.

Management

Do not attempt to correct the acute flexion. Complete rest, splinting if possible, and using padded POP slabs – NOT complete splints. Once the pain has stopped, shell casts are used and replaced weekly, with gradual correction of the flexion.

There is no possibility of effective aspiration. Surgical decompression is very rarely indicated. Use lots of factor.

Disseminated Intravascular Coagulation (DIC)

In its basics, DIC is simple to understand. The fundamental pathogenesis is as follows:

1. A noxious stimulus activates the procoagulant aspect of the hemostatic system **INTRAVASCULARLY**. This stimulus always involves damage to the endothelium. Physical trauma can also provoke DIC but only if it is very widespread with lots of tissue damage, especially if it is necrotic tissue. More commonly the stimulus is infection causing vascular damage due either to direct infection of the endothelium, the deposition of immune complexes, or other immune damage to the endothelium. Finally, cells normally foreign to the vascular tree, such as some types of malignant cells and products of conception, may be the offending stimulus.

2. In most cases, the mechanism by which the stimulus operates is via increased activity of tissue factor (TF). But usually this is not the normal perivascular TF but that produced pathologically by activated monocytes and macrophages (caused by pro-inflammatory cytokines) as well as induced increased expression by the endothelial cells; viruses can produce a DIC-like picture probably due to direct infection of the endothelial cells.

   Another important mechanism is access to the circulation of tissue thromboplastin, from trauma, obstetric emergencies, malignant disease, or an acute hemolytic transfusion reaction. DIC can complicate certain forms of acute myelogenous leukemia. DIC can also supervene in patients with massive blood loss.

   Finally, some snakebites can activate the coagulation system.

3. Once activated, widespread intravascular coagulation tends to occur. There are four very important sequelae:

   a. Intravascular coagulation consumes platelets and coagulation factors, resulting in bleeding, both purpuric-type and coagulation-defect type.
   b. The resultant fibrin strands damage the passing red cells, causing them to break, releasing hemoglobin into the plasma; the red cells tend to reform into fragmented and spherical entities that can be recognized morphologically.
   c. Secondary fibrinolysis occurs, with release of large amounts of fibrin degradation products. These further inhibit platelet function, aggravating the bleeding tendency.
   d. Impaired blood flow leads to organ damage.

Clinical Features

The most common presentation of DIC is an acute severe illness, with bleeding from orifices, drip-lines, and wounds. In these cases diagnosis is not usually a problem, especially if the underlying disorder is recognized. The FBC will show anemia with fragmented red cells, thrombocytopenia and usually neutrophilia with marked toxic changes. The HS will show abnormalities in all the tests; in addition D-dimers will be markedly raised.

In less severe cases the system may compensate quite extensively – sometimes the only clue to the diagnosis will be mild to moderate thrombocytopenia and fragmented red cells. The latter picture must be differentiated from

1. The picture that occurs with artificial heart valves and other intravascular prostheses.
2. Aortic aneurysms and giant hemangiomas.

There is however a more chronic form of DIC. This is more commonly found in malignancies, especially mucin-secreting adenocarcinomas. It will present very much like a partly compensated mild acute DIC. Some viruses, notably arboviruses, may present similarly.

Further Reading

Duthie RB, Rizza CR, Giangrande PLF, Dodd, CAF (eds) (1994). The Management of Musculoskeletal Problems in the Haemophilias. 2nd edn. Oxford University Press.

Lewis SM, Bain B, Bates I (2006). Dacie and Lewis Practical Haematology. 10th edn. Churchill Livingstone.

Hoffbrand AV, Catovsky D, Tuddenham EGD (eds) (2005). Postgraduate Haematology. 5th edn. Oxford: Blackwell Publishing.

Transfusion of blood and its components is an essential part of modern medicine. However, great circumspection must be practiced in prescribing them:

1. **THEY ARE VERY EXPENSIVE.**
2. **THEY ARE POTENTIALLY VERY DANGEROUS.** Ensuring safety for the recipient is not only the responsibility of the transfusion service – the responsible clinician has a very important role to play in this regard. He must be aware of the potential problems that may arise as well as various other aspects:

a) **COMPATIBILITY.** This is clearly a vitally important issue. Should the clinician submit the wrong tube of patient blood to the service for compatibility testing, for instance, the service can clearly not be held responsible for the often disastrous consequences. The responsibility of the clinician to ensure compatibility extends all the way through to the infusion of the components, and it concerns **THE NATURE OF THE COMPONENTS** going to be infused and **THE PATIENT** himself. With respect to the components issued by the service

   i. **BEFORE COMMENCING THE TRANSFUSION,** the component issued by the blood service should be verified either by a medical practitioner and a registered nurse or by two registered nurses (in this country, at any rate). It is important that certain procedures in this regard be followed:

   - All identification is carried out at the patient's bedside.
   - The information is read aloud by both people checking the data.
   - The patient's name and identification number on the component must be identical to that on the hospital record.

   - The identification number on the component must be the same as the component's number on the requisition form and/or label.
   - Make sure that the component's expiry date and time have not been reached.
   - The component and its container must be examined for abnormalities. The seal must be intact and show no evidence of being pierced after the container was filled.

   ii. **THE PATIENT** must be properly identified, using leading questions. The identification of the unconscious patient requires special care.

b) **THE HEALTH STATUS OF THE DONOR BLOOD.** Obviously, this is entirely the responsibility of the service, but it is important for the clinician to understand that this is not a trivial issue.

c) **ARISING FROM THE ABOVE,** it should be realized that conditions vary considerably in different countries, impacting on the safety of the components. For example, the incidence of HIV transmission via transfused components is <1:500,000 units in First World countries. This is relatively easy to achieve because

   i. They can afford the highly sophisticated testing that is necessary.
   ii. They can afford the highly sophisticated purification techniques.
   iii. They can afford very expensive recombinant technology.
   iv. The prevalence of HIV infection in the general population is very low; thus, the potential pool of donors is likely to be healthy and better informed, such that the answers to the questionnaires demanded by the service before accepting a donor are more reliable. In Third World

O.N. Beck, *Diagnostic Hematology*, DOI 10.1007/978-1-84800-295-1_19,
© Springer-Verlag London Limited 2009

countries the situation can be very different –
the prevalence of HIV infection is relatively
much higher resulting in a smaller pool of
potential healthy donors; and many of the
populace may find it difficult to understand
the import of the questionnaire. The sophisticated purification techniques are frequently not
available. Thus doctors working in Third World
countries may be constrained to be more than
usually circumspect in ordering blood components. These concepts apply to other transmis-
sible diseases as well.

d) **THE EFFECTS OF STORAGE ON COMPO-
NENTS** on their efficacy. Unless specifically moti-
vated, the service will issue blood or components
that are internationally recognized as within an
acceptable date of expiry. However, specific patient
conditions may be adversely affected by certain
components that are close to their expiry date. The
clinician must know what these circumstances are
and inform the service appropriately.

**The Effects on Blood Components of Bank
Storage**

1. Effects on red cells.

   a) *Potassium and lactate* tends to rise.
   b) *2,3-BPG* decreases to very low levels after
      about 1 week. Normally the patient can
      restore the levels within a few hours and in
      the short term can increase his cardiac out-
      put with some peripheral vasodilatation to
      maintain the oxygen supply to the tissues
      until the 2,3-BPG has been restored by the
      patient's own metabolism; in massive trans-
      fusion, this may be impossible, leading to
      decreased oxygen-carrying capacity. Conse-
      quently, patients with marginal cardiac
      reserves may not be able to cope.
   c) The deformability of the red cells decreases
      considerably. This means that the trans-
      fused cells have greater difficulty in nego-
      tiating the capillaries; this is generally only
      of significance where the capillaries are
      narrowed, usually due to endothelial swel-
      ling, leading to poor tissue perfusion and
      oxygenation. This often occurs precisely in
      clinical situations where increased perfusion
      is particularly needed. This is a potent
      source of acidemia and other problems in
      the critically ill.

2. Effects on platelets. *Platelets lose considerable
   viability* at the cold temperatures used for
   refrigeration. Recovery of viable platelets is
   about 20% after 72 h.
3. Effects on white cells. *Granulocytes lose functional viability* quite soon.

---

e) **ARISING FROM THE ABOVE,** the questionnaire
that most services require before **ISSUING** components also must be answered carefully. The service is
attempting to assist the users in minimizing any
adverse effects.

f) **THE TECHNIQUES OF ADMINISTRATION** of
the components are entirely the responsibility of the
clinician. Incorrect techniques may render the transfused components ineffective or dangerous. Relevant aspects of this are discussed later.

g) **MONITORING THE PATIENT FOR NEGA-
TIVE EFFECTS** too is entirely the responsibility
of the clinician. The nursing staff is usually very
competent, but in the event of a negative effect, it
is the responsible clinician who is held primarily
responsible, not the nurse.

The service is usually very keen on preventing
potential problems and goes out of its way to assist
the clinician. For this reason also the extensive
questionnaire that the service requires before issuing components should be answered as carefully as
possible.

It is convenient to describe the different components
available in terms of their indications, the possible complications that may arise, the possible adverse reactions,
the pathogenesis and clinical features, and their treatment
(in brief). Thus, a preliminary look at the **COMPLICA-
TIONS** and **REACTIONS** that may occur is necessary.

Complications of Transfusion of Blood Components

There are two groups of these: (1) acute or early complications and (2) delayed or long-term complications.

Acute or Early Complications

1. **THE COMPLICATIONS OF MASSIVE TRANSFU-
   SION.** Massive transfusion is defined as the infusion of

sufficient blood or components within 24 h that effectively replaces the total blood volume (approximately 5 l).

a) **CITRATE TOXICITY.** The importance of this complication is falling away, since newer anticoagulants contain no citrate. However, traditional anticoagulant contains citrate, and the infusion of a few units can usually be easily handled by the patient's metabolism (the Krebs cycle). With massive transfusion, the patient's capacity may be compromised, leading to acidosis.

b) **THE FORMATION OF MICRO-AGGREGATES.** Bits of fibrin with platelets and other material tend to form micro-aggregates. In massive transfusion, the capacity of the reticulo-endothelial system in clearing these may be exceeded. They are particularly dangerous in shock states and compromised pulmonary function.

c) **EFFECTS OF STORAGE.** The effects of storage have been mentioned earlier. Insofar as the red cells are concerned, they are really only of significance in massive transfusion. The decreased perfusion that may be found because of decreased red cell deformability is very difficult to quantify or even identify, since generally the patient is so ill with numerous serious clinical features.

d) **HYPOTHERMIA.** This is another effect of massively transfusing refrigerated components. These should be warmed properly, but only by means of the correct blood warmers – not on the radiator or in a microwave!

e) **SECONDARY BLEEDING.** Massive transfusion may lead to a bleeding tendency, by several possible mechanisms:

   i. **THE "WASHOUT" EFFECT.** It has been claimed that the coagulation factors and platelets are so diluted by massive transfusion that effective hemostasis is compromised. But it is thought that this mechanism is not the whole explanation.

   ii. **SOME PLASMA SUBSTITUTES,** particularly dextran, coat the platelets and impair their function.

   iii. **DISSEMINATED INTRAVASCULAR COAGULATION** (DIC). This causes the most severe bleeding disorders, especially in patients with extensive tissue damage plus prolonged shock and hence poor perfusion. Intravascular activation of hemostasis leads to consumption of platelets and coagulation factors, particularly factors V, VIII, II, and I. This is generally complicated by secondary hyperfibrinolysis which breaks down the fibrin formed, with release of fibrin-breakdown products that further inhibit coagulation and platelet plug formation. Note that it is currently thought that DIC, developing in the context of massive transfusion, is not primarily due to the transfusion itself but due to the underlying trauma or disease.

f) **HYPOCALCEMIA,** due to binding of calcium by citrate, is seldom a problem.

2. **CIRCULATORY OVERLOAD,** i.e., induced hypervolemia resulting in cardio-pulmonary decompensation.

Acute (and delayed) transfusion reactions are discussed separately, below.

Long-Term Complications

1. **IRON OVERLOAD.** It will be remembered that each ml of red cells contains about 1 mg of iron. Consequently, transfusion of red cells in any form leads to accumulation of iron, unless the patient is actively bleeding. Iron overload is further discussed in Chapter 20.

2. **TRANSMISSION OF DISEASES.** Modern technology has enabled the removal of very many infectious organisms from most blood components (except red cells and cryoprecipitate). None of these, however, is guaranteed to remove all. The important diseases that may be transmitted by infusion of all blood components are

   a) Retroviruses (HIV-1, HIV-2, HTLV-1, HTLV-2)
   b) Hepatitis A, B, and C.
   c) Syphilis (the spirochetes will die in blood stored for longer than 48 h).
   d) Malaria
   e) Chagas' disease.

Transfusion Reactions

These again can be divided into acute/early, occurring with a day or two, and delayed, usually occurring at 7–14 days. The acute/early reactions are potentially medical emergencies, and a few guidelines are necessary should they occur:

1. The transfusion should be stopped immediately, and the transfused component and the drip set are removed and replaced with a new drip set and crystalloid.

2. If the reaction is a mild febrile reaction (see below) and the patient feels otherwise reasonably well, the administration of an antipyretic should be monitored: if the

temperature settles down, the original unit can be started again. Should the reaction reoccur, that unit must be stopped permanently and the procedure outlined below followed.

3. The blood service must be informed and asked for advice.

Acute Transfusion Reactions

1. Febrile non-hemolytic reactions
2. Acute hemolytic reactions
3. Allergic and anaphylactoid reactions
4. Anaphylaxis
5. Transfusion-related acute lung injury (TRALI).

Febrile Non-hemolytic Reactions

1. These are the commonest of all transfusion reactions, caused by antibodies in the recipient's plasma that react with antigens on the surfaces of leukocytes (most commonly) and platelets.
2. They take the form within about 5 min of flushing, palpitations, and cough, often followed by an asymptomatic phase lasting for about 20 min, and then a rise in temperature with chills and sometimes rigors. They tend to occur more often in patients receiving regular transfusions and in women who have had multiple pregnancies.
3. Fever is the most prominent feature, with the temperature rising by at least 1°C; it is also most worrying, since the acute hemolytic reactions also are characterized by fever.
4. It is diagnosed by exclusion of a hemolytic reaction, and it usually responds well to antipyretics. Usually the transfusion does not have to be terminated.

Acute Hemolytic Reactions

1. These are the most dangerous and most feared reactions; the mortality is around 10%. They are most commonly due to incompatibility; occasionally, bacterial contamination of the blood is responsible.
2. The hemolytic reaction may be characterized by intravascular or by extravascular hemolysis (see Chapters 2 and 4).

   a) **INTRAVASCULAR HEMOLYSIS.** The most common acute hemolytic reaction to blood transfusion is intravascular and is most commonly due to ABO incompatibility. Occasionally, and atypically, other blood groups such as anti-Kell, anti-Kidd, and anti-Duffy are responsible, particularly if the patient has had repeated prior transfusions or multiple pregnancies. This form of hemolysis is characterized by the activation of complement. Note too that there is an element of extravascular hemolysis as well, due to the mopping up of opsonized red cells by the spleen and liver.

   b) **PURE EXTRAVASCULAR HEMOLYTIC TRANSFUSION REACTIONS** are usually due to anti-D, anti-E, and anti-Kell antibodies. Complement is not activated. These reactions are usually of the **DELAYED** type – see later.

3. **THE CLINICAL FEATURES** are a sudden onset of fever, chills, loin pain, pain at the infusion site, and hypotension. Hemoglobinuria and oliguria are common. Particular care must be taken when transfusing a patient under general anesthesia – the only signs of incompatibility may be an unexplained hypotension and excessive bleeding at the operation site.
4. If acute hemolysis is suspected, the transfusion must be stopped immediately, blood taken from the patient and submitted, together with the infused unit and the administration set, to the blood service.
5. Antigen–antibody complexes may activate both the coagulation mechanism and the fibrinolytic system, with a severe bleeding tendency.
6. It can be seen that differentiation from the febrile non-hemolytic reaction is critically important.

Allergic and Anaphylactoid Reactions

These reactions are caused by a protein constituent in the donor plasma. They constitute the second most common transfusion reaction. The reactions vary from pruritus to urticaria. **IT IS MOST IMPORTANT TO KNOW THAT PYREXIA IS ABSENT.** They are usually controllable with intravenous antihistamines. The particular unit being transfused must be stopped, the patient given antihistamines, and another unit started. The blood service must be informed. If it continues to occur, leukocyte-depleted components must be used, if available, else use a 30 μm filter. A common practice is to administer an antihistamine before the component is set up.

Anaphylactic Reactions

These are far more serious. They occur almost always in IgA-deficient recipients (IgA deficiency is the commonest of all immune deficiencies, with an incidence of 1:700 – see Chapter 22). Ten percent of IgA-deficient people develop anti-IgA antibodies and tend to develop severe anaphylactic reactions when infused components contain IgA.

Transfusion-Related Lung Injury (TRALI)

This condition is characterized by pulmonary infiltrates and pulmonary edema occurring within 4 h of the infusion of components containing antibodies that react with recipient leukocytes. The patients present with chest pain, cough, dyspnea, cyanosis, bloody sputum, and hypoxemia. They require ventilatory support.

Delayed Transfusion Reactions

These comprise delayed hemolytic and delayed non-hemolytic reactions.

1. **DELAYED HEMOLYTIC REACTIONS.** These are always extravascular and usually due to irregular antibodies. Generally, they are not picked up during cross-matching because their titer is so low; upon exposure to antigen in the recipient, they anamnestically increase. They usually present about 7–10 days after infusion, as typical extravascular hemolysis. It is thus clear that in any patient presenting with a typical extravascular hemolytic state, the history must include that of any recent transfusions.

2. **DELAYED NON-HEMOLYTIC REACTIONS**

   i. **POST-TRANSFUSION PURPURA.** This is rare and occurs 7–10 days after infusion. It often clears up without treatment; gammaglobulins may be necessary.

   ii. **GRAFT-VERSUS-HOST DISEASE.** This is due to transfused lymphocytes recognizing host tissues of the recipient. The patients develop fever, erythema, and bone marrow suppression with pancytopenia. It is clear that this complication can particularly be found when the donor is a first- or even second-degree relative, since the chances of HLA matching are so much greater. This is one of the arguments against "directed donation."

Directed Donation Many patients have decided that blood from a relative is safer and "better" than bank blood. Generally, this is a very mistaken view.

1. It has been found that donated blood is no safer than bank blood. Donors generally feel under some sort of moral pressure to donate, and as a result, they may conceal relevant information about their health status. There is thus possibly an *increased* risk of disease transmission.
2. Depending on the country's laws, such donors may lose the usual patient confidentiality.
3. There is an increased risk of graft-versus-host disease.

   The only real advantage is a decrease in anxiety on the part of the recipient!

   iii. **IMMUNOSUPPRESSION** is said to occur as a result of transfusion.

Components, Their Indications, and Their Dangers

Whole Blood

This is seldom used these days. The **ONLY** indication is where the patient requires both increased oxygen-carrying capacity and volume replacement. In these circumstances, it is cheaper and safer than using red cells and plasma separately. Note that **ANY** of the complications and reactions described above can occur.

Red Cells

These are provided in several different forms.

Red cell concentrates (RCC)

These are also called "packed cells."

Each unit essentially consists of whole blood with removal of plasma. In general, RCCs are indicated for any form of anemia that is severe enough and will not respond quite **RAPIDLY** to hematinics (as would be the case in most cases of megaloblastic anemia). One unit of RCC will raise the venous Hb by about 1 g/dl.

Indications for Use

In general terms, there are three indications for red cell transfusion:

1. Replacement of lost blood
2. Other forms of anemia
3. Replacement of abnormal cells. Sickle cells are a prominent example.

More specifically, the important question is, when is transfusion necessary in a patient with anemia? There are no absolute rules here, but a great deal depends on how rapidly the anemia developed; reasonable guidelines are

1. In an acute anemia, the patient has not had time to adapt (e.g., shift in the oxygen-dissociation curve), and oxygen requirements will generally be compromised with a Hb of about 8 g/dl. Chronic anemias can and do tolerate much lower Hbs. As a general rule, **ONE DOES NOT TRANSFUSE A HB LEVEL!**
2. An adult patient who is adjudged unlikely to be able to autonomously (physiologically) increase cardiac output or peripheral perfusion requires a Hb of at least **10 G/DL.**
3. All patients over the age of 65 years require a Hb of at least **10 G/DL.**
4. Post-operative patients with significant complications that will increase oxygen demand require a Hb of at least **10 G/DL.**
5. A patient for whom major surgery is contemplated will need a Hb of **8 G/DL,** although many surgeons prefer one a little higher.
6. Young to middle-aged patients who are basically healthy and have a well-compensated chronic anemia need a Hb of at least **6 G/DL.** However, most of these will complain of severe fatigue at this level, and will feel better at a Hb level of 8 g/dl. It has been observed that most of these patients will tell the doctor when they need a transfusion – and it turns out that their subjective acceptable level is always between 8 and 9 g/dl.
7. Patients on hypothermic cardio-pulmonary bypass require a minimum Hb of **6 G/DL.**
8. It is of interest that critically ill patients have better survival if the Hb is held **BELOW** 8 g/dl. There are several complex reasons for this.

Possible Reactions to RCC

Since RCC contain some plasma as well as leukocytes and platelets, any of the reactions listed above can occur.

ADVANTAGE OF RCC: minimal increase in blood volume.

DISADVANTAGE OF RCC: because of high viscosity, the infusion time is necessarily slow.

Washed Red Cells

These units are free of all plasma and 80% of leukocytes.

Specific Indications

The obvious indication for using this component is in those cases where plasma elements interact negatively with the red cells of the recipient. Paroxysmal nocturnal hemoglobinuria is a condition in which hemolysis is due to an acquired increased sensitivity of the red cell membrane to circulating complement, causing intravascular hemolysis. Since these patients usually need regular red cell transfusion, added plasma components in the transfusion would aggravate hemolysis and decrease the efficacy of the transfusion. Similarly, patients who are known to be hypersensitive to elements of the plasma proteins causing allergic reactions would benefit from plasma-free red cells, were they to require transfusion.

Ideally, preventing future reactions when using emergency group O blood by washing out the plasma would be very beneficial; however, washing the cells is a time-consuming job, and there is often not enough time. Note that washed RCC cannot be stored for longer than 24 h.

Other indications are the removal of micro-aggregates; this is important only in certain circumstances (see below).

Reactions That May Occur

1. Acute and early hemolytic reactions may occur.
2. Febrile non-hemolytic reactions are far less common, as are allergic and anaphylactic reactions.
3. TRALI may occur.
4. All the delayed reactions may occur.

Advantages of Washed RCC

1. Decreased febrile non-hemolytic reactions
2. Decreased micro-aggregates – this is especially important in patients with pulmonary dysfunction, cardiopulmonary bypass, and massive transfusion

Leukocyte-Depleted RCC

It can be seen that the leukocytes in transfused blood are responsible for a great many adverse events in transfusion (although the usual patient seems to do quite well with ordinary RCC). There are different techniques for achieving leukocyte depletion, with different outcomes.

1. **"BUFFY COAT" LEUKOCYTE DEPLETION AND BEDSIDE LEUKOCYTE FILTERS.** These will remove around 80% of leukocytes and may be sufficient to prevent mild febrile reactions.
2. **WITH THE MOST EFFICIENT TECHNIQUE** (which has to be done by the service), 99% of leukocytes are removed from such blood and 90% of the original red cells remain. It is thus an efficient method to minimize or remove the risk of leuko-agglutinin associated reactions.

It follows that when ordering the blood, the blood service should be informed as to the indication and clinical condition, since highly efficient leukocyte depletion is very expensive and may not be necessary.

Specific Indications

1. The most important indication is to prevent febrile non-hemolytic reactions.
2. It is probably advisable in patients requiring long-term transfusion to prevent HLA sensitization to leukocyte antigens.
3. It has also been shown to be effective in reducing refractoriness to platelet transfusion (see below).
4. Patients with aplastic anemia, who are potential stem cell transplant recipients, should receive leukocyte-depleted components from the beginning of the transfusion support.
5. Of note is that CMV cannot be transmitted without the presence of leukocytes. This is relevant when transfusing susceptible patients.

Reactions That May Occur

1. Acute and delayed hemolytic reactions
2. Some plasma remains. Thus all the other transfusion reactions may occur

Frozen Blood

This is a modern and very expensive technique, not universally available. The washed packed cells are treated with 45% glycerol and frozen. Obviously the blood must be deglycerolized before use.

Indications

1. Alloimmunized patients with a history of severe febrile non-hemolytic reactions
2. Anaphylactic responses in IgA-deficient patients
3. Patients requesting autologous transfusion (see later)

Advantages

1. **VERY** few leukocytes, platelets, plasma proteins, and viruses
2. No decrease in 2,3-BPG or ATP
3. It does not contain anticoagulant

Reactions That May Occur

1. Acute and delayed hemolytic reactions
2. All others are very rare

Irradiated Blood

This is primarily used for prevention of graft-versus-host disease in

1. Immune suppressed patients
2. Pre- and post-bone marrow transplant patients
3. Patients receiving blood from blood relatives

Note that it is only necessary to irradiate red cells and platelets.

Platelets

Platelet transfusions are often indicated in a number of bleeding disorders. The decision to transfuse platelets should not be made only by reference to the platelet count; clinical features play a large role in the decision. Similarly, the response to platelet infusion should be judged not only by the platelet count but by clinical improvement and the bleeding time. Note that platelet concentrates contain large amounts of factor V and are thus very useful in factor V deficiency, since factor V concentrates are not available.

Types of Platelet Product

There are two groups of product, depending on the method of preparation:

1. **RANDOM SINGLE DONOR UNITS.** These are prepared by centrifugation and contain about 5×10^{10} platelets in 50 ml of plasma. They have a 3–5-day survival. These are satisfactory for acute disorders such as DIC, and multiple units can be used. Over short periods, there is little danger of alloimmunization. Since it contains plasma, the allergic, anaphylactic, TRALI, and even post-tranfusional purpura may occur, although the latter is very uncommon. It should be borne in mind that random units are prepared from Rh-negative as well as Rh-positive donors; using Rh-positive units in Rh-negative recipients is acceptable if the clinician agrees. Because these units contain very few red cells, Rh immunization is unlikely to occur; however, in pre-menopausal women, it is advisable to use anti-D prophylaxis if Rh-positive units have to be used – use 500 IU of anti-D immunoglobulin for every six pooled random platelet units.
2. **PLATELETS PRODUCED BY APHERESIS.** These are obtained from a donor with the same ABO and Rh group as the patient, and are free of red cells and contain virtually no leukocytes. They contain ±300 × 10^9 platelets in 300 ml of plasma, with a shelf life of 5 days. They are recommended for patients requiring long-term platelet support, to minimize alloantibody formation.

Platelet Administration and Dosages

Platelets should be administered rapidly – over 15 min, else they will lose efficacy. The dosages depend on the type of platelets units being used:

1. Random single donor units (50 ml): 1 unit per 10 kg body weight
2. Apheresis unit (300 ml): 1 unit per average adult

Responses to Platelet Administration

It is important to evaluate the response to platelet transfusions; up to 10% of patients are refractory. Poor response ($<20 \times 10^9$/l) may be due to ITP, alloimmunization, infection, DIC, splenomegaly, and treatment with antibiotics and amphotericin. Higher dosages may be required if clinically necessary. Ultimately, if there is clinical improvement despite a poor increase in count, it may not be necessary to increase the dosage.

Evaluating Platelet Response In critical situations, such as the ICU and theater, it is often advisable to quantify the response to platelet infusion. There are two basic ways of doing this:

1. Corrected count increment (CCI):

$$CCI = \frac{(\text{Post-transfusion PC} - \text{Pre-transfusion PC}) \times \text{Surface area (m}^2)}{\text{Number of (single) units infused}}$$

Acceptable: CCI > 4,000–5,000
2. Percentage recovery. This formula should be used if there is splenomegaly.

$$\% = \frac{(\text{Post-transfusion PC} - \text{Pre-transfusion PC}) \times \text{Blood volume}}{\text{Total platelets infused} \times 2/3}$$

Expected recovery: 60% at 1 h; 40% at 24 h.

DISADVANTAGES OF PLATELET TRANSFUSIONS:

Possible Complications:

1. Bacterial contamination
2. Transmission of viruses and, since platelet units contain some red cells and thus possibly parasites
3. Pulmonary edema

Possible Adverse Reactions:

1. Because platelet units contain plasma, febrile non-hemolytic, allergic, and anaphylactic reactions may occur.
2. Because they contain some lymphocytes, graft-versus-host disease may occur in immuno-compromised patients.

Ideally, platelet units should be ABO cross-matched. HLA cross-matching is controversial – it is often very difficult to achieve, and 25% of fully HLA matched platelets are unsuccessful.

Plasma Components

NOTE: ALL PLASMA PRODUCTS ARE ANTIGENIC. HENCE, ALL THE TRANSFUSION REACTIONS DESCRIBED ABOVE DUE TO INTERACTIONS

BETWEEN PLASMA PROTEINS AND RECIPIENT CELLS CAN OCCUR. The following components are available:

1. Fresh frozen plasma (FFP)
2. Coagulation factor concentrates
3. Albumin
4. Stabilized serum
5. Immunoglobulins
6. A few miscellaneous other constituents

Fresh Frozen Plasma

This contains all the clotting factors in normal physiological concentrations. **FRESH FROZEN SINGLE DONOR PLASMA** carries the same risk of latent viral infection as a unit of red cell concentrate. Pooled plasma that has been virus-inactivated is available in most large centers. In addition, retested and quarantined FFP (to avoid the window period of many infections) is sometimes available.

Note also that FFP contains biochemicals from the original anticoagulant that need to be taken into account in certain cases, e.g., diabetes, hypertension, dehydration, shock states, and the elderly. Each unit contains, on average,

Glucose	24.8 mmol/l
Potassium	3.0 mmol/l
Sodium	165 mmol/l
Osmolarity	322 mmol/l
P_H	7.9.

Indications

1. Replacement of coagulation factor deficiencies if concentrates are not available. This includes vitamin K deficiency and liver disease with coagulation-type bleeding.
2. Immediate reversal of coumadin effect.
3. Acute DIC.
4. Thrombotic thrombocytopenic purpura (see Chapter 23)
5. Scoline apnea (FFP contains physiological quantities of choline esterase).

NOTE:

1. FFP is not to be used for hypovolemia or nutritional support.
2. FFP must be administered as rapidly as possible.

Coagulation Factors

While FFP contains all coagulation factors, there may not be enough to achieve hemostasis in severe deficiencies with severe bleeding, without overloading the patient. Factor concentrates are far more efficient. However, concentrates are generally not available for the rare deficiencies, when there is no option but to use FFP. There are three groups of these concentrates:

1. **CRYOPRECIPITATE.** Historically, this was the first concentrate available. It contains moderate amounts of factor VIII, von Willebrand factor, fibrinogen, and factor XIII, and it is thus suitable for treating deficiencies of these factors, although where factor VIII concentrates are available, they are far preferable since the levels are much higher and they are virus-inactivated (virus-inactivation cannot be done with cryoprecipitate).
2. **VIRUS-INACTIVATED FACTORS**

    a) **FACTOR VIII/VWF CONCENTRATE** (intermediate purity). Various size units are available, each containing 300, 500, or 1,000 IU factor VIII.
    b) **FACTOR IX COMPLEX,** containing factors II, VII, IX, and X (as a reminder, these are the vitamin K-dependent procoagulant factors). Each unit contains 500 IU of factor IX.
    c) **FACTOR IX CONCENTRATE** (intermediate purity). Each unit contains 500 IU of factor IX.

3. **RECOMBINANT FACTORS** VIII, IX, and VII.

Dosage in Hemophilia A

When a patient with hemophilia A is bleeding severely enough to require factor replacement, a number of relevant points should be noted:

1. It is possible to calculate the amount of factor required in a given patient. The formula is as follows:

$$\text{Factor VIII dose (in IU)} = \frac{\text{Patients mass (kg)} \times \text{Desired increase in factor level}}{2}$$

The problem now is to decide what the level should be. The following guidelines are generally acceptable:

a) Minor bleeds. Levels should be raised to 50% immediately and then kept at 25% for a day or so. So, assuming the patient has a basic factor VIII level of 1%, the desired increase would be 49% to start with.
b) Moderate bleeding, such as a hemarthrosis. Levels should be raised to 50% and kept there for 5 days after the bleeding has stopped.

c) Severe or very dangerous bleeding, such as major surgery or a head injury, immediately raise levels to 100% and maintain at 50% for 10 days.

The next decision is how to administer the factor. There are two basic methods: by continuous infusion and by bolus doses. With continuous infusion, one can usually get by with less total factor than with bolus treatment, but it requires careful monitoring.

Factor VIII has a half-life of 8–12 h. If the patient has pure factor VIII deficiency, the boluses are given every 8 h for the first 24 h, and then every 12 h. If the patient has von Willebrand disease, the infusion causes a more sustained rise in factor VIII and thus transfusions of factor VIII for vWD can be given daily.

2. Sometimes appropriate laboratory facilities are not available. Thus in a known factor VIII deficiency, empirical dosing can be used. Dosages in IU/kg body weight:

a) Minor bleeds, such as from lacerations: 10.
b) Moderate bleeds, such as in small joints or patients requiring dental surgery: 15.
c) Severe bleeds, as in large hemarthroses, soft-tissue hematomas: 20.
d) Pre- and post-operation: 50 as bolus immediately prior to surgery, then 20 every 12 h for 5 days, then 20 per day for 5 days.

3. Infusion of factor should be rapid – within 15 min.
4. Any suspicion of factor VIII inhibitors will require specialist consultation

Dosage in von Willebrand Disease

If DDAVP treatment has not been effective, one should start with factor VIII concentrate at a dosage of 30 IU/kg. Daily monitoring is satisfactory. If the response is unsatisfactory, use cryoprecipitate 15 IU/kg or random platelet concentrate (1 per 10 kg).

Dosage in Hemophilia B (Factor IX Deficiency)

There are two products available:

1. Factor IX complex. Since this contains factors II, VII, IX, and X, it has reportedly led to thrombotic complications when used for longer than about 5 days. It should therefore not be used longer than this.
2. Factor IX concentrate, for long-term use.

Note that the half-life of factor IX is longer than that of factor VIII; hence, daily dosing is sufficient.

The dosage can be calculated with the formula:

$$\text{Factor IX does in IU/kg} = \text{patient mass (in kg)} \times \text{desired increase} \times 1.2$$

If appropriate lab facilities are not available, use 15 IU/kg daily until hemostasis is achieved.

Dosage in Fibrinogen (Factor I) Deficiency (as well as Dysfunctional Fibrinogen)

Cryoprecipitate is used. The dosage depends on whether the condition is acquired or hereditary.

1. Acquired forms (e.g., DIC, massive transfusions): 4 g per average adult.
2. Hereditary forms: on average, 6 g will raise the fibrinogen levels to effective levels for about a week.

Patient Monitoring

Proper monitoring of the patient during the transfusion is clearly a fundamentally important part of patient care. This implies that the significance of the findings be properly interpreted.

1. It is absolutely essential that all findings be clearly recorded, in writing.
2. The patient's condition before transfusion commences should also be recorded, to facilitate the decision as to whether any changes noticed are new and thus potentially the result of the transfusion. As far as possible, the clinical status should be measured; clearly this includes all vital signs, particularly the temperature. In cases where there is a strong history of hemolysis or the patient already is jaundiced, we have found it useful to keep undisturbed a small tube of clotted patient's blood in the refrigerator; the red cells will settle and the supernatant is available for comparison with specimens taken during transfusion, should problems or suspicions arise. This is also of value in unconscious patients. Note that it can be very difficult to diagnose or even suspect a hemolytic reaction in a critically ill patient.
3. The intensity and frequency of monitoring depends on the basic condition of the patient:

a) The stable, "cold" case. The patient is observed closely for 30 min. Any suspicious features are noted, and where possible, measured. The most important clinical features to take note of are

i. Chills, rigors, sweating
ii. Urticaria
iii. Nausea and vomiting
iv. Dyspnea

The following features are recorded at 5, 15, and 30 min:

i. Temperature
ii. Pulse
iii. Blood pressure
iv. Respiratory rate
v. Symptoms of pruritus, loin pain, dyspnea, anxiety
vi. If urine is passed, it should be examined for bilirubin and blood.

Thereafter, in the absence of untoward features, the patient is monitored hourly.

b) The critically ill or unconscious patient. The patient features mentioned above should be monitored every 15 min throughout the transfusion.

Blood Substitutes

For several reasons, it is valuable to know something about blood substitutes. As has been said, blood components are very expensive, particularly because of the intensive testing that has to be done before release and then the cost of inactivating or eradicating possible infectious organisms. Blood components must be stored and transported under very carefully controlled conditions; this is frequently unpractical in many areas of the world. Blood is unquestionably dangerous and considerable research has gone into finding substitutes. Also, there are religious scruples.

Enormous amounts of research are being done into finding substitutes particularly for red cell substitutes.

Red Cell Substitutes

There are basically four types of red cell substitutes under development:

1. Perfluorocarbon emulsions
2. Stroma-free hemoglobin
3. Polymerized hemoglobin
4. Encapsulated hemoglobin

Perfluorocarbon Emulsions (PFCs)

These are organic polymers in which all the hydrogen atoms have been replaced by fluorine atoms. They have a half-life in the circulation of 13 h and a tissue half-life of 9 days. They have 20 times the solubility for oxygen (and carbon dioxide).

REPORTED SIDE EFFECTS:

1. Bronchospasm and pulmonary hypertension have been reported.
2. Oxygen toxicity – see below.
3. PFCs are retained by the liver and spleen.
4. Complement appears to be activated.

ADVANTAGES:

1. Contain no antigens; cross-matching is unnecessary.
2. Decreased viscosity of blood, hence better perfusion.
3. Do not carry infections.
4. Do not carry carbon monoxide – potentially of great value in the treatment of carbon monoxide poisoning.
5. Their small particle size permits oxygen carriage through compromised capillaries.

DISADVANTAGES:

1. Since oxygen has to be administered at the same time – up to 100%, there is a danger of oxygen toxicity.
2. Not been proven to be efficacious in severe anemia.

Stroma-Free Hemoglobin

This consists of hemoglobin with the bits of red cell membrane that are left after hemolyzing the cells removed completely.

ADVANTAGES:

1. Contains no antigens; cross-matching is unnecessary.
2. Does not carry infections.
3. Because of the high osmotic pressure it exerts, it is an excellent volume expander.
4. Decreased viscosity of the blood.
5. The small particle size permits oxygen carriage through compromised capillaries.

DISADVANTAGES:

1. It can activate the complement system.
2. It has a short circulatory half-life – <8 h.
3. Very high colloid osmotic pressure, with a tendency to retention of fluid in the circulation.
4. Unacceptably high oxygen affinity.
5. Potentially nephrotoxic.

Polymerized Hemoglobin

Currently this shows the most promise.

ADVANTAGES:

1. The oxygen carrying capacity is close to that of blood.
2. Does not affect the colloid osmotic pressure.
3. Can achieve a near-normal hemoglobin concentration.
4. A circulation half-life of 36 h.

DISADVANTAGES:

1. Nephrotoxicity, but probably less than with other preparations. Also, this is transient.
2. It may be immunogenic.

Encapsulated Hemoglobin

In this technology, free hemoglobin is encapsulated into some sort of artificial red cell. The original capsules were liposomes. Currently, micro-capsules containing hemoglobin and 2,3-BPG are receiving great attention, and show great promise.

Teaching Cases

CASE #87 (EXAMINE TABLE 19.1)

DISCUSSION:

1. The features were clearly that of a febrile non-hemolytic reaction, to the second unit of blood.
2. Bedside leukocyte filters are usually sufficient to prevent most cases of this complication.
3. The second unit was returned to the blood service. No evidence of incompatibility was found.
4. It was decided to use leukocyte-depleted cells prepared in the service in the future.

Table 19.1

Patient: Mr J V
The patient was recently diagnosed with a myelodysplastic syndrome, of the "refractory anemia" type. His Hb was 7.7 g/dl. He felt very weak and tired. The leukocyte and platelet counts were normal. The marrow showed no increase in blasts. He had never had a transfusion of any kind before. It was decided to transfuse him with 3 units of red cell concentrate. Since his basic condition was good and it could be expected that he would be a long-term recipient, it was decided to use a bedside leukocyte filter. His blood group was O Rh-positive; no irregular antibodies were found. The first unit was transfused without any problem. Ten minutes after the second unit commenced, he started feeling a bit peculiar, with mild palpitations and cough. His temperature was normal. The blood was stopped and replaced with crystalloid through a new drip set, to allow the patient either to settle down or show something more positive. He was given an antihistamine intravenously, despite there being no allergic symptoms. Ten minutes later his temperature was 39.2°C. He was given antipyretics, and the temperature and other symptoms settled down within 1 h. The third unit was then started, and this was transfused without any complications.

CASE #88 (TABLE 19.2)

Table 19.2

Patient: Miss J D, aged 12 years
This girl had been perfectly well until 8 days before, when she had her menarche. Her PV bleeding was very heavy and did not stop at all. Her family doctor had examined her very carefully and had attempted various measures without success. He even did a pregnancy test despite having noticed that she appeared to be virgo intacta; this was negative. The child was going into shock. He had started a blood transfusion but the bleeding continued. He referred the patient. Further questioning revealed no history of a bleeding tendency. She was clinically pale, very anxious, and somewhat hypotensive. Her basic condition, however, was very good. There was no evidence of infection, snakebite, or malignant disease. A number of tests were done.

The FBC showed the expected effects of acute blood loss. The morphology was normal.

A hemostatic screen was performed (Examine Table 19.3)

It is clear from Table 19.3 that there is a coagulation defect. To interpret this result, one could look at Table 18.4. When dealing with an emergency, such as this patient, one does not always have the table to hand. It is far better to be able to work out the answer from first principles, i.e., understanding the theory. If one were to

Table 19.3

Test	Value	Units	Reference range	
Bleeding time	3	Minutes	3	7
Platelet count	273	×10⁹/l	140	440
PT	**21**	Seconds	12	13
PTT	**77**	Seconds	23	36
D-Dimers	0.11	mg/l	0	0.25

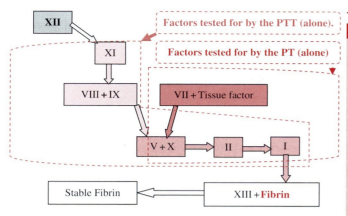

Fig. 19.1 The coagulation cascade (laboratory version)

look again at Fig. 19.1 (a reproduction of Fig. 2.30) and properly understand it, it should be easy to remember the essentials.

Thus, in Fig. 19.1, we see:

1. If both the PTT and PT are prolonged, it cannot mean a defect in factors VIII, IX, or XI, since in that case the PT would be normal.
2. If both the PTT and PT are prolonged, it cannot mean a defect in factor VII alone, since in that case the PTT would be normal.
3. Therefore, the defect must lie in factors V, X, II, or I. This narrows the extent of further investigations.

Deficiency of factor II alone is extremely rare. Isolated deficiency of factor I too is rare. Therefore, it was decided to do factor assays of factors V and X first. Factor X was normal but **THE FACTOR V LEVEL WAS 11%**

The patient was treated with FFP and 1 mega-unit of platelets (since platelet concentrates contain large amount of factor V). Within 30 min of commencing the above regime, the bleeding diminished and eventually ceased.

Prevention of this bleeding with subsequent menses was of course a major consideration. The patient was referred to a gynecologist.

CASE #89 (EXAMINE TABLES 19.4, 19.5, 19.6, AND 19.7)

DISCUSSION:

1. Clinically, the problem with most of these features of distress was that it was difficult to interpret them, in view of the patient's general condition and the fact that he was stuporose. The general impression was that this could be an allergic reaction. It is too soon for TRALI. The patient was given an intravenous

Table 19.4

Mr J S, aged 29 years.
The patient was brought to the emergency room with very severe injuries after an automobile accident. He smelt heavily of alcohol. He was severely shocked and "bled out," with a closed head injury, a crush injury to the chest, and fractures of both femurs, and he was actively bleeding from a lacerated femoral artery (evidently from a knife he was carrying in his belt). His blood pressure was all but unobtainable and the pulse was slow, thready, and irregular. The bleeding was stopped as far as possible with pressure and packs. Resuscitation was commenced with crystalloid and a starch-based plasma volume expander. Blood was drawn for compatibility testing as well as other tests. Several units of group O blood were ordered. He was taken to theater. As soon as the blood arrived, transfusion was started. It was only after 6 units were transfused as rapidly as possible through both arms and the CVP line that his BP responded sufficiently for surgery to begin. During the transfusion, he appeared to be reacting in a non-specific way – he became agitated and he was seen to be trying to scratch himself; a vesicular rash was present. His respiratory rate increased as did the pulse rate. There was no pyrexia. Table 19.5 shows the admission FBC, Table 19.6 the routine biochemistry, and Table 19.7 the hemostatic screen.

Table 19.5

	Value	Units	Reference range Low	Reference range High	Permitted range Low	Permitted range High
Red cell count	1.11	× 10¹²/l	4.77	5.83	1.08	1.14
Hemoglobin (Hb)	3.1	G/dl	13.8	18.0	3.0	3.2
Hematocrit (Hct)	0.10	l/l	0.42	0.53	0.09	0.10
Mean cell volume	88	fl	80	99	86.2	89.8
Mean cell Hb	27.9	pg	27	31.5	27.4	28.5
Mean cell Hb conc.	31.7	G/dl	31.5	34.5	31.1	32.4
Red cell dist. width	12.2	%	11.6	14	11.3	13.1
Retic. count	0.87	%	0.27	0.80	0.8	0.9
Retic. absolute (abs.)	9.7	× 10⁹/l	30	100	8.9	10.4
White cell count	8.34	× 10⁹/l	3.5	10	7.71	8.97
Corrected WCC	7.79	× 10⁹/l				
Neutrophils abs.	5.43	× 10⁹/l	1.5	7	5.02	5.84
Band cells abs.	0.00		0	0.00	0.00	0.00
Lymphocytes abs.	2.10	× 10⁹/l	1	3	1.94	2.26
Monocytes abs.	0.74	× 10⁹/l	0.2	1	0.69	0.80
Eosinophils abs.	0.03	× 10⁹/l	0.02	0.5	0.02	0.03
Basophils abs.	0.04	× 10⁹/l	0.02	0.1	0.04	0.04
Normoblasts	7	/100 WBC	0	0		
Platelet count	498.2	× 10⁹/l	150	400	448.4	548.0

antihistamine as well as hydrocortisone in case there was an element of anaphylaxis. Blood was drawn and spun down to see if the supernatant was hemolyzed; this was negative. Urine from the catheter was examined for Hb, bilirubin, and urobilin. These too were normal. These tests do not completely exclude hemolysis, but were sufficient for the transfusions to continue. (The difficulty of assessing patient responses to transfusion in the unconscious patient must be reiterated.)

Table 19.6

	Value	Units	Reference range Low	High
S-Urea	6.2	mmol/l	2.1	7.1
S-Creatinine	81.7	mmol/l	62	115
S-Urea:creatinine	75.9			
S-Sodium	141	mmol/l	136	145
S-Potassium	4.4	mmol/l	3.5	5.1
S-Chloride	**110.00**	mmol/l	98	108
S-Total CO_2	**18.2**	mmol/l	22	28
S-Anion Gap	**18.2**	mmol/l	5	14
S-Glucose	4.9	mmol/l	3.9	5.8
S-Osmolarity	277	mmol/l	275	295
S-Osmolality	287	mmol/kg	275	295
S-Osmolar Gap	10		–6	6
S-Bilirubin (total)	25.7	µmol/l	6.8	34.2
S-Bilirubin (direct)	8.1	µmol/l	1.7	8.6
S-Bilirubin (indirect)	17.6	µmol/l	5.1	25.6
S-ALP	101	IU/l	53	128
S-gGT	**58**	IU/l	8	37
S-ALT	**49**	IU/l	19	40
S-AST	**36**	IU/l	13	32
S-LDH	**219**	IU/l	90	180
S-Haptoglobin 20 yrs	0.19	g/l	0.16	2

Table 19.7

Test	Value	Units	Reference range	
Bleeding time	5	Minutes	3	7
Platelet count	**498.2**	$\times 10^9$/l	140	440
PT	13.4	Seconds	12	14
PTT	27	Seconds	23	36
D-dimers	0.21	mg/l	0	0.25

2. The FBC shows the marked anemia and the platelet response to acute hemorrhage.
3. The most prominent features of the biochemical tests are the hyperchloremic acidosis. Raised liver enzymes are disquieting.
4. The baseline hemostatic screen is normal, apart from the reactive thrombocytosis.

> It is a good policy to do a hemostatic screen on the admission of any patient who is likely to be needing massive amounts of blood.

Follow-up (Examine Table 19.8)

DISCUSSION OF TABLE 19.9:

1. The FBC report, particularly the morphological comment, was very revealing.

Table 19.8

Follow-up of case #89

Surgery was very difficult. The femoral artery lesion involved the groin. Upon exploration, further injuries were found in the pelvis. Eventually, he returned to the ICU and ventilation support continued. During the next few days, his condition remained critical but stable. On the third day his condition deteriorated, with respiratory insufficiency, hypotension, and full pulses. His urinary output decreased, he became jaundiced and mentally confused. He was not pyrexial. Biochemical studies confirmed renal insufficiency and both conjugated and unconjugated hyperbilirubinemia. His liver enzymes were considerably worse. A FBC at this time is shown in Table 19.9 and the hemostatic screen in Table 19.10.

Table 19.9

	Value	Units	Reference range Low	High	Permitted range Low	High
Red cell count	**2.41**	$\times 10^{12}$/l	4.77	5.83	2.34	2.48
Hemoglobin (Hb)	**7.1**	g/dl	13.8	18.0	6.9	7.3
Hematocrit (Hct)	**0.20**	l/l	0.42	0.53	0.19	0.20
Mean cell volume	81	fl	80	99	75.3	86.7
Mean cell Hb	29.5	pg	27	31.5	28.9	30.0
Mean cell Hb conc.	36.4	g/dl	31.5	34.5	35.6	37.1
Red cell dist. width	17.2	%	11.6	14	17.2	17.2
Retic. count %	2.1	%	0.27	1.00	2.0	2.2
Retic. absolute (abs.)	50.6	$\times 10^9$/l	30	100	49.1	52.1
White cell count	4.23	$\times 10^9$/l	4	10	3.91	4.55
Neutrophils abs.	2.28	$\times 10^9$/l	2	7	2.11	2.46
Band cells abs.	**0.38**		0	0.00	0.34	0.42
Lymphocytes abs.	1.21	$\times 10^9$/l	1	3	1.12	1.30
Monocytes abs.	0.31	$\times 10^9$/l	0.2	1	0.29	0.34
Eosinophils abs.	0.00	$\times 10^9$/l	0.02	0.5	0.00	0.00
Basophils abs.	0.04	$\times 10^9$/l	0.02	0.1	0.04	0.04
Normoblasts	0	/100 WBC	0	0		
Platelet count	**71.0**	$\times 10^9$/l	150	400	65.7	76.3
Sedimentation	**25**	mm/h	0	10	24	26
Morphology		The red cells are normochromic and show marked anisocytosis, with numerous target cells and stomatocytes and considerable fragmentation. The features are suggestive of a DIC.				

2. Otherwise the FBC picture is very much the sort of finding one can expect in these circumstances.

EXAMINE TABLES 19.10 AND 19.11
DISCUSSION OF TABLE 19.10:

1. Referral to Table 17.5 shows that the features are very much those of DIC, but also of liver failure and massive transfusion.

Table 19.10

Test	Value	Units	Reference range	
Bleeding time	9	Minutes	3	7
Platelet Count	71.0	× 10⁹/l	140	440
PT	21.2	Seconds	12	14
PTT	57	Seconds	23	36
D-Dimers	1.87	mg/l	0	0.25

Table 19.11

			Reference range	
	Value	Units	Low	High
S-Urea	9.7	mmol/l	2.1	7.1
S-Creatinine	189	mmol/l	62	115
S-Sodium	131	mmol/l	136	145
S-Potassium	5.7	mmol/l	3.5	5.1
S-Chloride	108.6	mmol/l	98	108
S-Total CO₂	20.5	mmol/l	22	28
S-Osmolality	287	mmol/kg	275	295
S-Bilirubin (Total)	45.7	µmol/l	6.8	34.2
S-Bilirubin (Direct)	12.1	µmol/l	1.7	8.6
S-Bilirubin (Indirect)	33.6	µmol/l	5.1	25.6
S-ALP	121	IU/l	53	128
S-Ggt	78	IU/l	8	37
S-ALT	61	IU/l	19	40
S-AST	45	IU/l	13	32
S-LDH	301	IU/l	90	180
S-Haptoglobin 20 yrs	0.16	g/l	0.16	2

2. Liver function tests would thus be of great value. These are shown in Table 19.11. Since one clinical possibility is multiple organ dysfunction (MODS), other tests also were warranted.

DISCUSSION ON TABLE 19.11

1. Renal and hepatic function have considerably deteriorated. These results lend credence to the idea of MODS in this patient, especially since his mental state had worsened a great deal.
2. DIC is a hemolytic state, which would partly explain the bilirubinemia and the raised LDH. The question can thus be raised – why is the haptoglobin normal? The problem is that haptoglobin is a positive acute phase reactant.

General Discussion

1. It should be clear that interpreting the first-line (and other) tests in the critical care situation can be enormously difficult. One is frequently reliant primarily on clinical expertise. The same difficulty occurs with attempting to interpret the hyperkalemia – although it is unlikely in this case to be due to multiple transfusion, since 4 days have elapsed since the transfusion; however, the transfusion may well have contributed to the problem.
2. The deteriorating pulmonary function could have many causes in this patient, one of which clearly is TRALI. Another is the possibility of fat embolism.
3. The point has been made before, that DIC after massive transfusion may well be due entirely to the underlying condition, in this case extensive trauma.
4. It is of interest that at no stage were any infective processes identified.

Exercise Case

CASE #90 (TABLE 19.12)

Table 19.12

Patient	Age	Sex	Race	Altitude
Mrs J.S	33 yrs	Female	Black	5,000 ft

This lady was P4G6 and had been admitted at 37 weeks with severe antepartum hemorrhage. She had not attended an antenatal clinic. There were signs of significant fetal distress. She was resuscitated and given 4 units of RCC, and an emergency C/S was performed, with a live infant. She was seen to be in a very poor general medical condition, with stomatitis and koilonychia. Physicians were consulted and after investigation she was put on treatment. She improved on good diet, specific therapy, and rest. She was on the point of being discharged on the eighth day when it was noticed that she was jaundiced. The hematology service was consulted. Table 19.12 displays her admission FBC.

	Value	Units	Reference range Low	Reference range High	Permitted range Low	Permitted range High
Red cell count	**2.43**	$\times 10^{12}$/l	4.03	5.09	2.36	2.50
Hemoglobin (Hb)	**7.4**	g/dl	12.7	15.9	7.1	7.7
Hematocrit (Hct)	**0.21**	l/l	0.38	0.49	0.21	0.22
Mean cell volume	88	fl	80	99	86.2	89.8
Mean cell Hb	30.5	pg	27	31.5	29.8	31.1
Mean cell Hb conc.	34.6	g/dl	31.5	34.5	33.9	35.3
Red cell dist. width	**19.4**	%	11.6	14	19.4	19.4
Retic. count	0.3		0.3	1.0	0.3	0.3
Retic. absolute (abs.)	**7.3**	$\times 10^9$/l	30	100	7.1	7.5
White cell count	**10.5**	$\times 10^9$/l	3.5	10	9.71	11.29
Neutrophils abs.	**8.13**	$\times 10^9$/l	1.5	7	7.52	8.74
Band cells abs.	0.00		0	0	0.00	0.00
Lymphocytes abs.	1.27	$\times 10^9$/l	1	3	1.18	1.37
Monocytes abs.	0.72	$\times 10^9$/l	0.2	1	0.67	0.78
Eosinophils abs.	0.30	$\times 10^9$/l	0.02	0.5	0.28	0.33
Basophils abs.	0.07	$\times 10^9$/l	0.02	0.1	0.07	0.08
Normoblasts	0	/100 WBC	0	0		
Platelet count	**58.0**	$\times 10^9$/l	150	400	50.2	67.8
Sedimentation	**41**	mm/h	0	20	39	43
Morphology	The red cells show anisochromia and anisocytosis with numerous small and large ovalocytes, tear-drop poikilocytes, target cells, elliptocytes, and some fragmented cells. The neutrophils show a prominent right shift.					

Questions

1. This FBC shows numerous changes. List and describe them. How would you state the anatomical diagnosis?

_____

_____

_____

_____

2. What are the possible general pathology diagnoses? Do you think that the changes can be ascribed to a single process? For example?

_____

_____

_____

3. Do you think the neutrophilia and thrombocytopenia could have other causes in this patient?

_____

4. Was the anemia sufficient to cause fetal distress?

_____

5. If you had seen the patient within the first few days, how would you have investigated and managed her?

_____

_____

_____

6. What do you think of the reticulocyte count?

_____

_____

7. What do you think of the raised ESR?

_____

Answers

1. Normocytic anemia with a moderately raised RDW and a very low reticulocyte count, mild neutrophilia and moderate thrombocytopenia.

   The anatomical diagnosis would necessarily be a description of the various changes, since the various changes need not be interrelated.

2. Trying to explain all the findings as part of one pathology should always be attempted first. In view of the clinical background, it is entirely possible that more than one process is at work. Considering the causes of a normocytic anemia, one possibility that springs immediately to mind is a combined deficiency of iron and vitamin B_{12} and/or folate; this is strongly supported by the morphology. What is against this, however, is the neutrophilia. And it would be dangerous automatically to assume that only one pathology is operating.

3. Neutrophilia is a normal finding in pregnancy. Thrombocytopenia could be due to gestational thrombocytopenia, HELLP syndrome, PET, or even ITP or TTP.

4. Yes.

5. Iron studies, red cell folate, and vitamin B_{12} levels in the first instance. In view of the complexity of the case, I would perform a bone marrow aspirate.

6. The poor reticulocyte response indicates that there is something wrong with the marrow, either anatomical or functional. In this case, it is probably due to chronic nutrient deficiency; the bone marrow aspirate should be of assistance.

7. A raised ESR can be normal in pregnancy. However, the level is probably too high for this to be the sole cause. It is probably due to a combination of factors: the pregnancy and the anemia.

Table 19.13 shows the FBC on the eighth day. The patient was noted to be jaundiced.

Table 19.13

	Value	Units	Reference range Low	Reference range High	Permitted range Low	Permitted range High
Red cell count	**3.55**	× 10^{12}/l	4.03	5.09	3.44	3.66
Hemoglobin (Hb)	**10.1**	g/dl	12.7	15.9	9.7	10.5
Hematocrit (Hct)	**0.32**	l/l	0.38	0.49	0.31	0.33
Mean cell volume	89	fl	80	99	87.2	90.8
Mean cell Hb	28.5	pg	27	31.5	27.9	29.0
Mean cell Hb conc.	32.0	g/dl	31.5	34.5	31.3	32.6
Red cell dist. width	**15.1**	%	11.6	14	15.1	15.1
Retic. count %	**4.1**	0.1	0.3		4e0	4.2
Retic. absolute (abs.)	**145.6**	× 10^9/l	30	100	141.2	149.9
White cell count	**14.1**	× 10^9/l	3.5	10	13.04	15.16
Neutrophils abs.	**9.45**	× 10^9/l	1.5	7	8.74	10.16
Band cells abs.	**0.42**		0	0.00	0.38	0.47
Lymphocytes abs.	2.82	× 10^9/l	1	3	2.61	3.03
Monocytes abs.	0.85	× 10^9/l	0.2	1	0.78	0.91
Eosinophils abs.	0.42	× 10^9/l	0.02	0.5	0.39	0.45
Basophils abs.	0.14	× 10^9/l	0.02	0.1	0.13	0.15
Normoblasts	0	/100 WBC	0	0		
Platelet count	**489.1**	× 10^9/l	150	400	440.2	538.0
Sedimentation	**29**	mm/h	0	20	28	30
Morphology	There is a dimorphic red cell picture with considerable auto-agglutination. There is a population of microcytic hypochromic cells with small ovalocytes and elliptocytes, and another of oval macrocytes with tear-drop poikilocytes.					

Questions

1. What do you think is the cause of the jaundice? Could it be as a result of the transfusion? If so, what would be the mechanism? What other causes are possible?

2. How would you go about confirming your suspicion – clinically and with laboratory tests?

3. Why do you think the hematology service was consulted for a case of jaundice?

4. Why is there a dimorphic red cell picture and auto-agglutination? Is the first FBC also not a dimorphic picture?

Answers

1. A delayed transfusion reaction is a strong possibility. The cause in this type of case is almost always an irregular antibody that was not detectable at the time of cross-match. The only transfusion-transmitted hepatitis virus that could possibly cause jaundice within a week is hepatitis A, but this virus is almost never transmitted by blood products.

2. Clinically I would search for an enlarged spleen. I would look for increased urobilin in the urine and have a Coombs test (direct antibody test or DAT) performed.

3. The obstetricians had immediately considered the possibility of a delayed transfusion reaction.

4. In this case, the dimorphic picture was clearly recognized as due to the presence of transfused cells. Mild auto-agglutination is common after a transfusion usually due to insignificant incompatibility. In this case, the auto-agglutination was far more prominent, in keeping with a more significant incompatibility. The first blood picture also was a dimorphic one, but in that case was recognizably different.

A DAT was performed and was positive for IgG and negative for C3. The blood bank identified an anti-Kell antibody. (This is one of the commoner blood groups responsible for this type of presentation.)

Further Reading

Clinical Guidelines for the Use of Blood Products (2001). South African National Blood Service.

Lewis SM, Bain B, Bates I (2006). Dacie and Lewis Practical Haematology. 10th edn. Oxford, Churchill Livingstone.

Hoffbrand AV, Catovsky D, Tuddenham EGD (eds) (2005). Postgraduate Haematology. 5th edn. Oxford, Blackwell Publishing.

As the name suggests, iron overload refers to a state (indeed potentially a disease state) where the total iron content of the body is increased. It is relevant particularly because iron cannot be got rid of without bleeding, or in the last few decades, with chelating agents.

Unless it is very severe, with obvious clinical sequelae, it is impossible to diagnose clinically. It may be possible to suspect the earlier, sub-clinical cases if a careful history, including a family history, is taken, and if certain commonly associated clinical disorders, such as porphyria cutanea tarda or thalassemia, are recognized. Confirmation is always, in the first instance, by blood tests.

As we have discussed before, iron cannot be eliminated from the body except by bleeding. Most of the problems from iron overload are due to deposition of iron in the tissues. However, which tissues are affected, with the attendant clinical sequelae, does depend on the cause of the iron overload. In days gone by, hemochromatosis was the term used for a hereditary condition where the iron was deposited in parenchymal tissues, and all other causes, with deposition in the reticulo-endothelial system (RES), were referred to as hemosiderosis. Subsequent studies have shown that this classification is incomplete, and currently, all cases of iron overload are referred to as hemochromatosis. This is perhaps a little confusing to the general reader, and it is as well for the pathology of the various disorders to be explained. Nor is this a trivial issue:

1. Chronic anemias are increasing all the time, including the myelodysplasias, and the use of red cell concentrates is increasing all the time.
2. There are many hemochromatosis genes, and they are very common in the population – 10% of whites carry the commonest of these genes.

Mechanisms of Iron Overload

There are two basic mechanisms:

1. **INCREASED ABSORPTION FROM THE GUT**. Here there are two possible processes responsible:

   a) **IN PERSONS WITH AN ESSENTIALLY NORMAL MARROW** with normal cellularity and plasma iron turnover, where there is increased absorption from the gut due to local disorders. The most important of these is **IDIOPATHIC HEREDITARY HEMOCHROMATOSIS**; however, it has been shown to occur in **PERSONS TAKING ORAL IRON FOR LONG PERIODS WHEN THEY HAVE NO NEED FOR IT.** When one considers that huge amounts of over-the-counter medications containing iron are sold every day, the potential dangers are obvious. Iron overload also tends to occur in alcoholism and porphyria cutanea tarda.
   b) **IN PERSONS WITH HYPERACTIVE AND INEFFECTIVE ERYTHROPOIESIS,** for example, thalassemia and sideroblastic anemia, where increased iron absorption is evidently mediated by a recently discovered protein from the liver called hepcidin (note that it is also implicated in anemia of chronic disorders).

2. **PARENTERAL ADMINISTRATION** – usually of red cells, but cases are known where it is due to over-enthusiastic and ill-considered iron injections or infusions.

Sometimes one may see reference made to the so-called iron-loading anemias. These essentially comprise both the persons with hyperactive and ineffective erythropoiesis and those receiving regular parenteral administration of red cells.

O.N. Beck, *Diagnostic Hematology*, DOI 10.1007/978-1-84800-295-1_20,
© Springer-Verlag London Limited 2009

Pathology and Resultant Clinical Features

There are two fundamentally different patterns of deposition of excess iron in the tissues, with significant clinical implications:

1. Where the excess iron derives from the parenteral route (i.e., due to repeated transfusions or iron infusions), the iron is deposited primarily in the RES, resulting eventually in hepatosplenomegaly but very little if any parenchymal involvement, perhaps until very late. This causes very little functional disturbance apart from hepatic dysfunction.
2. All other causes – i.e., due to increased absorption, from whatever reason – result in deposition in the parenchyma, notably the heart, liver, joints, pancreas, and other endocrine glands, eventually with significant functional abnormality. Note, however, that the development of overt clinical features usually takes decades to develop:

    a) The liver is one of the major sites for deposition, and this leads to fibrosis and often eventually to cirrhosis. Steatosis is a common finding.
    b) The heart is frequently affected, often presenting with arrhythmias. Ultimately cardiomyopathy and cardiac failure will supervene.
    c) The endocrine glands are frequently affected, presenting with diabetes mellitus, hypogonadism, etc.
    d) The joints are often involved, classically the first two metacarpo-phalangeal joints.
    e) The skin may be involved, producing a grayish, almost leaden appearance. This is seldom seen these days. The classic bronzing of the skin is very unusual.

In both types of deposition, the laboratory features are fairly classical.

1. Except in the so-called iron-loading anemias, the FBC is normal until complications occur – i.e., very late.
2. The serum iron levels are raised.
3. Transferrin levels are raised.
4. Iron Saturation of the transferrin is markedly increased.
5. Ferritin is markedly raised.
6. In addition, of course, one may find raised blood glucose levels, abnormal liver functions and so on.

Hemochromatosis

Despite the frequency of the iron-loading anemias and the overload that results from their treatment, hemochromatosis remains the commonest cause of iron overload among whites, especially those originating in northern Europe. Ten percent of this population carry one or other of the mutations responsible, and the prevalence of homozygous disease is probably around 1:300; this is a sobering statistic – it implies that the average family doctor, seeing say 200 patients a week, of whom at least 30% are going to be over 40 years of age, is going to see roughly one case (or miss one) every month! On average, men develop symptoms and are diagnosed between the ages of 30 and 55; women are usually diagnosed over the age of 50. (Note that there is an uncommon juvenile form presenting before the age of 30; there is even a neonatal form). There is no doubt, however, in our experience, that earlier presentation even with the classical mutations occurs quite often.

Because of the frequency of the disease and the frequency that it is misdiagnosed, we need to spend some time with the disease, to enhance awareness of this eminently treatable serious disease. It is thought that on average three doctors are consulted before the diagnosis is made.

Etiology

Several types of hemochromatosis have been described:

1. **TYPE I.** This can be regarded as the classic hemochromatosis. It is always due to mutations in the HFE gene. Over 20 different genetic mutations have been recognized, but only two are detectable in routine laboratories.
2. **TYPE II.** This is the juvenile form and is due to mutations of hemojuvelin or of hepcidin (see above).
3. **TYPE III.** This is due to a mutation in one of the transferrin receptors.
4. **TYPE IV.** This is due to a mutation in ferroportin (this protein works in a highly complex interaction with hemojuvelin and hepcidin to control iron absorption (and homeostasis).

Complications

Apart from cirrhosis, cardiac disease and so on, it should be realized that the incidence of hepatocellular carcinoma is about 15% in homozygous cases. The incidence in heterozygotes is not known for sure.

Clinical Variability in Type I Hemochromatosis

The clinically most serious type is due to homozygosity for the C282Y gene. A small number of heterozygotes appear to develop moderate liver and joint disease. It is very difficult to be sure, however, since double heterozygotes involving one of the rarer mutations cannot easily be detected, and it is thus possible that some of these so-called heterozygotes who are showing symptoms could be double heterozygotes.

Once tissue deposition is established, suspecting the diagnosis can be easy but can be a real conundrum. For example, cardiac arrhythmias are quite common, and most are not due to hemochromatosis, nor is the condition thought of in this case; the same might apply to the presentation of chronic liver disease.

The real challenge lies in identifying the early, easily treatable case. There is no question that in both cases a high index of suspicion should be maintained.

In effect, the real question is, on whom should screening iron studies be done? There is no real consensus. These tests are expensive, but it should be borne in mind that they only have to be done once in any male patient over the age of 30, and in any female patient over the age of 50. There is no doubt however that some young and significantly affected patients will slip through the cracks with this policy – please take careful note of Case #92.

The classic picture is

1. Iron saturation of transferrin >45%
2. Ferritin levels at least double the upper limit of the reference range

Once this picture is established, the following must be excluded:

1. The patient has not had repeated transfusions or iron infusions.
2. The patient does not have one of the so-called iron-loading anemias.
3. The patient shows no evidence of porphyria or alcoholism.
   If these are all negative, then PCR tests for the two common mutations should be requested. It is only when these are negative that a real diagnostic conundrum exists. These patients should all be referred. The decision will have to be made as to the value of liver and bone marrow biopsies. There is considerable controversy about this issue.

Teaching Cases

CASE #91 (TABLE 20.1)

Tables 20.3, 20.4, and 20.5 show follow-up reports and examples of blood findings at intervals.

Table 20.1

Patient	Age	Sex	Race	Altitude
Miss S A	20 yrs	Female	Indian	5,000 ft

This patient has been followed up for the last 17 years. She had been diagnosed as β-thalassemia major at the age of 1 year. She was treated with transfusions, but the highly educated parents had done some research and were concerned about iron overload. At the time of the first consultation she was found to be pale, sallow, and mildly jaundiced, as well as very disturbed emotionally. After a transfusion, the policy was adopted that, once the ferritin levels reached a level above normal, a subcutaneous pump would be arranged and desferrioxamine infusions started, initially for 6 h per day. The ferritin levels were monitored carefully, and as soon as it was established that the infusions were successful, a hypertransfusion policy was adopted, with the aim of keeping the Hb above 12 g/dl. The parents were also told to give the child tea and antacids with her meals and to avoid any vitamin/mineral preparation that contained iron. Table 20.2 shows the iron profile at the age of 2½ years.

Table 20.2

	Value	Units	Reference range Low	Reference range High
S-Ferritin	278.9	µg/l	14.0	233.1
S-Iron	16.8	µmol/l	11.6	31.3
S-Transferrin	2.07	g/l	2.12	3.60

Table 20.3

Follow-up #1 of case # 91. Interval 13 months (Table 20.3)

Clinically and physically the child was doing well; quite severe emotional problems were present throughout and the expert aid of a psychologist was employed.

	Value	Units	Reference range Low	Reference range High
Hemoglobin	11.5	g/dl		
S-Ferritin	389.9	µg/l	14.0	233.1
S-Iron	16.8	µmol/l	11.6	31.3
S-Transferrin	2.07	g/l	2.12	3.60
S-Fe saturation	32	%	15.0	35.0
Age	49	months		
Body mass	13.5	kg		
Total units of RCC	8			

Table 20.4

Follow-up #2 of case # 91. Interval 33 months (Table 20.4)

Clinically the child was still doing well and was beginning to accept the therapeutic regime.

	Value	Units	Reference range Low	Reference range High
Hemoglobin	11.5	g/dl		
S-Ferritin	929.2	µg/l	14.0	233.1
S-Iron	25.2	µmol/l	11.6	31.3
S-Transferrin	2.11	g/l	2.12	3.60
S-Fe saturation	47	%	15.0	35.0
Age	82	months		
Body mass	22	kg		
Total units of RCC	26			

Table 20.5

Follow-up #3 of case # 91. Interval 36 months (Table 20.5)				
Physically and emotionally the child was doing well				
			Reference range	
	Value	Units	Low	High
Hemoglobin	11.9	g/dl		
S-Ferritin	971.4	µg/l	14.0	233.1
S-Iron	27.5	µmol/l	11.6	31.3
S-Transferrin	2.01	g/l	2.12	3.60
S-Fe saturation	54	%	15.0	35.0
Age	10	years		
Body mass	29	kg		
Total units of RCC	42			

COMMENTS ON TABLE 20.3

Despite having received over 1.5 g of iron during the year, the ferritin had not risen proportionately, indicating

Table 20.6

Follow-up #4 of case # 91. Aged 20 years (Table 20.6)						
The patient was in general doing very well, playing soccer while wearing her pump, for example. It was noteworthy that she had developed no physical stigmata of thalassemia major, such as frontal bossing or maxillary prominence. She complained, however, of chronic backache and X-rays revealed osteopenia. Bone densitometry showed this to be very severe.						
			Reference range		Permitted range	
	Value	Units	Low	High	Low	High
Red cell count	4.54	× 10¹²/l	4.03	5.09	4.40	4.68
Hemoglobin (Hb)	11.9	g/dl	12.7	15.9	11.5	12.3
Hematocrit (Hct)	0.38	l/l	0.38	0.49	0.37	0.39
Mean cell volume	83	fl	80	99	81.3	84.7
Mean cell Hb	26.2	pg	27	31.5	25.7	26.7
Mean cell Hb conc.	31.6	g/dl	31.5	34.5	30.9	32.2
Red cell dist. width	16.9	%	11.6	14	16.9	16.9
Retic count %	0.7	0.1	0.3		0.7	0.7
Retic absolute (abs.)	31.8	× 10⁹/l	35	100	30.8	32.7
White cell count	6.87	× 10⁹/l	4	10	6.35	7.39
Neutrophils abs.	3.83	× 10⁹/l	2	7	3.55	4.2
Band cells abs.	0.00		0	0	0.00	0.00
Lymphocytes abs.	2.43	× 10⁹/l	1	3	2.25	2.61
Monocytes abs.	0.40	× 10⁹/l	0.2	1	0.37	0.43
Eosinophils abs.	0.14	× 10⁹/l	0.02	0.5	0.13	0.16
Basophils abs.	0.06	× 10⁹/l	0.02	0.1	0.06	0.07
Normoblasts	0	/100 WBC	0	0		
Platelet count	297.4	× 10⁹/l	150	400	267.7	327.1
Sedimentation	2	mm/h	0	20	2	2
			Reference range			
	Value	Units	Low	High		
S-Ferritin	1,105	µg/l	14.0	233.1		
S-Iron	27.5	µmol/l	11.6	31.3		
S-Transferrin	2.01	g/l	2.12	3.60		
S-Fe saturation	54	%	15.0	35.0		
Age	20	years				
Total units of RCC	131					

that the desferrioxamine infusions were at least partly successful. Increasing the time per day of the infusion was considered, but the psychologist advised waiting until she was a little older. (It must be emphasized that at that stage the infusions were a new development and none of us had much experience with them.)

COMMENTS ON TABLE 20.4

Iron overload was clearly becoming serious. It was decided to increase the infusion time to 12 h per day.

COMMENTS ON TABLE 20.5

Iron overload was significant but stable.
Table 20.6 shows her results at a recent visit.

COMMENTS ON TABLE 20.6

1. It is quite clear that subcutaneous desferrioxamine is very successful in preventing most of the serious complications of thalassemia major. However, it is by no means the complete answer. The ferritin level is very high, and one important complication of a chronically raised ferritin level – osteopenia – is present; it is likely to lead to more serious problems.
2. The question has been raised as to whether infusions should not have been started while the ferritin levels were still normal, and whether infusion time should not have been increased sooner. In retrospect, the answer is probably yes.
3. Note that the red cell count is normal.

Case #92 (Table 20.7)

Table 20.7

Patient	Age	Sex	Race	Altitude
Master G K	7 years	Male	White	5,000 ft

This boy's mother was very concerned about her family history; an uncle had been diagnosed with hemochromatosis at the age of 31 years, and had died of "heart failure" at the age of 36. The boy was an only child and the mother was already menopausal. She felt that the boy was not developing and insisted to the family doctor that he might have hemochromatosis. The doctor quite understandably was very skeptical. The only complaint the doctor picked up was of sore joints; he requested only a rheumatoid factor and anti-nuclear antibodies. The ANA was normal but the RF was raised 5 times normal. Nevertheless, rather than alienate the mother, he referred the boy. On examination the lad seemed quite normal and healthy, but for two reasons testing was agreed to: EKG examination showed a first-degree heart block; and the very strong family history.

Iron profile of Master G K				
			Reference range	
	Value	Units	Low	High
Hemoglobin	10.2	g/dl		
S-Ferritin	292.4	µg/l	14.0	233.1
S-Iron	27.8	µmol/l	11.6	31.3
S-Transferrin	1.8	g/l	2.12	3.60
S-Fe saturation	62	%	15.0	35.0

DISCUSSION

1. These results were quite frankly astonishing. The tests were repeated at another laboratory and found to be quite reproducible.
2. Further investigations were performed.

   a) PCR for hemochromatosis mutations showed the patient to be **HOMOZYGOUS** for the C282Y mutation.
   b) The FBC was completely normal, as were the liver functions.
   c) The raised RF remained unexplained. There was no clinical evidence of rheumatoid disease.

The patient was venesected (100 ml every 4 weeks) until the ferritin eventually came down to near normal. Thereafter, at follow-up, venesection was done as necessary, based on the iron studies. Of interest is that the heart block normalized.

At this age, even homozygous hemochromatosis hardly ever presents either with evident tissue damage or with such a markedly raised ferritin. Further investigation of the family origins revealed that the clan had originated in a remote valley in Central Europe, with a great deal of intermarriage. Extensive family studies were planned.

CASE #93 (EXAMINE TABLE 20.8)

The results of the PCR examination for hemochromatosis mutations revealed her to be heterozygous for the C282Y mutation.

The questions clearly were

1. Whether her clinical features were related to the iron status. A cardiologist's opinion was sought; he was uncertain but in view of her age and the family history, he felt that it was certainly possible. Extensive and sophisticated radiological and sonographic studies of her liver revealed no evidence of extensive iron deposition.
2. Whether to treat her. The patient was very anxious once her results became known. We clearly had no obvious guidelines, but she agreed that a limited number of venesections be carried out. This was done and the iron saturation settled down to around 33%. The situation is being watched very carefully. To date the dysrhythmia has not responded to venesection.

Table 20.8

Patient	Age	Sex	Race	Altitude
Mrs J D	29 yrs	Female	White	5,000 ft

This lady's father had been diagnosed with hemochromatosis at the age of 35, but had been well controlled with regular venesections. The family had been assured that the disease only presented later in life and had been given the suggestion that testing should be delayed until later. Recently, however, the father had been diagnosed with hepatocellular carcinoma. The daughter was well aware that this was a potential complication of hemochromatosis, and became very anxious.

Her history was unusual: she had recently begun experiencing palpitations and "missed beats," and she was getting vague pain and stiffness in the hands. These symptoms undoubtedly could be psychological in origin, but the overall impression of the young lady was of a very levelheaded person.

On examination, there was no obvious disorder in the hands. Numerous extrasystoles were palpated. All else was normal. EKG examination revealed a Wenckebach phenomenon with regular dropped beats. Blood tests were done. A subset of the FBC is shown.

	Value	Units	Reference range Low	Reference range High	Permitted range Low	Permitted range High
Red cell count	4.65	$\times 10^{12}$/l	4.03	5.09	4.51	4.79
Hemoglobin (Hb)	13.9	g/dl	12.7	15.9	13.4	14.4
Hematocrit (Hct)	0.42	l/l	0.38	0.49	0.41	0.44
Mean cell volume	91	fl	80	99	89.2	92.8
Mean cell Hb	29.9	pg	27	31.5	29.3	30.5
Mean cell Hb conc.	32.8	g/dl	31.5	34.5	32.2	33.5
Red cell dist. width	12.7	%	11.6	14	12.7	12.7
White cell count	7.87	$\times 10^9$/l	4	10	7.28	8.46
Platelet count	321.6	$\times 10^9$/l	150	400	289.4	353.8
Sedimentation	2	mm/h	0	20	2	2

	Value	Units	Reference range Low	Reference range High
S-Ferritin	229.7	µg/l	14.0	233.1
S-Iron	26.9	µmol/l	11.6	31.3
S-Transferrin	**2.10**	g/l	2.12	3.60
S-Fe saturation	**51**	%	15.0	35.0

CASE # 94 (EXAMINE TABLE 20.9)

Further investigations on urine and plasma were done for porphyrins. These revealed a pattern characteristic of porphyria cutanea tarda.

DISCUSSION

1. A number of findings should be evaluated:

   a) There is a mild normochromic anemia. This may be related to protein-calorie malnutrition but the RDW is suspiciously high. Morphological comment strongly suggests a combined iron deficiency and megaloblastosis. Iron, folate, and vitamin B_{12} studies were done. See Table 20.10. The results are somewhat peculiar.

Table 20.9

Patient	Age	Sex	Race	Altitude
Mr P T	47 yrs	Male	Black	5,000 ft

This patient was admitted in a state of mental confusion. No helpful history was obtainable. On examination he showed numerous clinical abnormalities apart from the mental confusion: the nutritional status was poor, and there was clinical evidence of pellagra; his skin was hyperpigmented and there was considerable hypertrichosis; there were atrophic scars on the forehead and hands; his liver was mildly enlarged and felt irregular. He was also mildly dehydrated. A preliminary diagnosis of pellagra plus porphyria cutanea tarda was made. Emergency nutritional support was commenced and then further investigations were carried out.

	Value	Units	Reference range Low	Reference range High	Permitted range Low	Permitted range High
Red cell count	4.11	$\times 10^{12}$/l	4.77	5.83	3.99	4.23
Hemoglobin (Hb)	11	g/dl	13.8	18.0	10.6	11.4
Hematocrit (Hct)	0.36	l/l	0.42	0.53	0.35	0.37
Mean cell volume	87	fl	80	99	85.3	88.7
Mean cell Hb	26.8	pg	27	31.5	26.2	27.3
Mean Cell Hb conc.	30.8	g/dl	31.5	34.5	30.1	31.4
Red cell dist. width	21.7	%	11.6	14	15.4	18.0
Retic count	1.1	%	0.27	0.80	1.0	1.2
Retic absolute (abs.)	45.2	$\times 10^9$/l	30	100	41.8	48.6
White cell count	3.61	$\times 10^9$/l	3.5	10	3.34	3.88
Neutrophils abs.	1.63	$\times 10^9$/l	1.5	7	1.51	1.75
Lymphocytes abs.	1.52	$\times 10^9$/l	1	3	1.41	1.63
Monocytes abs.	0.29	$\times 10^9$/l	0.2	1	0.26	0.31
Eosinophils abs.	0.14	$\times 10^9$/l	0.02	0.5	0.13	0.15
Basophils abs.	0.04	$\times 10^9$/l	0.02	0.1	0.03	0.04
Normoblasts	0	/100 WBC	0	0		
Platelet count	102.0	$\times 10^9$/l	150	400	91.8	112.2
Morphology	The red cells showed considerable anisocytosis and anisochromia, with large and small oval cells, target cells, and elliptocytes. There is a mild thrombocytopenia.					

i. Ferritin is raised while the iron saturation is decreased but not below the diagnostic 15% point. One can more or less rule out iron

Table 20.10

	Value	Units	Reference range Low	Reference range High
S-Ferritin	428.2	µg/l	14.0	233.1
S-Iron	8.2	µmol/l	11.6	31.3
S-Transferrin	2.01	g/l	2.12	3.60
S-Fe saturation	16	%	25.0	35.0
S-Vitamin B_{12}	311	pg/ml	193	982
S-Folate	2.1	ng/ml	3.0	17.0
RBC-Folate	67.2	ng/ml	93.0	641.0

deficiency. Iron malutilization as in ACD is possible. The raised ferritin could be the result of an acute (or chronic) phase response, although the level is very high for this. Alternatively it could be explained by the porphyria, possibly with associated alcoholism.

ii. Folate is decreased.

iii. These two features would explain the FBC appearances.

b) There is a mild thrombocytopenia. This could be related to liver disease. Liver functions were done and found to be moderately deranged. Ultrasound examination suggested and enlarged liver with a non-homogeneous pattern, and possibly indicating cirrhosis. This was later confirmed by biopsy.

2. Subsequent progress:

a) When the patient recovered full consciousness, he admitted to heavy alcohol abuse for years, and a very poor nutritional background. He had been losing weight for about 1 year and felt ill all the time. He had severe pain and paresthesiae in the legs and a sensory neuropathy was diagnosed. He also had chronic diarrhea: this could be ascribed to the pellagra or the folate deficiency. However, his general condition was very poor.

b) A chest X-ray revealed active tuberculosis. Further tests revealed him to be HIV positive. A CD4+ count was 61/mm^3.

c) Specific therapy was instituted. In addition 4 units of blood were removed over the next 4 months is Hb improved with time. The porphyric symptoms improved considerably.

d) The possibility that the microcytic component of his anemia was due to ACD was confirmed by bone marrow studies, which showed increased iron stores but decreased normal sideroblasts – there were however occasional pathological sideroblasts.

Comment It is interesting how well patients with porphyria cutanea tarda respond to the venesection of only a few units of blood. And the venesection does not have to be repeated for long – the improvement is relatively longlasting. Clearly the iron overload in this condition is metabolically unusual.

Further Reading

Andreoli TE, Bennett JC, Carpenter CCJ, Plum F (eds) (1997). Cecil Essentials of Medicine. 4th edn. Philadelphia: WB Saunders Company.

Bothwell TH, Charlton RW, Motulsky AG (1995). Hemochromatosis. In Scriver CR, Beaudet AL, Sly WS, Valle D (eds). The Metabolic and Molecular Basis of Inherited Disease. 7th edn. New York: McGraw-Hill.

Bulaj J, Griffen LM, Jorde LB, Edwards CQ, Kushner JP (1996). Clinical and Biochemical Abnormalities in People Heterozygous for Hemochromatosis. N. Engl. J. Med. 335: 1799.

The Hypercoagulable States

21

When it is considered that occlusive vascular disease is the greatest killer in First-World countries and that thromboembolic phenomena are by far the largest cause of these, the topic is clearly of vital importance. It is essential that the full context of vaso-occlusion not be forgotten, since there is a tendency to think only of thrombosis without realizing that vascular disease is often part and parcel of the problem. It is worthwhile to remember the famous Virchow triad. This identifies three crucial factors in the pathogenesis of vascular occlusion:

1. Decreased blood flow (i.e., stasis)
2. Disease in or around the vessels
3. Alterations in the blood itself (in modern terms, abnormalities in the balance of procoagulant, anticoagulant, and fibrinolytic processes).

While we will concentrate on the third of this triad, we must not lose sight of the inherent role played by the other two. In this regard, we can distinguish between arterial and venous occlusion:

1. In **VENOUS THROMBOSIS**, stasis plays a significant contributory role in many cases, and disease of the vessel wall is of minimal importance.
2. In **ARTERIAL THROMBOSIS**, stasis is seldom an issue, whereas disease of the vessel wall, primarily of the endothelium, is often a determining factor in the pathogenesis.

> WHILE THROMBOSIS CAN AND DOES OCCUR IN THE ABSENCE OF VASCULAR (MAINLY ENDOTHELIAL) DISEASE, IN MOST CASES EITHER STASIS OR AN UNDERLYING DEFECT IN A VESSEL PLAYS A SIGNIFICANT CONTRIBUTORY ROLE.

Note that the terms "hypercoagulability" and "thrombophilia" are used differently by different people. Traditionally, "thrombophilia" was used to indicate the inherited conditions, while "hypercoagulability" was used for the rest. Others use either term to refer to all of them. This is really just a matter of semantics, and for convenience, we will refer to all these pathologies as "hypercoagulability" or "the hypercoagulable states."

Before we discuss the features of arterial and venous occlusion separately, we will look at the basic mechanisms attributable to changes in the blood (i.e., the third of Virchow's factors). There is a very large number of blood changes that have clearly been identified as promoting thrombosis. For convenience, they are divided into primary (hereditary) and secondary (acquired) disorders.

The Primary Hypercoagulable States

Only a few of these were known prior to circa 1990, such as antithrombin deficiency (note that the term "antithrombin III" is no longer used). It is strongly recommended that Fig. 2.23 on page 37 be referred to again. It will be seen that the major natural anticoagulants are antithrombin, protein C, protein S, and tissue factor pathway inhibitor (TFPI), and clearly deficiency of these will predispose to inappropriate coagulation. However, there also are other causes:

1. Factor V_{Leiden}. Normally factors Va and VIIIa are neutralized by activated protein C, thus curtailing the thrombotic process. Factor V_{Leiden} is resistant to this; (the condition is also, probably not quite correctly, called activated protein C resistance). The disorder is now regarded as the commonest inherited disorder of hypercoagulability.

O.N. Beck, *Diagnostic Hematology*, DOI 10.1007/978-1-84800-295-1_21,
© Springer-Verlag London Limited 2009

2. Probably the second commonest hereditary disorder is an abnormal prothrombin – called prothrombin G20210A. This results in raised factor II levels and an increased risk of thrombosis. Protein C deficiency is possibly just as common. (Protein S deficiency and Antithrombin deficiency seem much less common).

3. Rarities include dysfibrinogenemia, hypoplasminogenemia, and raised plasminogen activator inhibitor release.

4. Finally, there are a few factors whose relevance is currently disputed, such as hyperhomocystinemia (except for carotid artery thrombosis) and lipoprotein (a).

A Note About Proteins C and S

It should be noted that these proteins also are vitamin K-dependent. Protein C has the shortest half-life of all the vitamin K-dependent factors; hence when a patient is started on warfarin therapy, there is a short period when the patient is **HYPERCOAGULABLE** due to an iatrogenic protein C deficiency. This is really only of significance in patients who are protein C deficient, but the practice of giving all patients 3 days of fractionated heparin while waiting for the warfarin to take effect is growing.

Note that protein C deficiency can be acquired, in septic shock and MODS. Both C and S can be deficient in vitamin K deficiency.

A Note About Antithrombin

Apart from the hereditary causes, there are a number of acquired causes of deficiency:

1. **NEPHROTIC SYNDROME**. The reason here is loss of natural anticoagulant proteins, especially antithrombin, in the urine.

2. **LIVER DISEASE** (poor synthesis).

3. **PREGNANCY, THE PILL AND HORMONAL TREATMENT** of Ca prostate (the effect of estrogens).

4. Since **HEPARIN THERAPY** works by counteracting the action of antithrombin, heparin therapy will lead to a deficiency.

5. **WIDESPREAD THROMBOSIS** will deplete antithrombin, and the interesting phenomenon of heparin resistance can occur as a result.

Secondary Hypercoagulable States

These can be considered in three groups:

1. A very large number of **GENERAL FACTORS** apparently predisposing to thrombosis have been identified,

mainly by extensive epidemiological studies. Many of these are the classical risk factors of coronary heart disease, such as obesity; raised LDL cholesterol especially if accompanied by normal or decreased HDL cholesterol levels; sedentary lifestyle; hypertension; smoking; and diabetes mellitus. Also pregnancy, stress, and immobilization are relevant.

2. A number of **MEDICAL CONDITIONS** are often associated with an increased incidence of thrombosis.

   a. Malignancy
   b. Sepsis
   c. Inflammatory bowel disease
   d. Nephrotic syndrome
   e. Pregnancy and hormone replacement therapy

3. A number of specifically **HEMATOLOGICAL DISORDERS** may also be associated with hypercoagulability.

   a. Factor XII deficiency
   b. Heparin-induced thrombocytopenia
   c. Acute promyelocytic leukemia
   d. Sickle cell disease
   e. Paroxysmal nocturnal hemoglobinuria (PNH)
   f. Paraproteins especially Waldenstrom macroglobulinemia
   g. Polycythemia vera and essential thrombocythemia. Note that secondary thrombocytosis has also been implicated in thrombotic events
   h. The antiphospholipid syndrome and lupus anticoagulant.

The Antiphospholipid Syndrome (APS)

This condition requires separate consideration since, unlike many of the others mentioned above, it has a fairly high incidence and can be responsible for serious mortality and morbidity. It is an autoimmune disease, with the antibodies directed against certain proteins which join with phospholipid elements to form specific complexes. Among the most important of these elements are some platelet receptors and the prothrombin–phospholipid complex. In vitro these prolong some of the coagulation times, but in vivo are responsible for a pro-thrombotic tendency.

Clinically, there are a number of unusual features, which if present tend to make the diagnosis relatively easy. Unfortunately, many cases present with only some features that in turn may be found in many other conditions.

1. **THROMBOSIS**. This may be arterial or venous and can involve any vessel. This may even include the micro-vasculature, resulting in widespread organ dysfunction and is termed "catastrophic APS." More

typically, however, deep vein thrombosis, pulmonary embolism, and stroke are found.

2. **FETAL LOSS.** Typically, one of three patterns may be found:

   a. Unexplained intrauterine death of a morphologically normal fetus at or beyond 10 weeks gestation.
   b. Three or more unexplained consecutive miscarriages before 10 weeks gestation.
   c. One or more premature births of a normal fetus before 34 weeks' gestation due to pre-eclampsia, eclampsia, or placental insufficiency.

3. **LIVEDO RETICULARIS.** A lacy rash mainly on the legs.
4. **MITRAL OR AORTIC VALVE INCOMPETENCE.**
5. **THROMBOCYTOPENIA.**
6. A tendency to **SEVERE ARTHRITIS.**

The condition may be associated with other autoimmune disease, notably systemic lupus erythematosis.

There are trends and tendencies with respect to whether an identified defect is particularly associated with venous thrombosis, with arterial thrombosis, or with both. Note, however, that no hard-and-fast rule can be given.

CONDITIONS MORE LIKELY TO BE ASSOCIATED WITH VENOUS THROMBOSIS

1. The Factor V_{Leiden} mutation
2. Protein C and protein S deficiency
3. Prothrombin G20210A mutation
4. Homocysteine levels over 18.5 µmol/l
5. Oral contraceptives, pregnancy, and hormone replacement therapy
6. Immobility and advancing age
7. Malignant disease
8. PNH

CONDITIONS MORE LIKELY TO BE ASSOCIATED WITH ARTERIAL THROMBOSIS

1. Polycythemia vera
2. Essential thrombocythemia
3. Sticky platelet syndrome
4. Sickle disease
5. Hypercholesterolemia
6. Diabetes

CONDITIONS THAT MAY BE ASSOCIATED WITH BOTH VENOUS AND ARTERIAL THROMBOSIS

1. Antiphospholipid syndrome
2. Antithrombin deficiency

3. Paraproteinemias
4. Factor XII deficiency
5. Dysfibrinogenemias
6. Essential thrombocythemia.

Venous Thromboembolic Disease (VTE)

It should be borne in mind that there are major difficulties with the statistics given with respect to VTE: the diagnosis is difficult; over 50% of cases of pulmonary embolism are initially undiagnosed; the traditional diagnostic methods have been shown to be very imprecise; a quarter of patients who are thought clinically to have VTE (in the best hands) do not in fact have it.

The epidemiological impact of VTE is enormous, with an annual incidence of about 70:100,000 population. Five percent of patients who develop pulmonary embolism will die.

It would appear that most patients with VTE do not have any abnormality of the hemostatic system. Certain presentations however do suggest the increased likelihood of an underlying disorder:

1. VTE occurring in a young person without any evidence of trauma, etc
2. VTE occurring in an unusual site: upper limb, mesenteric vein, etc
3. VTE occurring in a patient on anticoagulant therapy
4. A strong family history of excessive thrombosis.

However, it is important that secondary causes be excluded, such as pregnancy and immobilization.

Of the inherited causes of hypercoagulability, the following are particularly likely to result in VTE:

1. Proteins C and S deficiency
2. Factor V_{Leiden}
3. Prothrombin G20210A mutation.

Arterial Thrombosis

In the majority of cases of arterial thrombosis, there is underlying vascular disease. This causes the endothelial surface to be irregular and/or roughened, predisposing to platelet adhesion and activation.

The epidemiological impact of **ACUTE ARTERIAL THROMBOSIS** hardly needs emphasizing. There are numerous causes of arterial occlusion. By far the most common is atherosclerosis. Other causes include thromboangiitis obliterans (Buerger), connective tissue disorders, and some myeloproliferative disorders.

Hypercoagulability in acute arterial thrombosis is most commonly associated with the traditional risk factors, but the hereditary defects in the hemostatic mechanism and some acquired platelet disorders are coming to be seen more and more as significant role-players.

Many of the diseases affecting arteries, notably atherosclerosis, not only in themselves can compromise the circulation, but by damaging the intimal surface predispose to platelet adhesion and activation.

By contrast, the hereditary hypercoagulability disorders are virtually never involved in **CHRONIC ARTERIAL OCCLUSION**; the commonest causes here are arteriosclerosis obliterans (a complication of atherosclerosis), Buerger disease, and connective tissue diseases.

Making the Diagnosis

Again the point must be stressed: most of the causes listed above are rare, and some can be identified or suspected clinically or with the FBC. One needs specific motivation to order the (very expensive) special tests for hypercoagulability.

The following can often (or in some cases, always) be suspected clinically (this includes the presence of the classical risk factors). Since they are part of general medicine, no detail will be gone into:

1. Malignancy
2. Sepsis
3. Inflammatory bowel disease
4. Nephrotic syndrome
5. Pregnancy and hormone replacement therapy
6. Obesity
7. Hypercholesterolemia
8. Sedentary lifestyle
9. Hypertension
10. Smoking
11. Diabetes mellitus
12. Stress
13. Immobilization.

The following can be suspected, or indeed in some cases diagnosed, on the FBC.

1. Acute promyelocytic leukemia
2. Sickle cell disease
3. Polycythemia vera
4. Essential thrombocythemia
5. Paraproteinemias.

The following can be suspected, or indeed sometimes diagnosed, on the HS.

1. Factor XII deficiency – very rare indeed.
2. Hyperaggregable platelets and possibly a few other hypercoagulable states can sometimes be suspected with a significantly shortened PTT.

The following can be suspected by using various combinations of clinical features, the first-line tests, and biochemical/immunological tests (these tend to be the most difficult):

1. Heparin-induced thrombocytopenia
2. Paroxysmal nocturnal hemoglobinuria (PNH) – often a very difficult diagnosis indeed
3. Paraproteins especially Waldenstrom macroglobulinemia
4. The antiphospholipid syndrome and lupus anticoagulant.

Making the Diagnosis of Antiphospholipid Syndrome

Essentially one needs one clinical criterion and one laboratory criterion.

The clinical criteria that can be used are

1. Thrombosis
2. One of the types of fetal loss as described above.

The laboratory criteria are

1. At least moderate (> 30 GPL units) rise in anticardiolipin IgG or IgM antibodies
2. Lupus anticoagulant.

A Suggested Approach to Suspected Hypercoagulability

In practice, the following schema has been found the most useful:

1. The personal history
2. The family history
3. The clinical examination including specific search for risk factors.

Only now, if clinically warranted, does one proceed:

4. FBC and PTT
5. Liver and renal function tests; protein electrophoresis if indicated by other features
6. Appropriate imaging (Fig. 21.1).

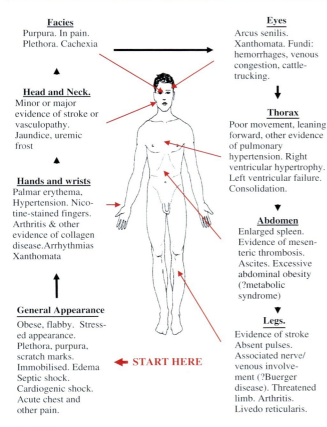

Facies
Purpura. In pain.
Plethora. Cachexia

Eyes
Arcus senilis.
Xanthomata. Fundi:
hemorrhages, venous
congestion, cattle-
trucking.

Head and Neck.
Minor or major
evidence of stroke or
vasculopathy.
Jaundice, uremic
frost

Hands and wrists
Palmar erythema,
Hypertension. Nico-
tine-stained fingers.
Arthritis & other
evidence of collagen
disease.Arrhythmias
Xanthomata

Thorax
Poor movement, leaning
forward, other evidence
of pulmonary
hypertension. Right
ventricular hypertrophy.
Left ventricular failure.
Consolidation.

Abdomen
Enlarged spleen.
Evidence of mesen-
teric thrombosis.
Ascites. Excessive
abdominal obesity
(?metabolic
syndrome)

General Appearance
Obese, flabby. Stress-
ed appearance.
Plethora, purpura,
scratch marks.
Immobilised. Edema
Septic shock.
Cardiogenic shock.
Acute chest and
other pain.

Legs.
Evidence of stroke
Absent pulses.
Associated nerve/
venous involve-
ment (?Buerger
disease). Threatened
limb. Arthritis.
Livedo reticularis.

◄ **START HERE**

Fig. 21.1 Examination in Possible Hypercoagulability

Making the Diagnosis of Deep Vein Thrombosis (DVT) and Pulmonary Embolism (PE)

These are among the most difficult and important diagnoses to make. Two of the most useful and practical schemas are those produced by Scarvelis and Wells[1] using a point system.

Deep Vein Thrombosis

Each of the following clinical features is allocated **1 POINT**:

1. Active cancer, with treatment within 6 months or using palliation
2. Paralysis or immobilization of the lower extremities
3. Bedridden for >3 days because of surgery within the last 4 weeks
4. Localized tenderness along the site of the deep veins
5. Swelling of the entire leg
6. Unilateral calf swelling of >3 cm compared with the other side, measured just below the tibial tuberosity
7. Unilateral pitting edema
8. Collateral superficial veins.

If there is an alternative diagnosis regarded at least as likely as DVT, **2 POINTS ARE SUBTRACTED** from the total.

Interpretation:

3 points or more: 75% risk of DVT being present (high-risk group).
1–2 points: 17% risk of DVT being present (moderate risk group)
<1 point: 3% risk of DVT being present (low-risk group).

Next, we look at the Wells probability tool for pulmonary embolism (PE).

Pulmonary Embolism

1. Each of the following features is allocated **3 POINTS:**

   a. Clinical features of DVT
   b. Other diagnosis less likely than PE

2. Each of the following features is allocated **1½ POINTS**

   a. Heart rate >100/min
   b. Immobilization, or surgery within the last 4 weeks
   c. Previous DVT or PE.

3. Each of the following features is allocated **1 POINT**.

   a. Hemoptysis
   b. Malignancy.

Interpretation:

6 points or more: 78.4% risk of PE being present (high-risk group)
2–6 points: 27.8% risk of PE being present (moderate-risk group)
<2 points: 3.4% risk of PE being present (low-risk group).

It will be realized that the real problem with both disorders lies with the moderate risk group, although even the low risk group poses some problems. Currently, the accepted test for confirming DVT is B-mode Doppler studies with compression; these are very dependent on local expertise and are expensive. Hence one looks for a test that will exclude DVT and PE with a high probability (i.e., high specificity), and that test is the D-dimer test. D-dimers have been discussed in Chapter 2.

The D-Dimer Test

The problem with the D-dimer test is its low specificity at mildly increased measured levels. Numerous causes of false and abnormal results have been demonstrated, and we only take notice of a D-dimer result if it is at least 2–3 times the upper limit of its reference range (i.e., 2.5). However, the major utility of the test with respect to DVT and PE is that if it is normal, they can be excluded with 97% certainly.

Otherwise, and only then, with clinical suspicion being present, is the patient submitted to specialized sonographic studies.

> Once the secondary causes of a thrombotic presentation have been excluded *and* there are sufficient suspicious features of hereditary hypercoagulability, can one proceed to investigate for these.

It has been a major problem to decide how far to go in investigating for suspected hereditary hypercoagulability disorders.

1. Many of them are very rare indeed, and from the economic point of view, testing for them has a yield that is quite unacceptably low.
2. A number of them can be picked up or suspected, and then specifically confirmed individually.
3. These specialized tests are all very expensive.

Consequently, the following consensus as to which screening tests are worth doing has been arrived at:

1. FBC
2. PTT, PT, and TT; occasionally the D-dimers if there is a suggestion of liver failure or DIC
3. Antithrombin assay
4. Protein C
5. Protein S
6. Factor V_{Leiden}
7. Prothrombin G20210A assay
8. Antiphospholipid antibodies.

The FBC in the Hypercoagulable States

The FBC in these conditions can provide a very strong pointer to the nature of the hypercoagulable presentation, and it may obviate proceeding to the further suggested tests.

1. **SICKLE CELLS.**
2. **SEVERE LIVER DISEASE.**
3. **PARAPROTEINEMIAS.** These may be suspected by the presence of marked rouleaux formation and the comment of "background staining" – the high protein

content of the plasma causes it to stain bluish with the standard FBC stains. Also a very high ESR would be suggestive.
4. **ACUTE PROMYELOCYTIC LEUKEMIA.**
5. **POLYCYTHEMIA VERA.**
6. **THE PICTURE OF DIC.**
7. **ESSENTIAL THROMBOCYTHEMIA.**
8. **THROMBOCYTOPENIA.** This may be relevant in the following cases:

   a. **HEPARIN-INDUCED THROMBOCYTOPENIA**
   b. **PARTLY COMPENSATED DIC**
   c. **THROMBOTIC THROMBOCYTOPENIC PURPURA** – see Chapter 22.

The Hemostatic Screen in the Hypercoagulable States

Here we discuss only the PT, PTT, thrombin time (TT), and the D-dimers. The platelet count has been discussed before.

1. **PTT.**

   a. **A PROLONGED PTT** may be indicative of five relevant conditions:

      i. Factor XII deficiency
      ii. Lupus anticoagulant
      iii. DIC
      iv. Liver disease
      v. Acute promyelocytic leukemia

   b. **A SHORTENED PTT** is sometimes observed as a non-specific feature in many hypercoagulable states.

2. **PT.** A prolonged PT may indicate three relevant conditions:

   a. Liver disease
   b. DIC
   c. Acute promyelocytic leukemia.

3. **TT.** This is sometimes noticeably shortened in many hypercoagulable states.
4. **D-DIMERS.** As indicated before, there are numerous non-specific causes of raised D-dimers. Significant rises always indicate a thrombotic process. The problem with interpreting the result is that it may rise secondary to thrombosis caused by other factors, or it may rise as a reflection of a primary cause, such as DIC.

Practical Point in Investigating Hypercoagulability It sometimes happens that a patient will present for consultation when he has already been placed on anticoagulant therapy. This clearly would interfere with many of the tests. It can be a very difficult decision to stop the treatment for the requisite time before the tests are done, since one may get into trouble should the patient have a thrombotic episode in the meantime. Sometimes one has no option, and probably the safest way is to do the tests that are not affected by the particular anticoagulant, then switching the treatment and doing the others. Many tests of course are not affected by anticoagulants.

Common tests that are affected by oral anticoagulants

1. Protein C
2. Protein S

Common tests that are affected by heparin (even fractionated heparin)

1. Antithrombin
2. Lupus anticoagulant (this should not theoretically be affected but we have seen this often in our unit)

Common tests that are not affected by anticoagulants

9. Factor V_{Leiden} by PCR
10. Prothrombin G20210A by PCR
11. Homocysteine
12. Anti-cardiolipin antibodies.

Table 21.1

Patient: Mrs E W, aged 47 years.				

The patient was referred by a pulmonologist whom she had consulted for recurrent attacks of pleuritic chest pain with dyspnea and cough. She also stated that she had had repeated episodes of what had been diagnosed as DVTs. Extensive investigation revealed a picture highly suggestive of recurrent pulmonary emboli. Of the tests for hypercoagulability, only antithrombin, protein C and protein S were done: protein C was decreased. The patient was anticoagulated. However, she continued to have recurrent pulmonary emboli and was referred.

Her family history was of a strong tendency to thrombotic disease. On examination, she was obese but otherwise looking quite well. The vital signs were normal. The chest and heart were clinically normal. No clear features of DVT were currently observable. The EKG revealed mild right ventricular strain. A V/Q scan revealed quite clearly a pattern of pulmonary emboli.

Test	Value	Units	Low	High
Platelet count	238	$\times 10^9/l$	140	440
PTT	30	s	26	37
PT	12.5	s	12	14
TT	10.1	s	9	11
Antithrombin	100	%	70	120
Protein C	**43**	%	70	140
Protein S	71	%	60	140
Factor V_{Leiden}	**Positive**		Negative	
Prothrombin G20210A	Negative		Negative	70
Anti-cardiolipin IgG	1	Units/ml	0	25
Anti-cardiolipin IgM	2	Units/ml	0	25
D-Dimers	**3.9**		0	2.5

Hence further tests were justified. The presence of two separate defects is rather uncommon, and in this regard, there is one important caveat: depending on the method of estimating protein C, the presence of a factor V_{Leiden} can produce a falsely low protein C. It is important that the laboratory does not use a clotting method for the estimation.

3. Inferior vena cavagram revealed numerous adherent clots below the level of the renal veins.
4. This type of patient represents a major therapeutic challenge. It was decided in consultation to have a Greenfield filter inserted into the IVC. This appeared to be successful, although it often is not in this type of case, since thrombi can form above it. It must be stated that many experts are not convinced about the value of the Greenfield and other vena caval filters.

Teaching Cases

CASE #95 (EXAMINE TABLE 21.1)

DISCUSSION

1. The raised D-dimers are compatible with but not diagnostic of the presence of thrombosis.
2. The recurrent emboli despite the patient being adequately anticoagulated is always a serious sign, strongly suggesting a hereditary hypercoagulability.

CASE #96 (EXAMINE TABLE 21.2)

DISCUSSION

The impact of hypercholesterolemia and indeed all the secondary acquired causes of hypercoagulability should never be forgotten.

Table 21.2

Patient: Mr T A R, aged 35years.
This patient presented to his family doctor with severe recent chest pain, and the diagnosis was made of angina. He performed a few blood tests; the fasting lipogram was markedly abnormal, with a total cholesterol of **16.3** mmol/l, HDL cholesterol of **0.5** mmol/l, and triglycerides of **6.0** mmol/l. Blood glucose was normal. He referred the patient to a cardiologist. An EKG revealed an intraventricular conduction delay as well as diffuse ischemic changes. An exercise EKG revealed severe ischemia. He was placed on a statin and aspirin, and his diet was corrected. His symptoms did not really improve, and further EKGs and echocardiography suggested that he was close to decompensating; it was decided to do a coronary bypass procedure. This was very successful.

CASE #97 (TABLE 21.3)

Table 21.3

Patient: Mrs du T, aged 40 years.
This patient was referred because of severe disturbances of sensation and headache. The headaches had many features suggestive of migraine, including the presence of fortification spectra and nausea. The disturbances of sensation were most peculiar in that they would be experienced either on the right or the left side of the body, but never both. The attacks were clinically similar, starting in the neck with what can best be described as formication, which spread down the arm, then the side of the body to the feet. At some time during this attack, which would last about 20 min, she would experience dimness of vision (on the affected side), the tongue would feel thick, and speech would become difficult. The arm and leg on that side would then become weak. At the time she was seen, however, there were no neurological deficits to be found.
On systematic enquiry, she complained of long-standing pain and swelling of the small joints with some morning stiffness. There was no evidence of other vascular abnormality, especially no thrombotic episodes. The family history was not contributory.
General examination revealed no abnormalities apart from mildly swollen and tender small joints.
MRI of the brain revealed high-intensity lesions in various parts, mostly posterior and in the corona radiata. CT scanning revealed linear structures in the vicinity of the posterior cerebral arteries, of uncertain significance. Doppler studies were normal. Further investigations were done. See Table 21.4.

Table 21.4

Test	Value	Units	Low	High
Platelet count	**98**	$\times 10^9/l$	140	440
PTT	32	s	26	37
PT	13	s	12	14
TT	10	s	9	11
Antithrombin	115	%	70	120
Protein C	100	%	70	140
Protein S	95	%	60	140
Factor V$_{Leiden}$	Negative		Negative	
Prothrombin G20210A	Negative		Negative	70
Anti-cardiolipin IgG	**55**	Units/ml	0	25
Anti-cardiolipin IgM	**21**	Units/ml	0	25
D-Dimers	**2.7**		0	2.5
Rheumatoid factor	10	Units	<40	
ANA	**1/160**	Titer	0	1/40
Anti-DNA	**6.6**	IU/l	0	4.2
Lupus anticoagulant	Negative			

2. There is not even certainty whether the neurological symptoms are caused by APS or by SLE, which is known to produce bizarre neurological features from time to time.

3. This case emphasizes the very large variety of clinical presentations of APS. There is no doubt that one should suspect APS in any and all cases of proven or suspected thrombosis, especially if there are atypical features.

4. Therapy of these cases is often a problem. Steroids are not indicated in this disease (being ineffective) unless there is "catastrophic" SLE with multiple organ failure. The only accepted treatment is warfarin anticoagulation – but with this caveat, the INR must be kept at or near 3.5, far higher than one normally aims for. This then is associated with a higher incidence of bleeding complications.

Further Reading

Lewis SM, Bain B, Bates I (2006). Dacie and Lewis Practical Haematology. 10th edn. Churchill Livingstone.

Hoffbrand AV, Catovsky D, Tuddenham EGD (eds) (2005). Postgraduate Haematology. 5th edn. Oxford: Blackwell Publishing.

Anderson DR, Kovacs MJ, Kovacs G et al. (2003). Combined use of clinical assessment and D-dimer to improve the management of patients presenting to the emergency department with suspected deep vein thrombosis (the EDITED study). J. Thromb. Hemost. 1: 645–651.

DISCUSSION

1. The diagnosis of the antiphospholipid syndrome is established. The real question, however, is whether the arthritis (possible SLE) plays any role – i.e., whether the APS is secondary or associated with the SLE. A big factor against this is the negative lupus anticoagulant. The thrombocytopenia too could be associated with the APS or SLE, were this proven.

This chapter covers three main groups of topics, some of them very briefly:

1. Immune deficiencies
2. The lymphomas and related conditions
3. Myeloma and related conditions

Diagnostic clinical immunology is a vast subject that will require a book of this size to handle adequately. Even the immune deficiencies are a very extensive and indeed a very difficult topic. Consequently, only certain aspects will be discussed here, of relevance only to clinical hematological practice.

Similarly, lymphomas are a very complex group of conditions, where the diagnosis with few exceptions always requires biopsy. They are thus of less significance in clinical diagnostic hematology at the general level.

The major thrust therefore of this chapter is on the myelomas and related conditions.

Immune Deficiencies

These days, the acquired immune deficiencies have achieved major prominence, particularly AIDS. This has been dealt with in Chapter 4. Note however that there are other causes of defective cellular immunity: cytotoxic and immunosuppressive therapy is very widely used these days; and certain nutritional deficiencies have been shown also to be implicated, notably of vitamin A, selenium, and zinc. Of the primary or hereditary deficiencies, there are three groups:

1. **SEVERE COMBINED IMMUNODEFICIENCIES**. These are rare and present in childhood. Of relevance though is that **LYMPHOPENIA** is a characteristic feature. In some of these syndromes,

THROMBOCYTOPENIA is characteristic (the Wiskott–Aldrich syndrome, for example). Many also predispose to the development of lymphoma.

2. **PRIMARY ANTIBODY DEFICIENCY**. There are only two conditions that need be mentioned:

   a. **IGA DEFICIENCY**. This is by far the commonest, affecting 1 in 700 people. It is of little significance except for the fact that about 10% of patients develop anti-IgA antibodies. These can be responsible for severe anaphylactic reactions during transfusion.
   b. **COMMON VARIABLE IMMUNODEFICIENCY**.

3. **DEFECTS IN COMPLEMENT**. These are very rare.
4. **DEFECTS IN PHAGOCYTE FUNCTION**. Functional disorders of phagocytes may occur at any stage in their normal activation (by microbes). These stages, very briefly are as follows:

   a. **LOCOMOTION.** The cells move along a chemotactic gradient, mediated by cell–cell adhesion. Numerous molecules are involved here.
   b. **DEGRANULATION.** Once the phagocytes have encountered the offending organisms, they degranulate either into lysozomes containing the engulfed organism or into the extracellular space.
   c. **KILLING.** This occurs by one of three mechanisms:

      i. The respiratory burst with the production of the OH· radical, which is microbiocidal.
      ii. Nitric oxide.
      iii. Anti-microbial proteins.

These functions are all mediated by two groups of molecules:

a. **CYTOKINES.** There is normally a complex web of cytokines operating to mediate and control the phagocytic response, such as IL-1, IL-2, Il-8, TNF, PAF.

O.N. Beck, *Diagnostic Hematology*, DOI 10.1007/978-1-84800-295-1_22,
© Springer-Verlag London Limited 2009

b. **CELL SURFACE RECEPTORS**, such as the selectins and integrins.

A number of rare hereditary conditions have been described.

The Lymphomas

These comprise Hodgkin disease (HD), non-Hodgkin lymphomas (NHL), hairy cell leukemia (HCL), and a number of peculiar conditions whose malignant status is in doubt. Chronic lymphocytic leukemia (CLL) is not really a lymphoma but sometimes needs to be distinguished from certain forms of lymphoma; it has been discussed previously.

The difficulties with the lymphomas are exemplified by the enormous complexity of their classification (there is an old joke that goes: there are three certainties in this life – death, taxes, and a new classification of the lymphomas). As was previously mentioned, diagnosis is always by biopsy (except sometimes in the case of HCL and of course in CLL). These diseases thus fall more under the purview of pathology than hematology. Consequently, we will only mention those issues that enter into routine clinical hematological practice:

1. **THE PROVISIONAL CLINICAL DIAGNOSIS OF LYMPHADENOPATHY**. This was covered in Chapter 5.
2. **THE EFFECTS OF THE LYMPHOMAS ON THE FBC**.

    a. **ANEMIA OF CHRONIC DISORDERS**. This is by far the commonest.

    b. **EFFECTS OF BONE MARROW INFILTRATION AND REPLACEMENT**. A number of possible presentations may thus occur:

      i. Pancytopenia
     ii. Leukoerythroblastic reaction

    c. **IRON-DEFICIENCY ANEMIA**, secondary to gastro-intestinal infiltration and mucosal erosion. Some lymphomas have a predilection for mucosal infiltration, such as the MALT lymphoma.

    d. **AUTOIMMUNE HEMOLYTIC ANEMIA**.

    e. **CERTAIN OTHER CHARACTERISTIC FBC APPEARANCES**.

3. **EFFECTS ON THE WHITE CELL COUNT**.

    a. **UP TO 20% OF HD PATIENTS WILL DEVELOP A MILD EOSINOPHILIA**.

    b. **LEUKOERYTHROBLASTIC REACTION** as mentioned above.

    c. **LYMPHOCYTOSIS**.

    d. Occasionally **LYMPHOPENIA**, as in some types of HD.

    e. **LEUKEMIC INFILTRATION** of the blood by "lymphomablasts."

Myeloma and Related Conditions

These conditions all are due to proliferation of malignant plasma cells (and are thus all of B-cell origin). The conditions to be discussed are as follows:

1. **MULTIPLE MYELOMATOSIS** (MM). There are several variants:

    a. Overt MM
    b. Smouldering MM
    c. Non-secretory MM
    d. Plasma cell leukemia
    e. Osteosclerotic myeloma

2. **PLASMACYTOMA** (solitary myeloma).
3. **WALDENSTRÖM MACROGLOBULINEMIA**.
4. **AMYLOIDOSIS**. Amyloidosis may be primary (characterized by M protein production) or secondary – to chronic inflammatory conditions.

There are a few rarities that will not be discussed.

AN ESSENTIAL (BUT NOT QUITE UNIVERSAL) CHARACTERISTIC is the tendency for the malignant plasma cells to produce excessive amounts of abnormal proteins, which are either complete immunoglobulins or parts of immunoglobulins (kappa (κ) or lambda (λ) chains, either of which constitutes Bence-Jones protein, or heavy chains. They are all referred to as M proteins. Since the production of M proteins is frequently a criterion for the diagnosis of myeloma and related conditions, it is necessary to understand that there are other, often non-malignant causes of M protein production (clearly of relevance in the differential diagnosis).

M Proteins Produced Regularly in the Course of a Disease

1. **OBVIOUSLY MALIGNANT CONDITIONS**

    a. Most multiple myeloma sub-types – excluding the non-secretory type
    b. Waldenström macroglobulinemia

c. Plasmacytoma very commonly

d. Primary amyloidosis

2. **STABLE CONDITIONS OF POSSIBLE MALIGNANT STATUS**

a. Monoclonal gammopathy of uncertain significance or MGUS

b. Chronic cold hemagglutinin disease (see Chapter 10)

The most important diagnostic characteristic of these M proteins is that they present as a sharp peak on electrophoresis – sharp because they represent the production of a single (usually malignant) clone of cells. They are thus called **MONOCLONAL PEAKS**; it is also a characteristic that the rest of the immunoglobulin production is decreased, referred to as **IMMUNOPARESIS**. This is in sharp contradistinction to the polyclonal wide peaks found due to the production of increased gammaglobulins derived from several different generations of plasma cells, as they produce increased numbers of antibodies as a response to infection and many types of inflammation not necessarily associated with infection.

The M proteins interfere with normal **RED CELL AGGREGATION**; thus there typically is marked rouleaux formation, accompanied by a markedly raised ESR.

These M proteins can have several other deleterious effects, the most important of which are the **HYPERVISCOSITY SYNDROMES** and **RENAL DYSFUNCTION** (there are other causes of renal dysfunction in myeloma as well, such a hypercalcemia, amyloidosis and dehydration). Amyloid proteins may be deposited in the nerve sheaths, causing neuropathy. The M proteins may also have **EFFECTS ON THE HEMOSTATIC SYSTEM**, due to various mechanisms:

1. **BLEEDING MAY RESULT FROM A NUMBER OF FACTORS**:

a. **COATING OF PLATELET SURFACES** by the M protein

b. **ADSORPTION ON TO THE SURFACE OF THE M PROTEINS OF COAGULATION FACTORS**, commonly factor X

c. **PERIVASCULAR AMYLOIDOSIS**

d. **THROMBOCYTOPENIA**

2. Occasionally **THROMBOSIS** may result from hyperviscosity or lupus anticoagulant.

ANOTHER IMPORTANT CHARACTERISTIC of many if not most of these conditions is that, since they originate from plasma cells and plasma cells are essentially marrow cells, the bone and bone marrow will be affected:

1. **LYTIC LESIONS IN BONES** where there is active marrow (it will be remembered that from adolescence onward, active (red) marrow gradually retreats from the long bones; hence lytic lesions are found only in the pelvis, ribs, vertebrae and the vertex of the skull). Alternatively there may be severe osteopenia. Severe bone pain is characteristic. This are accompanied by a **RAISED ALKALINE PHOSPHATASE** and a tendency to **HYPERCALCEMIA**, with its attendant polydipsia, polyuria, and constipation, and may contribute to renal failure. Characteristically there are > 30% myeloma cells in the marrow (but see under "Making the Diagnosis").

2. **BONE MARROW INFILTRATION BY MYELOMA CELLS**, resulting in various cytopenias and/or the leukoerythroblastic reaction. Myeloma cells can be very numerous and may be responsible for excessive amounts of uric acid – a contributory cause of renal failure.

3. **BONE MARROW FUNCTIONAL DISTURBANCE** due mainly to the production of enormous amounts of cytokines, resulting in conditions such as anemia of chronic disorders.

OVERT MULTIPLE MYELOMATOSIS

In this variety, by far the commonest, all the described features typically are present. Note that the prognosis is poor and treatment is essential.

SMOULDERING MYELOMATOSIS

These patients have a raised M protein and > 10% myeloma cells in the marrow but are asymptomatic and have no bony or renal lesions. They are not treated until and unless they progress.

NON-SECRETORY MYELOMA

These rare cases are very similar to overt myeloma except there is no M protein and consequently less renal involvement.

PLASMA CELL LEUKEMIA

In these rare cases, malignant plasma cells appear in the peripheral blood.

PLASMACYTOMA

Rarely a patient will present with a single mass (or occasionally a few masses) of myeloma cells, and which may be extraosseus. They may produce small amounts of M proteins. The prognosis is fair. There is a tendency for plasmacytomas to transform into disseminated disease.

WALDENSTRÖM MACROGLOBULINEMIA

This uncommon condition is characterized by the production of IgM M proteins with hyperviscosity and the presence in the marrow (and usually the blood) of plasmacytoid lymphocytes. It is generally regarded as a form of lymphoma.

AMYLOIDOSIS

A large number of abnormal proteins (called fibril precursor proteins) have been discovered. The "traditional" amyloidosis, occurring secondary to chronic inflammatory conditions, has a somewhat different anatomical distribution from the other, primary, types. These are described later.

MGUS

This is a condition characterized by the presence of an M protein in a patient without evidence of myeloma, amyloidosis, or macroglobulinemia. The following criteria must be met:

1. The M protein level must be < 35 g/l.
2. <10% plasma cells in the marrow.
3. No Bence-Jones protein.
4. No lytic lesions of bone.
5. No anemia.
6. No hypercalcemia.
7. No renal insufficiency (as a result of the disorder).

It is typically a disease of older people. The natural history is unpredictable. In long-term follow-up, a certain proportion (±10%) will eventually progress to myeloma, macroglobulinemia, amyloidosis, plasmacytoma or CLL. The cumulative risk for transformation is

1. 10% at 10 years after diagnosis
2. 20% at 20 years after diagnosis
3. 25% at 25 years after diagnosis

Making the Diagnosis

CLASSICAL OVERT MYELOMATOSIS

This condition is usually easy to suspect, and is not likely to be confused with any of the other disorders. Typically the patient presents with severe bone pain (>70% of cases), with pallor and often renal failure (>40% of cases). The FBC will show highly suggestive features (see below) and so will a number of biochemical tests.

NON-SECRETORY MYELOMA

This tends to present similarly to the classic types, except that renal failure is uncommon. In addition, the FBC will not show some of the characteristic features.

PLASMACYTOMA AND SMOULDERING MYELOMA

These are almost always discovered incidentally.

WALDENSTRöM MACROGLOBULINEMIA

In typical cases the condition is easy to suspect – it presents with a classical hyperviscosity syndrome:

1. Visual disturbances, with fundal hemorrhages, exudates, and sometimes cattle-trucking of the vessels

2. Mental confusion, various pareses, sensory disturbances, even stroke
3. Cardiac failure

Less typical cases may be difficult to suspect and are picked up incidentally.

AMYLOIDOSIS

There are two aspects to the problem of diagnosing amyloidosis:

1. Suspecting its presence
2. Identifying the type – primary or secondary

In this regard the anatomical distribution is often very helpful. In both types the liver, spleen, and kidneys will be involved. However, in the primary types, there is characteristically involvement of

1. The tongue causing macroglossia
2. The heart causing a cardiomyopathy
3. The peripheral nerves causing polyneuropathy **WITH PALPABLE NERVES**
4. The skin, especially the vessels, causing purpura, especially in the temporal region

MGUS

Since the condition per se is asymptomatic, it is always discovered on routine protein electrophoresis. Having been discovered, it is important that, at some stage or another (it is seldom urgent), the following tests must be done: FBC, bone marrow aspiration, renal function tests, serum calcium levels, Bence-Jones protein, skeletal survey.

Thereafter careful follow-up is required.

The Clinical Examination

Figure 22.1 offers suggestions on **SPECIFIC ASPECTS** of the examination of a patient in whom one of these conditions is known or suspected; clearly it is part of the overall examination is as is depicted in Fig. 5.4.

Diagnosis in Practice

It must be conceded that diagnosing these conditions is hardly a clinical activity unless some very obvious and characteristic features are present. The most striking clinical feature that must raise suspicion is **BONE PAIN**. In most cases the diagnosis will be suggested by the FBC, routine biochemistry, and occasionally by X-ray appearances.

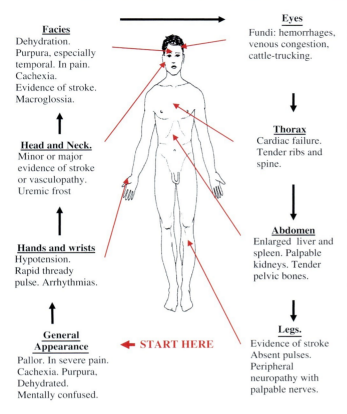

Facies
Dehydration.
Purpura, especially temporal. In pain.
Cachexia.
Evidence of stroke.
Macroglossia.

Head and Neck.
Minor or major evidence of stroke or vasculopathy.
Uremic frost

Hands and wrists
Hypotension.
Rapid thready pulse. Arrhythmias.

**General
Appearance**
Pallor. In severe pain.
Cachexia. Purpura,
Dehydrated.
Mentally confused.

Eyes
Fundi: hemorrhages, venous congestion, cattle-trucking.

Thorax
Cardiac failure.
Tender ribs and spine.

Abdomen
Enlarged liver and spleen. Palpable kidneys. Tender pelvic bones.

Legs.
Evidence of stroke
Absent pulses.
Peripheral neuropathy with palpable nerves.

← **START HERE**

Fig. 22.1 Possible lympho-plasma proliferative condition

Teaching Cases

CASE #98 (EXAMINE TABLE 22.1)

Table 22.2 shows the results of various biochemical investigations.

DISCUSSION

1. It will be observed that there is very little in the FBC to alert one to the possible diagnosis. The biochemical results are far more informative. Nevertheless, while extremely suspicious, one does not have enough for the diagnosis. The criteria for the diagnosis of multiple myeloma are: two major criteria, or one major plus one minor criteria, the following being the criteria.

MAJOR CRITERIA

  a. Plasmacytoma proven by biopsy
  b. Bone marrow infiltration with > 30% plasma cells
  c. Monoclonal peak of > 35 g/l (IgG) or > 20 g/l (IgA)

MINOR CRITERIA

  a. Bone marrow infiltration with > 10% plasma cells
  b. Monoclonal peak of less than defined above

  c. Lytic bone lesions
  d. IgM > 0.5 g/l, IgA > 1 g/l, IgG > 6 g/l

2. Accordingly, a marrow aspirate was performed. This, in summary, revealed 71% plasma cells, most of which were extremely abnormal and pleomorphic.

Comment Case #98 represents a very common and typical presentation of multiple myeloma. With a good index of suspicion the diagnosis should not be missed.

Table 22.1

Patient	Age	Sex	Race	Altitude
Mr J N	61 yrs	Male	Black	5,000 ft

This patient was referred by his family practitioner. The patient had consulted her about severe weakness and "general body pains." She had not found very much specific on examination, and had ordered a FBC and ESR. She noticed a mild normocytic anemia and a markedly raised ESR. As a result of this she ordered protein electrophoresis and immunoglobulins, and when the results were available she referred the patient.

When seen, the patient was in severe distress, with severe pain and bony tenderness in the dorsal spine and particularly the left scapula. He was pale and sallow. The vital signs were normal; there was no jaundice, purpura, bruising, splenomegaly, hepatomegaly or palpable kidneys. There was considerable peripheral neuropathy but no nerves were palpable.

	Value	Units	Reference range Low	Reference range High	Permitted range Low	Permitted range High
Red cell count	3.54	× 10¹²/l	4.77	5.83	3.10	3.98
Hemoglobin (Hb)	9.7	g/dl	13.8	18.0	9.4	10.0
Hematocrit (Hct)	0.30	l/l	0.42	0.53	0.30	0.31
Mean cell volume	86	fl	80	99	77.0	95.0
Mean cell Hb	27.4	pg	27	31.5	24.5	30.3
Mean cell Hb conc.	31.9	g/dl	31.5	34.5	31.2	32.5
Red cell dist. width	14.5	%	11.6	14	13.4	15.6
Retic count	0.21	%	0.27	0.80	0.0	0.0
Retic absolute (abs.)	19.7	× 10⁹/l	30	100	0.0	0.0
White cell count	9.45	× 10⁹/l	3.5	10	8.51	10.40
Neutrophils abs.	4.26	× 10⁹/l	1.5	7	3.84	4.69
Lymphocytes abs.	4.10	× 10⁹/l	1	3	3.69	4.51
Monocytes abs.	0.65	× 10⁹/l	0.2	1	0.59	0.72
Eosinophils abs.	0.34	× 10⁹/l	0.02	0.5	0.31	0.37
Basophils abs.	0.09	× 10⁹/l	0.02	0.1	0.09	0.10
Normoblasts	0	/100 WBC	0	0		
Platelet count	98.4	× 10⁹/l	150	400	86.1	110.7
Sedimentation	101	mm/h	0	10	100	102
Morphology	Rouleaux + + + Atypical lymphocytes +					

Table 22.2

	Value	Units	Reference range Low	High
S-Urea	**21.8**	mmol/l	2.1	7.1
S-Creatinine	**671.9**	mmol/l	62	115
S-Urea:creatinine	32.4			
S-Sodium	131	mmol/l	136	145
S-Potassium	**5.48**	mmol/l	3.5	5.1
S-Chloride	**111.00**	mmol/l	98	108
S-Total CO_2	**17**	mmol/l	22	28
S-Anion gap	8.5	mmol/l	5	14
S-Glucose	4.5	mmol/l	3.9	5.8
S-Osmolarity	274	mmol/l	275	295
S-Uric acid	**0.51**	mmol/l	0.21	0.42
S-Calcium (total)	**3.65**	mmol/l	2.2	2.55
S-Protein (total)	**91.4**	g/l	64	83
S-Albumin	**30,2**	g/l	34	48
S-Globulin	**51.2**	g/l	30	35
S-α1-globulin	1.1	g/l		1.9
S-α2-globulin	7.3	g/l	5	7
S-β-globulin	6.2	g/l	5	8
S-γ-globulin	**48.3**	g/l	6	10
S-Immunoglobulin G	**43.5**	g/l	2.5	12
S-Immunoglobulin M	0.09	g/l	0.19	1.93
S-Immunoglobulin A	0.03	g/l	0.07	0.94
C-Reactive protein	**33.2**	mg/l	0.0	10.0
Comment	There is a large monoclonal peak in the gamma region measuring 43.2 g/l, together with immune paresis.			

CASE #99 (EXAMINE TABLE 22.3)

Relevant biochemical results are shown in Table 22.4.

Plasma viscosity was performed. The result is shown in Table 22.5.

DISCUSSION

1. It is quite clear that there is severe hyperviscosity, due to massive amounts of IgM. Subsequent electrophoresis revealed the monoclonal nature of this protein. The morphology of the lymphocytes was in keeping with Waldenstrom macroglobulinemia.

2. There are some findings in the FBC that require comment:

   a. There is a significant absolute lymphocytosis, and the lymphocytes are atypical and plasmacytoid in form – however, they are not plasma cells as such, and these plasmacytoid lymphocytes are classical although not diagnostic of macroglobulinemia.

   b. The background staining reflects the raised serum proteins.

Table 22.3

Patient	Age	Sex	Race	Altitude
Mr H I	60 yrs	Male	White	Sea level

The patient was a visitor from overseas. He had hitherto been quite well and now he complained of fairly sudden blindness, coming on over a period of several hours (although on subsequent questioning he admitted to some intermittent slight blurring, with headache, lassitude, and exertional dyspnea for a few weeks).

A family doctor noticed extensive hemorrhages and exudates in the fundi; the disc was completely obscured. There was also horizontal nystagmus. An ophthalmologist felt that the features were in keeping with hyperviscosity and the patient was urgently referred. The patient was in mild cardiac failure and considerably confused mentally.

	Value	Units	Reference range Low	High	Permitted range Low	High
Red cell count	**4.21**	$\times 10^{12}$/l	4.5	5.5	4.08	4.34
Hemoglobin (Hb)	**12.1**	g/dl	13	17	11.7	12.5
Hematocrit (Hct)	**0.37**	l/l	0.4	0.5	0.36	0.38
Mean cell volume	87	fl	80	99	85.3	88.7
Mean cell Hb	28.7	pg	27	31.5	28.2	29.3
Mean cell Hb conc.	33.0	g/dl	31.5	34.5	32.4	33.7
Red cell dist. width	12.4	%	11.6	14	12.0	12.8
Retic count	0.74	%	0.25	0.75	0.7	0.8
Retic absolute (abs.)	31.2	$\times 10^9$/l	30	100	30.2	32.1
White cell count	9.98	$\times 10^9$/l	4	10	9.23	10.73
Neutrophils abs.	4.10	$\times 10^9$/l	2	7	3.79	4.41
Lymphocytes abs.	**4.76**	$\times 10^9$/l	1	3	4.40	5.12
Monocytes abs.	0.69	$\times 10^9$/l	0.2	1	0.64	0.74
Eosinophils abs.	0.28	$\times 10^9$/l	0.02	0.5	0.26	0.30
Basophils abs.	0.15	$\times 10^9$/l	0.02	0.1	0.14	0.16
Normoblasts	0	/100 WBC	0	0		
Platelet count	149.0	$\times 10^9$/l	150	400	137.8	160.2
Sedimentation	14	mm/h	0	10	13	15
Morphology	The red cells are normochromic and normocytic, with considerable rouleaux formation. There is intense background staining. There is a mild lymphocytosis with numerous plasmacytoid lymphocytes.					

c. The normal ESR is at first sight strange, since classically conditions with raised globulins have a raised ESR. The explanation is simple – the viscosity is so high that there is considerable interference with the settling of the red cells in the ESR tube. One would be interested in what the ESR would show once the raised globulins have been got rid of (see Table 22.5).

3. The patient was subjected to urgent plasmapheresis. He recovered his sight completely, the cardiac failure remitted and all the neurological and ophthalmologic findings reversed. A repeat FBC is shown in Table 22.6.

Table 22.4

	Value	Units	Reference range Low	Reference range High
S-Urea	6.4	mmol/l	2.1	7.1
S-Creatinine	94.2	mmol/l	62	115
S-Urea:creatinine	67.9			
S-Sodium	137	mmol/l	136	145
S-Potassium	4.4	mmol/l	3.5	5.1
S-Chloride	105	mmol/l	98	108
S-Total CO_2	22	mmol/l	22	28
S-Anion gap	14.4	mmol/l	5	14
S-Uric acid	0.33	mmol/l	0.21	0.42
S-Calcium (total)	2.32	mmol/l	2.2	2.55
S-Protein (total)	103.5	g/l	64	83
S-Albumin	41	g/l	34	48
S-Globulin	**62.5**	g/l	30	35
S-α1-globulin	1.1	g/l		1.9
S-α2-globulin	6.4	g/l	5	7
S-β-globulin	7.1	g/l	5	8
S-γ-globulin	47.9	g/l	6	10
S-Immunoglobulin G	11.2	g/l	2.5	12
S-Immunoglobulin M	**33.1**	g/l	0.19	1.93
S-Immunoglobulin A	0.8	g/l	0.07	0.94

Table 22.5

	Value	Units	Low	High
Plasma viscosity	**2.26**	mPa/s	1.16	1.33

Table 22.6

	Value	Units	Reference range Low	Reference range High	Permitted range Low	Permitted range High
Red cell count	4.58	$\times 10^{12}$ /l	4.5	5.5	4.44	4.72
Hemoglobin (Hb)	**12.9**	g/dl	13	17	12.4	13.4
Hematocrit (Hct)	0.40	l/l	0.4	0.5	0.39	0.42
Mean cell volume	88	fl	80	99	86.2	89.8
Mean cell Hb	28.2	pg	27	31.5	27.6	28.7
Mean cell Hb conc.	32.0	g/dl	31.5	34.5	31.4	32.6
Red cell dist. width	14.1	%	11.6	14	13.7	14.5
White cell count	9.47	$\times 10^9$/l	4	10	8.76	10.18
Neutrophils abs.	3.93	$\times 10^9$/l	2	7	3.64	4.22
Lymphocytes abs.	4.59	$\times 10^9$/l	1	3	4.25	4.94
Monocytes abs.	0.58	$\times 10^9$/l	0.2	1	0.53	0.62
Eosinophils abs.	0.29	$\times 10^9$/l	0.02	0.5	0.27	0.32
Basophils abs.	0.08	$\times 10^9$/l	0.02	0.1	0.07	0.08
Platelet count	159.9	$\times 10^9$/l	150	400	147.9	171.9
Sedimentation	**102**	mm/h	0	10	97	107

polycythemia, sickle disease, and some other disorders where the red cell shape is peculiar.

2. The Hb is higher than before. It should be realized that hyperviscosity syndromes, particularly those due to paraproteinemias, also cause an expansion of the plasma volume, resulting in a dilutional anemia.

The Hyperviscosity Syndrome The most important causes of the hyperviscosity syndrome are

1. The paraproteinemias
2. Polycythemia vera
3. Severe CML and CLL
4. Very marked hyperlipidemias

CASE #100 (TABLE 22.7)

Table 22.7

Patient	Age	Sex	Race	Altitude
Mrs E S	45 yrs	Female	White	Sea level

The patient was referred by a pulmonologist. He had seen her for recurrent chest infections which have responded poorly to antibiotics. During her latest admission she had been very ill, with a leukemoid reaction, deranged liver functions and a marked increase in acute phase proteins. In addition, a marked decrease in gammaglobulins was noted. The patient was referred.

By the time the patient was seen the pneumonia had resolved, but she complained of significant residual effects, such as very poor exercise tolerance. The current FBC was completely normal.

	Value	Units	Low	High
Total protein	**60.2**	g/l	63	78
Albumin	41.1	g/l	36	52
Globulin	**19.1**	g/l	20	36
IgG	**0.1**	g/l	8.0	18.0
IgM	**0.34**	g/l	0.6	2.5
IgA	**0.00**	g/l	0.9	4.5
Urine protein	<0.01	g/l	0.0	0.15
Bence-Jones protein	Absent			
Urine electrophoresis	Normal			
Urine immunofixation	Normal			
Comment	There is severe hypogammaglobulinemia without evidence of a paraproteinemia.			

DISCUSSION

1. Now that the excessive levels of paraprotein have been removed by plasmapheresis, the ESR has resumed at a level in keeping with a paraproteinemia. Other causes of a spuriously low ESR are iron-deficiency anemia,

To be on the safe side, a marrow aspirate was done: this proved to be completely normal.

CONCLUSION

The final diagnosis was combined variable agammaglobulinemia.

CASE #101 (TABLE 22.8)

Table 22.8

Patient	Age	Sex	Race	Altitude
Mr J J	18 yrs	Male	White	2,500 ft

This young man presented with a sudden onset of weakness, malaise, palpitations, and some vague pain in the loins. His mother noticed that he was very pale and a little yellow. He was seen by an internist who confirmed the pallor and jaundice. He found a tip of spleen palpable but otherwise the abdomen was quite normal. There were no glands palpable. His chest was clinically clear. As a first step he ordered a FBC and a Coombs test.

	Value	Units	Reference range Low	High	Permitted range Low	High
Red cell count	3.12	$\times 10^{12}$/l	4.64	5.67	3.03	3.21
Hemoglobin (Hb)	9.6	g/dl	13.4	17.5	9.3	9.9
Hematocrit (Hct)	0.30	l/l	0.41	0.52	0.29	0.31
Mean cell volume	97	fl	80	99	95.1	98.9
Mean cell Hb	30.8	pg	27	31.5	30.2	31.4
Mean cell Hb conc.	31.7	g/dl	31.5	34.5	31.1	32.4
Red cell dist. width	16.2	%	11.6	14	15.7	16.7
Retic count	5.99	%	0.26	0.77	5.8	6.2
Retic absolute (abs.)	186.9	$\times 10^9$/l	30	100	172.9	200.9
White cell count	9.89	$\times 10^9$/l	4	10	9.15	10.63
Neutrophils abs.	7.52	$\times 10^9$/l	2	7	6.95	8.08
Band cells abs.	0.49		0	0.00	0.45	0.54
Lymphocytes abs.	1.29	$\times 10^9$/l	1	3	1.19	1.38
Monocytes abs.	0.40	$\times 10^9$/l	0.2	1	0.37	0.43
Eosinophils abs.	0.20	$\times 10^9$/l	0.02	0.5	0.18	0.21
Basophils abs.	0.00	$\times 10^9$/l	0.02	0.1	0.00	0.00
Normoblasts	0	/100 WBC	0	0		
Platelet count	31.1	$\times 10^9$/l	150	400	28.8	33.4
Sedimentation	78	mm/h	0	10	74	82
Morphology	The red cells are normochromic and normocytic. Occasional spherocytes, fragmented cells and agglutinates are seen.					

The result of the Coombs test was as follows:

Anti-IgG   Positive + + +
Anti-C3   Negative

Table 22.9

Follow-up of case #101

The patient complained that he had been having spells of feverishness with slight cough for some weeks. He had not been out of his hometown for years.

The internist thus made the diagnosis of an immune hemolytic anemia, most likely autoimmune, since there was no history of drug ingestion. However, certain features of the FBC were disturbing and the patient was referred. Further findings are found in Table 22.9.

DISCUSSION

There are a number of puzzling features:

1. The thrombocytopenia
2. The markedly raised ESR, which seems too high for a primary immune hemolytic anemia

A chest X-ray revealed a large mass abutting the left ventricular border. Scanning revealed this to be a circumscribed mass arising from the mediastinum. Biopsy revealed this to be a nodular sclerosing Hodgkin disease.

CONCLUSIONS

1. This was a case of autoimmune hemolytic anemia secondary to Hodgkin disease.
2. The thrombocytopenia was most likely also due to the antibody – i.e., this was an Evan syndrome.
3. The very high ESR primarily reflected the Hodgkin disease and not the hemolysis.

Further Reading

Epstein RJ (1996). Medicine for Examinations. 3rd edn. Churchill Livingstone.

Hoffbrand AV, Pettit JE (2001). Essential Haematology. 4th edn. Oxford: Blackwell Science.

Hoffbrand AV, Catovsky D, Tuddenham EGD (eds) (2005). Postgraduate Haematology. 5th edn. Oxford: Blackwell Publishing.

Roitts I (1997). Essential Immunology. Berlin: Blackwell Wissenschaft-Verlag GmbH.

The previous cases in this book have been selected for the general reader, and in some cases simplified in the sense that frequent non-hematological aspects have been ignored or downplayed. It was necessary to do this but unfortunate in the sense that the reader does not get an insight into clinical complexities that often occur in practice. The few cases presented here provide a taste of some of the complex problems that can arise, as well as to provide those that are interested with more information.

CASE #102 (EXAMINE TABLE 23.1)

DISCUSSION:

The FBC provided several important clues. In summary, the findings are

1. A mild macrocytic anemia. However, the very wide RDW suggests the possibility of an associated microcytosis.
2. The low reticulocytes would be in keeping with a chronic nutrient deficiency.
3. However, the most significant and helpful finding is the pronounced eosinophilia. Putting together the clinical features with these findings suggested the possibility of a malabsorption syndrome, of the eosinophilic gastroenteropathy variety.

Further tests were done (Table 23.2):
These results tended to reinforce the diagnosis of malabsorption. Stool fats were measured and found to be considerably increased. The D-xylose test was performed, and this confirmed malabsorption. Finally, biopsy of the duodenal mucosa confirmed extensive eosinophilic infiltration.

Note that were it not for the eosinophilia, the differential diagnosis would have been large. For example, bacterial overgrowth may also present with unexplained diarrhea, steatorrhea, weight loss, and unexplained macrocytic anemia. This condition usually but not always occurs after abdominal surgery (it can, for example, occur in scleroderma).

Even once the eosinophilia is recognized, the diagnosis is not necessarily clear; certain parasitoses, notably Strongyloides stercoralis infestation, may cause malabsorption,

Table 23.1

Patient	Age	Sex	Race	Altitude
Mrs J M	42 yrs	Female	White	5,000 ft

This lady complained of progressive tiredness, weakness, vague abdominal pain, intermittent diarrhea, and muscular "spasms." On examination, she was pale and chronically ill looking. The vital signs were normal. Her mouth was painful and inflamed and there was bilateral ankle edema. It was extremely difficult to identify a pathology. A FBC was performed as a first step.

	Value	Units	Reference range Low	High	Permitted range Low	High
Red cell count	3.88	× 10¹²/l	4.77	5.83	3.86	4.10
Hemoglobin (Hb)	11.6	g/dl	13.8	18.0	11.2	12.0
Hematocrit (Hct)	0.41	l/l	0.42	0.53	0.39	0.42
Mean cell volume	102	Fl	80	99	94.9	109.1
Mean cell Hb	29.1	Pg	27	31.5	28.6	29.7
Mean cell Hb conc.	28.6	g/dl	31.5	34.5	28.0	29.1
Red cell dist. width	19.3	%	11.6	14	19.3	19.3
Retic count	0.21	%	0.27	1.00	0.2	0.2
Retic absolute (abs.)	8.4	× 10⁹/l	30	100	8.1	8.6
White cell count	13.11	× 10⁹/l	4	10	12.13	14.09
Neutrophils abs.	5.39	× 10⁹/l	2	7	4.98	5.79
Lymphocytes abs.	4.99	× 10⁹/l	1	3	4.62	5.37
Monocytes abs.	0.41	× 10⁹/l	0.2	1	0.38	0.44
Eosinophils abs.	2.25	× 10⁹/l	0.02	0.5	2.09	2.42
Basophils abs.	0.07	× 10⁹/l	0.02	0.1	0.06	0.07
Normoblasts	0	/100 WBC	0	0		
Platelet count	225.1	× 10⁹/l	150	400	208.2	242.0
Sedimentation	24	mm/h	0	10	23	25

O.N. Beck, *Diagnostic Hematology*, DOI 10.1007/978-1-84800-295-1_23,
© Springer-Verlag London Limited 2009

Table 23.2

	Value	Units	Reference range Low	Reference range High
S-Calcium (total)	**1.92**	mmol/l	2.2	2.55
S-Magnesium	**0.49**	mmol/l	0.66	1.07
S-Protein (total)	**61.1**	g/l	64	83
S-Albumin	26.5	g/l	34	48
S-Globulin	34.6	g/l	30	35
S-Ferritin female	57.1	µg/l	14.0	233.1
S-Iron	**9.6**	µmol/l	11.6	31.3
S-Transferrin	3.56	g/l	2.12	3.60
S-Fe saturation female	**10.8**	%	15.0	35.0
S-Vitamin B$_{12}$	542	pg/ml	193	982
S-Folate	**2.9**	ng/ml	3.0	17.0
RBC-folate	**78.1**	ng/ml	93.0	641.0

along with diarrhea and abdominal pain and associated with a marked eosinophilia, although most cases are asymptomatic. This infection is common in Southeast Asia and is found also in expatriates living in the area and soldiers who had served there. Its differentiation from eosinophilic gastroenteropathy can be very difficult, since stool examination for ova is not very sensitive. Note that in immune-compromised patients, the eosinophilia tends to disappear, making the diagnosis even more difficult.

To be on the safe side, the patient was given a course of albendazole, followed by a course of steroids. She responded dramatically.

CASE #103 (EXAMINE TABLE 23.3)

DISCUSSION:

1. The results expected in toxic shock syndrome are the neutrophilia, the thrombocytopenia, and the raised ESR. Note that eosinophilia is a common accompaniment of neutrophilia and need not mean anything specific.
2. What is concerning is the very high RDW. Taken in conjunction with the morphology, one would be suspicious of DIC. However, this is one of those cases where a classic appearance usually due to a single cause can be mimicked by numerous independent causes:

   a) Red cells are fragmented in burns by physical damage, partly direct damage to cells and partly by passage of normal red cells through burnt tissues
   b) Thrombocytopenia is an independent feature of toxic shock syndrome and does not necessarily imply DIC.

   Nevertheless, a hemostatic screen was advisable. It was normal at that time.
3. The diagnosis of toxic shock syndrome requires that there be no bacteremia or sepsis, apart from a staphylococcal infection. This can be difficult to exclude. Nevertheless, numerous blood cultures were ordered, all of which were

Table 23.3

Patient	Age	Sex	Race	Altitude
Mrs D T	43 yrs	Female	White	2,200 ft

This patient was referred from a rural facility where she had been admitted after suffering 40% burns (see case #71). She had been diagnosed as having developed toxic shock syndrome.

On admission to the ICU, she was seen to be extremely ill with a generalized erythroderma as well as petechiae, hypotension, jaundice, and mental confusion. There was no cardiac failure, and the lung fields were clear. The respiratory rate was normal. Her fluid status and hypotension were urgently addressed and then numerous blood tests were done.

	Value	Units	Reference range Low	Reference range High	Permitted range Low	Permitted range High
Red cell count	4.11	$\times 10^{12}$/l	3.91	4.94	3.99	4.23
Hemoglobin (Hb)	**11.1**	g/dl	12.4	15.5	10.7	11.5
Hematocrit (Hct)	**0.33**	l/l	0.37	0.47	0.32	0.34
Mean cell volume	81	fl	80	99	79.4	82.6
Mean cell Hb	27.0	pg	27	31.5	26.5	27.5
Mean cell Hb conc.	33.3	g/dl	31.5	34.5	32.7	34.0
Red cell dist. width	**20.1**	%	11.6	14	20.1	20.1
White cell count	**18.5**	$\times 10^9$/l	4	10	17.11	19.89
Corrected WCC	**17.96**	$\times 10^9$/l				
Neutrophils abs.	**12.01**	$\times 10^9$/l	2	7	11.11	12.91
Band cells abs.	**1.67**		0	0.00	1.50	1.83
Lymphocytes abs.	1.31	$\times 10^9$/l	1	3	1.21	1.41
Monocytes abs.	0.93	$\times 10^9$/l	0.2	1	0.86	0.99
Eosinophils abs.	**0.74**	$\times 10^9$/l	0.02	0.5	0.68	0.80
Basophils abs.	0.19	$\times 10^9$/l	0.02	0.1	0.17	0.20
Blasts		%	0	0		
Promyelocytes	**2**	%	0	0		
Myelocytes	**3**	%	0	0		
Metamyelocytes	**4**	%	0	0		
Normoblasts	**3**	/100 WBC	0	0		
Platelet count	**87.0**	$\times 10^9$/l	150	400	78.3	95.7
Sedimentation	**57**	mm/h	0	20	54	60
Morphology	The red cells are normochromic and show considerable anisocytosis with numerous fragmented and crenated cells.					

negative. In addition, extensive search was made for a deep-seated infection (as the source of the staphylococci). Most commonly toxic shock syndrome is secondary to the use of tampons. This was excluded in this case.

Her subsequent progress is detailed in Table 23.4.

DISCUSSION:

1. The very low Hb in the absence of bleeding and in the context of the clinical features suggest very strongly a hemolytic state.
2. The drop in neutrophils suggests that the marrow is becoming exhausted. This tends to strengthen the possibility of sepsis and therefore of DIC. Table 23.6 shows the hemostatic screen results.

Table 23.4

Case #103: Subsequent progress.
The patient remained very ill but stable for 5 days. Thereafter, a serious complication set in – she developed a serious nosocomial gram-negative infection. The first pointers to this were a drop in blood pressure, increased respiratory rate, and a drop in arterial Po$_2$. Over the next 36 h, she deteriorated and developed jaundice and severe pallor. It was noticed that she bled easily from skin punctures. At this stage, it was noted that she had developed a marked neutrophilia with a severe left shift – the neutrophilia gradually decreased but the neutrophil precursors increased. It was also noted that the Hb was dropping very rapidly. Tables 23.5 and 23.6 show her FBC and other results 56 h later.

Table 23.6

Test	Value	Units	Reference range	
Bleeding time	9	Minutes	3	7
Platelet count	21	$\times 10^9$/l	140	440
PT	17	Seconds	12	13
PTT	44	Seconds	23	36
D-Dimers	0.39	mg/l	0	0.25

Table 23.7

	Value	Units	Reference range Low	High
S-Bilirubin (total)	51.9	µmol/l	6.8	34.2
S-Bilirubin (direct)	17.1	µmol/l	1.7	8.6
S-Bilirubin (indirect)	34.8	µmol/l	5.1	25.6
S-ALP	179	IU/l	53	128
S-gGT	65	IU/l	8	37
S-ALT	54	IU/l	19	40
S-AST	33	IU/l	13	32
S-LDH	871	IU/l	90	180
Haptoglobin	0.1	g/l	0.16	2

Table 23.7 show the results of some biochemical investigations.

3. It can be seen that the features are undoubtedly in keeping with hemolysis, but if there is a DIC it is rather mild (note the D-Dimers being only mildly raised), probably not enough to explain the drop in Hb. The possibility of another hemolytic mechanism should be considered. This was extensively investigated, including the family and past history for one of the hereditary hemolytic syndromes (negative); the Coombs test for immune hemolysis (negative); she had had no blood transfusions up to the time that the problem started. Subsequent transfusions could have partly been responsible. The blood service was asked to investigate and it found an irregular antibody in one of the post-transfusion specimens, but was uncertain how relevant this was.

Table 23.5

	Value	Units	Reference range Low	High	Permitted range Low	High
Red cell count	1.76	$\times 10^{12}$/l	3.91	4.94	1.71	1.81
Hemoglobin (Hb)	5.1	g/dl	12.4	15.5	4.9	5.3
Hematocrit (Hct)	0.17	l/l	0.37	0.47	0.17	0.18
Mean cell volume	97	fl	80	99	95.1	98.9
Mean cell Hb	29.0	pg	27	31.5	28.4	29.6
Mean cell Hb conc.	29.9	g/dl	31.5	34.5	29.3	30.5
Red cell dist. width	19.3	%	11.6	14	19.3	19.3
Retic count	17.9	%	0.25	0.75	17.1	18.5
Retic absolute (abs.)	315	$\times 10^9$/l	30	100	305	324
White cell count	4.12	$\times 10^9$/l	4	10	3.81	4.43
Neutrophils abs.	1.77	$\times 10^9$/l	2	7	1.64	1.90
Band cells abs.	0.37		0	0.00	0.33	0.41
Lymphocytes abs.	0.82	$\times 10^9$/l	1	3	0.76	0.89
Monocytes abs.	0.37	$\times 10^9$/l	0.2	1	0.34	0.40
Eosinophils abs.	0.16	$\times 10^9$/l	0.02	0.5	0.15	0.18
Basophils abs.	0.00	$\times 10^9$/l	0.02	0.1	0.00	0.00
Blasts		%	0	0		
Promyelocytes	2	%	0	0		
Myelocytes	5	%	0	0		
Metamyelocytes	8	%	0	0		
Normoblasts	0	/100 WBC	0	0		
Platelet count	21.0	$\times 10^9$/l	150	400	18.9	23.1
Sedimentation	68	mm/h	0	20	65	72
Morphology	The red cells show severe anisocytosis with numerous poikilocytes, including extensive fragmentation					

COMMENT Anemia in the critically ill patient is frequently a conundrum. There are many possible causes, and because of the serious condition of most of these patients, many tend to coexist. Possible causes are

1. Blood loss. Apart from the obvious causes, it should be remembered that the average patient in ICU loses 70 ml per day for diagnostic testing. This amounts to one unit of blood per week and 450 mg of iron.
2. Deficiency of nutrients. TPN is sometimes not well tolerated. Folate deficiency is a particular problem in the patient who is having nasogastric suction.
3. Hemolysis is the other major cause. It may be due to

   a. Immune hemolysis, including from blood transfusions.
   b. Drugs and chemicals.
   c. Sepsis, either directly or via DIC.
   d. Existing hereditary (and other) hemolytic conditions that normally either are well compensated or are not manifest if not being stressed: for example, some forms of G6PD

deficiency are asymptomatic until the patient is exposed to certain drugs or toxins.

It is often very difficult to make the precise diagnosis. One point to bear in mind is that bone marrow studies are seldom useful, and indeed can be dangerous, in septic patients.

CASE #104 (TABLE 23.8)

Table 23.8

Patient	Age	Sex	Race	Altitude
Mrs T K	41 years	Female	White	5,000 ft

This patient presented with a sudden onset of a grand mal seizure. She recovered very slowly and was later found to be stuporose with an upper motor lesion affecting mainly the legs; there was also a disorder of conjugate gaze. An urgent CSF examination revealed only a mild increase in protein; cells were normal. An urgent MRI showed only mild diffuse evidence of poor perfusion. The clinical picture was very suggestive and some blood tests were done – see Tables 23.9 and 23.10

Table 23.9

	Value	Units	Reference range Low	Reference range High	Permitted range Low	Permitted range High
Red cell count	4.11	$\times 10^{12}$/l	4.03	5.09	3.99	4.23
Hemoglobin (Hb)	12.9	g/dl	12.7	15.9	12.4	13.4
Hematocrit (Hct)	0.37	l/l	0.38	0.49	0.36	0.39
Mean cell volume	91	fl	80	99	89.2	92.8
Mean cell Hb	31.4	pg	27	31.5	30.8	32.0
Mean cell Hb conc.	34.5	g/dl	31.5	34.5	33.8	35.2
Red cell dist. width	**18.3**	%	11.6	14	18.3	18.3
Retic count	**2.9**		0.3	0.9	2.8	3.0
Retic absolute (abs)	**119.2**	$\times 10^9$/l	30	100	115.6	122.8
White cell count	7.98	$\times 10^9$/l	4	10	7.38	8.58
Neutrophils abs.	4.07	$\times 10^9$/l	2	7	3.76	4.38
Lymphocytes abs.	3.15	$\times 10^9$/l	1	3	2.92	3.39
Monocytes abs.	0.45	$\times 10^9$/l	0.2	1	0.41	0.48
Eosinophils abs.	0.25	$\times 10^9$/l	0.02	0.5	0.23	0.27
Basophils abs.	0.06	$\times 10^9$/l	0.02	0.1	0.06	0.07
Platelet count	**5.9**	$\times 10^9$/l	150	400	5.3	6.5
Morphology	The red cells are normochromic and show marked anisocytosis, with considerable fragmentation and occasional microspherocytes. There is a marked thrombocytopenia.					

DISCUSSION:

1. In summary, the picture shows the following salient features:

   a. Significant CNS disturbance
   b. Severe thrombocytopenia
   c. Evidence of red cell fragmentation
   d. Evidence of mild renal dysfunction
   e. Evidence of mild hemolysis.

2. In this very typical presentation, it was fairly easy to suggest the diagnosis of thrombotic thrombocytopenic purpura (TTP) (although this patient did not show purpura). A minority of patients present less acutely and in them it can be very difficult to suspect the diagnosis.

3. A bone marrow aspirate showed the expected megakaryocytic hyperplasia.

4. Note once again the importance of a raised RDW with otherwise normal red cell counts.

5. The patient was successfully treated with repeated sessions of plasmapheresis. Note that steroids are largely of no benefit.

6. Note that there is another condition that in many ways is similar to TTP – hemolytic-uremic syndrome (HUS). The two conditions are currently thought to be on the same pathogenetic spectrum. The major differences are that in HUS:

   a) Renal involvement is pronounced, whereas central nervous system involvement is minimal.

Table 23.10

	Value	Units	Reference range Low	Reference range High
S-Urea	**8.5**	mmol/l	2.1	7.1
S-Creatinine	**123**	mmol/l	62	115
S-Potassium	4.9	mmol/l	3.5	5.1
S-Bilirubin (total)	**47.8**	μmol/l	6.8	34.2
S-Bilirubin (direct)	**9.1**	μmol/l	1.7	8.6
S-Bilirubin (indirect)	**38.7**	μmol/l	5.1	25.6
S-ALP	112	IU/l	53	128
S-gGT	46	IU/l	8	37
S-ALT	44	IU/l	19	40
S-AST	27	IU/l	13	32
S-LDH	301	IU/l	90	180
S-Haptoglobin	**0.21**	g/l	0.35	1.75

   b) The hemolytic element is more pronounced.
   c) Most cases of HUS have been identified as being caused by a specific strain of **E. COLI**.

CASE #105 (EXAMINE TABLE 23.11)

DISCUSSION:

1. The obvious microcytic anemia with a background of significant hemoglobinuria and the absence of any chronic disease is strongly suggestive of iron

Table 23.11

Patient	Age	Sex	Race	Altitude
Mr W de K	20 yrs	Male	White	5,000 ft

The patient is a third-year medical student. He has always enjoyed excellent health. Recently he noticed that, particularly in the mornings, he was passing very dark urine. He himself tested his urine in a training laboratory and found that it contained large amounts of hemoglobin. He applied to the hematology department for consultation.

On systematic enquiry, there was no evidence of any specific disease. The family history was unremarkable. He was a big lad, and fairly pale, but otherwise no abnormal clinical features were found. Specifically, there was no evidence of purpura or repeated infections.

	Value	Units	Reference range Low	Reference range High	Permitted range Low	Permitted range High
Red cell count	**4.09**	$\times 10^{12}$/l	4.77	5.83	3.97	4.21
Hemoglobin (Hb)	**9.9**	g/dl	13.8	18.0	9.6	10.2
Hematocrit (Hct)	**0.31**	l/l	0.42	0.53	0.30	0.32
Mean cell volume	**76.5**	fl	80	99	71.1	81.9
Mean cell Hb	**24.2**	pg	27	31.5	23.7	24.7
Mean cell Hb conc.	31.6	g/dl	31.5	34.5	31.0	32.3
Red cell dist. width	**15.3**	%	11.6	14	15.3	15.3
Retic count	**4.4**	%	0.27	1.00	4.3	4.5
Retic absolute (abs.)	**180.0**	$\times 10^9$/l	30	100	174.6	185.4
White cell count	4.11	$\times 10^9$/l	4	10	3.80	4.42
Neutrophils abs.	2.02	$\times 10^9$/l	2	7	1.87	2.17
Lymphocytes abs.	1.64	$\times 10^9$/l	1	3	1.52	1.77
Monocytes abs.	0.25	$\times 10^9$/l	0.2	1	0.23	0.27
Eosinophils abs.	0.15	$\times 10^9$/l	0.02	0.5	0.14	0.16
Basophils abs.	0.05	$\times 10^9$/l	0.02	0.1	0.04	0.05
Normoblasts	0	/100 WBC	0	0		
Platelet count	167.0	$\times 10^9$/l	150	400	154.5	179.5
Morphology	There is a mild microcytic and hypochromic anemia, with numerous small oval cells and some elliptocytes and target cells.					

deficiency. This was confirmed by the iron studies. One would then think of various possible renal causes of significant hematuria. It was thus essential that the nature of the blood in the urine be precisely identified, since the possible differential diagnosis would be very different were the "blood" due to red cells and not hemoglobin. Accordingly, several fresh morning specimens were examined (if urine is left standing, red cells in it may hemolyse, producing a spurious impression of hemoglobinuria). Hemoglobinuria was repeatedly confirmed; in addition, tests for hemosiderinuria were positive. Hemosiderinuria is produced by the following mechanism: some of the hemoglobin in the renal tubules is reabsorbed by the tubular epithelial cells where it is degraded into globin and iron. The iron persists in the cell in the form of granules. When those cells eventually desquamate, the siderotic

granules can be demonstrated in the urine by microscopy using special stains. Hemosiderinuria can occur in any intravascular hemolytic state if severe enough – i.e., if the amount of hemoglobin released exceeds the capacity of haptoglobin and related molecules to "mop" it up.

2. However, there are some oddities in this FBC: the reticulocytosis is prominent. One could think that this is purely secondary to the bleeding. This unlikely since the platelet and white cell counts are normal – indeed the WCC and neutrophil count are close to the lower limit of normal.

3. There being nothing to suggest another cause of intravascular hemolysis, the diagnosis of paroxysmal nocturnal hemoglobinuria (PNH) was entertained. This was confirmed by the Ham test and later by flow cytometry.

Paroxysmal Nocturnal Hemoglobinuria In many ways, this is a mysterious disease. There are several possible elements, not all of which always are present:

1. Intravascular hemolysis. This is due to an acquired membrane defect of a population of red cells (i.e., not of all the red cells), resulting in the cells being unduly sensitive to circulating complement.

2. Tendency to thrombosis, particularly arterial thrombosis.

3. Tendency to aplasia of the marrow. Indeed, aplastic anemia may transform into PNH, and vice versa. It has a far better prognosis than aplastic anemia.

4. A lot of the clinical features appear to depend on how large is the population of affected cells, and how rapidly this is growing.

5. Treatment. A small proportion of patients respond to androgens or corticosteroids. Treatment is otherwise entirely symptomatic. Note that washed red cells must be used for transfusion, to eliminate any complement.

CASE #106 (EXAMINE TABLE 23.12)

The following comments plus the results of follow-up investigations were supplied by the laboratory (Table 23.14)

The results of protein electrophoresis on concentrated urine are found in Table 23.15

Table 23.12

Patient	Age	Sex	Race	Altitude
Mr G S	47 years	Male	White	5,000 ft

This patient had been cared for and extensively investigated by an experienced family practitioner. He had numerous problems and was frequently symptomatic. He had had severe hepatitis as a child and still complained of "liverishness," with fluctuating bilirubinuria. A radio-isotopic scan suggested poor hepatic function although liver function tests were otherwise normal. No gallstones were found on CT scanning. He also had chronic prostatitis. He complained of episodes of diarrhea, exhaustion, and night sweats, with possible fever. He also mentioned "impotence." She was also treating him for quite severe hypertension. The doctor eventually did several other tests in the hope of finding something. Two important findings were the following: a monoclonal peak on protein electrophoresis and raised ferritin levels. Test for Bence-Jones protein was negative. Renal function was normal. She referred the patient, partly because of these results and partly for assistance in sorting out his various problems.

Of his extensive medical history, two possibly relevant facts emerged: he lived on a farm, and at one stage, a few years before had used unpasteurized milk extensively; and there were huge numbers of ticks, causing a major problem with livestock. There was no bleeding tendency. He complained of episodes of flushing with tinnitus. He had had a blood transfusion years ago after an accident and had experienced severe reactions, with hypotension.

On examination, he was somewhat obese and ill looking. His color was normal and there was no lymphadenopathy. The blood pressure was 160/110. The heart was normal in size and the heart sounds were closed, but with an accentuated A2. There was no evidence of cardiac failure. Fundoscopy revealed a grade II retinopathy. The rest of the examination was non-contributory. A number of tests were done, both for his general problems and the hematological ones. The results of selected biochemical tests are found in Table 23.13.

Table 23.13

	Value	Units	Reference range Low	Reference range High
S-Calcium (total)	2.51	mmol/l	2.2	2.55
S-Phosphate	1.1	mmol/l	0.87	1.45
S-Protein (total)	73	g/l	64	83
S-Albumin	42	g/l	34	48
S-Globulin	31.0	g/l	30	35

Table 23.14

Comment on protein electrophoretic studies:
There is a monoclonal band in the early gamma region measuring 12 g/l. There is a degree of immune paresis.

DISCUSSION:

1. One important question is the relevance of the monoclonal peak. The laboratory opinion on there being

Table 23.15 (of case #106)

U-Protein (total)	94	Unit
U-Albumin	39.3	mg/l
U-α1-globulin	6.5	mg/l
U-α2-globulin	17.2	mg/l
U-β-globulin	14.7	mg/l
U-γ-globulin	16.3	mg/l
Comment		There is a tubular excretion pattern. A small monoclonal peak is present in the gamma region. Immunofixation of the serum peak showed that it was a monoclonal IgG and kappa protein. Immunofixation of the urine peak showed that it was an intact monoclonal IgG kappa molecule.

immune paresis may well be correct, in which case the M protein is significant despite it being small. On the other hand, there is unquestionable decrease in IgA but not in IgM. The question arises as to whether this is not a hereditary absence of IgA. This possibility is reinforced by the blood transfusion reaction he had suffered. Normal renal function does not of course exclude a significant paraproteinemia, but it is against it.

2. Bone marrow aspiration was therefore done. This showed less than 5% plasma cells, and was otherwise normal except for increased iron stores.

3. It was decided that provisionally the paraproteinemia would be treated as a MGUS and followed up.

4. However, three more aspects of this patient's presentation required investigation: the iron overload state and possible complications, the hypertension and the possibility of a chronic infection.

The Iron Overload

Blood was sent for hemochromatosis mutations. The C282Y mutation was negative but the H63D was heterozygous positive. Once again the question arose as to its

Table 23.16

	Value	Units	Reference range Low	Reference range High
S-ACTH	<9	ng/l	0.0	46.0
S-Cortisol	138	nmol/l	38	690
S-T4	13.4	pmol/l	9.1	23.8
S-TSH	2.67	mIU/l	0.49	4.67
S-Testosterone male 50	7.1	nmol/l	7.4	25.7
S-DHEAS	2.2	nmol/l	2.2	15.2
S-SHB globulin male	20.5	nmol/l	13.0	71.0
Free testosterone	0.34	nmol/l	0.4	0.8

Table 23.17

Patient	Age	Sex	Race	Altitude
Mrs J F	23 yrs	Female	White	5,000 ft

This woman was 31 weeks pregnant. She was seeing her obstetrician regularly but went to her family doctor for what she thought was a mild viral infection; she had malaise, nausea, mild epigastic discomfort, and headache. The blood pressure was normal, and there was no proteinuria. The doctor was concerned about mild right upper quadrant tenderness but treated her symptomatically and told her to return if not better in a few days. Instead she deteriorated, with severe vomiting and right shoulder-tip pain. Thinking she might have developed acute cholecystitis, acute fatty liver of pregnancy, TTP or HUS, he ordered various blood tests and referred her to her obstetrician.

	Value	Units	Reference range Low	Reference range High	Permitted range Low	Permitted range High
Red cell count	4.29	$\times 10^{12}$/l	4.03	5.09	4.16	4.42
Hemoglobin (Hb)	13.3	g/dl	12.7	15.9	12.8	13.8
Hematocrit (Hct)	0.40	l/l	0.38	0.49	0.39	0.41
Mean cell volume	93	fl	80	99	91.1	94.9
Mean cell Hb	31.0	pg	27	31.5	30.4	31.6
Mean cell Hb conc.	33.3	g/dl	31.5	34.5	32.7	34.0
Red cell dist. width	**17.4**	%	11.6	14	14.4	14.4
White cell count	7.89	$\times 10^9$/l	4	10	7.30	8.48
Neutrophils abs.	4.19	$\times 10^9$/l	2	7	3.88	4.50
Lymphocytes abs.	2.95	$\times 10^9$/l	1	3	2.73	3.17
Monocytes abs.	0.47	$\times 10^9$/l	0.2	1	0.43	0.50
Eosinophils abs.	0.20	$\times 10^9$/l	0.02	0.5	0.18	0.21
Basophils abs.	0.09	$\times 10^9$/l	0.02	0.1	0.08	0.09
Platelet count	**56.2**	$\times 10^9$/l	150	400	50.6	61.8
Morphology	The red cells are normochromic and normocytic and show marked anisocytosis, with spherocytes and fragmented cells. There is a thrombocytopenia. DIC, TTP, and HUS should be excluded.					

Table 23.18

	Value	Units	Reference range Low	Reference range High
S-Urea	5.3	mmol/l	2.1	7.1
S-Creatinine	71	mmol/l	62	115
S-Urea:creatinine	74.6			
S-Sodium	136	mmol/l	136	145
S-Potassium	4.2	mmol/l	3.5	5.1
S-Chloride	104.00	mmol/l	98	108
S-Total CO$_2$	24	mmol/l	22	28
S-Anion gap	12.2	mmol/l	5	14
S-Glucose	4.1	mmol/l	3.9	5.8
S-Osmolarity	271	mmol/l	275	295
S-Uric acid	0.41	mmol/l	0.21	0.42
S-Bilirubin (total)	28.9	µmol/l	6.8	34.2
S-Bilirubin (direct)	8.2	µmol/l	1.7	8.6
S-Bilirubin (indirect)	20.7	µmol/l	5.1	25.6
S-ALP	104	IU/l	53	128
S-gGT	**98**	IU/l	8	37
S-ALT	**321**	IU/l	19	40
S-AST	**216**	IU/l	13	32
S-LDH	**309**	IU/l	90	180
U-Bilirubin	" + "	" + "		
U-Urobilin	" + "	" + "		

Table 23.19

Test	Value	Units	Low	High
PTT	33	Seconds	26	37
PT	14	Seconds	12	14
TT	10	Seconds	9	11
D-Dimers	**4.9**		0	2.5
Fibrinogen	323	mg/dl	200	400
Haptoglobin	**0.04**	g/l	0.16	2

significance. The orthodox view is that it is not in itself significant, but as has been shown in Chapter 20, a small percentage of heterozygous patients unquestionably have complications. In this present case, the history of impotence is troubling. Accordingly, some further tests were done. See Table 23.16. Note that the CRP is negative – it is always wise to do an activity test when considering a raised ferritin, since it is an acute phase protein (although this level of ferritin is really too high to be explained by a phase reaction.)

DISCUSSION:

While there is evidence of hypogonadism, this is not necessarily due to iron overload, despite iron granules being demonstrated by MRI in the hypothalamus. The effect of regular venesection will be observed in the long term.

The Blood Pressure

On frequent occasions, it was noticed that BP fluctuated considerably. In view of this and the history of flushing, tests for pheochromocytoma were carried out. These were negative.

The Possibility of a Chronic Intracellular Infection

The TMX tests were all negative. Specific Brucella antibodies too were negative. The possibility of a organism like Ehrlichia was considered, being tick borne. No diagnostic test was available, and the effect of a 6-week course of doxycycline would be observed.

CASE #107 EXAMINE TABLES #23.17 AND #23.18

By the time the obstetrician saw her, she was extremely ill, and he had her admitted to the ICU. When seen there, she was seriously confused mentally. She was clearly in extreme pain in the abdomen, and her blood pressure had risen moderately. After stabilization, a number of further tests were requested (Table 23.19).

The diagnosis of the HELLP syndrome was made. She was placed on high doses of methylprednisolone with supportive and antihypertensive therapy. With great difficulty, she was carried through to 34 weeks, and since she was still very ill, a live infant was delivered by caesarean section.

Steroid therapy was maintained post-partum until it was clear that she was recovering.

In this chapter, a few exercise cases are presented to provide an opportunity to test your knowledge and especially your understanding of some essential hematological principles, particularly methodological and logical principles. There are two groups of cases presented:

1. **GENERAL.** These cases are aimed at students and family practitioners as well as some specialists who are only peripherally involved with blood diseases.
2. **ADVANCED.** These cases are aimed at internists, intensive care practitioners, and other specialists who may find themselves facing difficult hematological problems.

General Hematological Problems

CASE #108 (TABLE 24.1)

Table 24.1

Patient	Age	Sex	Race	Altitude
Miss J M	13 yrs	Female	White	2,500 ft

This girl from a small country town presented with tiredness, poor concentration, and poor performance at school sports. She stated that people had commented that she looked ill and pale and a bit yellow. She had hitherto always been well. She had never had a blood transfusion or indeed any blood tests. She stated that a maternal aunt had had a "blood disease" that had been cured by an operation. On examination, she was almost certainly anemic and jaundiced. Table 24.2 is her FBC from her local laboratory.

Table 24.2

	Value	Units	Reference range Low	Reference range High
Red cell count	**3.11**	$\times 10^{12}/l$	3.91	4.94
Hemoglobin (Hb)	**9.9**	g/dl	12.4	15.5
Hematocrit (Hct)	**0.27**	l/l	0.37	0.47
Mean cell volume	86	fl	80	99
Mean cell Hb	**31.8**	pg	27	31.5
Mean cell Hb conc.	**37.0**	g/dl	31.5	34.5
Retic count	**4.5**	%	0.25	0.75
Retic absolute (abs.)	**140.0**	$\times 10^9/l$	50	100
White cell count	7.3	$\times 10^9/l$	4	10
Neutrophils abs.	3.43	$\times 10^9/l$	2	7
Band cells abs.	**0.37**		0	0.00
Lymphocytes abs.	2.70	$\times 10^9/l$	1	3
Monocytes abs.	0.44	$\times 10^9/l$	0.2	1
Eosinophils abs.	0.29	$\times 10^9/l$	0.02	0.5
Basophils abs.	0.07	$\times 10^9/l$	0.02	0.1
Platelet count	278.0	$\times 10^9/l$	150	400
Sedimentation	14	mm/h	0	20

Questions:

1. Do you have enough evidence to suggest an anatomical diagnosis? If not, what are the possibilities? Discuss these. What further clinical features would you like to know about, and why?

_____
_____
_____
_____

2. What further laboratory results would you like to see, and why?

_____
_____

Answers:

1. No. There are a few possibilities based on the data:

   a. Megaloblastic anemia
   b. Hemolytic anemia.

Megaloblastic is unlikely given the normal MCV, unless there is an associated disorder of iron metabolism. Hemolytic anemia by exclusion therefore seems the most likely.

I need to know whether the spleen is enlarged. An enlarged spleen would tend to eliminate megaloblastosis and be very much in favor of hemolysis.

2. First, liver functions to assess the bilirubinemia and to exclude hepatitis. Second, haptoglobin levels and urine bile pigments to assess hemolysis.

Table 24.3 shows some further results.

Table 24.3

	Value	Units	Reference range	
			Low	High
S-Bilirubin (total)	**54.1**	μmol/l	6.8	34.2
S-Bilirubin (direct)	7.7	μmol/l	1.7	8.6
S-Bilirubin (indirect)	**46.4**	μmol/l	5.1	25.6
S-ALP	**141**	IU/l	53	128
S-gGT	32	IU/l	8	37
S-ALT	36	IU/l	19	40
S-AST	21	IU/l	13	32
S-LDH	351	IU/l	90	180
S-Haptoglobin	**0.08**	g/l	0.16	2
U-Bilirubin		"+"		
U-Urobilin	**"+ + +"**	"+"		

Further Questions:

3. What can you conclude from these results?

_____

_____

4. Can you now suggest a general diagnosis? What else do you need to be more certain?

_____

Answers:

3. There is no evidence of hepatitis. The raised alkaline phosphatase reflects her age. The haptoglobin and urobilinuria strongly suggest hemolysis.
4. The features strongly suggest a chronic extravascular hemolytic anemia. I need to know the size of the spleen.

See Table 24.4

Table 24.4

Further findings in case #108.

The spleen was 1 cm enlarged and slightly tender.

Further Questions:

5. What can you now conclude?

_____

_____

6. What are the specific diagnostic possibilities? What further would you like to know to assist you in this?

_____

_____

_____

Answers:

5. The features are very strongly in favor of a chronic extravascular hemolysis.
6. There are many possibilities: membrane disorders such as hereditary spherocytosis; enzyme deficiencies; and hemoglobinopathies such as HbC disease. The red cell morphology could be most revealing.

Scrutiny of the blood smear revealed the presence of spherocytes.

Further Questions:

7. What specific disease is therefore a strong possibility? How would you confirm the diagnosis?
8. Name some important possible complications of this disease?

Answers:

7. Hereditary spherocytosis. The traditional method of confirmation is by osmotic fragility. Newer methods are available. Consult the laboratory.
8. Complications include

   a. Pigment gallstones presenting as acute cholecytitis or bile duct obstruction.
   b. Aplastic crisis. The chronically hyperplastic marrow (in compensation) is particularly susceptible to infection with the parvovirus B19, which can

cause severe aplasia. It can be foreseen that the FBC (and clinical) picture would change dramatically.

c. Hemolytic crisis, where the rate of hemolysis increases dramatically. This is rare in hereditary spherocytosis, being much more common in sickle disease.

CASE #109 (TABLE 24.5)

Table 24.5

Patient	Age	Sex	Race	Altitude		
Mrs H G	28 yrs	Female	White	5,000 ft		

This patient had been diagnosed with acute severe rheumatoid arthritis at the age of 23 years. She had responded but slowly to treatment and required NSAIDS plus methotrexate (plus analgesics) to achieve a reasonable response. About 4 months ago, she had once again deteriorated, and gold salts had been added to her regime. This afforded some improvement. However, recently she complained of worsening malaise and severe infections of her mouth. On examination, she was both acutely and chronically ill. There was severe acute periodontal disease.

	Value	Units	Reference range Low	Reference range High	Permitted range Low	Permitted range High
Red cell count	**3.89**	× 10¹²/l	4.03	5.09	3.77	4.01
Hemoglobin (Hb)	**10.1**	g/dl	12.7	15.9	9.7	10.5
Hematocrit (Hct)	**0.30**	l/l	0.38	0.49	0.29	0.31
Mean cell volume	**77.1**	fl	80	99	75.6	78.6
Mean cell Hb	**26.0**	pg	27	31.5	25.4	26.5
Mean cell Hb conc.	33.7	g/dl	31.5	34.5	33.0	34.3
Red cell dist. width	16.2	%	11.6	14	16.2	16.2
Retic count	1.2	%	0.7	1.2	1.2	1.2
Retic absolute (abs.)	46.7	× 10⁹/l	30	100	45.3	48.1
White cell count	**3.11**	× 10⁹/l	4	10	2.88	3.34
Neutrophils abs.	**0.47**	× 10⁹/l	2	7	0.43	0.50
Band cells abs.	0.00		0	0	0.00	0.00
Lymphocytes abs.	2.39	× 10⁹/l	1	3	2.21	2.57
Monocytes abs.	0.21	× 10⁹/l	0.2	1	0.20	0.23
Eosinophils abs.	**0.01**	× 10⁹/l	0.02	0.5	0.01	0.01
Basophils abs.	0.03	× 10⁹/l	0.02	0.1	0.03	0.03
Platelet count	**453.0**	× 10⁹/l	150	400	407.7	498.3
Sedimentation	**41**	mm/h	0	20	39	43

Questions:

1. What is your first-stage diagnosis of the FBC, taking the clinical features into account? If uncertain, what are the possibilities? Discuss these. What further clinical features would you like to know about, and why?

_____

_____

2. What further laboratory results would you like to see, and why?

_____

_____

Answers:

1. There is a microcytic anemia, a severe neutropenia, and a thrombocytosis.

   a. The microcytic anemia may be due either to ACD, iron deficiency, or both.
   b. The neutropenia may be due to drugs or Felty syndrome, in the first instance.
   c. The thrombocytosis may reflect the acute on chronic disease.

   I need to know whether the spleen is enlarged. An enlarged spleen would be in favor of a Felty syndrome (or large granular lymphocytosis); this would be unlikely however since the patient is on methotrexate.

2. Iron studies would be of value in assessing the nature of the microcytosis.

Further Question:

How would you go about managing this problem?

Answer:

Assuming there is no iron deficiency, I would immediately stop the gold therapy and institute filgastrim therapy. A periodontist's assistance would be invaluable.

CASE #110 (EXAMINE TABLE 24.6)

Questions:

1. Can you make a first-stage diagnosis? Do you think there is a helpful pattern?

_____

_____

Table 24.6

Patient	Age	Sex	Race	Altitude
Miss B T	11 yrs	Female	Black	Sea level

This girl from a rural and remote subtropical coastal region was brought to a local clinic with a history of marked lassitude, mental dullness, lack of interest in schoolwork and evident weakness. On examination, she was found to be chronically ill and underweight. She was pale but there was no jaundice, purpura, lymphadenopathy, or splenomegaly.

			Reference range	
	Value	Units	Low	High
Red cell count	2.99	$\times 10^{12}$/l	3.8	4.8
Hemoglobin (Hb)	5.8	g/dl	12	15
Hematocrit (Hct)	0.21	l/l	0.36	0.46
Mean cell volume	69	fl	80	99
Mean cell Hb	19.4	pg	27	31.5
Mean cell Hb conc.	28.1	g/dl	31.5	34.5
Red cell dist. width	15.1	%	11.6	14
Retic count	0.9	%	0.25	0.75
Retic absolute (abs.)	26.9	$\times 10^9$/l	30	100
White cell count	4.8	$\times 10^9$/l	4	10
Neutrophils abs.	2.26	$\times 10^9$/l	2	7
Band cells abs.	0.19		0	0.00
Lymphocytes abs.	1.20	$\times 10^9$/l	1	3
Monocytes abs.	0.34	$\times 10^9$/l	0.2	1
Eosinophils abs.	0.82	$\times 10^9$/l	0.02	0.5
Basophils abs.	0.00	$\times 10^9$/l	0.02	0.1
Normoblasts	0	/100 WBC	0	0
Platelet count	158.0	$\times 10^9$/l	150	400
Sedimentation	38	mm/h	0	20
Morphology	The red cells are microcytic and hypochromic, with small oval cells, elliptocytes, target cells, and pencil cells. The neutrophils show a right shift.			

2. What further laboratory results would you like to see, and why? Explain your rationale.

_____

_____

Answers:

1. There are two clear abnormalities: microcytic anemia and mild eosinophilia. This does constitute a pattern but an unusual one.
2. In the first instance, iron studies to identify the nature of the microcytosis. It is essential to do this since any further investigations would be strongly influenced by the results.

Question:

Because of the distance from a laboratory capable of doing iron studies, a preliminary diagnosis would need to be made so as to institute treatment. On the basis of the clinical features, a further lab test was ordered which provided the answer. What was this lab test and what did it show?

Answer:

Stools were examined for ova. Numerous hookworm ova were seen. The iron studies are shown in Table 24.7

Table 24.7

			Reference range	
	Value	Units	Low	High
S-Ferritin female	3.1	µg/l	14.0	233.1
S-Iron	7.3	µmol/l	11.6	31.3
S-Transferrin	4.1	g/l	2.12	3.60
S-Fe saturation female	1	%	15.0	35.0

CASE # 111 (TABLE 24.8)

Table 24.8

Patient	Age	Sex	Race	Altitude
Mrs J S	31 yrs	Female	White	5,000 ft

This patient had enjoyed good health until one morning 2 days ago when she went for her morning bath and noticed large numbers of bluish-black spots on her skin. She had no other symptoms. On examination, she had extensive purpura but no pallor, jaundice, pyrexia, lymphadenopathy, or splenomegaly. There was no history of any drug ingestion, of joint pains or mental or psychological symptoms. She was not pregnant.

			Reference range		Permitted range	
	Value	Units	Low	High	Low	High
Red cell count	4.78	$\times 10^{12}$/l	4.03	5.09	4.64	4.92
Hemoglobin (Hb)	13.2	g/dl	12.7	15.9	12.7	13.7
Hematocrit (Hct)	0.42	l/l	0.38	0.49	0.40	0.43
Mean ell volume	87.2	fl	80	99	85.5	88.9
Mean cell Hb	27.6	pg	27	31.5	27.1	28.2
Mean cell Hb conc.	31.7	g/dl	31.5	34.5	31.0	32.3
Red cell dist. width	12.6	%	11.6	14	12.6	12.6
White cell count	5.34	$\times 10^9$/l	4	10	4.94	5.74
Neutrophils abs.	2.58	$\times 10^9$/l	2	7	2.39	2.78
Lymphocytes abs.	2.03	$\times 10^9$/l	1	3	1.88	2.19
Monocytes abs.	0.49	$\times 10^9$/l	0.2	1	0.45	0.53
Eosinophils abs.	0.18	$\times 10^9$/l	0.02	0.5	0.16	0.19
Basophils abs.	0.05	$\times 10^9$/l	0.02	0.1	0.05	0.06
Platelet count	4.3	$\times 10^9$/l	150	400	3.9	4.7
Sedimentation	17	mm/h	0	20	16	18

Questions:

1. What is your first-stage diagnosis?

   _____

2. What, in your opinion, are the general pathology possibilities?

   _____

   _____

   _____

   _____

Answers:

1. Thrombocytopenia.
2. No answer will be given at present to your chosen answers for question 2. They will be discussed next, in the form of further questions.

Further Questions:

1. If you suggested ITP, could this occur without any evidence of a recent viral infection?
2. If you suggested a spurious thrombocytopenia (as described in Chapter 6), what clinical features are completely against this diagnosis?
3. If you suggested psychogenic purpura, how likely do you think this is?
4. If you suggested early myelodysplasia, how likely do you think this is?
5. If you suggested bone marrow infiltration, what would be strongly against this diagnosis?
6. Would you be happy to go ahead and treat this as an ITP?
7. Or would you do a bone marrow examination?
8. Can you think of a possible cause that has not been mentioned?

Answers:

1. Yes. By no means are all cases of ITP preceded by an infection.
2. No. The patient has thrombocytopenia.
3. Most unlikely. The patient appears well integrated.
4. In the absence of morphology, this is difficult to answer. MDS presenting as an isolated thrombocytopenia is very uncommon.

5. Most unlikely. The most common appearances of this are pancytopenia and the leukoerythroblastic reaction, neither of which is present.
6. This is a contentious question. Many would go ahead and do just that.
7. Again a controversial issue.
8. Early aplastic anemia (remember that the platelets have among the shortest of life spans, and that therefore changes in the white and especially the red cells will manifest much later). Note also that a marrow examination done at this time will not help you much.

Further Question:

However, there is one important test that was not done and could help considerably in answering the question as to aplasia. What is that? There is also something else that needs done. What is that?

Answer:

The reticulocyte count. Even if the RCC is still normal, the presence of aplasia will undoubtedly show up in a decreased reticulocyte count. Secondly, blood film morphology is very important.

The reticulocyte count was done, and the absolute count was $9.1 \times 10^9/l$. The morphological examination showed normal appearances.

Consequently, aplastic anemia was suspected. The FBC was repeated several times over the next few weeks. The RCC and WCC steadily dropped. Eventually, a marrow examination revealed classic aplastic anemia.

CASE 112 (EXAMINE TABLES 24.9 AND 24.10)

Questions:

1. What was the referring doctor's anatomical diagnosis?
2. Do you think he proceeded correctly in investigating this?
3. Why did he order a C-reactive protein?
4. Do you think he was correct in being puzzled?

Answers:

1. Microcytic anemia.
2. Yes.

Table 24.9

Patient	Age	Sex	Race	Altitude
Master J de B	14 yrs	Male	White	5,000 ft

This lad was referred because of a FBC done while he had bronchopneumonia some weeks previously, and an unexpected picture was seen. This had been investigated routinely and no clear answer was forthcoming. Clinically, there was nothing specific to suggest an etiology. The referring doctor confirmed that the patient had not been taking iron medications. Tables 24.9 and 24.10 show the results in question.

	Value	Units	Reference range Low	High	Permitted range Low	High
Red cell count	**4.31**	$\times 10^{12}$/l	4.77	5.83	4.18	4.44
Hemoglobin (Hb)	**11.1**	g/dl	13.8	18.0	10.7	11.5
Hematocrit (Hct)	**0.32**	l/l	0.42	0.53	0.32	0.33
Mean cell volume	**75.4**	fl	80	99	70.1	80.7
Mean cell Hb	**25.8**	pg	27	31.5	25.2	26.3
Mean cell Hb conc.	34.2	g/dl	31.5	34.5	33.5	34.8
Red cell dist. width	12.1	%	11.6	14	12.1	12.1
Retic count	0.96	%	0.27	1.00	0.9	1.0
Retic absolute (abs.)	41.4	$\times 10^9$/l	30	100	40.1	42.6
White cell count	7.21	$\times 10^9$/l	4	10	6.67	7.75
Neutrophils abs.	4.04	$\times 10^9$/l	2	7	3.74	4.35
Lymphocytes abs.	2.45	$\times 10^9$/l	1	3	2.27	2.64
Monocytes abs.	0.42	$\times 10^9$/l	0.2	1	0.39	0.45
Eosinophils abs.	0.24	$\times 10^9$/l	0.02	0.5	0.22	0.26
Basophils abs.	0.06	$\times 10^9$/l	0.02	0.1	0.05	0.06
Platelet count	303.0	$\times 10^9$/l	150	400	280.3	325.7
Sedimentation	5	mm/h	0	10	5	5
Morphology	The red cells are microcytic and hypochromic. Possible causes include iron deficiency and chronic disease.					

Table 24.10

	Value	Units	Reference range Low	High
C-Reactive protein	4.1	mg/l	0.0	10.0
S-Ferritin male	178.3	µg/l	20.0	250.0
S-Iron	19.1	µmol/l	11.6	31.3
S-Transferrin	2.56	g/l	2.12	3.60
S-Fe saturation male	30	%	20.0	50.0

3. In case the etiology was ACD and the ferritin result was normal or even raised, he wanted to be able to discount this.
4. Yes. A microcytic anemia with completely normal iron studies is strange. His question with respect to iron medication indicated that he understood iron ingestion could interfere with the interpretation of the iron studies.

Further Question:

What should be the next step?

Answer:

This is really a specialist procedure. Several further tests were done and ultimately the disease was identified as HbE disease. This is very rare among whites, and the object of presenting this case was not to teach about HbE disease but to make clear that

1. There are unusual causes of common presentations.
2. Peculiar patterns should be recognized as such and identified. This is important, since medical treatment may be inappropriate otherwise – for example, in this case prescribing iron therapy would be contra-indicated.

Advanced Cases

CASE #113 (EXAMINE TABLES 24.11 AND 24.12)

The results in Table 24.12 accompanied the patient and had been ordered by his doctor about 2 weeks before.

Note that in Table 24.12, abnormal results have deliberately not been highlighted.

Questions:

1. With respect to the FBC, what is your first-stage diagnosis?

_____

_____

2. What are the general pathology possibilities, taking into account the biochemical results? Evaluate them in terms of probability.

_____

_____

_____

_____

_____

_____

Table 24.11

Patient	Age	Sex	Race	Altitude
Mr K M	37 yrs	Male	White	5,000 ft

This patient was a hard-driving businessman and had been feeling increasingly weak over a period of weeks. He consulted his doctor who told him his problem was low blood pressure. A FBC and routine biochemical tests were done but no comment was made about them, except that the ESR was raised and there might therefore be an underlying chronic inflammatory or infective disease, for which however he found no evidence. The patient tried various measures and eventually decided to try to ignore the problem. One day at work he suddenly collapsed. In consultation, he was found to be very hypotensive. Because of suspicions raised by the blood tests, certain clinical features were carefully looked for; these will be discussed shortly. We will first look at the FBC that shows changes typical of his disease.

	Value	Units	Reference range Low	Reference range High	Permitted range Low	Permitted range High
Red cell count	**3.96**	$\times 10^{12}/l$	4.77	5.83	3.84	4.08
Hemoglobin (Hb)	**11.3**	g/dl	13.8	18.0	10.9	11.7
Hematocrit (Hct)	**0.35**	l/l	0.42	0.53	0.34	0.36
Mean cell volume	87.8	fl	80	99	81.7	93.9
Mean cell Hb	28.5	pg	27	31.5	28.0	29.1
Mean cell Hb conc.	32.5	g/dl	31.5	34.5	31.9	33.2
Red cell dist. width	12.7	%	11.6	14	12.7	12.7
Retic count	0.71	%	0.27	1.00	0.7	0.7
Retic absolute (abs.)	**28.1**	$\times 10^9/l$	30	100	27.3	29.0
White cell count	7.87	$\times 10^9/l$	4	10	7.28	8.46
Neutrophils abs.	4.42	$\times 10^9/l$	2	7	4.09	4.75
Lymphocytes abs.	2.21	$\times 10^9/l$	1	3	2.05	2.38
Monocytes abs.	0.48	$\times 10^9/l$	0.2	1	0.44	0.52
Eosinophils abs.	0.70	$\times 10^9/l$	0.02	0.5	0.65	0.75
Basophils abs.	0.06	$\times 10^9/l$	0.02	0.1	0.05	0.06
Normoblasts	0	/100 WBC	0	0		
Platelet count	289.1	$\times 10^9/l$	150	400	267.4	310.8
Sedimentation	**28**	mm/h	0	10	24	26

Table 24.12

	Value	Units	Reference range Low	Reference range High
S-Urea	8.7	mmol/l	2.1	7.1
S-Creatinine	113	mmol/l	62	115
S-Urea:creatinine	76.7			
S-Sodium	129	mmol/l	136	145
S-Potassium	5.4	mmol/l	3.5	5.1
S-Chloride	109.7	mmol/l	98	108
S-Total CO_2	23	mmol/l	22	28
S-Anion gap	1.7	mmol/l	5	14
S-Glucose	4.7	mmol/l	3.9	5.8
S-Osmolarity	262	mmol/l	275	295
S-Calcium (total)	2.43	mmol/l	2.2	2.55
S-Magnesium	0.69	mmol/l	0.66	1.07
S-Phosphate	1.2	mmol/l	0.87	1.45
S-Protein (total)	74	g/l	64	83
S-Albumin	41	g/l	34	48
S-Globulin	33.0	g/l	30	35
S-α1-globulin	1.1	g/l		1.9
S-α2-globulin	5.2	g/l	5	7
S-β-globulin	6.1	g/l	5	8
S-γ-globulin	8.9	g/l	6	10
S-Bilirubin (total)	28.5	μmol/l	6.8	34.2
S-Bilirubin (direct)	8.1	μmol/l	1.7	8.6
S-Bilirubin (indirect)	20.4	μmol/l	5.1	25.6
S-ALP	67	IU/l	53	128
S-gGT	31	IU/l	8	37
S-ALT	34	IU/l	19	40
S-AST	24	IU/l	13	32
S-LDH	170	IU/l	90	180
C-Reactive protein	4.1	mg/l	0.0	10.0
S-Ferritin male	189.2	μg/l	20.0	250.0
S-Iron	21.6	μmol/l	11.6	31.3
S-Transferrin	2.78	g/l	2.12	3.60
S-Fe saturation male	30	%	20.0	50.0
S-Vitamin B_{12}	512	pg/ml	193	982
S-Folate	7.9	ng/ml	3.0	17.0
RBC-folate	345.1	ng/ml	93.0	641.0

3. What do you think is the significance of the reticulocyte count and the ESR?

_____

_____

_____

_____

4. How would you proceed? What clinical features were searched for on the basis of the laboratory findings? What result in the FBC, deliberately not highlighted, strongly suggests the diagnosis? Which biochemical tests support this diagnosis?

Answers:

1. There is a normocytic anemia with a decreased reticulocyte count and a raised ESR.

2. The possibilities are

   a. Renal failure. Probably not, with a normal creatinine.

   b. Combined megaloblastosis with defective iron metabolism. Most unlikely in view of the normal RDW and normal LDH. However, there is no morphological comment available.

   c. Hemolytic disease. Most unlikely in view of the normal LDH and bilirubin.

   d. ACD. Most unlikely: the MCV is a little high for this and the iron studies are normal.

e. Hypersplenism. Possible. One would need to know the size of the spleen.

f. Pure red cell aplasia. Certainly possible.

g. Endocrine deficiency. Possible.

3. The low retic count suggests an underactive erythropoiesis, compatible in this case with red cell aplasia and endocrine deficiency. The ESR is completely explainable by the anemia.

4. The mild eosinophilia cannot be ignored. While it may indicate any number of causes, in this case, there are a number of associated features that suggest the diagnosis: mild normocytic anemia, hyponatremia, mild hyperkalemia, hypotension, and weakness all suggest Addison disease. The additional features looked for as a result of this suspicion were

a. Hyperpigmentation. This was absent except for a few patches inside the mouth.

b. Craving for salt. This was present.

Indeed a more detailed history and exhaustive physical examination may have permitted the diagnosis sooner. However, the blood tests would still be necessary. Addison disease was proven biochemically.

CASE #114 (EXAMINE TABLE 24.13)

Questions:

1. How would you characterize the first-stage diagnosis from the hematological point of view?

_____

_____

2. Although these have not been discussed in the text, what general pathology possibilities can you suggest for this diagnosis? More specifically, what possibilities arise with this patient and what tests should be done to investigate?

_____

_____

_____

3. Do you think there are any clues as to the final diagnosis? What are they and what could be the diagnosis? How would you go about confirming this?

_____

_____

_____

_____

Table 24.13

Patient	Age	Sex	Race	Altitude
Miss J J	29 yrs	Female	White	5,000 ft

The patient is a nightclub hostess. She complained of recurrent chronic abdominal pain. The pain was mainly periumbilical, cramping, and worse after meals. The abdomen was soft between attacks and without guarding; no masses were palpable. Antacids proved of no value. Gastroscopy was negative. *Helicobacter pylori* was found, however, and she was placed on triple therapy, but this caused no improvement in her symptoms. One night, she developed an acute abdomen and was referred to a surgeon. He found her in severe pain; the abdomen remained soft and without any rigidity. Endoscopic and radiological studies all proved negative. He ordered a mesenteric arteriogram, and it was reported that the superior mesenteric and celiac arteries were obstructed by thrombus. Urgent laparotomy was performed and ±60% of infarcted small bowel was resected. The patient was admitted to the ICU and further consultation was sought.

A brief history was obtained from the boy friend. She had a miscarriage at 10 weeks pregnancy some years before and had taken great care not to become pregnant again, using a combination contraceptive pill. She had also complained recently of joint pains, mainly affecting the small joints; the family doctor had prescribed NSAIDS without much improvement.

On examination, her lungs were clear and ventilation was satisfactory. Mild general swelling of the MP and IP joints of both hands was noted. A faint reticular rash was observed on her legs. In consequence of the whole clinical picture, certain further tests were ordered.

Table 24.13 shows a FBC, and Table 24.14 shows some biochemical tests that were done shortly before consulting the surgeon. Table 24.15 shows the results of some current tests.

	Value	Units	Reference range Low	Reference range High	Permitted range Low	Permitted range High
Red cell count	4.65	$\times 10^{12}$/l	4.03	5.09	4.51	4.79
Hemoglobin (Hb)	13.7	g/dl	12.7	15.9	13.2	14.2
Hematocrit (Hct)	0.42	l/l	0.38	0.49	0.41	0.44
Mean cell volume	91	fl	80	99	89.2	92.8
Mean cell Hb	29.5	pg	27	31.5	28.9	30.1
Mean cell Hb conc.	32.4	g/dl	31.5	34.5	31.7	33.0
Red cell dist. width	13.5	%	11.6	14	13.5	13.5
Retic count %	1.1	0.1	0.3		1.1	1.1
Retic absolute (abs.)	51.2	$\times 10^9$/l	30	100	49.6	52.7
White cell count	14.9	$\times 10^9$/l	4	10	13.78	16.02
Neutrophils abs.	11.32	$\times 10^9$/l	2	7	10.47	12.17
Band cells abs.	1.04		0	0.00	0.914	1.15
Lymphocytes abs.	1.19	$\times 10^9$/l	1	3	1.10	1.28
Monocytes abs.	0.75	$\times 10^9$/l	0.2	1	0.69	0.80
Eosinophils abs.	0.45	$\times 10^9$/l	0.02	0.5	0.41	0.48
Basophils abs.	0.15	$\times 10^9$/l	0.02	0.1	0.14	0.16
Platelet count	153.0	$\times 10^9$/l	150	400	137.7	168.3
Sedimentation	43	mm/h	0	20	41	45

Table 24.14

	Value	Units	Low	High
S-ALP	198	IU/l	53	128
S-Amylase	421	IU/l	25	125

Table 24.15

Test	Value	Units	Low	High
PTT	**24**	Seconds	26	37
PT	13.2	Seconds	12	14
TT	**8.6**	Seconds	9	11
Antithrombin	105	%	70	120
Protein C	90	%	70	140
Protein S	86	%	60	140
Factor V$_{Leiden}$	Negative		Negative	
Prothrombin G20210A	Negative		Negative	70
Anti-cardiolipin IgG	**59**	units/ml	0	25
Anti-cardiolipin IgM	**31**	units/ml	0	25
Lupus anticoagulant	**Positive**			
D-dimers	**7.3**		0	2.5

4. Why are the S-ALP and S-Amylase raised?

_____

_____

Answers:

1. Possible hypercoagulable tendency.
2. Virchow's triad is an excellent place to start. With reference to this patient, the one very suggestive possible causative feature is that she is on the pill. Another is a vague suggestion with reference to her lifestyle – it would probably be wise to test her for HIV, since one known complication of HIV infection is the lupus anticoagulant (see Chapter 4).
3. Yes, apart from the points raised above.

   a. The reticular rash on the legs could be suspicious of livedo reticularis – characteristic of the antiphospholipid syndrome.
   b. She has arthritis of the small joints of the hand – this too could be a feature of APS.
   c. She had a miscarriage at 10 weeks once before. This may mean nothing but could fit in with the APS.
   d. Blood should be sent for lupus anticoagulant and anti-cardiolipin antibodies.

4. These enzymes are characteristically raised in mesenteric thrombosis since they are present in the tips of the villi and are released with severe ischemia.

Further Investigations:

The test for HIV was negative.

Questions:

5. Do you think you have enough evidence for the diagnosis of the APS?

_____

6. What long-term problems can be expected with this patient?

_____

_____

7. The PTT and TT are shortened. Do you think that this is a reliable indicator of hypercoagulability?

_____

Answers:

5. Yes.
6. Malabsorption.
7. No.

CASE #115 (TABLE 24.16)

Table 24.16

Patient	Age	Sex	Race	Altitude
Mr J L	78 yrs	Male	White	5,000 ft

This patient was referred to an internist because of severe anemia. There was very little relevant in the history, apart from tiredness and weakness with some loss of weight. On examination, there was nothing relevant to find.

	Value	Units	Reference range Low	Reference range High	Permitted range Low	Permitted range High
Red cell count	**2.12**	× 10^{12}/l	4.77	5.83	2.06	2.18
Hemoglobin (Hb)	**7.1**	g/dl	13.8	18.0	6.9	7.3
Hematocrit (Hct)	**0.23**	l/l	0.42	0.53	0.22	0.23
Mean cell volume	**107**	fl	80	99	99.5	114.5
Mean cell Hb	**33.5**	pg	27	31.5	32.8	34.2
Mean cell Hb conc.	**31.3**	g/dl	31.5	34.5	30.7	31.9
Red cell dist. width	**16.9**	%	11.6	14	16.9	16.9
Retic count	**10.3**	%	0.27	1.00	10.0	10.6
Retic absolute (abs.)	**218.4**	× 10^9/l	30	100	211.8	224.9
White cell count	**2.78**	× 10^9/l	4	10	2.57	2.99
Neutrophils abs.	**1.59**	× 10^9/l	2	7	1.47	1.71
Lymphocytes abs.	**0.81**	× 10^9/l	1	3	0.75	0.87
Monocytes abs.	0.25	× 10^9/l	0.2	1	0.23	0.27
Eosinophils abs.	0.09	× 10^9/l	0.02	0.5	0.08	0.10
Basophils abs.	0.04	× 10^9/l	0.02	0.1	0.04	0.04
Normoblasts	0	/100 WBC	0	0		
Platelet count	**54.7**	× 10^9/l	150	400	50.6	58.8

A number of blood tests and bone marrow aspiration and trephine biopsy were requested.

Bone Marrow Examination

Bone marrow aspiration and biopsy (in summary) showed a mildly hypercellular marrow with dysplasia involving all three lineages. No abnormal non-hemopoietic cells were seen. There was no increase in fibrous tissue or reticulin.

Questions:

1. The first-stage diagnosis is complex. Try to state it. What do you think the possibilities are?
   _____
   _____
   _____

2. Do you think the marrow appearances are diagnostic of a myelodysplastic syndrome?
   _____

3. How would you proceed?
   _____
   _____
   _____

Table 24.17

	Value	Units	Reference range Low	Reference range High
S-Urea	6.9	mmol/l	2.1	7.1
S-Creatinine	103	mmol/l	62	115
S-Urea:creatinine	67.0			
S-Protein (total)	71	g/l	64	83
S-Albumin	40	g/l	34	48
S-Globulin	31.0	g/l	30	35
S-Bilirubin (total)	28.5	μmol/l	6.8	34.2
S-Bilirubin (direct)	6.1	μmol/l	1.7	8.6
S-Bilirubin (indirect)	22.4	μmol/l	5.1	25.6
S-ALP	97	IU/l	53	128
S-gGT	27	IU/l	8	37
S-ALT	33	IU/l	19	40
S-AST	26	IU/l	13	32
S-LDH	154	IU/l	90	180
S-Ferritin male	151	μg/l	20.0	250.0
S-Iron	21.2	μmol/l	11.6	31.3
S-Transferrin	2.98	g/l	2.12	3.60
S-Fe saturation male	22.3	%	20.0	50.0
S-Vitamin B_{12}	451	pg/ml	193	982
S-Folate	9.8	ng/ml	3.0	17.0
RBC-folate	389.7	ng/ml	93.0	641.0
S-Haptoglobin 60 yrs	1.4	g/l	0.35	1.75
U-Protein	70	mg/l	10	140
U-Bence-Jones protein	N	"+"	Negative	Negative
U-Bilirubin	"−"	"+"		
U-Urobilin	"+"	"+"		
Direct Coombs anti-IgG	Negative			
Anti C3	Negative			

Answers:

1. There is a pancytopenia with macrocytic red cells and a moderate reticulocytosis, in the presence of a hyperactive marrow. General possibilities are

   a. Marrow dysfunction due to nutrient deficiency (vitamin B_{12} and/or folate, because of the macrocytosis). Unlikely because of the reticulocytosis, unless there is an independent cause.
   b. Marrow dysfunction due to clonal abnormality of precursors (e.g., myelodysplasia). **WITH ONE EXCEPTION,** this is unlikely because of the reticulocytosis unless there is an independent cause.
   c. Acute hemorrhage, hemolysis, or hypoxia in a preexistent pancytopenia from any cause.
   d. Hypersplenism.

2. Dysplastic changes can be secondary to many other bone marrow/blood diseases, although in this case, trilineage dysplasia is very suggestive of primary disease.

3. Check for evidence of nutrient deficiency; look for cytogenetic evidence of a primary myelodysplastic syndrome; look for evidence of hemolysis; an enlarged spleen; and look for a source of chronic bleeding. Table 24.17 shows the results of diverse tests.

Further Questions:

4. How have these results helped you?
   _____
   _____

5. In view of the blood results, there is one important point that was not elicited in the history. What is that, and why could this be relevant?
   _____
   _____
   _____

6. We mentioned an exception in (1b) above. What do you think this is?

_____

_____

Answers:

4. They show that hemolysis, chronic hemorrhage, liver and renal disease, and vitamin B_{12} and folate deficiency are hardly likely.
5. It was not established whether the patient had been taking chemotherapeutic agents. Many of these interfere with folate metabolism and can cause a macrocytosis with normal folate levels, and can of course cause bone marrow depression directly. The current hyperactive marrow could be early regeneration. In fact the patient had never been treated with any form of cytotoxic drug.
6. Paroxysmal nocturnal hemoglobinuria (PNH). This condition has already briefly been described. One classical presentation is pancytopenia with a hyperactive marrow and reticulocytosis. Indeed, this was the provisional diagnosis made in this case at this stage.

Tests for PNH were done: Ham's test, CD55, and CD59. These were all negative. We were now faced with a conundrum.

In the meantime, sonography of the abdomen showed a normal-sized spleen; colonoscopy revealed no pathology; but gastroscopy revealed severe erosive oesophagitis with several bleeding points. Nevertheless, in view of the normal iron studies, it was concluded that this could not have been the cause of the pancytopenia and the dysplasia (unless of course there was a co-existing iron-loading anemia).

However, examine the post-transfusion FBC (Table 24.18).

Further Questions:

7. What do you make of this FBC? Can you give a name to this appearance? What can it mean?

_____

_____

Table 24.18

	Value	Units	Reference range Low	Reference range High	Permitted range Low	Permitted range High
Red cell count	3.43	$\times 10^{12}$/l	4.77	5.83	3.33	3.53
Hemoglobin (Hb)	9.3	g/dl	13.8	18.0	9.0	9.6
Hematocrit (Hct)	0.34	l/l	0.42	0.53	0.33	0.35
Mean cell volume	99.1	fl	80	99	92.2	106.0
Mean cell Hb	27.1	pg	27	31.5	26.6	27.7
Mean cell Hb conc.	27.4	g/dl	31.5	34.5	26.8	27.9
Red cell dist. width	15.9	%	11.6	14	15.9	15.9
Retic count	6.32	%	0.27	1.00	6.1	6.5
Retic absolute (abs.)	216.8	$\times 10^9$/l	30	100	210.3	223.3
White cell count	3.43	$\times 10^9$/l	4	10	3.17	3.69
Corrected WCC	2.50	$\times 10^9$/l				
Neutrophils abs.	1.21	$\times 10^9$/l	2	7	1.12	1.30
Band cells abs.	0.24		0	0.00	0.22	0.26
Lymphocytes abs.	1.06	$\times 10^9$/l	1	3	0.98	1.14
Monocytes abs.	0.35	$\times 10^9$/l	0.2	1	0.33	0.38
Eosinophils abs.	0.07	$\times 10^9$/l	0.02	0.5	0.07	0.08
Basophils abs.	0.02	$\times 10^9$/l	0.02	0.1	0.02	0.02
Blasts	1	%	0	0		
Promyelocytes	2	%	0	0		
Myelocytes	4	%	0	0		
Metamyelocytes	7	%	0	0		
Normoblasts	37	/100 WBC	0	0		
Platelet count	34.4	$\times 10^9$/l	150	400	31.8	37.0

Answers:

This is a classical leukoerythroblastic reaction (marked left shift plus normoblasts). It is sometimes found in any acutely stimulated marrow, e.g., hemolysis, but generally suggests an infiltrative condition. The problem was that the marrow biopsy did not show this.

A radionuclide bone scan was done and numerous lesions strongly suggestive of secondary deposits were seen. One of these was biopsied by an orthopedic surgeon, and anaplastic adenocarcinoma was diagnosed. Note that secondary dysplastic changes can occur in the marrow with metastatic malignancy.

CASE #116 (TABLE 24.19)

Table 24.19

Patient	Age	Sex	Race	Altitude
Mr J T	47 yrs	Male	Black	2,500 ft

The patient is a rural subsistence farmer. He consulted a doctor because of increasing weakness and buzzing in the ears, and a feeling of fullness in the abdomen. He was a heavy smoker. He had consulted a traditional healer to no avail. The doctor found a large mass on the left side of the abdomen, extending to below the left costal margin. The mass had a notch and moved slightly with respiration. He diagnosed splenomegaly and suspected a blood disease; he ordered a FBC. He made a provisional diagnosis of chronic myelocytic anemia and referred the patient. During a thorough examination, the consultant found the patient to be pyrexial, and made a clinical finding that strongly contradicted the above diagnosis.

	Value	Units	Reference range Low	Reference range High
Red cell count	6.59	$\times 10^{12}/l$	4.64	5.67
Hemoglobin (Hb)	19.3	g/dl	13.4	17.5
Hematocrit (Hct)	0.53	l/l	0.41	0.52
Mean cell volume	81	fl	80	99
Mean cell Hb	29.3	pg	27	31.5
Mean cell Hb conc.	36.2	g/dl	31.5	34.5
Red cell dist. width	16.7	%	11.6	14
Retic count	1.1	%	0.26	0.77
Retic absolute (abs.)	72.5	$\times 10^9/l$	30	100
White cell count	12.56	$\times 10^9/l$	3.5	10
Neutrophils abs.	7.03	$\times 10^9/l$	1.5	7
Band cells abs.	0.63		0	0.00
Lymphocytes abs.	1.76	$\times 10^9/l$	1	3
Monocytes abs.	1.00	$\times 10^9/l$	0.2	1
Eosinophils abs.	0.50	$\times 10^9/l$	0.02	0.5
Basophils abs.	0.13	$\times 10^9/l$	0.02	0.1
Blasts		%	0	0
Promyelocytes	1	%	0	0
Myelocytes	3	%	0	0
Metamyelocytes	8	%	0	0
Normoblasts	1	/100 WBC	0	0
Platelet count	489.0	$\times 10^9/l$	150	400
Sedimentation	15	mm/h	0	10

Questions:

1. Do you agree with the doctor's questioning of the diagnosis? Are there any features of this count that you find odd? Can you think of any other possible explanation?

———————————————————————

———————————————————————

———————————————————————

———————————————————————

———————————————————————

2. What did the consultant find that profoundly changed the diagnosis?

———————————————————————

Answers:

1. CML is possible: large spleen plus leukocytosis with a marked left shift. Erythrocytosis and thrombocytosis may accompany the leukocytosis in CML (see case #67 in Chapter 16). There are, however, a few difficulties with this conclusion:

   a. There is no basophil leukocytosis.
   b. One would expect the WCC to be much higher with a spleen of this size.
   c. The erythrocytosis is disproportionately high in comparison with the leukocytosis. Indeed, if the spleen were normal in size or only mildly enlarged, polycythemia should have been the point of departure.

   The only alternative suggestions would be

   a. Myelofibrosis either resulting from a transformation from P vera, or, rarely, a primary myelofibrosis that is transforming into P vera.
   b. A chronic infection (e.g., schistosomiasis) plus an independent cause for erythrocytosis, e.g., smoking.

2. The mass in the abdomen was not a spleen. Upon turning the patient prone, he found that he could not get a fingertip between the lateral border of the erector spinae and the mass; this indicated that the mass was retroperitoneal (i.e., not a spleen).

CT scanning of the abdomen revealed features consistent with a huge renal adenocarcinoma, with considerable necrosis. This would explain the pyrexia, the leukocytosis, and the thrombocytosis.

Further Questions:

What further investigation would you order to explain the erythrocytosis?

Answers:

Erythropoietin levels.
   EPO levels were markedly raised, strongly suggesting origin from the carcinoma.

Appendix A: Drugs, the First-Line Tests, and Blood Diseases

Drug ingestion by patients is a potent source of problems in hematology:

1. By causing blood diseases.
2. By causing changes in the first-line tests that may complicate the diagnosis both by the laboratory and the clinician. It is thus important that the relevant drugs be included in the request forms for hematological tests.

By far, the commonest side effects of drugs on the blood are cytopenias of one kind or another. There are several possible mechanisms that are known:

1. **DIRECT DAMAGE** to the marrow or the circulating cells.
2. **IMMUNE-MEDIATED DAMAGE**. This in turn can be by one of three mechanisms:

   a. **DRUG DEPENDENT.** Here the drug is firmly bound to the cell membrane, and antibodies produced as a response directly damage the membrane. Damage to the cells tends only to develop after prolonged, especially high-dosage therapy. The antibody is an IgG. Such antibody tests that are available are only positive in the presence of the offending drug.
   b. **PASSIVE AGGLUTINATION.** The drug acts as a **HAPTEN**. When antibodies are produced, immune complexes are formed which then attach themselves to the cell membrane, with activation of complement. Damage to the cells only occurs on the second or third exposure to the drug, and then the cytopenia often develops extremely abruptly. It is an IgG or IgM antibody.
   c. **THE FORMATION OF AUTOANTIBODIES.** Such antibody tests that are available are positive without the drug being present, and can remain positive for years.

Four additional points must be made:

1. Drugs that normally would produce few or no reactions in normal subjects may do so in the presence of (perhaps hitherto unrecognized) metabolic disorders of the cells.
2. Patients who have experienced hypersensitivity previously often seem more prone to respond negatively to drugs in general.
3. In the following lists, we mention only those drugs that frequently are associated with the side effect. It is a good rule however that with any change in a test that cannot conveniently be explained otherwise the drug regime be looked at, suspected and if necessary (and if possible) stopped, even if such drugs are not "officially" listed as causing the effect.
4. In the lists, we cannot use trade names, especially since these can be different in different parts of the world.

Aplastic Anemia

1. Chloramphenicol
2. Quinacrine
3. Trimethadione
4. Methylphenylhydantoin
5. Phenylbutazone
6. Gold compounds.

Neutropenia

1. **CHEMOTHERAPEUTIC AGENTS**. These almost all cause neutropenia by direct damage to the marrow precursors.
2. **OTHERS**. These again may act directly or via immune mechanisms.

   a. Semi-synthetic penicillins (only after several weeks of continued high dosage).
   b. Cephalosporins (±10% incidence).
   c. Sulphonamides, especially when combined with trimethoprim, and particularly in a vulnerable bone marrow, e.g., one recovering after an aplastic crisis.

d. Phenothiazines (tending to occur after ±6 weeks of therapy or when the total dose has exceeded 5 g).
e. NSAIDS especially phenylbutazone and related compounds.
f. Gold compounds.
g. Antithyroid drugs: ±10% incidence.
h. Anti-arrhythmic drugs, especially quinidine and procainamide. The neutropenia can occur up to 12 weeks after therapy has been started.
i. Clozapine.

Thrombocytopenia

1. Quinidine and quinine
2. Sulphonamides especially with trimethoprim
3. Heparin
4. Gold.

Hemolytic Anemia

1. **DRUG-DEPENDENT TYPE.** Quinine and quinidine
2. **IMMUNE COMPLEX TYPE**

    a. Penicillin
    b. Cephalosporins
    c. Erythromycin
    d. Tolbutamide
    e. Chlorpromazine
    f. Chlorpropamide

3. **AUTOANTIBODIES.** Methyldopa is the only reasonably common cause of this side effect. Fifteen percent of patients on the drug develop a positive Coombs test, but only 1% will develop overt hemolysis. Other drugs include

    a. Levodopa
    b. Mefenemic acid
    c. Procainamide

4. **IN THE PRESENCE OF AN UNSTABLE HEMO-GLOBIN OR G6PD DEFICIENCY**, a number of drugs can cause often devastating hemolysis:

    a. Primaquin
    b. Paraquin
    c. Pamaquin
    d. Quinacrin

e. Nalidixic acid
f. Nitrofurantoin
g. Some sulpha drugs

Miscellaneous

1. **DRUGS AFFECTING PLATELET FUNCTION** (and consequently will affect platelet function tests):

    a. Aspirin
    b. NSAIDS
    c. High-dose beta-lactams, especially carbenicillin.

2. **METHEMOGLOBINEMIA**

    a. **NITRITES.** Included is amyl nitrite in high doses (as often used for "recreational" purposes)
    b. **PHENACETIN**
    c. Acetaminophen
    d. Some sulpha drugs
    e. Nitroprusside (used especially in the emergency intra-arterial treatment of malignant hypertension)
    f. Local anesthetics.

3. **NEUTROPHILIA**

    a. **ADRENERGIC DRUGS**
    b. **STEROIDS.**

4. **EOSINOPHILIA**

    a. Halothane

5. **INTERFERENCE WITH FIBRINOLYTIC TESTS.**

    a. ε-Amino-caproic acid (**EACA**) – an anti-plasmin drug.

6. Drugs causing malabsorption

    a. Tetracycline: **IRON** (by chelation)
    b. Antacids: **IRON** (by binding)
    c. Phenytoin: **FOLATE** (by competitive binding)
    d. Alcohol:

        i. **FOLATE** (toxic effect on mucosa)
        ii. **VITAMIN B$_{12}$** (toxic effect on mucosa)

    e. Methotrexate: **FOLATE** (competition for binding site)
    f. Colchicine: **VITAMIN B$_{12}$** (mucosal damage)
    g. Metformin: **VITAMIN B$_{12}$** (mucosal damage).

Appendix B: Likelihood Ratios and the Fagan Nomogram

In Chapter 2, a number of basic concepts with respect to likelihood ratios were discussed. In this appendix, we shall show you how to use the ratios plus your pre-test diagnostic hypothesis to reach a level of certainty as to how much further to take the diagnostic process. To recapitulate very briefly:

Having seen a patient, we form a preliminary hypothesis as to the diagnosis. This is achieved by the results of the clinical history and examination, and informed by the extent of your knowledge, experience, and the prevalence of the possible diseases in the community.

We want to know by how much a specific diagnostic test will assist us in reaching a level of post-test certainty. This we achieve by applying existing knowledge of the likelihoods of

1. The test being positive in proven cases of the suspected disease.
2. The test being positive in cases were the disease is absent.

From these, we derive a likelihood ratio. We then use the Fagan nomogram to find out what the post-test certainty is. Depending on the result, we either

1. Do nothing except reassure the patient and send him home.
2. Act promptly and decisively in treating the condition.
3. Balance up the pros and cons (the patient's age, and general status, the economic implications of doing further tests or instituting treatment, and any special

facts peculiar to the individual) to decide how far to go. This latter aspect is frequently ignored. A recent case illustrates the importance:

A mother lost her eldest son to a fatal huge pulmonary embolus. No diagnosis had been made as to the presence of a hypercoagulability state since the PE was quite unexpected. The remaining son (the only remaining child in fact), aged 9 years, was tested and found to be heterozygous for factor V_{Leiden}. The father had also been positive and had died of a myocardial infarction at the age of 41; the mother's family had a fairly strong history of thrombotic-related incidents. The mother wanted him anticoagulated; the laboratory insisted that there was no evidence that he was at an increased risk. In consultation, this was an impossible situation, and prompted wide consultation with numerous clinical experts; they were unanimous in agreeing to anticoagulation. Whether this was right or wrong, nobody can tell, and it is true that we were treating the mother rather than the boy, yet who is to say that she was wrong? Doubtless many would disagree – in the end, you have to use your best knowledge, insight, and wisdom in dealing with these problems.

Let us look at a very banal example, merely to illustrate the principles. Consider that you have a patient with a microcytic anemia. Is a ferritin level a good first choice in following this up? You find a good review that tells you that

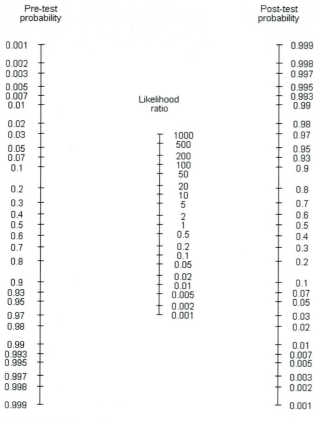

Fig. B.1 The Fagan Nomogram

1. Of 211 patients with proven iron deficiency, 197 had a decreased ferritin level. Thus the positive likelihood = 0.93.
2. Of 185 patients in whom it was proven that there was no iron deficiency, 9 had a ferritin below normal. Thus the negative likelihood = 0.05

This gives us a likelihood ratio of 0.93/0.05 = 18.6. How then are we to interpret this? As a general guideline:

1. LR > 10 or LR < 0.1 is highly likely to make a significant difference to the pre-test probability
2. LR < 2 or LR = 0.5–1 are most unlikely to add to one's pre-test diagnosis.
3. LR = 2–5 or LR = 0.5–0.2 sometimes will add to the pre-test diagnosis.
4. LR = 5–10 and LR = 0.1–0.2 often will lead to changes in the pre-test diagnosis.

How then do we get to the post-test level of certainty, once armed with all this data?

Refer now to the Fagan nomogram (Fig. B.1). Place a ruler to intersect the pre-test probability and the LR (in the middle column). Now read off the post-test level of certainty in the third column and proceed accordingly. You will see that this has produced a post-test level of certainty of 0.1 – a good guide that you should proceed to investigate.

Reference

Jaeschke R, Guyatt GH, Sackett DL (1994). Users' Guide to the Medical Literature: How to Use an Article About a Diagnostic Test. JAMA 271(9): 703–707.

Appendix C: Emergency Tests of Hemostasis

You may sometimes find yourself working in primitive situations far from any kind of modern laboratory and are presented with a patient who is bleeding and you are uncertain as to whether it is a bleeding disorder, or alternatively you know there is a bleeding disorder but need some means of monitoring your treatment.

You will find that a simple bleeding time and whole blood coagulation time will take you a long way.

The Bleeding Time (Duke's)

1. Apply a blood pressure cuff and pump it up to 40 mmHg.
2. Swab the ventral surface of the forearm.
3. Prick the skin firmly with a lancet in three places.
4. Suck up the resulting blood with the torn edge of a piece of blotting or filter paper. Do not wipe the wound.
5. Measure the time until the bleeding stops in each puncture.
6. Average the times.
7. The normal is 3–6 min. Anything longer than this will indicate one (or more) of

   a. A vascular lesion such as scurvy
   b. Thrombocytopenia
   c. Platelet dysfunction, as in von Willebrand disease.

8. If you feel confident enough and have the necessary equipment, you can make a blood smear with fresh blood, stain it, and look at the platelets. They may be obviously decreased, or they may show obvious lack of spontaneous aggregation. In addition, you may see marked fragmentation of red cells with microspherocytes, which may permit you to make a provisional, and under the circumstances, treatable diagnosis of DIC.

The Whole Blood Coagulation Time (Lee and White)

1. Prepare some sort of water-bath containing water at roughly body temperature (a clinical thermometer is fine).
2. Take some blood from a vein into a glass syringe and place ±0.5 ml of blood into each of three glass tubes, preferably 0.5 cm bore. Note the time when the blood enters the syringe.
3. Place all three into your water-bath and leave strictly alone for 5 min.
4. At the end of 5 min, remove one tube, partially invert it **ONCE**, check for a clot, and replace it in the water.
5. Repeat every 30 s. Once it has clotted, note the time and repeat with each of the other tubes in sequence.
6. You end up with 3 times. Take the average, and that is your WBCT.
7. The normal is 5–11 min. Anything longer than this will indicate a condition where the PTT, if it could have been done, would be more than ±20–30% above normal.

Reference

Lewis SM, Bain B, Bates I (2006). Dacie and Lewis Practical Haematology. 10th edn. Churchill Livingstone.

Index